Gynecologic Surgery

second edition

Gynecologic Surgery

second edition

edited by

Luis E. Sanz

M.D., F.A.C.O.G.
Professor and Chief
Division of Gynecology and Obstetrics
Director, Gynecologic Urology and Pelvic Relaxation Clinic
Department of Obstetrics and Gynecology
Georgetown University Medical Center
Washington, DC

b
Blackwell
Science

Blackwell Science

EDITORIAL OFFICES:

238 Main Street, Cambridge,
    Massachusetts 02142, USA
Osney Mead, Oxford OX2 OEL, England
25 John Street, London WC1N 2BL,
    England
23 Ainslie Place, Edinburgh EH3 6AJ,
    Scotland
54 University Street, Carlton,
    Victoria 3053, Australia
Arnette Blackwell SA, 1 rue de Lille,
    75007 Paris, France
Blackwell Wissenschafts-Verlag
    GmbH, Kurfürstendamm 57,
    10707 Berlin, Germany
Blackwell MZV,
    Feldgasse 13,
    A-1238 Vienna, Austria

Acquisitions: Victoria Reeders
Development: Coleen Traynor
Production: Lee Medoff
Manufacturing: Kathleen Grimes
Typeset by BookMasters, Inc., Ashland, Ohio
Printed and bound by Braun-Brumfield, Inc.

© 1995 by Blackwell Science, Inc.
Printed in the United States of America
95 96 97 98 5 4 3 2 1

Notice: The indications and dosages of all drugs in this book have
been recommended in the medical literature and conform to the
practices of the general medical community. The medications described do not necessarily have specific approval by the Food
and Drug Administration for use in the diseases and dosages
for which they are recommended. The package insert for each
drug should be consulted for use and dosage as approved by the
FDA. Because standards of usage change, it is advisable to keep
abreast of revised recommendations, particularly those concerning new drugs.

DISTRIBUTORS:

North America
Blackwell Science, Inc.
238 Main Street
Cambridge, Massachusetts 02142
(Telephone orders: 800-759-6102 or 617-876-7000)

Australia
Blackwell Science Pty Ltd
54 University Street
Carlton, Victoria 3053
(Telephone orders: 03-347-5552)

Outside North America and Australia
Blackwell Science, Ltd.
c/o Marston Book Services, Ltd.
P.O.Box 87
Oxford OX2 ODT
England
(Telephone orders: 44-865-791155)

Library of Congress Cataloging-in-Publication Data
Gynecologic surgery / edited by Luis E. Sanz. — 2nd ed.
        p.   cm
    Includes bibliographical references and index.
    ISBN 0-86542-341-5
    1. Generative organs, Female — Surgery.   I. Sanz, Luis E.
    [DNLM: 1. Genitalia, Female — Surgery.   WP 660 G9973 1995]
RG104.G954   1995
618.1'059— dc20
DNLM/DLC
for Library of Congress   94-10997
                                                            CIP

To
My wife Miriam and my daughter Monica
for their help and support
And to Raymond T. Holden, M.D.
my friend, mentor, and surgical teacher.

Contents

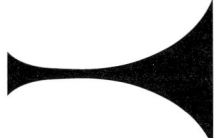

Contributors

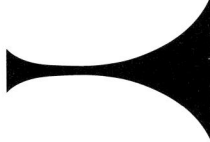

Albert Altcheck MD *Clinical Professor of Obstetrics, Gynecology, and Reproductive Science, Chief of Pediatric and Adolescent Gynecology, Mount Sinai School of Medicine, Obstetrics-Gynecology Staff, Lenox Hill Hospital, New York, New York*

Shawky Z. A. Badawy MD *Department of Obstetrics and Gynecology, Division of Reproductive Endocrinology, State University of New York, Health Science Center, Syracuse, New York*

Michael S. Baggish MD *Department of Obstetrics and Gynecology, Good Samaritan Hospital, Cincinnati, Ohio*

Willard A. Barnes MD *Director, Division of Gynecologic Oncology, Department of Obstetrics and Gynecology, Georgetown University Medical Center, Washington, DC*

James F. Barter MD *Associate Professor, Department of Obstetrics and Gynecology, Division of Gynecologic Oncology, Georgetown University Medical Center, Washington, DC*

Lutwin Beck MD *Professor and Chairman, Department of Obstetrics and Gynecology, The University of Dusseldorf, Dusseldorf, Germany*

Hans Georg Bender MD *Professor, Department of Gynecology and Oncology, Frankfurt University Medical Center, Frankfurt, Germany*

Kenneth Blank MD *Department of Obstetrics and Gynecology, Georgetown University Medical Center, Washington, DC*

Richard V. Brenner MD *Department of Surgery, Division of General Surgery, Georgetown University Medical Center, Washington, DC*

John F. Bresette MD *Columbia Hospital for Women, Washington, DC*

Brendan Burke MD *Assistant Professor, Department of Obstetrics and Gynecology, Georgetown University Medical Center, Washington, DC*

Alexander F. Burnett MD *Associate Professor, Department of Obstetrics and Gynecology, Division of Gynecologic Oncology, Georgetown University Medical Center, Washington, DC*

Stephen H. Cruikshank MD, FACOG, FACS *Chief, Department of Obstetrics and Gynecology, Hennepin County Medical Center, Professor and Vice Chairman, Department of Obstetrics and Gynecology, University of Minnesota Medical School, Minneapolis, Minnesota*

Gregorio Delgado MD *Professor and Chairman, Department of Obstetrics and Gynecology, Loyola University Medical Center, Stritch College of Medicine, Maywood, Illinois*

Christina M. Drollette MD *Department of Obstetrics and Gynecology, Division of Reproductive Endocrinology, State University of New York, Health Science Center, Syracuse, New York*

Stephen R. T. Evans MD, FACS, FACOG *Department of Surgery, Division of General Surgery, Georgetown University Medical Center, Washington, DC*

William F. Feller MD *Professor, Department of Surgery, Georgetown University Medical Center, Washington, DC*

Victor Gomel MD *Professor and Head, Department of Obstetrics and Gynecology, University of British Columbia, Vancouver, British Columbia, Canada*

Edward A. Graber MD *Professor Emeritus, Cornell University Medical School, Department of Obstetrics and Gynecology, Honorary Attending in Obstetrics and Gynecology, New York Hospital-Cornell Medical Center, New York, New York*

William A. Growdon MD *Association of Gynecologic Laparoscopy, Santa Monica, California*

B. Frederick Helmkamp MD *Clinical Professor, Department of Obstetrics and Gynecology, George Washington University Medical Center, Washington, DC, Co-director, Gynecologic Oncology, The Fairfax Hospital, Annandale, Virginia*

Edward C. Hill MD *Department of Obstetrics and Gynecology, University of California Medical Center, San Francisco, California*

Patricia M. Hoyne MD *Department of Obstetrics and Gynecology, Georgetown University Medical Center, Washington, DC*

W. Glenn Hurt MD *Professor, Department of Obstetrics and Gynecology, Medical College of Virginia, Richmond, Virginia*

Jacqueline C. Johnson MD *Assistant Professor, Department of Obstetrics and Gynecology, Division of Gynecologic Oncology, Georgetown University Medical Center, Washington, DC*

Nicholas Kadar MD *Director of Gynecology, Oncology, and Laparoscopic Surgery, Jersey Shore Medical Center, Neptune, New Jersey, Clinical Associate Professor of Obstetrics and Gynecology, UMD-Robert Wood Johnson Medical School, Piscataway, New Jersey*

Larry C. Kilgore MD *Assistant Professor, Department of Obstetrics and Gynecology, Division of Gynecologic Oncology, University of Alabama School of Medicine, Birmingham, Alabama*

S. R. Kovac MD, FACS, FACOG *Department of Obstetrics and Gynecology, Hennepin County Medical Center, Department of Obstetrics and Gynecology, University of Minnesota, Minneapolis, Minnesota, Vaginal Surgeon, St. John's Mercy Hospital, St. Louis, Missouri*

Hans-B. Krebs MD *Clinical Professor, Department of Obstetrics and Gynecology, George Washington University Medical Center, Washington, DC, Gynecologic Oncology Center, The Fairfax Hospital, Annandale, Virginia*

Thomas B. Lebherz MD *Department of Obstetrics and Gynecology, University of California, Los Angeles, California*

Raymond A. Lee MD *Department of Obstetrics and Gynecology, Mayo Clinic, Rochester, Minnesota*

Thomas C. Lee MD, FACF, FACOG *Assistant Professor, Department of Surgery, Division of General Surgery, Georgetown University Medical Center, Washington, DC*

Dan C. Martin MD *Reproductive Surgeon, Baptist Memorial Hospital, Clinical Associate Professor, University of Tennessee, Memphis, Tennessee*

Robert S. Neuwirth MD *Director of Gynecologic Endoscopy, Columbia Presbyterian Medical Center, New York, New York*

David H. Nichols MD *Department of Obstetrics and Gynecology, Massachusetts General Hospital, Boston, Massachusetts*

Miles J. Novy MD *Oregon Regional Primate Research Center, Beaverton, Oregon*

Donald R. Ostergard MD FACOG *Professor, Department of Obstetrics and Gynecology, University of California at Irvine, Associate Medical Director of Gynecology, Women's Hospital, Long Beach Memorial Medical Center, Long Beach, California*

James A. Patterson MD *Associate Professor, Chief, Division of Gynecology and Obstetrics, Department of Obstetrics and Gynecology, Loyola University of Chicago, Stritch College of Medicine, Maywood, Illinois*

Stephen F. Ponchak MD FACOG *Salem Women's Health Associates, Salem, Massachusetts*

John C. Riggs MD *Assistant Director, Gynecology Clinic, West Jersey Health System, Voorhees, New Jersey*

Joseph A. Riggs MD *Clinical Professor of Obstetrics and Gynecology, Jefferson Medical University Hospital, Philadelphia, Pennsylvania*

Jacques-E. Rioux MD, MPH *Professor, Department of Obstetrics and Gynecology, Le Centre Hospitalier de l'Universite Laval, Ste-Foy, Quebec, Canada*

Jack R. Robertson MD *Department of Obstetrics and Gynecology, Valley Community Hospital, Santa Clara, California*

Timothy C. Rowe MD *Professor, Department of Obstetrics and Gynecology, University of British Columbia, Vancouver, British Columbia, Canada*

Preston C. Sacks MD *Center for Fertility and Reproductive Endocrinology, Columbia Hospital for Women, Clinical Instructor, Department of Obstetrics and Gynecology, Georgetown University Medical Center, Washington, DC*

Luis E. Sanz MD *Professor and Chief, Division of Obstetrics and Gynecology, Director, Gynecological Urology and Pelvic Relaxation Clinic, Department of Obstetrics and Gynecology, Georgetown University Medical Center, Washington, DC*

Young K. Shin MD *Associate Professor, Department of Anesthesia, Georgetown University Medical Center, Washington, DC*

Hugh M. Shingleton MD *J. Marion Simms Professor, Department of Obstetrics and Gynecology, University of Alabama School of Medicine, Birmingham, Alabama*

Richard Soderstrom MD *Department of Obstetrics and Gynecology, University of Washington, Seattle, Washington*

Steven E. Swift MD *Clinical Instructor, Department of Obstetrics and Gynecology, University of California at Irvine, Women's Hospital, Long Beach Memorial Medical Center, Long Beach, California*

John B. Wheelock MD *Gynecologic Oncology Associates of Nashville, P. C., Nashville, Tennessee*

James P. Youngblood MD, FACOG *Professor and Chairman, Department of Obstetrics and Gynecology, Truman Medical Center, University of Missouri, Kansas City, Missouri*

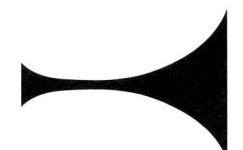

Foreword

Gynecologic surgery has a magnificent tradition in the United States, stretching back more than 100 years into the late 1800s. But it was during the first years of this century that the foundation of this discipline was built. Daring and resourceful operators developed many reliable procedures that have stood the test of time and are still widely used today—the abdominal intrafascial hysterectomy, for example, and vesicourethral suspensions for stress incontinence. To these were added innovative vaginal techniques that decreased morbidity and improved patients' chances for a quick recovery.

Then came World War II. Medicine responded to the exigencies of the battlefields with another series of rapid advances—improved anesthetic techniques, refined blood banking, and broad-spectrum antibiotics. Over the next two decades, armed with these new weapons and the experience of their predecessors, gynecologists were able to dramatically reduce mortality and morbidity associated with pelvic operations. Gynecologic surgery took its place in hospital training programs, and proficiency in its art became a standard expectation for ob-gyn residents.

About 1970 another burst of technologic advances began to extend the reach of the gynecologic surgeon even more. Foremost among these advances were surgical scopes. First came the laparoscope to help the operator sharpen diagnosis, avoid unnecessary laparotomies, and provide ingenious low-risk therapy. Then the colposcope enabled the gynecologist to direct cervical biopsies to the most productive sites, and thereby improve the diagnostic yield and often avoid cone biopsy. At the same time, the hysteroscope opened the door to investigation of intrauterine pathology. Finally, the operating microscope paved the way for delicate infertility therapy and other marvels of microsurgery.

Many other important developments also fueled this revolution. Diagnostic ultrasound and plasma β-hCG studies facilitated the early diagnosis of ectopic pregnancy and probably decreased the likelihood of future infertility. The laser helped decrease operative morbidity; while it has not revolutionized gynecologic surgery, it certainly has refined it.

These advances have combined to establish the high-tech character of gynecologic surgery. But one thing has not changed: success still depends on careful adherence to the general surgical principles laid down earlier in this century. Every gynecologist must enter the operating room with a clear understanding of anatomy and physiology, not to mention full mastery of surgical technique. Failure to do so can only invite a poor outcome.

Now we are taking gynecologic surgery with its high-tech capabilities into a new era. We are entering the era of managed care. This means fewer operations, shorter hospital stays, switching from inpatient to outpatient surgery. As managed care moves to capitated care there will be a trend to assign surgeries to the gynecologists with the best "report cards." Those with the short stays, short operating times, and fewest complications and transfusions will have an advantage.

As the population ages, there will be special needs. The aging women will have had fewer children and fewer vaginal deliveries. The relatively high cesarean section rates should result in fewer instances of relaxed vaginal outlet, but since women will live considerably longer there will be a need for urogynecology. Hormone replacement therapy, postmenopausal bleeding and new challenges such as complications of tamoxifen therapy will increase. Gynecologists will need to continue to learn new techniques to manage the problems of this aging female population.

Still, we face a future in which there will almost certainly be more gynecologists and fewer surgical cases. Proper training and rigorous CME will be even more necessary in the coming years. Some gynecologists may find they are doing so little surgery that they can't maintain proficiency. For most, it will be a major effort to keep their knowledge and operative skills at superior levels. With these needs in mind, Dr. Luis Sanz has organized and edited this book. He has enlisted the specialty's top authorities to share their experiences. Anatomy, physiology, and surgical principles are carefully explained. Both vaginal and abdominal techniques and their complications are described concisely, step by step, with the help of excellent and accurate illustrations. There is a special section on infertility surgery.

Overall it is a superb compilation, designed in the most practical way to help the gynecologic surgeon perform with confidence and skill. I am sure it will be used regularly as a standard reference.

John T. Queenan, M.D.
Professor and Chairman
Department of Obstetrics and Gynecology
Georgetown University School of Medicine

Preface

The ever changing field of gynecologic surgery requires the updating of the highly successful first edition of *Gynecologic Surgery*. The primary change has been in the field of endoscopic surgery, which has revolutionized gynecologic procedures. However, with its steep learning curve, endoscopic surgery will demand high proficiency on the part of the surgeon and a need to perform many cases so as to become an expert in the field of pelvic surgery. This second edition draws on the expertise of leading general and gynecologic surgeons from universities around the country and continues to provide authoritative and up-to-date coverage of innovative surgical procedures

It is important in a new edition not only to update all of the chapters but also to add totally new chapters and new authors. We have been able to accomplish all of these goals so that we can bring to you the most recent surgical techniques. The text is supported by detailed line drawings and other illustrations to reinforce key points and to document important procedural steps. We have added new chapters in laparoscopic hysterectomies by Drs. Sanz and Kadar, management of episiotomies, abdominal incisions, paravaginal repairs of USI by Dr. Youngblood, management and prevention of pelvic adhesions and geriatric gynecologic surgery, among others.

Gynecologic Surgery, second edition has extensive sections on pelvic anatomy, wound management, general surgery, vaginal and urological surgery, infertility surgery, endoscopic surgery and an important section on the management of gynecologic complications. The management of gynecologic complications is well covered by Drs. Shingleton and Wheelock. There are multiple chapters with extensive coverage of wound management and suture materials to add a scientific background to this very important area that is very seldom covered in other books. These sections are divided into 46 chapters to allow for easy review of each particular topic. Areas of general surgery that are relevant to the gynecologic surgeons such as appendectomy, hernia repair and management of breast masses are expertly discussed by Drs. Evans and Feller.

There is a large section on vaginal surgery with many chapters by Dr. David H. Nichols, an internationally-known expert in vaginal reconstruction. The surgical management of rectovaginal fistulas, enterocele, vaginal prolapse, anal incontinence, and other commonly encountered problems that can be repaired vaginally are well covered. This section on vaginal surgery is very important since it is one type of surgery that only the well-trained gynecologic surgeon can perform. Unfortunately, many of our residents are finishing the residency without the expertise to perform complicated vaginal surgery.

There are also sections on urologic surgery and infertility surgery that are pertinent to the gynecologic surgeon. The management of ectopic pregnancy is extensively covered. I expect that this extensive update of the first edition will help residents and gynecologic surgeons and that it will also be used as a source of reference when an uncommon surgical procedure has to be performed. But my most important expectation is that this book will improve the outcome when surgery is required in our female patients who deserve the best results from us.

ACKNOWLEDGMENTS

Ten years ago Dr. Queenan encouraged me to edit a book on gynecologic surgery that would cover recent surgical techniques. Fortunately, I followed his advice, and, as a result, the first edition of *Gynecologic Surgery* was very well received. I appreciate Dr. Queenan's guidance and encouragement throughout both editions. I am indebted to the expert and very professional staff at Blackwell Science. I want to thank Dr. Victoria Reeders for asking me to do the second edition. Coleen Traynor has made this possible by working with me since the inception of the book. Throughout all this work she was always helpful and constantly encouraged me when things were difficult. Thank you Coleen!

I also want to thank my daughter Monica, a student at my alma mater Georgetown University, for typing my chapters so that I could update them. I am grateful and indebted to the many well-known gynecologists and surgeons who have taken time to write new chapters and update previous chapters for this second edition of *Gynecologic Surgery*. Their superb contributions have made this book possible. To all my patients who have had faith in my ability to take care of them throughout the years, and to my parents for inspiring and encouraging me during my career. To my wife Miriam for her assistance while in college and medical school. Finally, to the many residents and students of Georgetown University School of Medicine, whom I have had the privilege of teaching: their motivation, dedication, and enthusiasm in their care of patients have been great sources of inspiration for me.

Luis E. Sanz, M. D.
Georgetown University School of Medicine
Washington, D.C.

Gynecologic Surgery

second edition

Part 1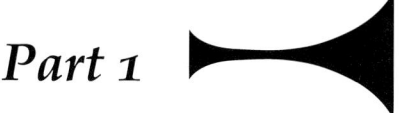

Anatomy: Principles of Surgery and General Surgery

Chapter 1

Anatomy of the retroperitoneum

Edward C. Hill

The retroperitoneum contains the bladder, rectum, cervix, vagina, and ureters, as well as ligaments, large blood vessels, nerves, and lymph nodes. Also within it are six avascular openings—the prevesical, vesicovaginal, rectovaginal, presacral, paravesical, and pararectal spaces. Knowing how to negotiate these areas will enable one to avoid injuring the ureters, nerves, or blood vessels.

Relation of ligaments to avascular spaces

Strands of fibrous connective tissue enclose the cervix and radiate from it laterally as the cardinal, anteriorly as the vesicouterine, and posteriorly as the uterosacral ligaments (Fig. 1-1). Dissection is easiest to perform on the retroperitoneal periphery, where the ligaments are thinnest and the avascular spaces are located.

Connective tissue also surrounds the ureters, nerves, blood vessels, and avascular spaces. By developing the avascular spaces, one can approach the lymph nodes, isolate large blood vessels, and safely dissect the ureters.

How to locate the ureter

To enter the retroperitoneum, make an incision in the parietal peritoneum over the psoas muscle at a point lateral to the infundibulopelvic ligament. Gently tease apart the areolar tissue to expose the psoas muscle, genitofemoral nerve, lymph nodes surrounding the external iliac vessels, and pelvic ureter as it crosses the bifurcation of the common iliac artery.

The ureter, found on the peritoneum's medial leaf posterior to the ovarian vessels, is identified by the small curlicue blood vessels in its adventitia (Fig. 1-2). To confirm its identity, look for peristalsis or roll the tube between thumb and index finger to elicit the characteristic tactile snap.

Developing the paravesical space

To approach the paravesical space, dissect through an avascular plane between the external iliac vessels and the hypogastric artery's anterior division lateral to the bladder. First expose the external vessels near their entrance to the femoral canal. This is best done by dividing the round ligament near the internal inguinal ring.

Note where the circumflex iliac vein crosses the external iliac artery (Fig. 1-3). The anterior hypogastric artery lies just medial.

The paravesical space is areolar down to the pelvic floor, or to the superior fascia of the levator ani muscle. On its medial boundary are the bladder and vagina, both extremely vascular. On its lateral side is the obturator fossa, containing the obturator nerve and blood vessels encased in fat-bearing lymph nodes.

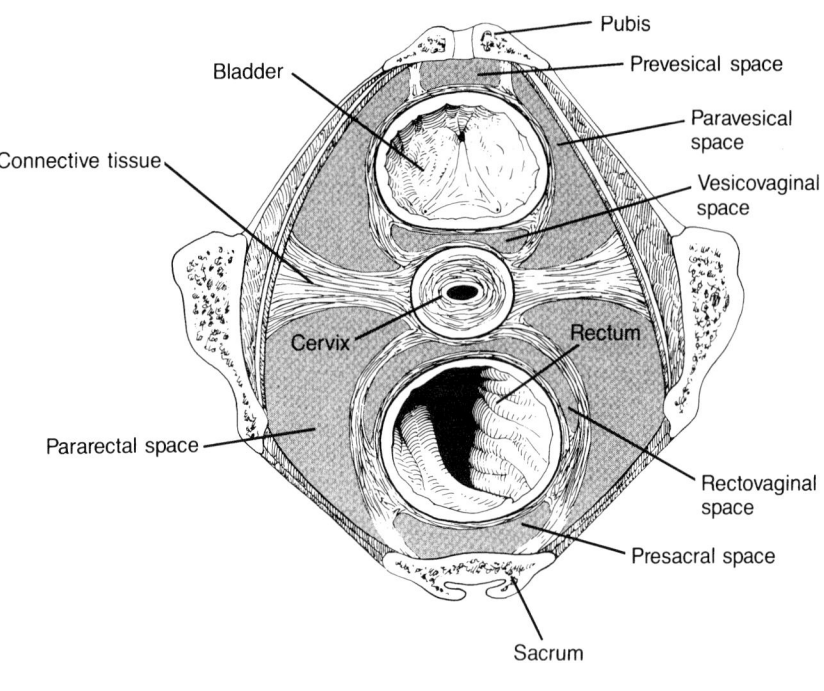

Pubis
Prevesical space
Bladder
Paravesical space
Connective tissue
Vesicovaginal space
Cervix
Rectum
Pararectal space
Rectovaginal space
Presacral space
Sacrum

Fig. 1-1 Avascular spaces. A connective tissue matrix in the retroperitoneum surrounds the bladder, cervix, rectum, and avascular spaces.

Approaching the pararectal space

To best develop the pararectal space, dissect between the first portion of the hypogastric artery's anterior division laterally and the ureter medially. It is important to remain close to the rectum to avoid the hypogastric vein and its pelvic sidewall tributaries.

The web, or cardinal ligament's peripheral segment, divides the paravesical and pararectal spaces (Fig. 1-4). Across its superficial portion can be found—and, if neces-

sary, ligated and divided—the uterine artery after it branches from the hypogastric artery.

A small branch of the uterine artery supplies the ureter, which is encased in the cardinal and vesicouterine ligaments. Freeing it requires entering the ureteral tunnel.

Access without blood loss is usually possible via areolar tissue in the middle of the vesicouterine ligament's deep part, beneath the ureter as it swings medially to join the

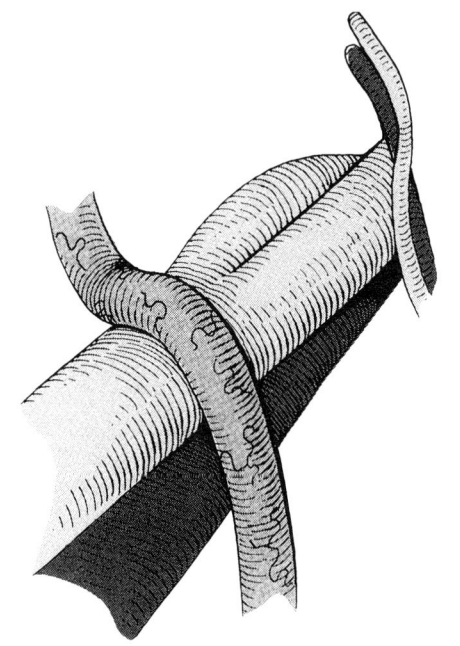

Fig. 1-2 Small curlicue blood vessels in the adventitia serve to distinguish the ureter.

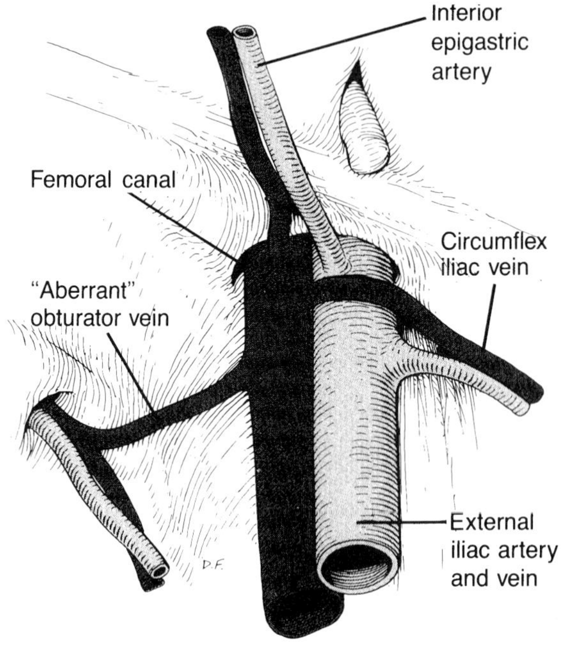

Inferior epigastric artery

Femoral canal

Circumflex iliac vein

"Aberrant" obturator vein

External iliac artery and vein

Fig. 1-3 Paravesical space's blood vessels. In developing the paravesical space, beware of the circumflex iliac vein as it crosses the external iliac artery to drain into the external iliac vein.

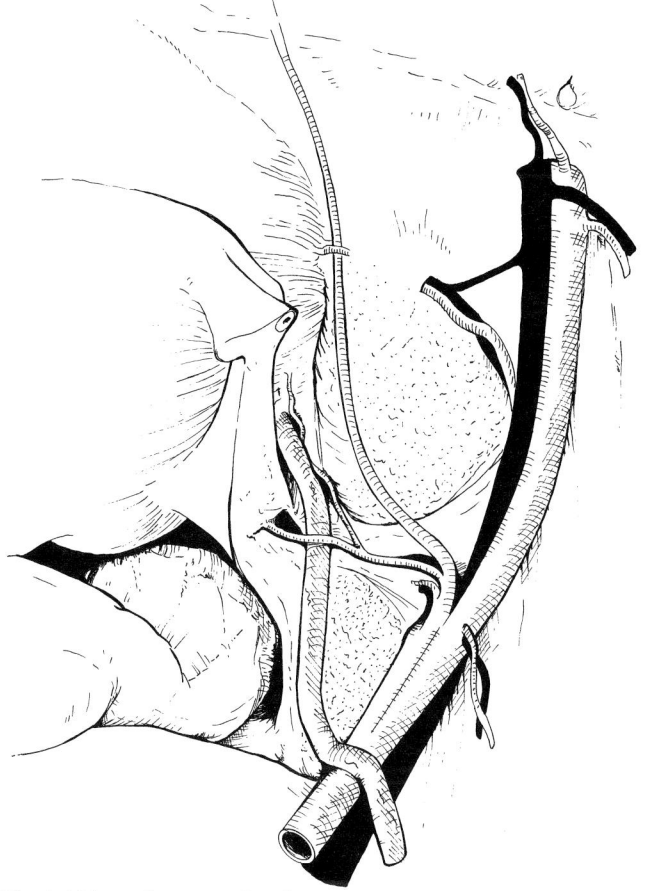

Fig. 1-4 The web, or peripheral segment of the cardinal ligament, is shown with adjacent structures.

bladder. Avoid other ligament areas, which contain tributaries of the uterine artery's descending branch and corresponding veins.

Vesicovaginal space techniques

To enter the vesicovaginal space, incise the vesicouterine peritoneal fold transversely. Development techniques vary from pushing the bladder down bluntly with a sponge stick to sharp dissection. I prefer to use Metzenbaum scissors to dissect areolar tissue while elevating the bladder with a pair of smooth thumb forceps.

A common error is to dissect too close to the cervix and fail to get into the proper plane. In dissecting toward the bladder muscle's soft, meaty red fibers, one encounters increased vascularity. Although the smooth, white, shiny fascia over the cervix is avascular, entering the cervix can cause bleeding. Be aware of the vesicouterine ligaments laterally. These are very vascular and contain the distal ureter, which curves medially to join the bladder.

Rectovaginal space may be altered

One can enter the rectovaginal space by incising the peritoneum between the insertion of the uterosacral ligaments.

At the vaginocervical junction the space becomes areolar, permitting dissection of the rectum away from the posterior vaginal wall.

Dividing the superficial portions of the uterosacral ligament's attachment to the cervix may simplify dissection. Remember, however, that the ureters are just lateral to these ligaments.

Anatomy of both the vesicovaginal and rectovaginal spaces may be considerably altered by previous cesarean section, endometriosis, pelvic infection, leiomyomata, or malignancy. In such instances, developing the paravesical and pararectal spaces first is very helpful.

Prevesical and presacral spaces

To enter the prevesical space, gently dissect the areolar tissue immediately posterior to the symphysis pubis. This provides access to the anterior bladder wall, vesical neck, urethra, and anterior vaginal wall. Watch for azygos veins.

Access to the presacral space is through an incision in the overlying parietal peritoneum. One may displace the sigmoid colon to the left. Inside this space, encased in fat, is the sympathetic nerve plexus (presacral nerve). Also found here, within the presacral fascia, are the middle sacral artery and vein. Take care not to sever the presacral vein, as bleeding from it is difficult to control.

Know the pelvic blood vessels

Opposite the lumbosacral joint, the right and left common iliac arteries divide into the right and left external iliac and internal iliac, or hypogastric, arteries, respectively (Fig. 1-5). Crossing both sets of common iliac vessels are the ovarian vessels, ureters, and sympathetic nerves. On the left are the mesocolon's sigmoid portion and the inferior mesenteric vessels.

The inferior epigastric artery arises from the external iliac artery just before it enters the femoral canal (Fig. 1-3). Frequently, too, a so-called aberrant obturator vein arises from the posterior external iliac vein near the canal. It is important to watch for it when dissecting into the obturator fossa.

The hypogastric artery dips into the pelvis and crosses the lumbosacral plexus, often giving off a small medial branch to the ureter. Approximately 3.5 cm from its origin arises its posterior division. This division supplies the parietal tissues through its ileolumbar, lateral sacral, and superior gluteal branches.

The hypogastric artery's anterior division, a continuation of the main artery, gives rise to the obturator, uterine, and superior vesical arteries superficially and the internal pudendal, vaginal, and middle hemorrhoidal branches deeper in the pelvis. Because none of the anterior division's

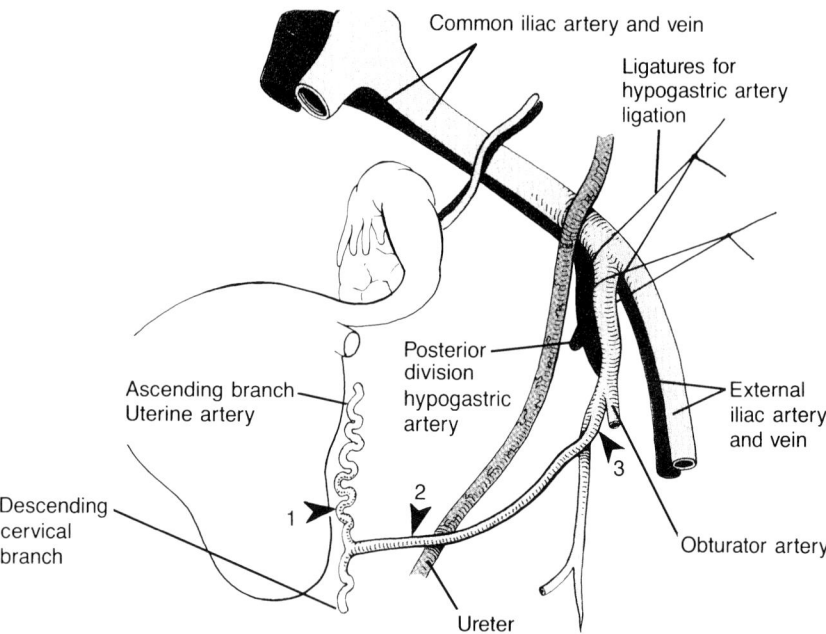

Common iliac artery and vein

Ligatures for
hypogastric artery
ligation

Posterior
division
hypogastric
artery

Ascending branch
Uterine artery

External
iliac artery
and vein

Descending
cervical
branch

1   2   3

Obturator artery

Ureter

Fig. 1-5 Hypogastric and uterine artery ligation. To tie off the hypogastric artery, pass two heavy ligatures around it as close to the bifurcation of the common iliac artery as possible. Where the uterine artery is ligated after hysterectomy depends on whether the procedure was (1) simple, (2) extended, or (3) radical.

branches arise anteriorly, one usually can develop it with little blood loss by staying on top of it.

Ligating the hypogastric arteries

To control hemorrhage, it may be necessary to ligate the hypogastric arteries. Prophylactic ligation, too, may be wise when a procedure involving considerable blood loss is anticipated.

Ligation is best carried out in the hypogastric artery's proximal portion, near the bifurcation of the common iliac artery (Fig. 1-5). First, identify the external iliac artery and vein, the hypogastric vein, and the ureter. Then elevate the artery with a Babcock clamp and carefully dissect between it and the vein. Risk of injuring the vein is reduced by dissecting from lateral to medial.

The next step is passing two heavy ligatures around the vessel. Tie them as near the bifurcation as possible, to minimize the chance of thrombus formation in a blind lumen and embolization of the lower extremity.

Uterine artery ligation

Performing a hysterectomy involves clamping, dividing, and ligating the uterine artery. Where on the artery this is done depends on the radicality of the operation (Fig. 1-5):
• For a simple hysterectomy, first develop the bladder flap, incise the posterior peritoneal leaf down to the insertion of the uterosacral ligaments, and, finally, skeletonize the ascending branch.
• For an extended hysterectomy, divide and ligate the vessel as it crosses the ureter about 1.5 cm lateral to the cervix.
• For a radical hysterectomy, divide the vessel at its origin. Both extended and radical hysterectomy require identify-

ing the ureter at the point where it passes beneath the uterine artery.

Pelvic and abdominal nodes

The external iliac nodes are encased in fatty areolar tissue surrounding the external iliac vessels. They receive afferent channels from the inguinofemoral and hypogastric nodes, external genitalia, deeper portions of the anterior abdominal wall, and pelvic viscera. They drain into the common iliac, hypogastric, and para-aortic nodes.

The hypogastric, or obturator, nodes are in the fat filling the obturator fossa posterior to the external iliac vessels. Because the obturator vessels and nerve are also in this area, care must be taken to avoid them when dissecting the nodes. The hypogastric nodes receive afferent vessels from the uterus, vagina, bladder, rectum, tubes, and ovaries. Drainage is to the external, common iliac and para-aortic nodes.

A parametrial, or ureteral, lymph node is one occurring near the point where the uterine artery crosses the ureter. Such a finding is common.

The para-aortic nodes are found in the fat pad anterior and lateral to the aorta. Those of concern to the gynecologist lie below the second portion of the duodenum and have the inferior vena cava on the right, the inferior mesenteric artery on the left, and the ovarian vessels and ureters on both sides (Fig. 1-6).

Locating key somatic nerves

The genitofemoral nerve runs along the psoas muscle lateral to the external iliac vessels and sends cutaneous branches to the vulva. Be sure to look out for it when dissecting the external iliac nodes.

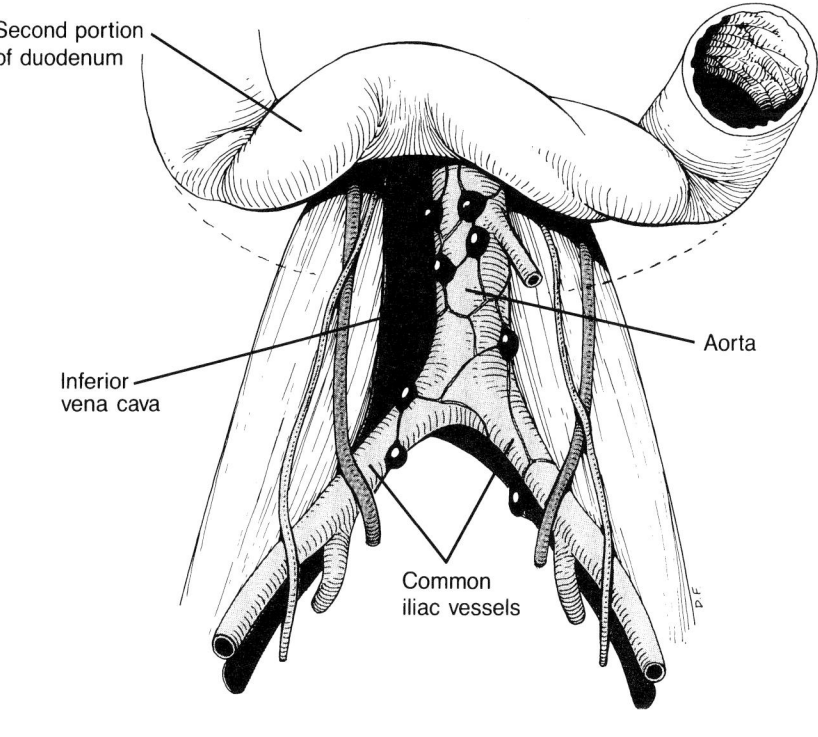

Fig. 1-6 Para-aortic nodes. The upper limit of nodal dissection for the gynecologist is the second portion of the duodenum.

The femoral nerve arises from vertebral levels L2, L3, and L4, descending in the angle between the psoas and iliacus muscles. There it is subject to ischemic damage from lateral abdominal retraction. It sends motor fibers to the rectus femoris and three vastus muscles of the anterior thigh, as well as sensory fibers to the front of the leg and ankle. Damage to the femoral nerve causes partial loss of extension of the leg and loss of sensation in the cutaneous distribution.

The obturator nerve, which is encased in the fat posterior to the external iliac vessels, passes downward in the obturator fossa along the pelvic lateral wall and exits through the obturator canal. This nerve supplies the adductor muscles of the thigh.

The common peroneal nerve, which is a major branch of the sciatic nerve, winds around the neck of the fibula to sup-

ply the leg's peroneal muscles. In addition, it sends cutaneous branches to the dorsum of the ankle and to the third, fourth, and fifth toes. Stirrup pressure injury to the nerve often produces foot drop and loss of sensation in the corresponding sensory distribution.

Suggested Readings

McCall ML, Bolten KA, eds. Martius' gynecological operations with emphasis on topographic anatomy. Boston: Little, Brown, 1956.

Netter FH. The Ciba collection of medical illustrations, reproductive system, vol 2. West Caldwell, NJ: CIBA Medical Education Division, 1965.

Novak F. Surgical gynecologic techniques. New York: Wiley, 1978.

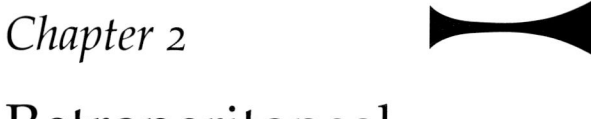

Chapter 2

Retroperitoneal approaches to pelvic surgery

Willard A. Barnes and Gregorio Delgado

Retroperitoneal dissection, although commonly used during surgical treatment of malignant disease, can be invaluable for managing benign conditions such as endometriosis, chronic pelvic inflammatory disease or tubo-ovarian abscess, large or interligamentous leiomyomata, and resection of residual ovaries, or for hypogastric artery ligation. The ability to utilize a retroperitoneal approach to the pelvic viscera should be an integral part of the gynecologic surgeon's armamentarium. To operate confidently and safely on the retroperitoneum, the surgeon must have a thorough understanding of the major retroperitoneal structures and avascular planes of the pelvis. This chapter briefly reviews surgical anatomy of the female pelvis along with techniques for retroperitoneal exploration.

Entering the retroperitoneum

When retroperitoneal dissection is anticipated, a preoperative excretory pyelogram is recommended to identify patients with preexisting genitourinary abnormalities, especially complete ureteral duplication. If the surgery is to be confined strictly to the pelvis, a transverse abdominal incision may be utilized; however, if the possibility of an extended operation exists, a vertical incision is preferable.

Once the pelvis has been exposed adequately, the retroperitoneal space can be entered in a variety of locations. If the pelvic lesion allows identification of the round ligament, a retractor may be placed to give upward traction on the round ligament, which may then be grasped with a Kelly clamp and elevated well away from the external iliac vessels (Fig. 2-1). From this position, a transfixing suture can be placed through the avascular portion of the broad ligament and the lateral portion of the round ligament. The broad ligament should be incised sharply in its lateral portion overlying the psoas muscles (Fig. 2-2) because a medial incision is more likely to result in vascular injury of the utero-ovarian plexus. The peritoneum can then be incised in a cephalad direction, lateral and parallel to the ovarian vessels. A combination of sharp and blunt dissection may then expose the retroperitoneal structures. If the uterus is displaced medially, the alveolar tissue may be grasped with atraumatic tissue forceps, gently elevated, and divided using fine scissors. Blunt dissection may be accomplished digitally or with the aid of moist sponge sticks, and should be performed by a gentle sweeping motion in the longitudinal axis rather than with a lateral-to-medial motion. The initial dissection should be bounded by the posterior leaf of the broad ligament and ureter medially and by the iliac vessels and pelvic sidewall laterally. Care should be taken not to dissect in a more lateral plane, as injury to the sidewall vessels may result.

Identifying the ureter

At this point some major retroperitoneal structures may be identified. The ureter can be seen crossing into the pelvis on

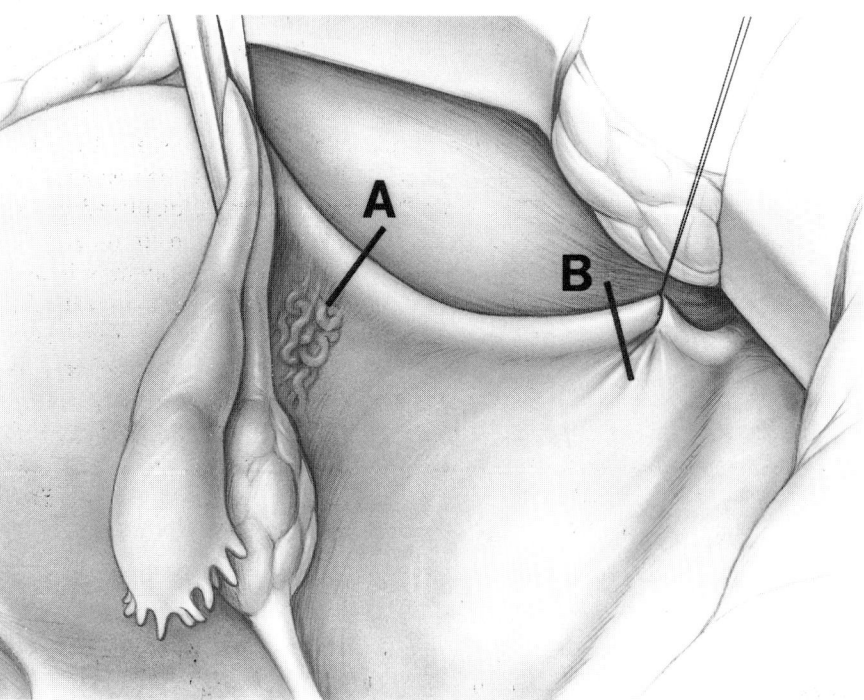

Fig. 2-1 Upward retraction of the round ligament will provide a point of easy entry into the retroperitoneal space.

the posterior aspect of the broad ligament at the bifurcation of the common iliac artery (Fig. 2-3). This crossing point is a consistent landmark and may be used routinely to locate the ureter. As it descends into the pelvis, the ureter remains intimately attached to the broad ligament peritoneum and can be located by gentle blunt dissection or by palpation. The ovarian vessels will also be found retroperitoneally near the ureter as it crosses the pelvic brim. Direct visualization of the ureter will allow safe ligation of the ovarian vessels and is particularly important whenever large pelvic masses or previous surgery distort the pelvic anatomy.

Using a paracolic approach

If the pelvic anatomy is severely distorted and the round ligament not easily identified, or if the pelvis is occupied with a mass, alternative approaches may be used to enter the retroperitoneal space. A paracolic approach is particularly useful when there are large pelvic lesions (Fig. 2-4). With this method, the paracolic peritoneum can be elevated and incised. Blunt and sharp dissection can then be used to mobilize medially the cecum or sigmoid colon, or both, in order to visualize the ureters before they enter the true pelvis.

The retroperitoneal dissection can be continued down into the pelvis, using the ureter as the landmark around which both the ovarian and the iliac vessels may be identified. The retroperitoneal space may also be entered by means of a lateral approach directly over—or even lateral to—the psoas muscle.

With any retroperitoneal approach to the pelvis that may require blunt dissection in an area of limited exposure and

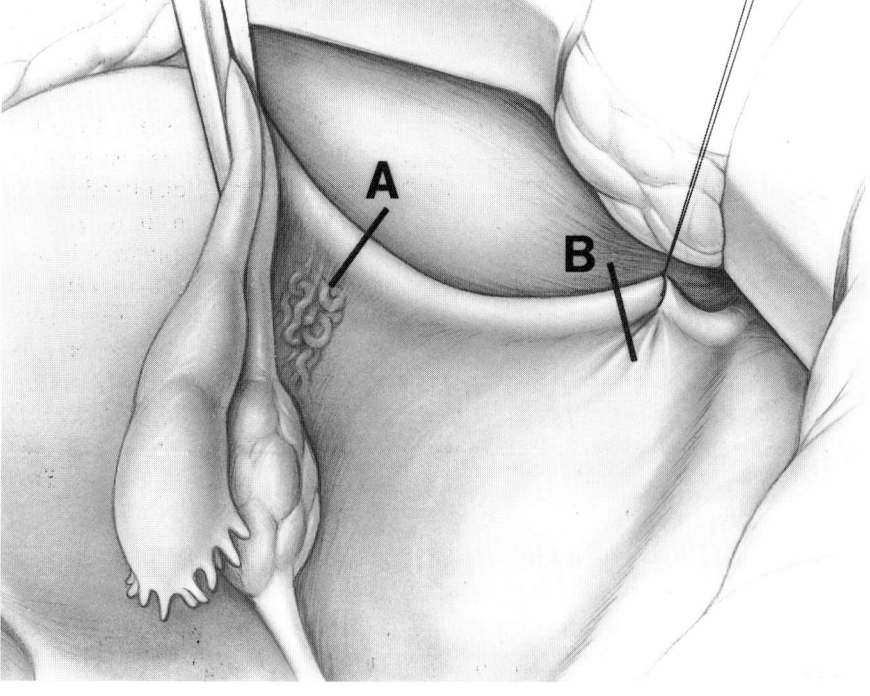

Fig. 2-2 Medial division of the round ligament (A) should be avoided; lateral transection of the round ligament (B) provides easier and safer access into the retroperitoneal space.

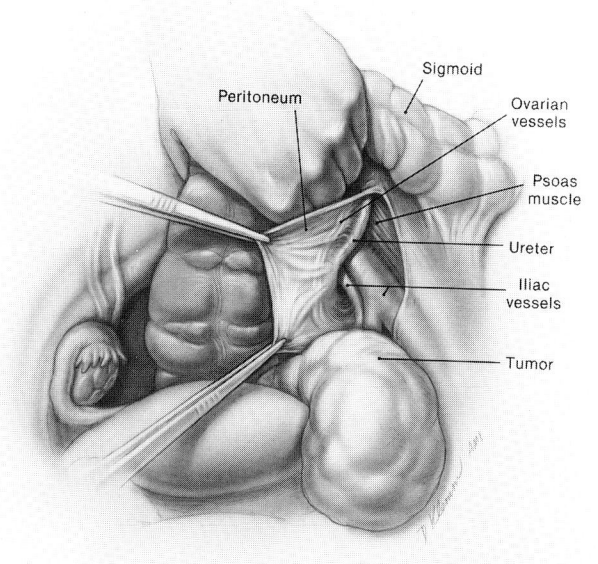

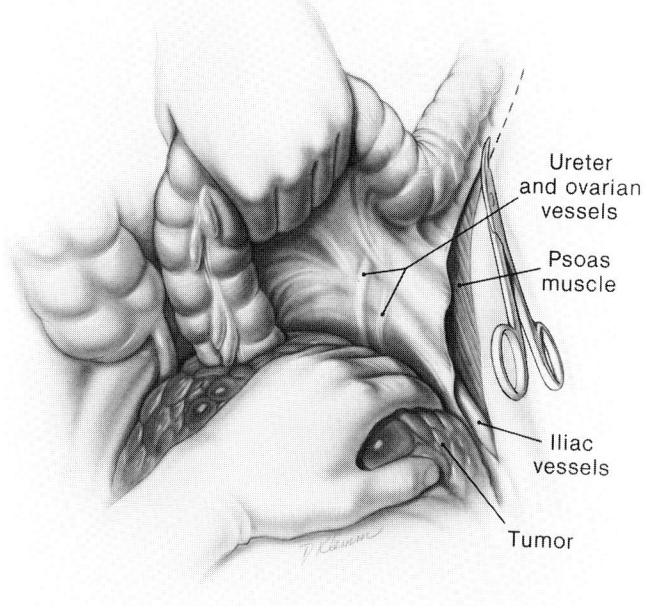

Fig. 2-3 The ureter passing into the pelvis is located near the bifurcation of the iliac vessels.

Fig. 2-4 To enter the retroperitoneum via the paracolic peritoneum, begin the incision over the psoas muscle, lateral to the ureter and ovarian vessels.

visibility, it is critical that the dissection begin and stay medial to the iliac vessels (Fig. 2-5). Inadvertent lateral dissection that enters the space between the psoas muscle and iliac blood vessels is quite possible and can lead to major blood vessel injury. The pelvic veins are particularly susceptible to avulsive injury (Fig. 2-6).

The initial retroperitoneal dissection can be invaluable because it provides some pelvic mobility and permits visualization of the ureter and major vessels. It also allows the surgeon to operate in a more pristine area than may be found intra-abdominally. These benefits alone can often result in safe removal of the otherwise onerous pelvic lesion.

Using the avascular pelvic planes

Further mobility, as well as visualization and definition of deep pelvic structures, can be obtained by using various avascular planes of the pelvis (Fig. 2-7). These planes are potential spaces that border the pelvic viscera, its fascial support, and blood supply. By properly developing the avascular spaces, the surgeon may approach any area of the pelvis without causing excessive morbidity.

The most anterior of these avascular planes is the prevesical space (of Retzius), which is commonly used during abdominal procedures for urinary stress incontinence. This space usually can be entered and easily developed primarily by blunt dissection of the bladder from the overlying symphysis pubis. The retrorectal space, the most posterior avasacular plane in the pelvis, is of value when dealing with a pelvic mass involving the sigmoid; it may also be used to gain access to the other presacral structures. This space may be entered by incising the peritoneum lateral to

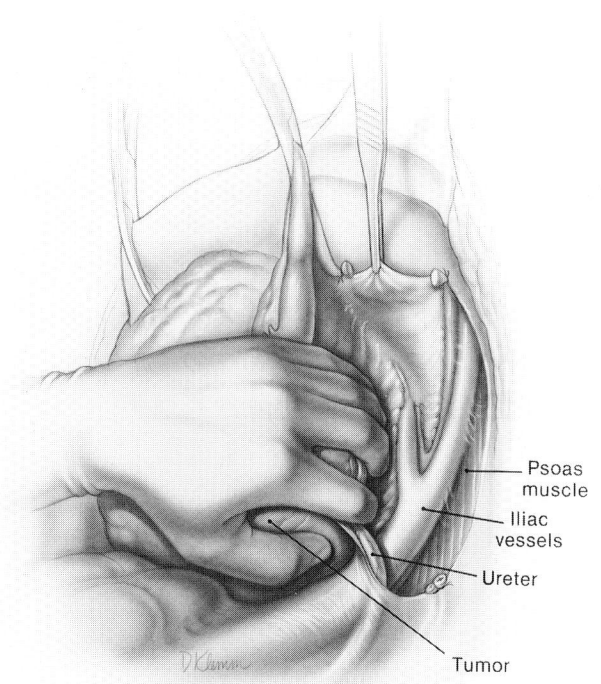

Fig. 2-5 When exposure is limited, develop the retroperitoneal space medial to the iliac vessels.

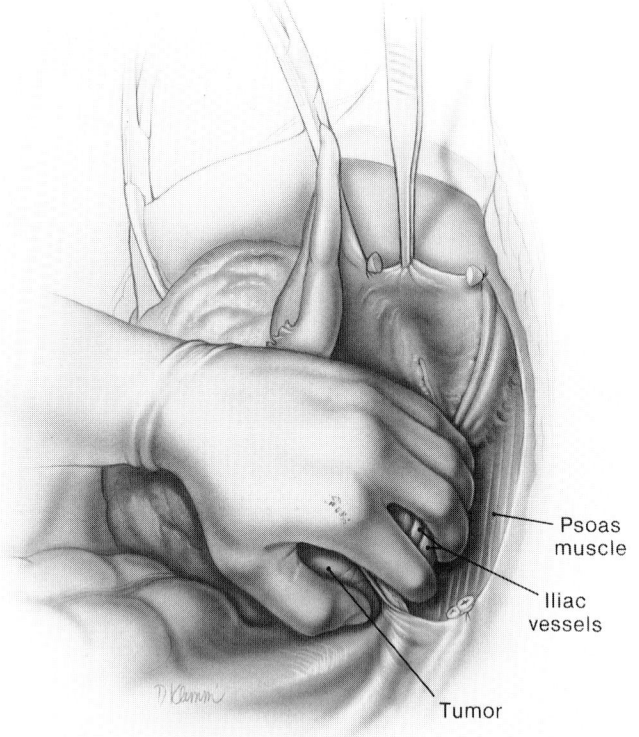

Fig. 2-6 Lateral dissection can lead to major vascular injury. The pelvic veins are especially vulnerable.

the sigmoid colon and its mesentery; blunt dissection is most commonly used to develop this space fully. Care must be taken, however, not to traumatize the sacral venous plexus. Its valveless array of interconnecting veins, if injured, can produce serious bleeding.

Of particular interest to the gynecologic surgeon are the avascular planes that encompass the uterus, its vascular and fascial support, and the pelvic ureter. As illustrated in Figures 2-7 and 2-8, these are the pararectal, paravesical, and rectovaginal spaces medially; they are routinely used during the course of any extended hysterectomy and can be of tremendous value during deep pelvic exploration and surgery. The paravesical space can be entered by elevating and dividing the connective tissue between the superior vesical artery medially and the external iliac vessels laterally. Blunt dissection following the inward pelvic slope can be continued to the pelvic diaphragm. The pararectal space is entered between the ureter and hypogastric artery and is developed in a similar fashion, again keeping dissection well medial to the pelvic sidewall and its vessels. To enter the rectovaginal space, the peritoneum at the base of the pouch of Douglas is divided, and the vagina is bluntly dissected from the rectum by sweeping the palm along the posterior vaginal wall. Should sharp dissection be required for adherent areas of the vagina and rectum, dissection should be against the vagina to minimize the possibility of enterotomy.

The vesicovaginal space is developed to a greater or lesser degree during the course of any hysterectomy; to develop this space more fully, sharp dissection may be continued down the anterior cervix and vagina, keeping medial to the vascular bladder pillars. Proper development

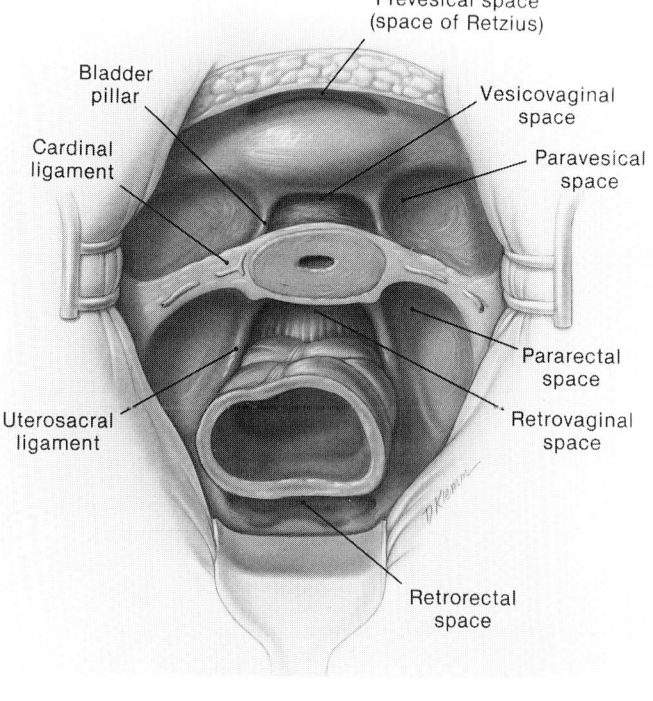

Fig. 2-7 Avascular spaces. Maneuvering within the retroperitoneum's avascular spaces during an operation can help reduce morbidity. *Prevesical or retropubic space (of Retzius):* bounded by the posterior surface of the symphysis pubis and the dome of the bladder. This space provides access to the bladder neck, urethra, and retroperitoneal portion of the bladder. *Vesicovaginal space:* bounded posteriorly by the cervix and the vagina, anteriorly by the bladder, and laterally by the bladder pillars. Development of this space gives access to the vesicouterine ligament, which contains the ureter as it passes to the bladder. *Paravesical space:* bounded medially by the superior vesical artery, laterally by the external iliac vessels and obturator nerve, and posteriorly by the uterine artery. The levator ani muscle forms the floor of the space. *Pararectal space:* bounded medially by the ureter and rectum, laterally by the hypogastric artery and pelvic wall, anteriorly by the uterine artery, and posteriorly by the sacrum. The levator ani forms the floor of the space. *Rectovaginal space:* bounded anteriorly by the vagina and posteriorly by the rectum. Lateral boundaries are the uterosacral ligaments and rectal pillars, which contain the middle hemorrhoidal arteries. *Rectorectal or presacral space:* bounded posteriorly by the sacrum and anteriorly by the rectum, with the uterosacral ligaments forming the lateral boundaries.

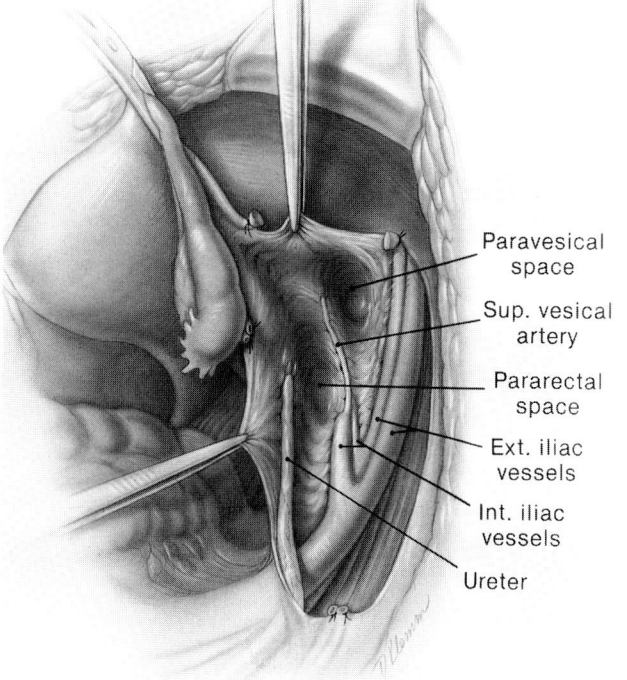

Fig. 2-8 Develop the paravesical, pararectal, and rectovaginal spaces to outline the cardinal and uterosacral ligaments and adjacent structures.

and exploration of these spaces should not result in significant operative morbidity or vascular compromise of the pelvic viscera. Moist gauze packing will usually control any slow venous bleeding encountered during dissection of these spaces.

Important anatomic relations

Following the development of the avascular planes, several important anatomic relations should be appreciated and used to guide further dissection (Figs. 2-7 and 2-8). The uterosacral ligament and ureter are located very near each other, between the rectovaginal and pararectal spaces. Awareness of the proximity of the ureter and its anatomic relation to these two avascular spaces is the key to avoiding ureteral injury when dissecting in this area of the pelvis. The ureter continues along the medial aspect of the pararectal space until it is crossed by the uterine artery and cardinal ligament, which, along with the superior vesical artery, lie between the pararectal and paravesical spaces. The ureter then remains close to the cervix as it transverses Wertheim's canal and enters the bladder. In this more complex area of the pelvis, meticulous dissection and careful identification of the surrounding structures are required and are best accomplished only after full development and proper use of the surrounding avascular spaces.

By fully utilizing the avascular planes of the pelvis, the surgeon can circumscribe most pelvic lesions without sacrificing any major structures or committing to further

surgery. Figure 2-9 illustrates how deep pelvic exploration may be accomplished laterally by taking advantage of the paravesical and pararectal spaces on each side. This type of exploration will allow identification of the lateral extent of a mass and permits its safe dissection and removal. Figure 2-10 illustrates how the same type of approach may be used

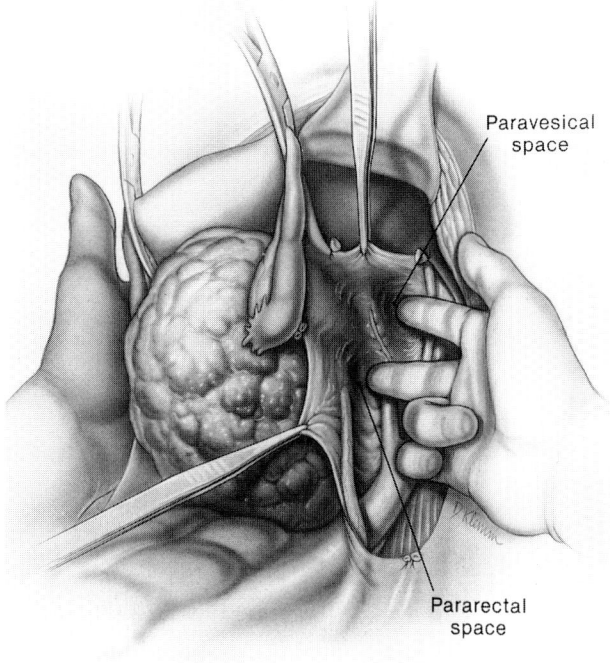

Fig. 2-9 By using the avascular planes, a large lesion can be completely circumscribed laterally.

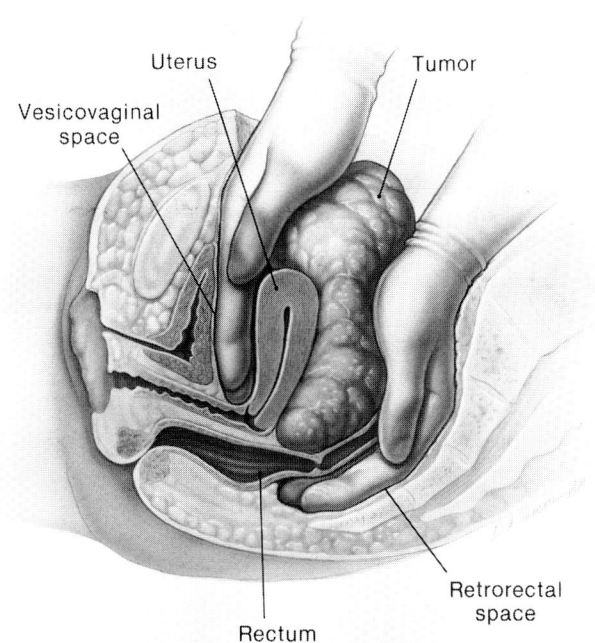

Fig. 2-10 The anterior and posterior extent of a large pelvic lesion can be encompassed retroperitoneally.

in the anteroposterior dimension of the pelvis. By combining these two maneuvers, the surgeon may grasp the pelvic viscera for examination and exploration. Once the extent of the operation has been delineated, the individual fascial and vascular structures may be approached retroperitoneally, dissected, and divided safely by utilizing various avascular spaces to provide exposure and anatomic perspective.

Summary

In summary, a variety of surgical approaches to the pelvis can be effected retroperitoneally. The approach is dictated by the lesion encountered and the operation anticipated. In most cases, the round ligament may be divided and the peritoneum lateral to the infundibulopelvic ligament incised without difficulty when the pelvic mass is small to moderate in size. When larger pelvic lesions or more severe anatomic distortion of the pelvis are encountered, a paracolic or lateral psoas muscle approach may be required for initial entry.

Once the peritoneum has been entered by one of these maneuvers, the ureter and iliac artery may be identified by combining palpation with sharp and blunt dissection. As these landmarks are exposed, they may be used to guide the surgeon into the various avascular planes of the pelvis, which then may be developed as needed to allow exploration and safe dissection of any area required. A retroperitoneal approach to the pelvic viscera can produce gratifying surgical results when dealing with a variety of pelvic pathology. There is no substitute for the exposure, mobility, anatomic display, and flexibility in approach offered by use of the retroperitoneal space and avascular planes of the pelvis.

Suggested Readings

Gray H. Gray's anatomy of the human body, 37th ed. New York: Churchill Livingstone, 1989.

Meigs JV, ed. Surgical treatment of cancer of the cervix. New York: Grune and Stratton, 1954.

Chapter 3

Selection of sutures in gynecologic surgery

Luis E. Sanz

As long there have been wounds to close, surgeons have sought the perfect suture material—one that would be ideal for all situations. This material would be easy to handle, maintain good knot security, and have low tissue drag and lasting tensile strength. It would also be nonallergenic and would retain its holding power even in the presence of infection. Finally, it would be absorbed in a predictable way throughout the wound-healing process. Obviously, this miraculous, all-purpose material remains undiscovered. No suture currently available has all the desired qualities; however, some have many of them. The surgeon's task is to understand the properties of each material and to select the one most appropriate for the job at hand.

The goal of wound closure is to help the patient's own repair mechanism restore normal anatomic relations. Toward this end, choice of suture material is just as important as proper incision and closure techniques in achieving good cosmetic results and preventing such complications as dehiscence and infection (1). The choice has widened since the end of World War II, with the appearance of synthetics offering superior strength, durability, and predictability. These advances in suture design have combined with advances in surgical technique and instrumentation to improve the surgeon's chances of success.

Sutures currently available—whether natural or synthetic, single-stranded or braided, coated or uncoated—fall into two broad types: absorbable and permanent (Table 3-1). As the name suggests, absorbable sutures are those that through either hydrolysis or proteolysis are eventually absorbed by the healing tissue. Nonabsorbable sutures are those that remain in the tissue forever (2). This chapter discusses the structure and uses of each.

Natural absorbable material

Plain catgut

One of the earliest sutures, dating back to the nineteenth century, is still called "catgut," though its source is actually the sheep. To make this material, submucosa of sheep jejunum and ileum is sliced into longitudinal ribbons. These are treated with a dilute formaldehyde that alters their collagen structure to increase tensile strength and resistance to enzymatic lysis. Two or more ribbons are twisted together to develop the desired caliber. The resulting strand is then dried under tension, polished, cut into appropriate lengths, attached to a needle, and sterilized by cobalt-60 irradiation.

Plain catgut, because it is derived from a naturally occurring substance, acts like a foreign body in the wound and can elicit a marked tissue reaction. Moreover, it is quickly degraded by the acid proteases of inflammatory cells and maintains tensile strength for only 4 to 5 days. For these reasons, it should not be used to close abdominal layers or other tissues that heal slowly.

Table 3-1 Classification of suture material

	Generic name	Raw material	Trade names
Absorbable			
Natural collagen	Plain catgut	Submucosa of sheep intestine	—
	Chromic catgut	Catgut plus buffered chromicizing	—
Synthetics	Polyglycolic acid	Homopolymer of glycolide with or without poloxamer 188 coating	Dexon, Dexon-S, Dexon-Plus
	Polyglactin	Copolymer lactic and glycolic acid, with or without calcium stearate coating	Vicryl, Coated Vicryl, Polysorb
	Polydioxanone	Monofilament	PDS
	Polyglyconate	Monofilament	Maxon
	Poliglecaprone 25	Monofilament	Monocryl
Nonabsorbable			
Natural fiber	Surgical cotton	Twisted natural cotton	—
	Surgical silk	Braided protein naturally spun by silkworms	Sofsilk
Synthetic	Nylon	Polyamide polymer	Bralon
		Monofilament	Dermalon, Ethilon, Monosof
		Multifilament	Neurolon
		Multifilament–silicone treated	Surgilon
	Polypropylene	Polymer of polypropylene	Surgipro
		Monofilament	Surgilene, Prolene
	Polybutester	Monofilament	Novafil
	Polyethylene	Thermoplastic synthetic resin	Dermalene
	Polyester	Polyethylene terephthalate–multifilament	
		Braided–plain	Dacron, Mersilene, Surgidac
		Braided–silicone treated	Ti-Cron
		Braided–polybutilate coated	Ethibond
		Braided–PTFE (Teflon)-coated	Polydek, Ethiflex
		Braided–heavily PTFE impregnated	Tevdek
Metal	Stainless steel wire	Ferrous alloy	—
		Twisted multistrand	Flexon
		Monofilament strand	—

Chromic catgut

Treating plain catgut with basic chromium salts creates a suture material that is stronger and more resistant to absorption. Chromic catgut maintains tensile strength for 14 to 21 days depending on its diameter and is suitable for use on visceral, serosal, and vaginal surfaces that heal rapidly. It is not recommended for slower healing wounds (3).

Like untreated catgut, chromic catgut is absorbed by proteolysis, a process that can produce marked inflammation. One should therefore never use chromic catgut on the skin, where it may serve as a nidus for bacterial infection and cause enough inflammation to leave significant scar-

ring. However, because it dissolves quickly, it is the suture of choice for the Pomeroy tubal ligation procedure. A longer-lasting suture might allow a fistula to form between the two ends of the bisected tube, increasing the likelihood of ligation failure.

Absorbable synthetics

Polyfilaments

Devised to overcome the shortcomings of catgut, polyglycolic acid (Dexon) became available in 1970 and polyglactin (Vicryl) in 1975. Polyglycolic acid, a high molecular weight linear copolymer of glycolic acid, is synthesized, melted, stretched into filaments, and similarly braided into sutures (4).

Polyglycolic acid and polyglactin have almost identical biological properties. They do not rely on cellular processes for absorption but are degraded by slow hydrolysis. These sutures cause inflammation and are absorbed at a reliable and constant rate. Neither undergoes much degradation during the first 10 days in animal tissue. Absorption begins between 10 and 15 days and is completed in 28 to 70 days, depending on suture size.

The initial tensile strength of Dexon and Vicryl is greater than that of catgut, a benefit they owe to their braided structure. Moreover, they stand up well. Each retains approximately 55% of its original tensile strength at 14 days and 20% at 20 days. In comparison, after 14 days, chromic catgut retains only 34% of its original strength and plain catgut is entirely absorbed (5). Another suture is Polysorb, a braided synthetic suture of lactomer 9-1 that handles like silk and is similar to Dexon and Vicryl although it has a lower drag coefficient and a slightly higher initial tensile strength.

Knot security is an important consideration in choosing a suture material. This refers to the material's resistance to slippage under tension after being tied into a square knot. The ability to hold a knot correlates with the material's coefficient of friction, which in the case of natural sutures can be lowered by tissue fluids. Dexon and Vicryl are less subject to these influences than catgut is and maintain good knot security in vivo (6). The length of the cut end, type of knot, and surgical technique also influence knot security.

One drawback of synthetic absorbable sutures is that they generally do not handle as well as natural ones. To reduce this difficulty, manufacturers have introduced coated versions (Dexon-Plus, Coated Vicryl) that have less memory than the uncoated type and lie easier. Dexon-S, another option, is constructed of finer filaments that are woven tightly to form a smoother, more manageable braid. The improved feel of these modified synthetic absorbable sutures has been achieved at some expense to knot security. Because knots with these newer materials tend to slip when not properly thrown, the manufacturers recommend adding two additional square knots with longer tails when using them.

Monofilaments

A newer class of synthetic absorbable suture is represented by the monofilaments polyglyconate (Maxon) and polydioxanone (PDS) (7). These single-stranded sutures are similar to the polyfilaments in tensile strength, knot security, and ability to curtail tissue inflammatory response.

Like all sutures, Maxon and PDS cause initial inflammation. However, this response is short-lived. Seldom, if ever, does subsequent chronic inflammation occur with these materials, because their monofilament structure contains no interstices to serve as a nidus for bacterial invasion and infection.

Maxon and PDS maintain tensile strength longer than Dexon and Vicryl. They retain as much as 95% of their initial tensile strength by postoperative day 10 and about 50% by postoperative day 28 (40% with Maxon and 50% with PDS). This property is particularly beneficial in situations of delayed wound healing, as in patients who have diabetes or infection or who are undergoing chemotherapy or corticosteroid therapy (Fig. 3-1).

The synthetic absorbable monofilaments are also preferable in wounds involving the fascia, because they can support the incision adequately for more than 6 weeks. One should not, however, attempt subcuticular skin closure with Maxon or PDS sutures unless they will be removed within 7 to 10 days. These sutures take so long to be absorbed that some material will be rejected from the incision site if left in longer. It is therefore better to use fine sutures (4-0 or 5-0) of Vicryl, Dexon, or poliglecaprone 25 (Monocryl) for subcuticular closures (8).

Monocryl, a new monofilament synthetic with the same characteristics as PDS and Maxon but with a faster absorption rate, is a great aid to the gynecologic surgeon. Monocryl handles better than PDS and Maxon because it has less memory. It is absorbed in 21 to 28 days. In the future, this will be one of the most commonly used sutures in obstetrics and gynecologic surgery.

Because they cause less tissue inflammation and have greater tensile strength than catgut materials, Maxon, PDS, and Monocryl are also excellent for pelvic and vaginal surgery. Like all monofilaments, however, these sutures require special attention with respect to knotting and handling. Knots must be properly placed with the standard surgical technique of flat and square ties, and with additional throws as indicated by circumstances. Particular care is needed when a continuous suture is used to ensure that the knot will not open. To avoid damaging the monofilament structure during handling, do not grip the strands with a needle holder or any other instrument unless one is grasping the free end of the suture. Abrasions left by such instruments can seriously weaken the suture and increase the risk that it may break down later. This is especially important when using the Smead-Jones closure technique, because any crack in the material will produce a dehiscence or an incisional hernia (9).

Nonabsorbable sutures

Silk, cotton, nylon, polyester, polypropylene, polybutester, and stainless steel constitute the currently available nonabsorbable suture materials. Polypropylene (Prolene and Surgipro) and polybutester (Novafil) are available in monofilament form; silk, cotton, and polyester are available in polyfilament form; and nylon and stainless steel are available in both monofilament and polyfilament form.

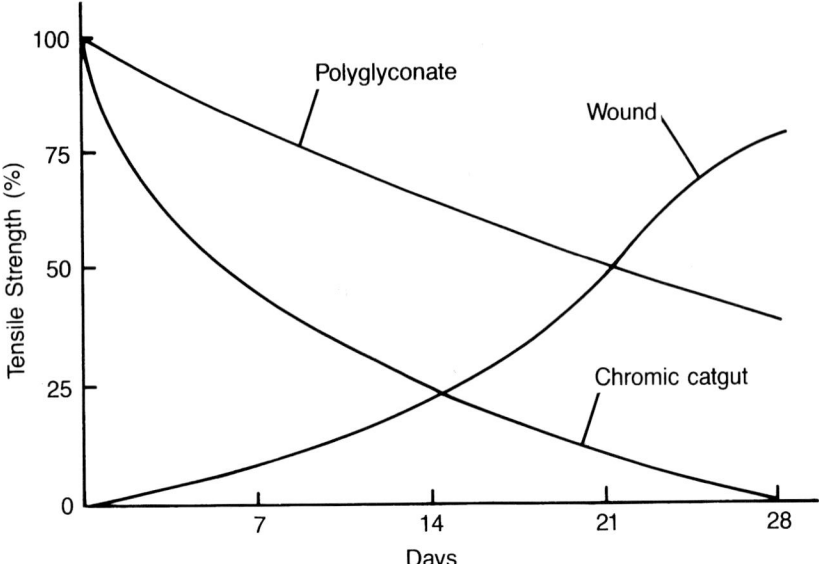

Fig. 3-1 Wound and suture tensile strengths. Over time, wound tensile strength increases and suture tensile strength decreases. Polyglyconate, a synthetic material, retains its tensile strength better than chromic catgut.

Surgical silk is derived from the naturally occurring fiber and, like catgut, has a long history of surgical use. It is classified as nonabsorbable because it retains most of its tensile strength for more than 60 days; it loses approximately 50% after one year and most of it after 2 years. Although it is stronger than cotton, it is weaker than the synthetic nonabsorbable sutures. Silk has low memory—that is, it does not tend to recoil to its original form after being bent or twisted. It therefore offers good knot security and is easy to handle. Its current lack of popularity stems from the significant amount of inflammation it can initiate. This reaction is unavoidable, because silk is a naturally occurring protein that can elicit an immune response. No other nonabsorbable suture causes as much tissue reaction in certain patients.

Cotton, the only other natural nonabsorbable suture material currently available, is rarely used. Like silk, it handles easily and causes a great deal of tissue reaction, but it is weaker. Because wet cotton is 10% stronger than dry cotton and also handles better, it is helpful to moisten cotton before use.

Braided polyfilament nylon (Neurolon, Surgilon, and Bralon) and monofilament nylon (Dermalon, Ethilon, and Monosof) are nonabsorbable materials composed of synthetic polymer fibers. They have an initial tensile strength similar to that of silk, but they lose only 20% of this initial strength (through hydrolysis) after one year and none thereafter. Because it is a synthetic material, nylon induces less tissue reaction than naturally occurring silk or cotton. The monofilament nylons incite even less reaction than their polyfilament counterparts, so they are more desirable for suturing contaminated wounds and closing skin and fascia. All nylon sutures are easy to handle, but they have a greater tendency toward knot slippage than do the polyester materials. Close attention to surgical technique and additional square knots are required for adequate knot security.

Polyester sutures possess greater initial tensile strength than nylon, silk, or polypropylene; only stainless steel is stronger. Dacron polyester, a braided material, causes less tissue reaction than silk but is equally manageable, easy to tie, and unlikely to slip its knot. A wide variety of polyester formulations is available. The plain uncoated types (Mersilene, Dacron, and Surgidac) offer the best knot security; those coated with polytetrafluoroethylene (PTFE or Teflon), such as Polydek, Ethiflex, and Tevdek, handle better. Ethibond, coated with polybutilate, is also easy to handle and provokes less tissue reaction than other polyesters. In contrast, Tevdek and the silicone-coated suture Ti-Cron, although easy to handle, cause comparatively more inflammation and have poorer knot security. Moreover, because they are braided, they must be removed if an infection develops.

Stainless steel wire, made from a ferrous alloy, provides more tensile strength and knot security than any other nonabsorbable or absorbable suture and can therefore be used to repair wound disruption, evisceration, and infected sites. However, the newer sutures of polypropylene or polybutester are preferable. Stainless steel provokes less tissue reaction than nylon or polyester materials but is difficult to handle, tending to fatigue, kink, and deform at points of stress and fracture. Some of these shortcomings have been corrected by twisting multiple strands of fine steel wire into a single suture (Flexon). However, this material must be handled carefully, as it has a tendency to puncture gloves and tissue. Special instruments are required to cut stainless steel suture, and it is seldom used.

Which suture to use?

In the early postoperative days, wounds display a mild inflammatory reaction, characterized by migration of polymorphonuclear cells (10). During this lag phase and until the proliferative phase of healing begins, tissue tensile strength remains low. As collagen is synthesized and deposited, wound tensile strength increases proportionately. During the lag phase and early proliferative phase, sutures are needed to hold the wound together.

Choice of suture material is therefore based on how rapidly the affected tissues will heal and how much strength will be needed to support them while they are healing. Because visceral organs and peritoneal or vaginal surfaces generally heal quickly, wounds in these tissues can be managed with sutures that maintain tensile strength relatively briefly. Chromic catgut or Monocryl is appropriate for these wounds because it retains strength long enough to endure through the critical healing phase and is absorbed rapidly thereafter. One can also use Vicryl and Dexon, but only in fine diameters (3-0 or 4-0); with larger calibers, some suture may remain after the wound has healed.

By contrast, sutures in the skin and fascia, which heal more slowly, must provide longer-term tensile strength. Durability is particularly important in fascia, which regains only 25% of its original strength after 20 days of healing. Wounds will dehisce or herniate if the fascial layer is closed improperly or with the wrong material. Probably the best sutures for closing fascia are the long-lasting monofilament absorbables Maxon and PDS. Dexon and Vicryl retain tensile strength longer than chromic suture, but are quickly absorbed after 30 days—too soon to be effective for fascial repair unless a larger diameter, such as No. 0 or 1, is used. Prolene, Surgipro, and Novafil, synthetic monofilaments that are strong and dependable, are also used frequently in fascial and Smead-Jones closures. Maxon and PDS sutures, however, are permanent.

Before synthetic sutures appeared, fascia was generally closed with interrupted sutures. This approach was recommended primarily because the absorption rate of the suture then used, chromic catgut, was sometimes unpredictable. With the availability of more predictable materials like Maxon and PDS, most fascial closures can be accomplished with a continuous technique.

Risk of inflammation and infection is still a prime concern in choosing a suture material. The polyfilament absorbable sutures Dexon and Vicryl and the polyfilament nylon sutures provoke minimal inflammation except when infection is present. With these polyfilament sutures, significant inflammation associated with infection has been attributed to the ability of bacteria to invade and colonize the braids' interstices. The evoked inflammatory response from the surrounding tissue is unable to eradicate these bacteria because granulocytes and macrophages are too large to migrate within the tightly woven braid. Monofilament sutures like Monocryl do not provide such a nidus for infection. Infection slows the absorption of Dexon and Vicryl sutures but does not prolong retention of their tensile strength; the two qualities do not correlate. Hence, most of the holding power of Dexon and Vicryl is lost in infected tissue after 30 days, even though much material may remain unabsorbed.

Synthetic monofilament nonabsorbable sutures, such as Prolene and Novafil, are the materials of choice for closing infected tissue. This is particularly true in cases of infected abdominal wall fascia, in which tensile strength is crucial and chronic inflammation is least desirable.

Surgical needles

Surgical needles are made of high-quality stainless steel alloy that is heated to increase its strength. The needles undergo electropolishing, and some have a microthin silicone finish that decreases tissue drag and trauma. The less trauma to the tissues, the less chance of wound infection. The selection of the needle depends on the type of tissue to be sutured, the size of the suture material, and the location of the injured site. Surgical needles have the resilience to bend 45 degrees before breaking; otherwise, breaking of the needles could be a much more common event.

All needles have three parts: the point, the body, and the eye. The point can be cutting, tapercut, tapered, or blunt. Cutting needles should be avoided unless necessary because they can cut vessels and increase the bleeding. In gynecologic surgery, they are usually needed for subdermal closures; very seldom are they needed in the fascia, as tapered needles are strong enough to penetrate it. The most common needle used in gynecology is the tapered point. The body of the needle is the needle-grasping area, which can be oval, round, triangular, side-flattened rectangular, or trapezoidal. The longitudinal shape of the body can be half-curved, straight, curved, or compound curved. The eye of the needle can be French (the end is split), closed eye, and swaged. Some of the swaged needles have a control release mechanism, which makes them excellent for interrupted sutures because the needle can be pulled from the suture without cutting.

Summary

The judicious choice of proper surgical materials will assist the patient's healing process and ensure a good cosmetic result. In selecting suture material and surgical needles, the surgeon must consider the type of operation to be done and the tissues involved, as well as the patient's history and medical complications. Although one ideal suture for all situations may never be forthcoming, the variety of materials available offers the operator ample opportunity to choose one that is likely to produce optimal results.

References

1 Sanz LE. Choosing the right wound-closure technique. Contemp Ob Gyn 1983;21(Surg):142.
2 Peacock EE. Wound repair, ed 3. Philadelphia: WB Saunders, 1984.

3 Greenburg AG, Saik RP, Peskin GW. Wound dehiscence: patho-physiology and prevention. Arch Surg 1979;114:143.

4 Yu GV, Cauqliere R. Suture materials—properties and uses. J Am Podiatr Assoc 1981;73:57.

5 Sanz LE, Smith S. Mechanism of wound healing, suture material, and wound closure. In: Buchsbaum HJ, Walton LA, eds. Strategies in gynecologic surgery. New York: Springer-Verlag, 1986:53–76.

6 Trimbus JB. Security of various knots used in surgical practice. Obstet Gynecol 1984;64–274.

7 Sanz LE, Patterson JA, Kamath R, et al. Comparison of Maxon suture with Vicryl chromic gut PDS sutures in fascial closure in rats. Obstet Gynecol 1988;71–73.

8 Stillman RM, Bella FJ, Seligman SJ. Skin wound closure methods on susceptibility to infection. Arch Surg 1980;115:674.

9 Wallace D, Hernandez W, Schlaerth J, et al. Prevention of abdominal wound disruption utilizing the Smead-Jones closure technique. Obstet Gynecol 1980;56:226.

10 Sanz LE. Wound management: matching materials and methods for best results. Contemp Obstet Gynecol 1987;30:86.

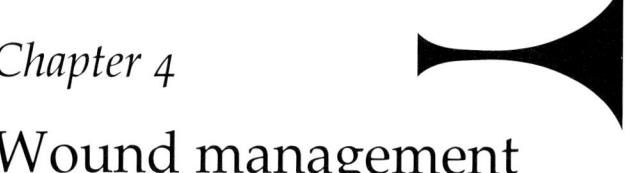

Chapter 4

Wound management

Luis E. Sanz

The goal of surgical wound closure is to help the patient's own repair mechanisms restore normal anatomic relations. Selecting the proper incision method, suture material, and closure technique will prevent such complications as dehiscence and infection while ensuring good cosmetic results. To choose correctly, and consequently decrease morbidity and mortality, one must thoroughly understand the physiology of wound healing.

How the body repairs wounds

The four phases of wound healing are inflammation, migration, proliferation, and maturation. The inflammatory response, occurring initially in all wounds, serves to dispose of all foreign materials, dying tissue, and bacteria so repair may begin (1). Cellular and vascular processes occurring in this phase are identical regardless of the type of injury (2). At this early phase neutrophils infiltrate the injured site to eliminate bacteria. However, if infection occurs, this first inflammatory phase is prolonged. This will cause continued activation of complement and further tissue injury and delayed healing. It also prevents proliferation of epithelial cells to approximate the wound, therefore increasing scar formation (3). Wound contamination and foreign bodies may cause chronic inflammation, granuloma formation, and some other associated complications.

Migration of fibroblasts along fibrin strands in the wound initiates the second phase of healing. Fibroplasia, which increases tensile strength and parallels the rate of collagen synthesis, then occurs (4). Simultaneously, basal layer epithelial cells migrate toward one another until contact inhibition takes place. However, this event can be a problem in the peritoneal surface of the abdomen because it can create adhesions. The peritoneum consists of a single layer of mesothelial cells. Underneath this layer there are many infection-fighting cells like lymphocytes, macrophages, plasma cells, mast cells, and fibroblasts. Adhesions are formed when there is excessive inflammation and increased fibrin formation (5). This may lead to adhesions and their sequelae of pain, bowel obstruction, and infertility. Plasminogen activator present in this mesothelium aids in the lysis of early fibrinous attachments and therefore prevents adhesion formation through the process of fibrinolysis. Other chemical factors in adhesion formation are the cytokines and prostaglandins. This is why it is important to minimize damage to both parietal and visceral peritoneum during surgery (4). Tissue ischemia is another important factor in decreasing fibrinolysis because tissue vascularity is critical for proper healing (6). Thus one must avoid closing the peritoneum under tension or with interlocking sutures. Many studies have shown that there are fewer adhesions when the peritoneum is left open because the peritoneum heals mainly by metaplasia. According to Rosenberg, the main cause of peritoneal adhesions are trauma, ischemia, foreign bodies, bleeding, and raw surfaces (7). Therefore minimizing trauma to the tissues and good hemostasis are important for good healing.

In the skin, once migration stops, the epithelial layer becomes thicker. Wound contamination is prevented by the epithelial layer 24 to 48 hours after migration begins. Proliferation, a continuation of migration, serves to increase the wound's tensile strength.

Maturation produces the wound's final cosmetic appearance, in which the initial red, firm scar becomes white and soft. Remodeling of the scar is an important dynamic process involving collagen breakdown and proliferation. In those few persons in whom collagen production exceeds degradation, a bulkier scar, or keloid, may form. If there is no rejection of suture material and collagen destruction exceeds production, a softer, less conspicuous scar will form.

Is the incision method relevant?

Abdominal wound disruption is a serious postoperative complication, with mortality occurring in approximately 20% of cases (range 11%–35%) (8). Despite advances in surgical technique, the incidence of fascial dehiscence has remained between 0.5% and 5% generally, and between 0.3% and 0.7% for gynecologic procedures specifically. The slightly lower rates of dehiscence in gynecologic surgery have been attributed to infraumbilical and low transverse incisions, lower average patient age, less postoperative physical activity, lower infection rates, and fewer bowel-related procedures (9). Abdominal wall elasticity resulting from pregnancy has also helped decrease dehiscence.

Although studies had indicated that transverse abdominal wall incisions were stronger than vertical ones, these conclusions were later questioned on the grounds that the studies might not have been performed under appropriately randomized conditions. Because vertical incisions allow faster access to the abdominal cavity, they were probably performed in sicker patients. In 95% of cases, I prefer to use a transverse incision, either a Pfannenstiel or a Maylard incision. There is no question that it is stronger and cosmetically satisfying for the patient.

Recent experiments have not supported the theory that transverse incisions are under comparatively less tension. Suture material, surgical technique, and the patient's general condition are better predictors of wound healing than incision type. Many mechanical, biologic, and technical factors contribute to perioperative wound dehiscence (Table 4-1). In general, it can be said that wound disruption occurs most commonly between postoperative days 5 and 12, with postoperative day 8 being the mode. The technique used to make the abdominal incision, particularly in the fascia, has significant influence on wound integrity. One study reported that six of eight dehiscences were associated with the use of electrocautery for incising the fascia. In most of these cases, aseptic necrosis was found at the site of wound approximation.

Table 4-1 High-risk factors for wound dehiscence

Preoperative

Advanced age

Chemotherapy

Chronic cough

Chronic illness

Malignant disease

Poor nutrition

Obesity

Previous abdominal surgery

Prior radiotherapy

Pulmonary disease

Steroid therapy

Intraoperative

Improper selection of incision, suture material, or closure technique

Postoperative

Ileus

Intestinal obstruction

Vomiting

Wound infection

Suture choice also plays a large part in ensuring wound integrity. If the suture is absorbed too rapidly, tensile strength is lost from the healing wound and breakdown occurs. Suture material such as chromic catgut is frequently incriminated in these wound disruptions. Although breakage is uncommon, it can occur, particularly if the suture is tied incorrectly. Furthermore, knots may untie or slip (10). For this reason, it is essential that properly applied surgical knots always be used in wound closure. Clinically, the most common cause of wound dehiscence is the intact suture cutting through the tissue in which it has been placed (11). One study reports this problem alone as responsible for 88% of disrupted wounds (12). Large bites with thick suture material are less likely to slice tissue than small bites with thin suture material. One should tie sutures relatively loosely to avoid tissue ischemia, which contributes to weakening of the suture line (Fig. 4-1) (13).

Finally, general closure technique strongly influences wound integrity. Several studies show that mass closure, when indicated, is mechanically more sound because it allows for the 30% increase in abdominal distention that occurs postoperatively. Midline incisions with mass closure (Smead-Jones) are three times as resistant to dehiscence as paramedian incisions with layer-by-layer closure, twice as resistant as layer-by-layer closures within the linea alba, and 1.7 times as resistant as layer-by-layer closures of a transverse supraumbilical incision.

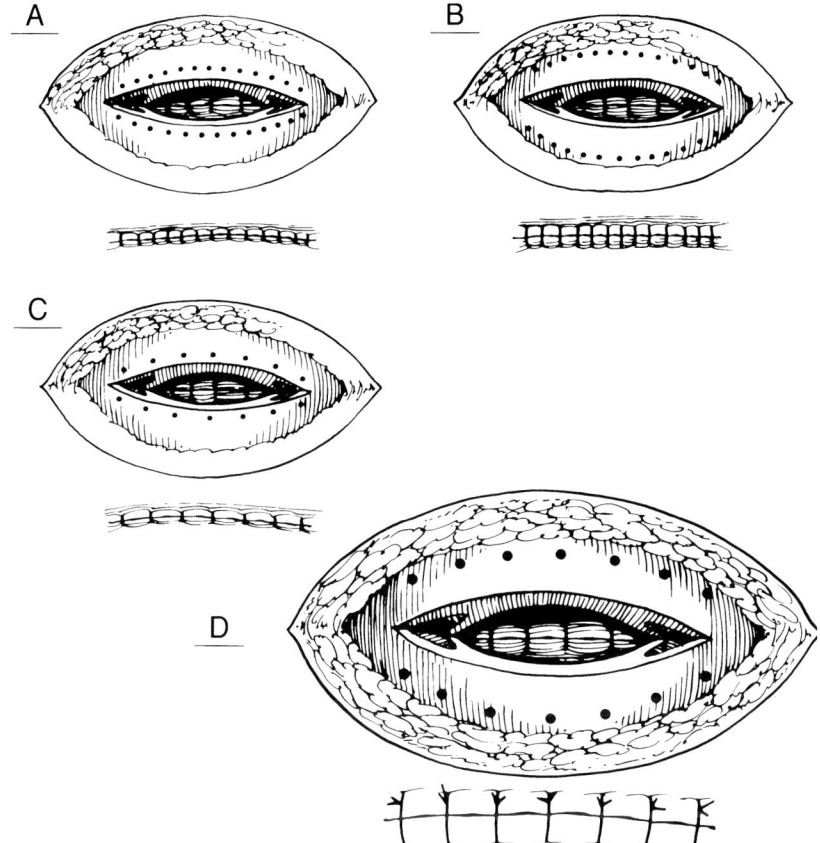

Fig. 4-1 Sanders and colleagues report that closure is stronger when sutures are placed 1 cm from the fascial edge and tied loosely (16). Techniques shown in A, B, and C are wrong; D is correct.

Many surgeons believe that interrupted sutures provide greater tensile strength than continuous suturing; however, this view is not well documented. More likely, tissue bites and diameter of suture material have greater influence on wound security. Patients at low risk of wound dehiscence will tolerate layer-by-layer closure, but mass closure is recommended for high-risk patients. External retention sutures are not used very often, as they are painful, cosmetically unattractive, and more likely than internal mass closure to serve as a nidus for wound infection.

Layer-by-layer closure

Before closing the peritoneum, one should accomplish hemostasis and wash the pelvic cavity several times with warm saline to remove debris, decrease opportunity for infection, and reduce likelihood of adhesion formation. Then one should close individually the layers of the abdomen, parietal peritoneum, fascia, subcutaneous tissue, and skin. A large randomized trial by Elkins (5) showed no difference in rates of dehiscence between patients who underwent peritoneal closure and those who did not. If the peritoneum is to be closed, one should use small-diameter absorbable suture, such as No. 3-0 poliglecaprone 25 (Monocryl). Maintenance of the suture material's tensile strength is required for only 24 to 48 hours, as peritoneum heals rapidly. One

should leave minimal amounts of suture material within the peritoneal cavity. Care also must be taken to avoid peritoneal ischemia, which can decrease tissue lysis of fibrin and interfere with wound healing.

Closure of the fascial layer is crucial to proper recovery. As fascia provides most of the wound's tensile strength, it is extremely important that it be approximated appropriately and for a sufficient time. In patients at low risk of dehiscence, continuous sutures of No. 0 or No. 1 polydioxanone (PDS) or polyglyconate (Maxon) are the best choice, as these synthetic monofilament absorbable sutures will cause the least tissue reactivity and serve to enhance wound strength (Fig. 4-2).

One should place sutures 1 cm from the wound edge. Closely placed sutures initially add to wound strength but ultimately weaken the fascial layer. Sutures should be tied loosely to approximate but not strangulate tissue (Fig. 4-1). In transverse incisions, fascia can be closed with continuous synthetic monofilament absorbable sutures.

The subcutaneous tissue, containing fat, blood, serum, and debris, is an excellent medium for bacterial invasion and proliferation. One must close this dead space to avoid such complications and controlled capillary bleeding. Small-caliber absorbable sutures, such as No. 3-0 polyglycolic acid (Dexon), Monocryl, or polyglactin (Vicryl), are a good choice, as they cause little tissue reactivity. A contin-

Table 4-2 Indications for delayed primary wound closure

Patient

Chronic or debilitating disease

Diabetes

Human or animal bites

Immunosuppression

Malnutrition

Obesity

Disease process

Infection

    Clinical endometritis or amnionitis

    Diverticulitis

    Intraperitoneal abscess

    Pelvic inflammatory disease

    Prolonged rupture of membranes

Malignancy

Surgical procedure

"Above and below" procedures such as radical vulvectomy or ure-throvesical sling

Break in aseptic technique

Excessively moist wound

Opened bowel

Any incision when infection is endemic in the hospital

Adapted from Brown SE, Allen WH, Robins RN. The use of delayed primary closure in preventing wound infections. Am J Obstet Gynecol 1977;127:713.

uous suture of 3-0 Monocryl or Vicryl placed within the subcutaneous fat suffices for closure. For skin closure, cosmetic considerations determine the choice of suturing method. Subcuticular placement of absorbable synthetic monofilament small-caliber (No. 5-0) material provides the best results (Fig. 4-3). In patients who tend to form keloids, continuous pullout subcuticular suturing with No. 4-0 polypropylene (Prolene) or polybutester (Novafil) is preferred. One may remove these sutures 7 to 10 days after surgery to lessen inflammation. Sterile strip adhesive tape reduces tension on subcuticular sutures. One may also use staples but should replace them with tape 5 days after surgery to decrease scarring. Prolene, Novafil, or monofilament nylon should be used if one chooses interrupted suturing for skin closure. In such cases, care is necessary to produce eversion of the approximated skin edges. A new stapler by Auto Suture, the SQS-20 Disposable subcuticular stapler made of absorbable staples of polyglactin (Polysorb), will revolutionize surgical skin closure. It will

be faster, very cosmetically appealing, and convenient because the staples do not have to be removed. Finally, surgeons should be aware of the various techniques of interrupted suture placement, such as horizontal mattress, vertical mattress, and simple placement, that are described in most standard surgery textbooks.

Skin edge tension will be increased by early postoperative edema, resulting in cutting of the skin. Permanent skin suture marks may result, especially if sutures are left in place for longer than 7 days. If the wound is closed at right angles to muscle pull or if excessive tissue is removed beneath the wound, lateral skin pull may occur. This problem can be reduced by first placing subcutaneous sutures to reduce tension on skin edges.

Mass closure

Patients at high risk of wound dehiscence should undergo mass closure. Smead-Jones, or far-near mass closure, which has a wound dehiscence incidence of approximately 0.1%, is highly recommended (Fig. 4-4) (1,14). In Smead-Jones closure, the anterior fascia serves as the second portion and the muscle is the first. A variation is to place interrupted sutures within the fascia to reinforce mass closure. Fascial edges are

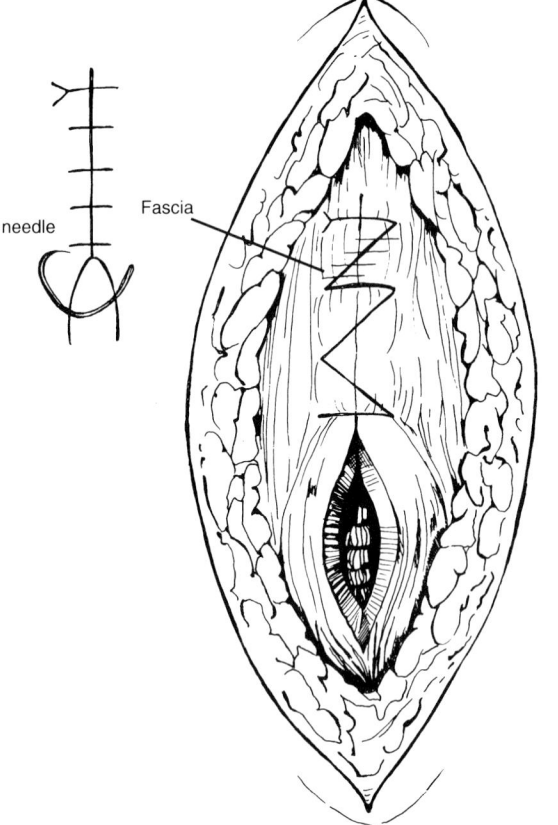

Fig. 4-2 Single-layer closure. End result of fascial closure with continuous technique. Sutures are loose, with big bites.

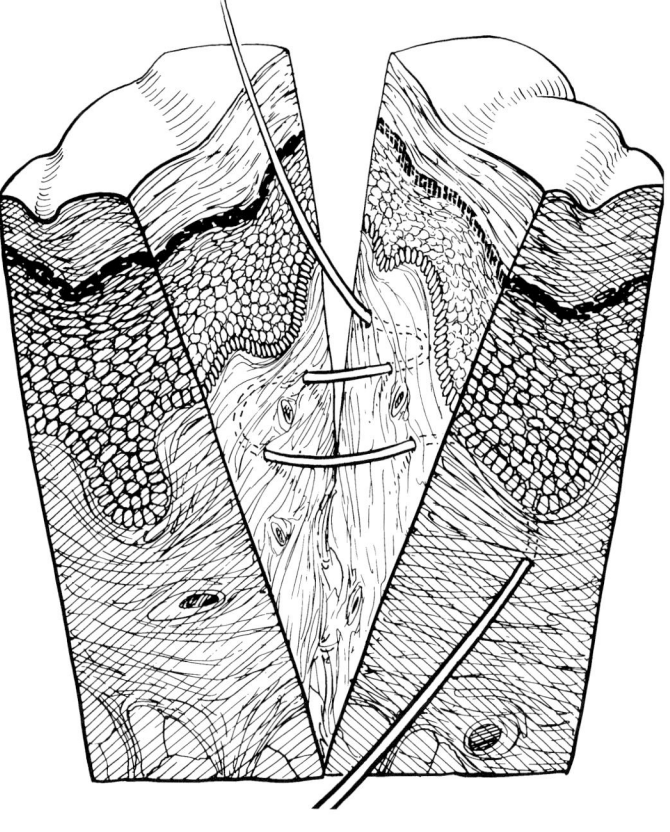

Fig. 4-3 Subcuticular skin closure. For best appearance, use a continuous subcuticular No. 4-0 or 5-0 suture, such as polyglycolic acid or polyglactin. The alternative is a continuous pullout subcuticular closure, with a nonabsorbable monofilament suture, such as polypropylene. The latter must be removed in 7 to 10 days.

then more closely approximated, reducing the likelihood of incisional hernias. Monofilament nonabsorbable suture material is best for mass closure. Excellent results have been obtained using polybutester; Maxon or PDS would be better choices among absorbable sutures because they last longer. Place sutures 2 cm apart and 2.5 cm from the fascial edge. Loose approximation of tissue edges will minimize devascularization of muscle and fascia. However, a modification of the Smead-Jones closure is done more and more often with identical results. Sutton and Morgan report on a large series of gynecologic-oncology patients in whom a running looped monofilament suture was used with results comparable to those obtained with the Smead-Jones technique. It is still a mass closure method but done in a continuous fashion instead of interrupted like the Smead-Jones. They used a monofilament absorbable suture (15). The key to both procedures of mass closure is not to produce ischemia in the tissues, which will devascularize the tissues and weaken them (16,17).

Delayed primary closure

A surgical incision in which the wound is reapproximated by a standard closing technique is said to heal by primary intention, whereas one in which epithelialization and granulation are relied on to fill the gap between unopposed edges is said to heal by secondary intention (Fig. 4-5). In third intention, or delayed primary closure, the wound is

temporarily kept partially open to prevent wound infection and abscess formation.

Closure by third intention (delayed primary closure) has been recognized by military surgeons for many years as a way to manage contaminated wounds. It also has been found useful in surgery involving gynecologic cancer, morbid obesity, bowel contamination, tubo-ovarian abscess, and suppurative appendices (Table 4-2) (18). For example, the incidence of wound infection in patients with perforating appendices has declined from 34.1% to 2.3% with the use of delayed primary closure (19).

Healing by delayed primary closure can be valuable because exudation into a wound is maximal during the first 24 postoperative hours and decreases rapidly over the subsequent 48 hours. Therefore, any contaminated wound closed by first intention traps bacteria, exudate, blood clots, and debris (20). Bacteria cultured from these wounds are usually the same as those found intraoperatively, whereas infections that occur after delayed closure are generally acquired through nosocomial mechanisms. Moreover, tissue tensile strength is not adversely affected by delayed primary closure because significant collagen synthesis does not usually occur until postoperative day 5. Wounds can be classified according to their infection risk as clean wounds, clean-contaminated wounds, contaminated wounds, and dirty or infected wounds.

To accomplish delayed closure, one closes the peritoneum and fascia (Fig. 4-6), irrigates the wound with ster-

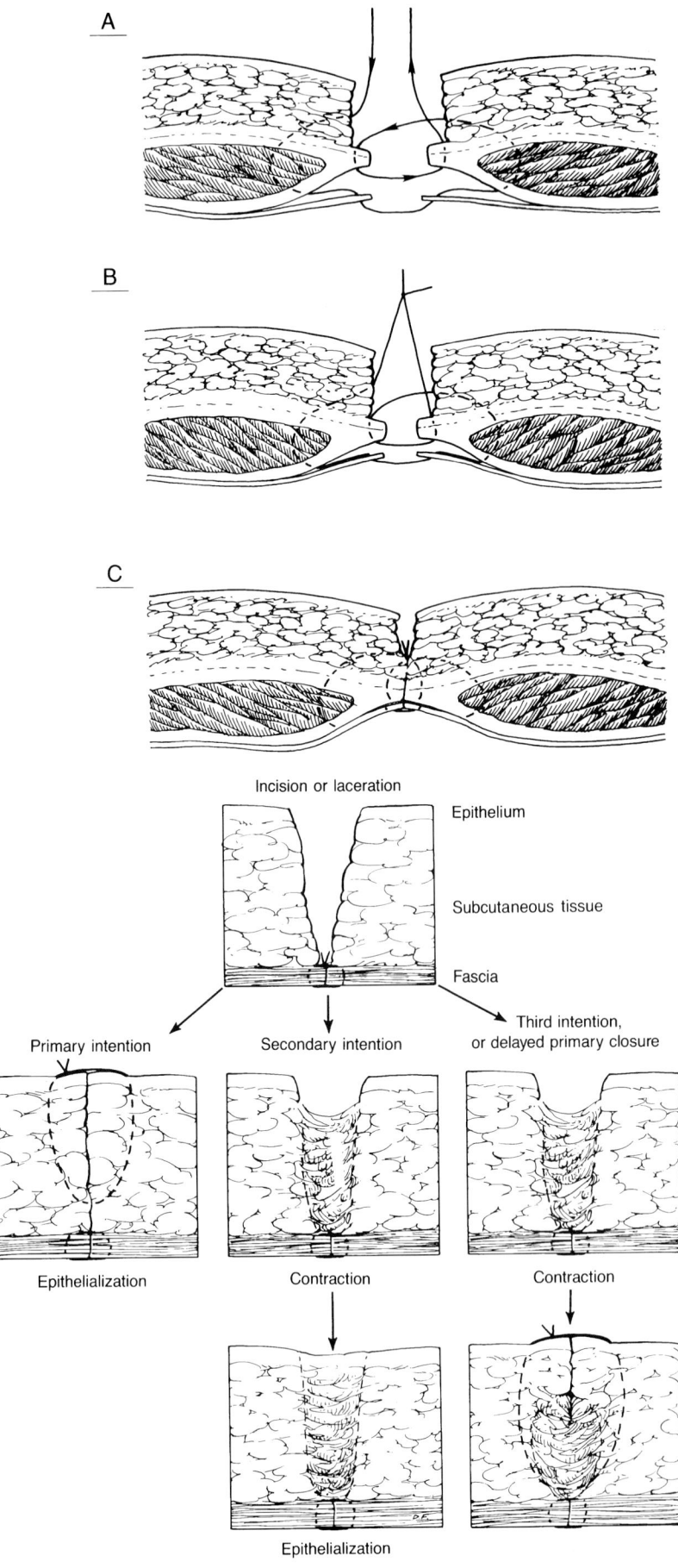

Fig. 4-4 Modified Smead-Jones closure. In this approach, only 1 cm of the peritoneum is enclosed by the suture, to prevent entrapment of the bowel by the large intra-abdominal loop. (A) Suture going through the anterior and posterior fascia should be at least 2.5 cm from the edge of the fascia. (B) Minimize the amount of suture material inside the abdominal cavity. (C) Approximate the edge loosely to prevent ischemia and necrosis.

Incision or laceration

Epithelium

Subcutaneous tissue

Fascia

Primary intention

Secondary intention

Third intention, or delayed primary closure

Epithelialization

Contraction

Contraction

Epithelialization

Epithelialization

Fig. 4-5 Types of healing.

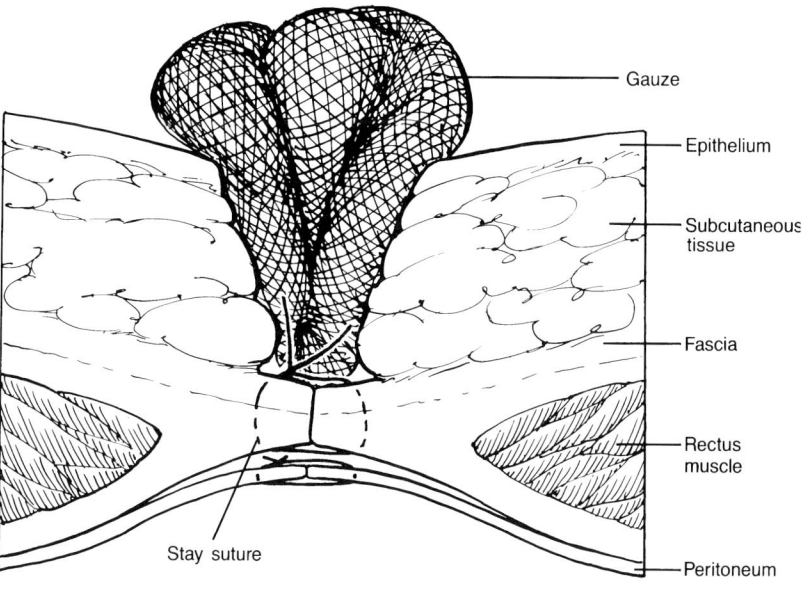

Gauze

Epithelium

Subcutaneous tissue

Fascia

Rectus muscle

Stay suture

Peritoneum

Fig. 4-6 Delayed primary closure. Leave the wound open above the fascia and irrigate it twice daily. Place gauze soaked with povidone-iodine (Betadine) inside the wound and cover it with a dressing. On day 5 to 7 close the wound with the permanent monofilament stay sutures.

ile saline, and places untied vertical interrupted skin mattress sutures, preferably of monofilament nonabsorbable material, at 2 cm intervals, leaving skin and subcutaneous tissue open. Sterile gauze soaked with very dilute povidone-iodine (Betadine) solution is placed in the wound to cover subcutaneous tissue down to the fascia, and a dry dressing covers the incision. One should examine the wound daily and clean it with peroxide. If no infection develops, the surgeon ties the sutures at the bedside on postoperative day 5 under local anesthesia or intravenous sedation. The surgeon can also place the skin sutures at this time.

Delayed primary closure is simple, safe, and effective in minimizing infections and complications of wound healing. It does not increase hospital stay or adversely affect wound strength (20). In cases of superficial skin and subcutaneous dehiscence, it is better to close the wound after proper debridement and a wait of 4 to 5 days than to wait for closure by secondary intention (21). Closure by secondary intention is reserved for heavily contaminated wounds to prevent chronic infections.

Familiarity with the properties of the various suture materials is necessary to ensure proper healing and good cosmetic results. It also is necessary to understand when to use mass closure and layer-by-layer closure, as well as to grasp the relative benefits of delayed and primary closure.

References

1 Sanz LE. Choosing the right wound-closure technique. Contemp Ob/Gynecol 1983;21(Surg):142.

2 Peacock EE. Wound repair, ed 3. Philadelphia: WB Saunders, 1984.

3 Summers Paul R, Sharp HT. Enhancing surgical wound healing. Clin Adv Treatment Infections 1992;6:1.

4 Drollette CM, Badawy SZ. Pathophysiology of pelvic adhesions. J Reprod Med 1992;37:107.

5 Elkins TE, Stovall TG, Warren J. A histological evaluation of peritoneal injury and repair: implication for adhesion formation. Obstet Gynecol 1987;70:225.

6 Masterson BJ. Taking steps to promote wound healing. Clin Ob/Gynecol 1988;(31)3:736–743.

7 Rosenberg SM. Can we achieve adhesion free surgery? The female patient 1990;15:59.

8 Greenburg AG, Saik RP, Peskin GW. Wound dehiscence: pathophysiology and prevention. Arch Surg 1979;114:143.

9 Sanz LE, Smith S. Mechanism of wound healing, suture material, and wound closure. In: Buchsbaum HJ, Walton LA, eds. Strategies in gynecologic surgery. New York: Springer-Verlag, 1986:53–76.

10 Trimbus JB. Security of various knots used in surgical practice. Obstet Gynecol 1984;64:274.

11 Sanz LE, Patterson JA, Kamath R, et al. Comparison of Maxon suture with Vicryl chromic gut PDS sutures in fascial closure in rats. Obstet Gynecol 1988;71–73,418–422.

12 Wallace D, Hernandez W, Schlaerth J, et al. Prevention of abdominal wound disruption utilizing the Smead-Jones closure technique. Obstet Gynecol 1980;56:226.

13 Greenburg AG, Saik RP, Peskin GW. Wound dehiscence: pathophysiology and prevention. Arch Surg 1979;114:143.

14 Gorman ML, Veidenheimer MC. Controlled clinical trials of three suture materials for abdominal wall closure after bowel operations. Am J Surg 1981;141:510.

15 Sutton G, Morgan S. Abdominal wound closure using a running, looped monofilament polybutester suture: comparison to Smead-Jones closure in historic controls. Obstet Gynecol 1992;80:650.

16 Sanz LE. Wound management: matching materials and methods for best results. Contemp Ob/Gynecol 1987;30:86.

17 Sanders RJ, DiClementi D, Ireland K. Principles of abdominal wound closure. II. Prevention of wound dehiscence. Arch Surg 1977;112:1184.

18 Stillman RM, Bella FJ, Seligman SJ. Skin wound closure methods on susceptibility to infection. Arch Surg 1980;115:674.

19 Dodson MK, Everett MF, Meeks GR. A randomized comparison of secondary closure and secondary intention in patients with superficial wound dehiscence. Obstet Gynecol 1992;80:321.

20 Brown SE, Allen WH, Robins RN. The use of delayed primary closure in preventing wound infections. Am J Obstet Gynecol 1977;127:713.

21 Walters MD, Dombrosky RA, Davidson SA, et al. Reclosure of disrupted abdominal incisions. Obstet Gynecol 1990;76:597.

Chapter 5

Abdominal incisions

Jacqueline C. Johnson and

Willard A. Barnes

Gynecologic surgical procedures may be performed through a wide variety of abdominal incisions. Choosing the appropriate incision is an important step in any successful surgical procedure. Adequate exposure of the intra-abdominal pathology is essential. The choice of incision should take into consideration the planned procedure, the expected disease process or pathology, as well as the patient's body habitus, previous surgical history, and special medical conditions. Attention to good surgical technique when making the abdominal incision will help prevent postoperative wound complications.

Anatomic considerations

The abdominal wall is composed of layers of muscles and fascia that overlie the parietal peritoneum and encase the abdominal contents. The large rectus abdominus muscles extend from the xiphoid process and adjacent costal cartilages to the pubic tubercle on either side of the midline, making up the major muscles anteriorly. Laterally, the three flat abdominal wall muscles—the external oblique, transversus abdominus, and internal oblique—make up the sidewalls of the abdomen. Their fascia stretches anteriorly to form an aponeurosis that forms the rectus sheath, surrounding the rectus muscles anteriorly and posteriorly with a thick layer of fascia. Between the rectus muscles lies the linea alba, a relatively avascular plane and the thinnest point in the abdominal wall. This line represents the coalescence of fascia from all of the abdominal wall muscles.

The blood supply to the anterior abdominal wall originates from the anterior thoracic artery, a branch of the subclavian artery, giving rise to the superior epigastric and musculophrenic arteries, which directly supply the anterior abdominal wall. The lateral and lowermost portions of the abdominal wall are supplied by the inferior epigastric and deep circumflex iliac arteries, branches of the external iliac artery. The inferior and superior epigastric arteries run at the lateral edges on the underside of the rectus abdominal muscles, forming an anastomosis between the external iliac and subclavian arterial systems (1). Extensive collateral circulation within the anterior abdominal wall allows for ligation of the epigastric branches when performing muscle-splitting transverse abdominal incisions without compromise of the blood supply (Fig. 5-1).

The nerve supply of the abdominal wall is provided by the anterior branches of the lateral cutaneous nerves, which pierce the rectus muscles and anterior sheath. These nerves arise from T7 through T12 vertebral levels, with T10 supplying the area at the level of the umbilicus. In the lower abdomen, the iliohypogastric and ilioinguinal nerves course between the external and internal oblique muscles, and can be encountered when making abdominal incisions. The iliohypogastric nerve is the highest branch of L1, and passes toward the skin at the lateral edge of the rectus muscle just

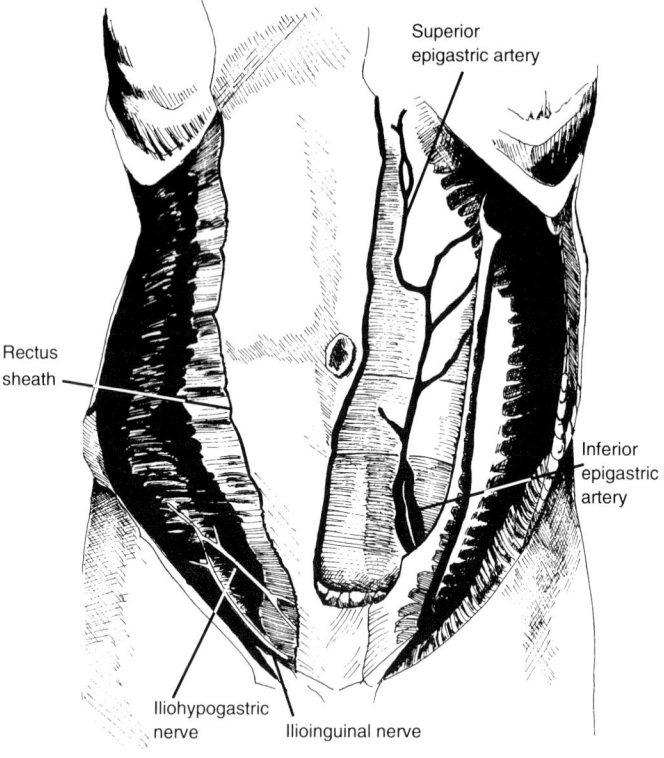

Fig. 5-1 Abdominal wall structures.

above the superficial inguinal ring, where it may be damaged during transverse incisions. Entrapment of the nerve may result in paresthesia or anesthesia in the area below the incision into the mons pubis, or development of a painful neuroma at the incision site. These complications can be resolved by excision of the neuroma or scar at the site of entrapment (2). The ilioinguinal nerve lies more caudally and more laterally, making it less likely to be injured by transverse abdominal incisions. Injury to the ilioinguinal nerve may result in anesthesia or paresthesia in its area of sensory supply, the skin overlying the inguinal canal and the labia majora (Fig. 5-1).

Types of incisions and indications

Incisions commonly used for gynecologic procedures include the low transverse abdominal incision (Pfannenstiel), the transverse muscle-splitting incision (Maylard), the muscle-releasing incision (Cherney), the vertical midline incision, the paramedian incision, and the high transverse incision. Each is appropriate for a given clinical situation (Fig. 5-2, 5-3).

Vertical incisions

The midline is the most versatile abdominal incision, allowing extension from pubis to xiphoid. This incision allows exposure to any abdominal or pelvic pathology and is essential when access to the upper abdomen is needed for

staging and treatment of ovarian cancer, for an upper abdominal procedure such as cholecystectomy or splenectomy, and for removal of abdominopelvic masses (3). The linea alba provides a relatively avascular plane of entry into the abdominal cavity through the thinnest point in the anterior abdominal wall. The midline incision, the most rapid entry into the peritoneal cavity, is usually used when a patient with known hemoperitoneum is hemodynamically unstable, or when the cause of the bleeding is unknown. A midline incision should also be used for acute abdominal pain of unknown etiology, bowel obstruction, or free air in the peritoneal cavity on upright abdominal x-ray, as access to all abdominal viscera may be needed. A preexisting incisional hernia can also be an indication for midline incision to allow repair of the hernia and reinforcement of the abdominal wall at the time of surgery.

Paramedian incisions have many of the same indications as do midline incisions, but are not as rapid, and are used less frequently for gynecologic procedures. They also involve penetration of the rectus muscles with potential injury to the epigastric vessels and hematoma formation. A variation of the paramedian incision is the pararectus incision, which is made just lateral to the border of the rectus muscles.

Transverse incisions

Transverse incisions include the Pfannenstiel or low transverse incision (and its modifications), the Maylard incision, or transverse muscle-splitting incision, and the Cherney incision, in which the rectus muscles are detached from their insertion on the pubic symphysis. They are cosmetically acceptable and provide suitable access to the pelvis when pathology is known to be confined to the pelvic organs. The Maylard incision can also provide limited access to the upper abdomen and para-aortic node region.

Indications for Pfannenstiel incisions are uterine myomata confined to the pelvis, tubal surgery, known ectopic pregnancy in hemodynamically stable patients, hysterectomy for benign disease, cervical dysplasias, and benign ovarian or tubal conditions. Transverse muscle-splitting incisions can be effective for myomectomy or hysterectomy in the larger myomatous uterus, or in cases of endometrial carcinoma in which staging may be necessary, radical hysterectomy for carcinoma of the cervix, tubo-ovarian abscesses, extensive endometriosis, or in any situation that requires generous exposure of the pelvis.

The Pfannenstiel incision, initially described in 1900, is the most common incision used in obstetrics and gynecology. It provides a low transverse skin incision and a transverse fascial incision, preserving the integrity of the rectus muscles (4). The curvilinear skin incision is made about 2 cm above the pubic symphysis at the midline. The incision's length can be increased for further exposure of the pelvic cavity, although exposure is generally limited laterally by the rectus muscles. The subcutaneous tissues and fascia are

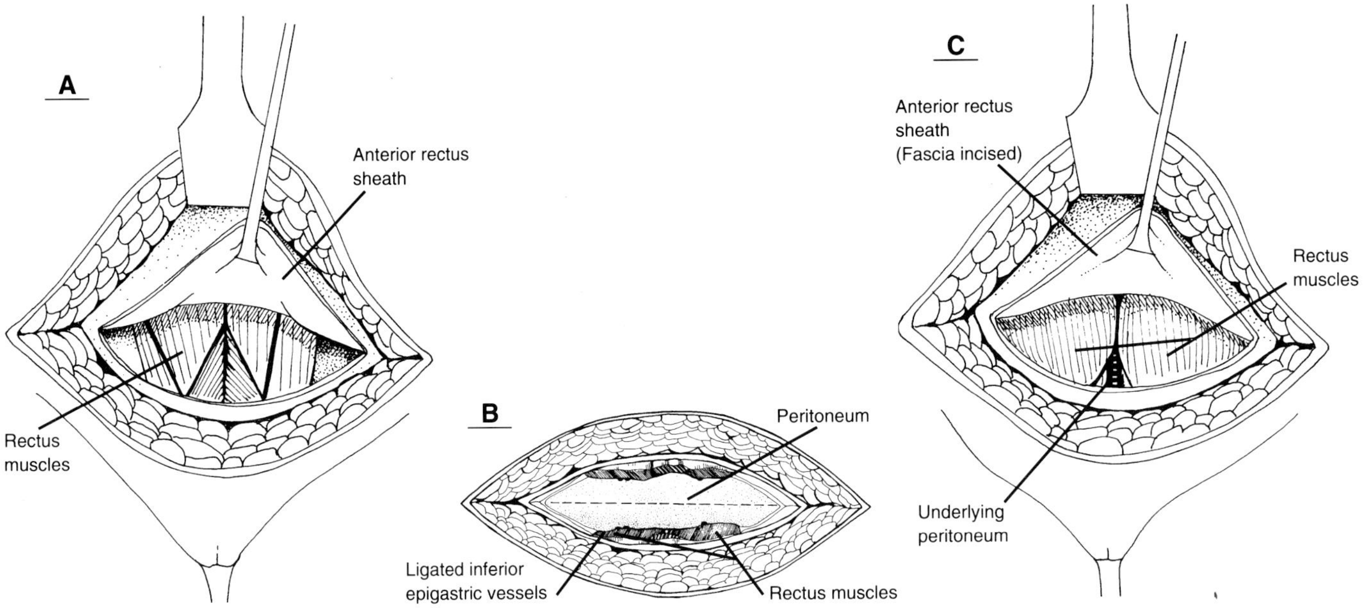

Fig. 5-2 (A) Cherney, (B) Midline/Maylard, and (C) Pfannenstiel incisions.

divided in the same direction as the skin incision, extending the ends of the incision upward from the midline. The fascia is then carefully separated from the underlying rectus muscles with sharp and blunt dissection, taking care to ligate or cauterize perforating vessels. The rectus muscles are bluntly separated in the midline, and a midline incision is made in the peritoneum. Modifications of the Pfannenstiel include transverse peritoneal incision, which causes little change in exposure but may cause injury to the epigastric vessels as the muscles are retracted from the midline and peritoneum, or a midline fascial entry, which can severely limit the exposure provided by the incision and calls for increased dissection in the subcutaneous space above the fascia. Care should be taken during the midline incision of the peritoneum to identify and avoid the dome of the bladder and any structures which may be adherent to the peritoneum.

The transverse muscle-splitting incision, or Maylard incision, provides increased operative exposure of the pelvis and can give limited exposure to the midabdomen, making it appropriate for more difficult pelvic procedures such as radical hysterectomy (5,6). Pelvic sidewall exposure may be more direct with this incision than with a traditional midline incision. The Maylard is a slightly higher transverse abdominal skin incision that is less curvilinear in shape than the Pfannenstiel, and is near the same level on the skin surface as the anterior superior iliac spines. The subcutaneous tissues and rectus sheath are divided transversely, exposing the anterior rectus sheath. The rectus muscles are then divided, using the cautery to divide them layer by layer, lifting them from the peritoneal surface to avoid inadvertent entry into the peritoneal cavity below. The inferior epigastric vessels, which will be encountered while dividing the muscles, should be separately clamped and ligated. These vessels arise from the external iliac arteries in the pelvis and are at their most lateral position at the lower portion of the rectus muscle. They lie more medially in the upper abdominal wall. Once the muscles have been divided and the epigastric vessels are secure, a large area is exposed for the peritoneal incision, which may be made either transversely or longitudinally. As with the Pfannenstiel, care should be taken to avoid the bladder dome and other underlying structures on the midline peritoneal incision, although the bladder is more likely to be encountered with the lower Pfannenstiel approach. A modification of the Maylard calls for incision of the fascia and muscle layers intact, leaving the recti within their sheath. The epigastric vessels must also be ligated with this technique; however, the muscles remain attached to the fascia, and reapproximation of the muscles occurs when the fascia is reapproximated. Some surgeons prefer to suture the muscles together with mattress sutures when closing a Maylard incision; however, the muscles will come together whether or not they are sutured, as the fascial layer above them is closed. Subfascial suction drains may be placed to prevent hematoma formation in the subfascial space.

The Cherney incision combines the low transverse skin incision used for the Pfannenstiel with a transverse detachment of the rectus muscles from their insertion onto the pubic tubercle (7). A skin and subcutaneous incision is made as with the Pfannenstiel, about 2 cm above the symphysis. The fascia is incised transversely and reflected off the underlying muscles. The rectus muscles and pyramidalis muscles are then separated from their bony insertion, usually in the tendinous portion, close to the bone. Some surgeons prefer to incise the muscles a few centimeters higher

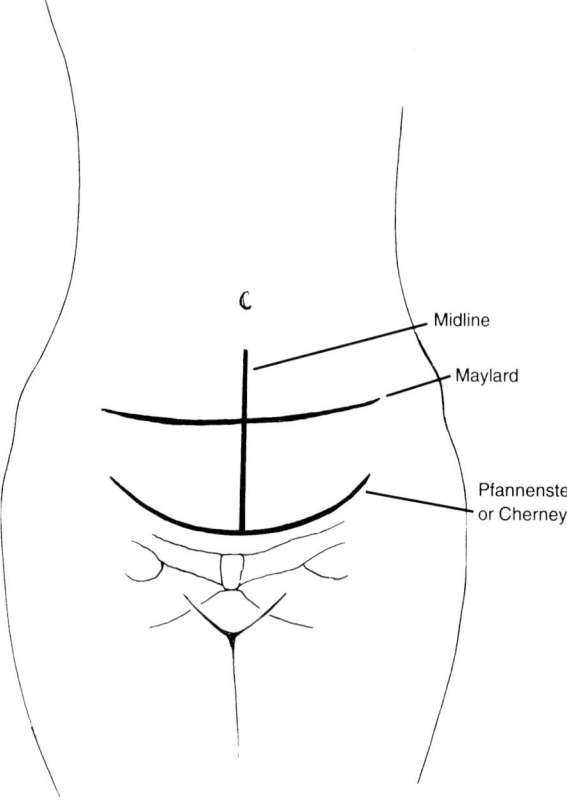

Fig. 5-3 Abdominal incisions.

to avoid the risk of inflammation at the pubic symphysis. The epigastric vessels are unlikely to be encountered near the symphysis; however, if the incision is made substantially higher, these vessels must be identified and ligated. The muscles are then retracted upward. The prevesical space of Retzius may be easily developed if necessary at this time. Care must be taken, if the peritoneal cavity is entered at this point, not to injure the bladder (which will be particularly close at this level) as the incision is made through the transversalis fascia and peritoneum.

The incision is closed by reapproximating the fascia, as with a Maylard. The ends of the muscles themselves need not be sutured together, although some authors suggest suturing the muscles to the overlying fascia. A suction drain may be used in the space of Retzius. Exposure to the lower pelvis and bladder is enhanced with the Cherney incision; however, exposure to the upper pelvis is diminished by the retracted muscles, and midabdominal exposure is poor. Hernias have been reported in the parapubic space through defects left by this type of low incision, and an effort should be made to close the fascia securely.

Limited upper abdominal exposure may be obtained through a high transverse muscle-splitting incision, similar to the Maylard, but placed high on the abdominal wall, usually near the umbilicus, although cosmesis is poorer than with a low transverse approach. Cosmesis may be improved by making a curvilinear low transverse skin incision, developing a superficial skin flap, and making the fascial incision above the level of the iliac crests. This incision may be made to incorporate a previous low transverse skin incision.

Ovarian cancer staging has been accomplished in some select cases through a high transverse abdominal incision; however, McGowan and others showed that 71% of patients with ovarian cancer were inadequately staged when a transverse incision was used (8,9). Studies are currently being designed to examine the use of the laparoscope for staging of gynecologic cancers, although no information from these trials will be available for several years. Laparoscopy has been used under certain specified conditions to assess a patient's response to chemotherapy, usually in a research setting. The current standard for the staging and surgical treatment of ovarian cancer is complete surgical staging through an adequate midline incision.

Complications

Hematomas

All surgical incisions are subject to possible complications. Wound hematomas and seromas are common occurrences and are usually easily resolved by opening the skin and subcutaneous tissues, allowing the seroma to drain or evacuating the hematoma, and continuing wound cleansing and irrigation while allowing healing by secondary intention or by secondarily closing the wound. Healing will not occur unless evacuation or drainage is complete, and antibiotics are not generally required once the wound has been opened and cleaned. Irrigation with normal saline is adequate to maintain wound cleanliness as healing occurs. Ultrasound of the abdominal wall can be used to localize and follow hematomas, although most will leak through the incision line, preventing healing of the skin until they are evacuated. Closed suction drains may be used in the subfascial space in muscle-splitting incisions, which incur a greater risk of hematoma formation.

Infections

Several factors have been associated with high risk of wound infection. Steroid use and immune suppression are well-known risk factors for poor healing and wound disruption. Other high-risk factors are age over 60, obesity, diabetes mellitus, and malnutrition (10).

The question of reclosing abdominal wounds that have required drainage is a controversial one. Two recent reports described reclosure of disrupted abdominal incisions after drainage and debridement of seromas, hematomas, or wound infections. There was a high success rate (85%) for healing after secondary closure. The authors noted no reinfected wounds and a significantly decreased time to healing in reclosed wounds, as much as 35 days shorter than those allowed to heal by secondary intention. Reclosure was carried out in an *en bloc* fashion incorporating the full thickness of subcutaneous fatty tissue from fascia to skin, and one study in infected wounds used intravenous administration of antibiotics (11,12).

Abdominal incisions for infected cases are often left open and then closed by delayed primary closure several days after the initial surgery as a means of preventing wound infection. This technique is advocated for all cases of infection, such as ruptured tubo-ovarian abscesses, and in some clean-contaminated cases in patients at high risk of wound infection (10).

Wound separation or dehiscence

Several factors have been associated with increased incidence of wound dehiscence. Among those significantly associated in one study are wound infection, contaminated cases, vertical incision, male sex, and age over 50. This study was unable to show a relation between dehiscence and type of closure, hypoproteinemia, reoperation, obesity, increased intra-abdominal pressure, steroid use, or race (13). Other studies have found that patients with excessive coughing or vomiting postoperatively, wound infections, or abdominal distention develop dehiscence at a higher rate than those who do not have these postoperative complications (14).

Some feel that midline incisions are the most prone to wound separations and dehiscence. Incidence of wound dehiscence has been reported to be 2% to 3% for midline incisions versus 0.3% to 0.68% for transverse abdominal incisions (13,15). However, randomized prospective trials have shown no difference in wound complications between transverse and vertical (both midline and paramedian) incisions (16,17). In addition, a prospective randomized trial found no difference in wound complications in midline incisions when the incision was made through the umbilicus rather than around it (18). Likewise, no differences have been found between paramedian and midline incisions (13,16).

Most likely the perceived difference in morbidity is related to the fact that transverse incisions are more often used for limited pelvic pathology, and midline incisions for complicated and high-risk patients. The higher rate of wound infections and dehiscence may result from the types of patients who receive vertical incisions.

The incidence of mortality from wound dehiscence with evisceration has been reported to be 15% to 25%. Dehiscence is uncommon in gynecologic surgery, with one large report of 2500 gynecologic laparotomies showing 8 dehiscences (0.3%) (14). Dehiscence can be guarded against by strict attention to surgical technique in wound closure, use of nasogastric tubes to avoid abdominal distention in high-risk patients, and leaving the skin and subcutaneous tissues open in contaminated cases to prevent wound infection.

Hernias

Incisional hernias occur more often with vertical incisions. The development of incisional hernias is increased in cases involving an older age group, male sex, obesity, bowel surgery, wound infection, and abdominal distention (19). Incisional hernias can occur in any type of incision that is reopened (up to 12%) (20). Studies have shown incisional hernias in 6.7% to 7.4% of vertical incisions combining a paramedian and vertical (19,21). Incisional hernias in transverse incisions are rare; however, hernias have been reported in the parapubic area after detachment of the rectus muscle tendons from their insertion into the pubic symphysis as would be performed in the Cherney incision (22). It is also reported that the incidence of incisional hernia is decreased when a more lateral paramedian incision is used. This incision is made more than two-thirds of the width of the rectus muscle from the midline and showed significantly fewer hernias than either traditional paramedian incisions (about 2 cm from midline) or midline incisions (21).

Special considerations

Weighing several factors may lead the surgeon to choose one particular incision. One example is the patient with pulmonary disease. In a study comparing incisions below the umbilicus, respiratory function was less impaired by transverse abdominal incisions than by vertical incisions (23). Patients' ventilatory function was better in the transverse incision group and improved faster than in the midline group. Another study comparing upper abdominal transverse and midline incisions also found fewer pulmonary complications in the transverse group (24). It therefore seems that the patient at high risk of pulmonary complications would benefit from a transverse incision.

Obese patients are often difficult surgical challenges. The optimal incision in the obese patient creates as little "dead space" and as little opportunity for fluid and blood collection in the subcutaneous space as possible, while providing adequate access to the peritoneal cavity and pelvis. Frequently, these patients are opened through transverse incisions which lessen the risks of hernia formation, respiratory morbidity, and pain. In markedly obese patients, the external umbilicus is carried downward with the panniculus while the umbilical attachment on the fascia remains in its anatomic position, midway between the symphysis and the xiphoid under the subcutaneous fatty layer. The skin incision may be made above the panniculus to avoid cutting through redundant adipose tissue. For transverse incisions the panniculus is retracted downward and the incision is made above it, either above or below the external position of the umbilicus. Exposure to the pelvis will be more direct than the skin incision would indicate and will approximate the fascial position on a low transverse incision in the nonobese patient (25). A midline incision can also be made in the periumbilical area, avoiding the panniculus and the mons fat pad. Although periumbilical on the skin surface, the incision will gain access to the abdominal or pelvic cavity below the annulus umbilicalis on the fascia and allow for optimal exposure to the pelvis for procedures such as hysterectomy.

All patients undergoing exploration for a pelvic mass, regardless of age, should understand that malignancy is a possible finding and that proper staging is important and requires access to the upper abdomen facilitated by a midline incision. When there is suspicion of ovarian cancer, a patient has an abdominopelvic mass, or a patient with a pelvic mass is over age 40 and the etiology of the mass is not known, the midline incision is the procedure of choice (8).

Patients with incisional hernias who require further abdominal or pelvic procedures are candidates for reopening the initial incision and hernia repair. Although reoperation through an incision generally increases the risk of hernia formation, attention to reconstruction of the abdominal wall can resolve this problem. A double-layer graft of synthetic mesh can be used to strengthen the abdominal wall and the incision, which is closed with interrupted permanent sutures in an imbricating fashion, with a hernia recurrence rate of 10% (26).

Certain situations predispose to skin complications and abdominal wall necrosis. For example, parallel incisions, such as a paramedian and midline, can cause devascularization of the intervening space and lead to necrosis of skin, subcutaneous tissues, and fascia, causing morbidity and even death (27).

Rarely, complications occur in patients with extensive vascular disease of the aortoiliac region who depend on collateral circulation for vascular supply to the lower extremities. In these patients, flow in the epigastric vessels may be reversed, and the blood supply from the subclavian artery into the superior epigastric vessels through anastomoses to the inferior epigastric vessels may provide much of the blood supply to the lower extremities when the iliac vessels are diseased. Disruption of the inferior epigastric vessels by transverse incisions may lead to claudication and ischemia in these patients. Patients with severe vascular disease should be evaluated by a vascular surgeon before abdominal surgery, and if epigastric vessels are an important source of collateral blood flow, incisions should be planned to spare them (28).

Consideration must also be given to the epigastric vessels in terms of the supply of the rectus muscles. In gynecologic malignancies, the rectus muscles are sometimes used in musculocutaneous flaps for vulvar reconstruction. In addition, treatment of breast cancer, which now strikes one in nine American women, may require mastectomy. The rectus muscles are an important source for myocutaneous flaps used in breast reconstruction. In women who are at risk of breast cancer or who have gynecologic (vulvar or vaginal) malignancies, attention should be given to spar-

ing the inferior epigastric vessels to maintain rectus abdominus blood supply. Muscle-splitting transverse incisions are best avoided.

Wound closure and suture materials are covered specifically elsewhere in this text (see Chapters 3 and 4). In general, mass closures with either absorbable or permanent sutures are effective when proper knot-tying and surgical techniques are observed, and can decrease anesthesia time. Subcutaneous drains, sutures, and retention sutures have no proven effect on wound healing and the prevention of wound complications.

Summary

Familiarity with the muscular anatomy and blood supply of the abdominal wall is important in making abdominal incisions. Injuries to vessels and nerves can be avoided with good incision planning and anatomic knowledge. Both transverse and vertical incisions can be used safely and effectively in gynecologic surgery. Choosing the appropriate incision requires consideration of the patient's indications for surgery, medical and surgical history, and body habitus. Complications such as wound infections, hernias, wound hematomas, and dehiscence can be minimized with appropriate surgical techniques. Special considerations such as obesity, poor pulmonary function, previous incisions, or vascular disease may influence the choice of incision in some patients.

Choosing the appropriate abdominal incision is important for successful pelvic and abdominal surgery. With strict attention to surgical technique and to factors that place a patient at high risk of wound complications, the surgeon can safely cross the abdominal wall and ensure smooth postoperative wound healing.

References

1 Christopherson WA. Abdominal incisions and their anatomic basis. Contemp Obstet Gynecol 1988;38–56.

2 Grosz CR. Iliohypogastric nerve injury. Am J Surg 1981;142(5):628.

3 Mattingly RF, Thompson JD. TeLinde's operative gynecology. Philadelphia: JB Lippincott, 1985:159–168.

4 Pfannenstiel J. Ueber die vortheile des suprasymphyaren fascienquerschnitts fur die gynakologischen koliotomien zugleich ein beitragzu der indikationsstellung der operationswege. Samml Klin Votr (Leipzig) 1900;268:1736–1755.

5 Helmkamp BF, Krebs HB. The Maylard incision in gynecologic surgery. Am J Obstet Gynecol 1990;163(5):1554–1557.

6 Maylard AE. Direction of abdominal incisions. Br Med J 1907; 2:895–901.

7 Cherney LS. A modified transverse incision for low abdominal operations. Surg Gynecol Obstet 1941;72:92–95.

8 McGowan L. Abdominal incisions and staging in ovarian cancer. Arch Surg 1986;121:800–802.

9 Barnes WA, Delgado G, Petrilli E. An alternative approach to the vertical midline abdominal incision for staging in ovarian carcinoma. Gynecol Oncol 1987;28:129–132.

10 Verrier ED, Bossart KJ, Heer FW. Reduction of infection rates in abdominal incisions by delayed wound closure techniques. Am J Surg 1979;138(1):22–28.

11 Hermann GG, Bagi P, Christoffersen I. Early secondary suture versus healing by secondary intention of incisional abscesses. Surg Gynecol Obstet 1988;167:16–18.

12 Walters MD, Dombroski RA, Davidson SA, Mandel PC, Gibbs RS. Reclosure of disrupted abdominal incisions. Obstet Gynecol 1990;76(4):597–602.

13 Keill RH, Keitzer WF, Nichols WK, Henzel J, Deweese MS. Abdominal wound dehiscence. Arch Surg 1973;106:573–577.

14 Pratt JH. Wound healing—evisceration. Clin Obstet Gynecol 1973;16:126–134.

15 Mowat J, Bonnar J. Abdominal wound dehiscence after cesarean section. Br Med J 1971;2:256–257.

16 Ellis H, Coleridge-Smith PD, Joyce AD. Abdominal incisions—vertical or transverse? Postgrad Med J 1984;60:407–410.

17 Stone HH, Hoefling SJ, Strom PR, Dunlop WE, Fabian TC. Abdominal incisions: transverse versus vertical placement and continuous vs interrupted closure. South Med J 1983;76(9):1106–1112.

18 Paes TRF, Stoker DL, Ng T, Morecroft J. Circumbilical versus transumbilical incision. Br J Surg 1987;74:822.

19 Ellis H. Commentary—midline abdominal incisions. Br J Ob/Gynecol 1984;91:1–2.

20 Lamont PM, Ellis H. Incisional hernia in re-opened abdominal incisions: an overlooked risk factor. Br J Surg 1988;75:374–376.

21 Guillou PJ, Hall TJ, Donaldson DR, Broughton AC, Brennan TG. Vertical abdominal incisions—a choice? Br J Surg 1980;67:395–399.

22 Benadavid R. Incisional parapubic hernias. Surgery 1990;108 (5):898–901.

23 Elman A, Langonnet F, Dixsaut G, et al. Respiratory function is impaired less by transverse than by median vertical supraumbilical incisions. Intensive Care Med 1981;7:235–239.

24 Becquemin J-P, Piquet J, Becquemin M-H, Melliere D, Harf A. Pulmonary function after transverse or midline incision in patients with obstructive pulmonary disease. Intensive Care Med 1985;11:247–251.

25 Krebs H-B, Helmkamp BF. Transverse periumbilical incision in the massively obese patient. Obstet Gynecol 1984;63:241–245.

26 Usher FC. The repair of incisional and inguinal hernias. Surg Gynecol Obstet 1970;131:525–530.

27 Pillgram-Larsen J, Normann E, Raeder M. Skin necrosis between parallel abdominal incisions. Acta Chir Scand 1979;145:277–278.

28 Krupski WC, Sumchai A, Effeney DJ, Ehrenfeld WK. The importance of abdominal wall collateral blood vessels. Arch Surg 1984;119:854–857.

Chapter 6

Use of surgical staplers in gynecologic surgery

James Barter, Luis E. Sanz, and

Alexander F. Burnett

History

Dr. Homer Hültl engineered and used the first staple instrument in Budapest, Hungary in 1908 (1). This instrument looked like a gastrointestinal anastomosis (GIA) instrument, but gave two staple lines with a space in between. Scissors were then needed to cut between the staple rows. The B configuration of the staples compressed the tissue, allowing hemostasis, but did not totally occlude small vessels, preventing distal ischemic necrosis. This theory of staple compression without strangulation persists in modern staple designs. Hultl reported a series of stapled gastrostomies in which staple instruments caused less tissue trauma, less blood loss, and saved time compared with hand suturing (1). In the 1950s, the Russians further developed staple instruments. In the late 1960s, Steichen and Ravitch introduced staple products into the United States. During the 1970s and 1980s, staples virtually replaced hand suturing for most gastrointestinal procedures. Over the last few years, staple products have been designed to expedite gynecologic procedures (2). With continued cost reduction and instrument refinements, staples may replace conventional hand suturing in gynecologic procedures, as well (Fig. 6-1).

Current staple composition

Currently, staples are composed of two different materials. Permanent staples are made of the light, but strong metallic element titanium. Titanium does not interfere with future magnetic resonance imaging. Malleability allows a totally compressed staple (clips and ligate-divide-staple [LDS] instruments), or the B-shaped configuration (GIA and thoracoabdominal anastomosis [TA]). Previous staple metal alloys caused a "starburst" effect on computed axial tomography scans, but this does not occur with titanium (3). Differing staple sizes are available for different instruments, and this must be understood for error-free surgery. For titanium staples, the measurement refers to the precompression leg length, and it is given in millimeters.

The second staple material is Polysorb, an absorbable lactomer copolymer of blended polylactic and polyglycolic acids. These staples break down into carbon dioxide and water, causing very little tissue reaction (4). This material is not malleable, and requires a different staple shape. Polysorb staples are composed of an arched staple with pointed ends that fix into a staple base or retainer. The arch allows compression, ensuring hemostasis, yet preserves distal microcirculation, so that there is not anoxic tissue beyond the staple line. As with titanium, different staple sizes are available for different instruments. The measurement is from the staple top to the bottom of the leg, where it attaches to the fastener. As opposed to titanium, this measurement is given in tenths of an inch (i.e., 60 corresponds to a 0.060-inch staple length).

Internal stapler types

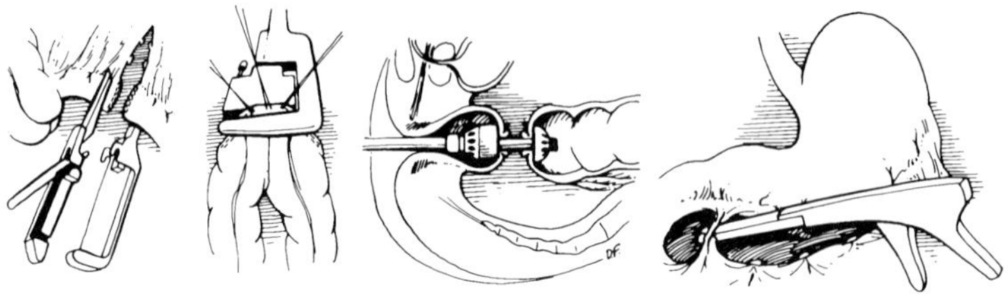

Manufacturer	Basic design and function			
Auto Suture Company	GI anastomosis (GIA)	Thoracoabdominal (TA)	End-to-end anastomosis (EEA)	Ligate–divide–staple (LDS)
American V. Mueller	Inverted linear anastomosis (ILA)	Pneumointestinal (PI)	—	—
Ethicon	Proximate linear cutter (PLC)*	Reloadable (RL)*	Intraluminal stapler (ILS)	—

Fig. 6-1 Internal stapler types.

The proximate linear cutter and reloadable types are disposable as well as reloadable.

Staple products can simplistically be divided into three prototypical instruments: the clip, the GIA, and the TA types of apparatus. There are several instruments in each of these categories.

Clips and ligate-divide-staple instruments

The simplest staple product is the occlusive clip, used to secure blood vessels. Four clip sizes are available, with the larger clips being in the longer instruments. The clip applier we find most helpful is the "medium clip," which is housed in an 11.5-inch apparatus (Fig. 6-2). Initial clip products were not correctly designed and would squeeze the vessel or tissue out of the clip during compression. These initial automatic clip appliers were not successful or well accepted. Current clips close in a distal-to-proximal direction, entrapping the vessel and thus correcting the previous inadequacy (5,6).

The LDS is a most helpful modification of the simple clip. It provides two curvilinear occlusive staples and a knife that cuts between them (Fig. 6-3). The occluded staples measure 8 mm in length. This instrument is particularly helpful with omentectomies, adhesions, and bowel mesenteric vessels. Incorrect LDS use may dull the knife, precluding hemostasis. Each vessel must be skeletonized before LDS application. The vessel is cradled in the bottom of the LDS chamber before firing, ensuring that clips and knife traverse the tissue perpendicularly. Crossing at skewed angles may prevent hemostasis. The instrument requires two-hand stabilization, as there is a modest recoil.

Disregarding this results in jerking, which may tear tissue or vessels.

GIA-type instruments

Gastrointestinal anastomosis

The GIA is the "workhorse" of intestinal surgery (7) (Fig. 6-4). Like Hultl's 1908 instrument, current GIAs give staggered double-staple rows. Each titanium staple has the B configuration, allowing microcirculation beyond the staple line. Unlike Hultl's instrument, current GIAs have an internal knife simultaneously cutting the tissue as the staple rows are formed.

GIAs come in lengths of 60 or 80 cm, with the shorter length for small bowel, and the larger for large bowel. For each apparatus, there are different titanium staple sizes for different situations. A pediatric 2.5-mm staple does not have much applicability for gynecology, whereas the 3.8- and 4.8-mm lengths do. Generally, for the bowel (large or small) the 3.8-mm length is most suitable. Occasionally, one may need a 4.8-mm staple length for distal thickened sigmoid or rectum. The 3.8-mm staples are in blue cartridges, and the 4.8-mm staples are in green. For any instrument's varying staple size, the lighter color denotes a smaller staple. It is imperative to use the correct staple size; otherwise, failed anastomoses or bleeding may result. The disposable GIA instrument carrier can be reloaded seven times (eight total firings). Each cartridge unit has a fresh internalized blade, allowing a new knife for each firing. The sheathed

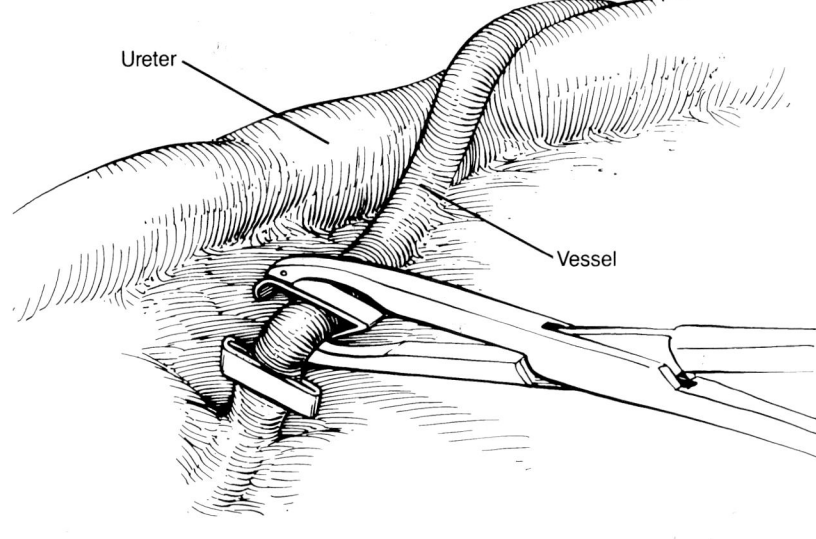

Ureter

Vessel

Fig. 6-2 Single clip vessel ligation. Here, a single clip is applied to a vessel with the ureter in close proximity.

blade virtually eliminates accidental injury during cartridge changing.

End-to-end anastomosis

The end-to-end anastomosis (EEA) is an ingenious device. It provides two circular B-shaped staggered titanium staple lines and a circular knife that cuts just inside the inner staple line. This instrument allows very low rectal reanastomosis and can also restore intestinal continuity elsewhere in the gastrointestinal tract. The instrument comes in sizes of 25, 28, or 31 mm, with the size referring to the outer instrument diameter. Instruments use 4.8-mm staples.

Cesarean-section stapler

Modifications of "knife-carrying" instruments have been developed for obstetric-gynecologic use. The Poly C/S 57 (cesarean-section stapler) is 57 mm in length and provides two Polysorb absorbable staple lines and a knife that cuts between them. Emerging data show the cesarean-section stapler results in less infection, blood loss, operative time, and postoperative hospital days compared with conventional suturing techniques (8–11). For gynecologic purposes, the stapler may be applied across the rectus muscles in Maylard incisions, which may be less traumatic and quicker than Bovie electrocoagulation.

Importantly, there are two staple sizes for the cesarean-section instrument. The 140 (0.140-inch length) is for thinner muscle, and the 170 (0.170-inch staple) is for thicker muscles. Using the wrong size precludes hemostasis.

Poly-GIA

The poly-GIA is a GIA-type instrument giving four staggered Polysorb staple lines, with an internal knife simulta-

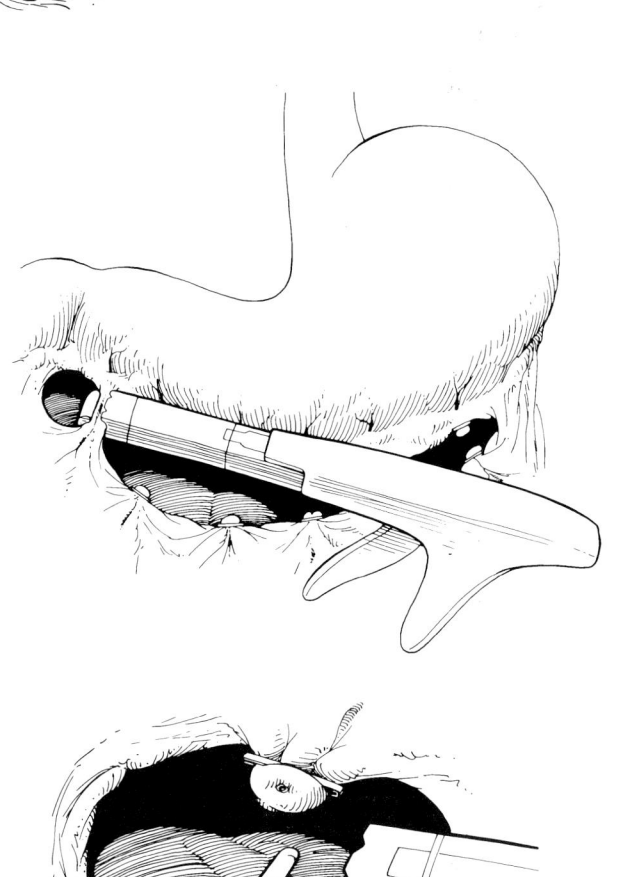

Fig. 6-3 A noteworthy use of the ligate-divide-staple instrument is for performing omentectomy.

neously cutting between the second and third rows. Its one specific gynecologic use is for the utero-ovarian ligament. This thick ligament contains the blood vessels and connective tissue between the uterus and the ovary, the fallopian tube, and the round ligament. Rather than free tying and suture ligating this broad pedicle into a rounded mass, this instrument flattens the ligament and applies multiple compressing hemostatic absorbable staples across it. Flattening this thick ligament and securing hemostasis at multiple linear points seems safer and more physiologic than circularly tying it off into a large pedicle. The Poly-GIA is also used on bowel for continent or noncontinent urinary conduits. The absorbable Polysorb eliminates the nidus for stone formation and infection that permanent metal staples can cause.

Endo-GIA

The Endo-GIA 30 is the laparoscopic stapler making many intra-abdominal procedures feasible. The 30-mm instrument applies six staggered rows of fine B-shaped titanium staples with space in the middle for a knife blade simultaneously to cut the secured tissue. Row staggering allows hemostasis without strangulation. Two staple sizes are available, 2.5 mm (white cartridge) and 3.5 mm (blue cartridge). The measurement, again, refers to the precompression leg length. It is imperative to measure tissue thickness with the endogauge to adjudicate correct staple size.

Choosing the wrong staple size results in bleeding. The Endo-GIA 60 is a recently released 60-mm laparoscopic GIA that comes with staples of 2.5, 3.5, or 4.8 mm. This instrument will encourage laparoscopic intestinal surgery, especially simplifying appendectomies.

TA type instruments

TA prototype staplers give a staple line (which may have one to three staple rows in it)—nothing less, nothing more. There is no internal knife system (Fig. 6-5).

Thoracoabdominal instrument

The specific TA instrument gives two staggered titanium staple rows and is very helpful with lung resections, low sigmoid resections (in which a GIA cannot negotiate the pelvic confines), and enterotomy closures. The instrument comes in lengths of 30, 55, or 90 mm. The 30 and 55-mm instruments are roticulated, allowing placement in narrow surgical areas. For each instrument there are two staple

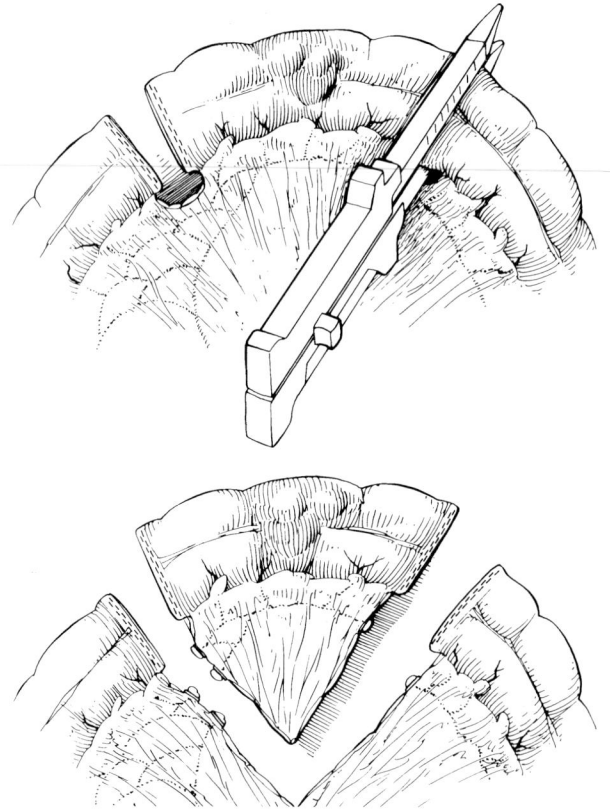

Fig. 6-4 Resection of the bowel segment is done with the gastrointestinal anastomosis (GIA) stapler.

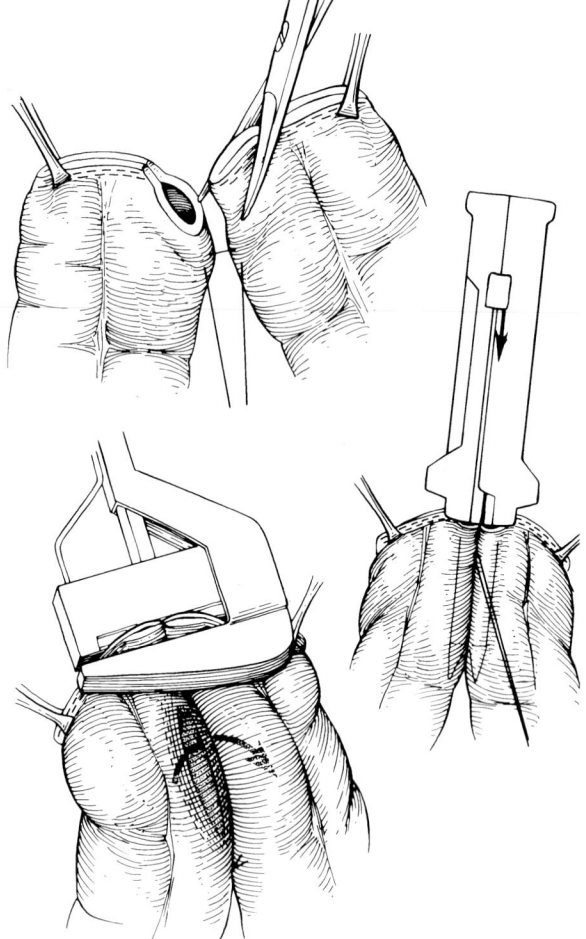

Fig. 6-5 Here, a functional end-to-end anastomosis is completed by closure with the thoracoabdominal (TA) device.

sizes, 3.5 mm (blue cartridge) and 4.8 mm (green cartridge). Generally, the 3.5-mm length is used for most small and large bowel, reserving the 4.8-mm length for thickened sigmoid or unusually thick tissue.

The 30-V-3

The 30-V-3 is a TA-type instrument giving three staggered rows of 2.5-mm titanium staples. The staple size and row staggering achieve hemostasis, even though each individual staple assumes the B configuration after the instrument is fired. This presumably allows persistent distal microcirculation, as opposed to a constricting circular free tie suture and stitch. This instrument is also used in thoracic cases for the pulmonary artery. In gynecology, the 30-V-3 is used for the infundibulopelvic ligament. A "back-clamp" is necessary to prevent retrograde ovarian bleeding, and a knife or scissors is necessary to cut the pedicle. The 30-V-3 must be released slowly and under control to avoid jerking the ligament and staple line. The instrument is most helpful in securing infundibulopelvic ligaments where carcinoma is coating the nearby peritoneum.

The Roticulator-55

The Roticulator 55 is a roticulate TA-type instrument fired across the upper vagina as the final step of a hysterectomy (12–14) (Fig. 6-6). After the bladder flap is created, the instrument is placed across the upper vagina and fired, squeezing the cervix cephalad (15–17). One must know the location of the ureters before firing this instrument to avoid bilateral ureteral transection. Two staggered rows of Polysorb staples are formed, closing off the vagina. The vagina is then cut with Jorgenson scissors, and the specimen is removed from the operative field. The stapler takes the place of suturing the vaginal cuff (18–20). There are two staple sizes. The 170 (0.170-inch) is used for thinner, postmenopausal vaginal tissue, and the larger 200 (0.200-inch) for thicker, premenopausal tissue. Using the wrong size prevents proper tissue compression, resulting in bleeding. For uterine procedures, the surgeon must know the details of pelvic anatomy and be meticulous in dissecting vessels before stapling. Confidence in handling the stapler will help avoid injury to nearby structures. Difficult cases involving pelvic masses, adhesions, endometriosis, or malignancy in obese patients should not be undertaken by the uninitiated, as the potential for injury is high. In one series, 2 (3.6%) of 56 patients who had vaginal cuff closures by stapling needed reoperation for ureteral injuries. In experienced hands, however, the advantages of stapling for the operator are also great: there is minimal tissue manipulation, and the vagina is never entered. Metal staplers should never be used in the vaginal cuff, as dyspareunia, male and female, can follow.

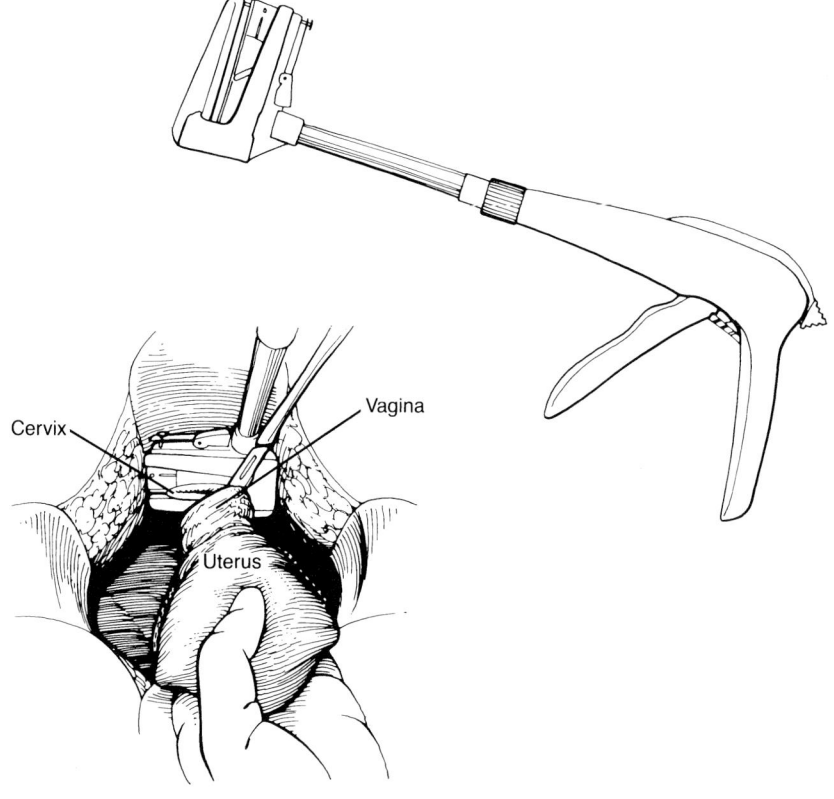

Fig. 6-6 The flexible-head stapler of the Roticulator 55 may expedite closure of the vaginal cuff.

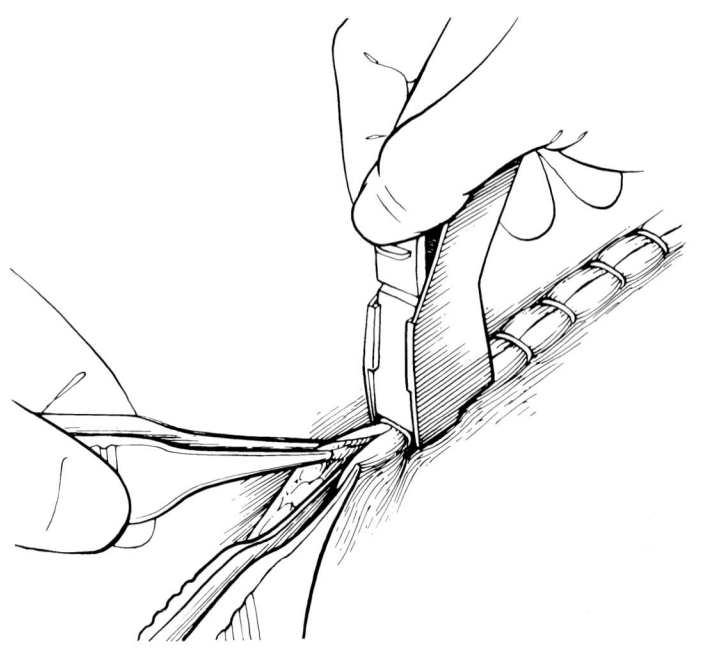

Fig. 6-7 Fine tissue forceps for reapproximation. The skin edges are everted before the surgeon begins to place the staples.

Endo-TA

A laparoscopic TA, the Endo-TA has recently been released. It gives three staggered titanium staple rows and comes in lengths of 30 or 60 millimeters. The 30-mm instrument has staple lengths of 2.5 and 3.5 mm, whereas the 60-mm length also has a 4.8-mm staple available. This instrument will allow more laparoscopic intestinal surgery and may also be used for the cardinal ligament in laparoscopically assisted hysterectomies.

Working on the skin and the fascia

In deciding on a skin closure method, the surgeon must consider cosmetic results, possible complications, patient comfort, ease of postoperative care, and speed of wound closure (Fig. 6-7). Staples are an excellent alternative for skin closures. They may be more expensive than sutures, but they can be placed more quickly and easily than sutures. Infection rates are lower, and tissue reactions occur less after stapling than after suturing (Table 6-1). A continuous subcuticular suture produces better cosmetic results than stapling, but it takes longer. However, there is a new stapler, the SQS-20 disposable subcuticular stapler made of absorbable staples of Polysorb (Fig. 6-8). This will revolutionize surgical skin closure because it will be faster, very cosmetically appealing, and convenient in that the staple does not have to be removed because it is placed subcuticularly. A large choice of external staples is available. The major characteristics to check are alignment and placement of the staples, comfort of the device in the hand, mechanical features, and cost.

Fascial devices that use nonabsorbable staples are now available, and absorbable staples are in the research and

Table 6-1 Skin stapler considerations

Alignment and placement
Staple-release mechanisms
Staple placement visible
Locating arrow and center line
Operator's fingers away from wound
Comfort
Balance and stability
Hand comfort
Trigger force to operate
Serrated handle
Mechanical features
No-jam ratchet
Staple counter
Cost

development stage. Nevertheless, until more data are available, it is better to depend on standard methods of fascial closure.

To summarize, these instruments may be very helpful in the appropriate setting. Understanding their mechanism, appropriate uses, and limitations is essential. The use of staplers in gynecology is growing rapidly because they can decrease blood loss, minimize tissue reaction, and save time. Nevertheless, their use cannot bypass careful dissection; bypassing these steps will result in surgical errors. The operator unfamiliar with these devices should read extensively about their applications and gain experience first on

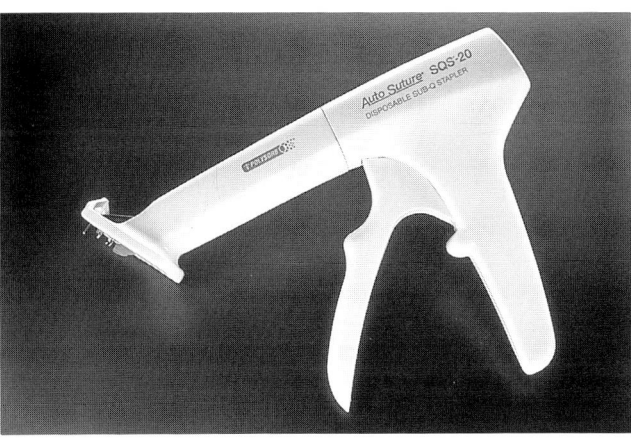

Fig. 6-8 Auto Suture, U.S. Surgical, the SQS-20 disposable subcuticular stapler.

models and laboratory animals. Use in patients should be very selective initially. These tools cannot replace basic tenets of surgery, but can add neatness, precision, and speed if properly applied.

References

1 Hültl H. Il Kongress der Ungarischen Geseheschaft fur Chirurgie, Budapest, May 1908. Pester Med Chin Presse 1909;45:108–110, 121–122.

2 Barter JF, Sanz LE. Surgical staplers. In: Sanz L, ed. Contemporary gynecologic surgery. Oradelle, NJ: Medical Economics, 1988:39–50.

3 Laakman RW, Kaufman B, Han JS, et al. MR Imaging in patients with metallic implants. Radiology 1985;157(3):711.

4 Steckel RR, Jann HW, Kaplan D, et al. Experimental evaluation of absorbable copolymer staples for hysterectomy. Obstet Gynecol 1986;68:404–410.

5 Burke G. The corrosion of metals in tissues: an introduction to tantalum. Can Med Assoc J 1940;43:125.

6 Samuels PB, Roedling H, Katz R, Cincotti JJ. A new hemostatic clip: two-year review of 1007 cases. Ann Surg 1966;163(3):427.

7 Steichen FM, Ravitch MM. Mechanical sutures in surgery. Br J Surg 1973;60(3):191.

8 Faro S, Martens MG, Maccato M. Use of an absorbable uterine stapling device in cesarean section. Presented at the 36th Annual Clinical of the American College of Obstetricians and Gynecologists, Boston, May 22–25, 1988.

9 Bond SJ, Harrion MR, Slotnick RN, et al. Cesarean delivery and hysterotomy using an absorbable stapling device. Obstet Gynecol 1989;74:25.

10 Burkett G, Jensen LP, Lai A, et al. Evaluation of surgical staples in cesarean section. Am J Obstet Gynecol 1989;161:540.

11 Martens MG. Reduction of infectious morbidity with uterine stapling device. Adv Therapy 1990;7:105.

12 Kahn E. Auto-suture in abdominal hysterectomy. Obstet Gynecol 1968;31:852–854.

13 Albert RO. Use of automatic stapler in vaginal hysterectomy, anterior colpoplasty, and posterior colpoperineoplasty. Tex Med 1974;70:66–76.

14 Messit J. Dyspareunia from auto suture staples. Obstet Gynecol 1977;49:369.

15 Zerner J, Miller B, Nelson B. Unusual complications following abdominal hysterectomy: dyspareunia and consort glans laceration after vaginal cuff stapling. J Maine Med Assoc 1980;71:169.

16 Wolf D. Abdominal hysterectomy: comparison of closed cuff, open cuff, and staple closure techniques. J IAOA 1980;79:625.

17 Brun G, Spautz F, Girard P, Cossard F. Mechanical vaginal sutures after hysterectomy. Surg Clin North Am 1984;64:609–618.

18 McTammany JR. Vaginal cuff closure during abdominal hysterectomy using absorbable staples. Berks County Med Record 1986;77:35–36.

19 Buka NJ. Absorbable staples in abdominal hysterectomy. Surg Gynecol Obstet 1988;166:174–176.

20 Kalbefleisch RE. Prospective randomized study to compare a closed vault technique using absorbable staples at the time of abdominal hysterectomy versus open vault technique. Surg Gynecol Obstet 1992;175:337.

Chapter 7

Application of surgical drains

B. Frederick Helmkamp and Hans-B. Krebs

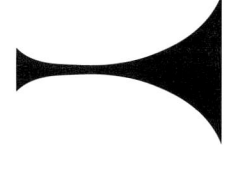

Although surgical drainage was introduced in 400 B.C. by Hippocrates, who used drains to treat empyema, significant controversy still persists concerning the indications for drainage and the type of drain to be used (1–3). Drains may be used therapeutically for a documented fluid collection, or as prophylaxis against a potential accumulation of fluid. Therapeutic indications include abscess, hematoma, and enteric fistula. The use of drains in these conditions has led to few problems. Most of the controversy regarding surgical drainage has to do with the use of prophylactic drains.

Prophylactic drainage of surgical sites has been promulgated to prevent infection and to minimize the risk of hematoma or seroma formation. Altemeier (4) and McIlreth and associates (5) have shown that removing accumulating tissue fluid and blood by suction tubes will expedite healing; and the elimination of dead space is a basic surgical principle, as Halstead emphasized more than 100 years ago (6). However, Cruse and Foord (7), in a 5-year study of more than 20,000 wounds, and Higson and Kettlewell (8) showed the lowest clean-wound infection rate in wounds that had no drainage at all.

Types of drains

Drains may be either passive or active. Passive drains function primarily by overflow, assisted occasionally by gravity or capillary action, and establish a tract, or path of least resistance (1). Active drains are connected to either low-pressure (30–50 cm H_2O) or high-pressure (100 cm H_2O) suction reservoirs.

Passive drains

Penrose

The passive drain invented by Charles Bingham Penrose is still one of the most popular and widely used (9). Penrose initially used glass tubes, rubber sheets, and gauze, either alone or in combination, for surgical drainage. However, these methods led to a high incidence of complications and infection. In 1897, he devised a new drain by cutting the end from a condom and placing gauze inside the tube that remained. Modifications of this drain bear Penrose's name today (3). Because Penrose drains have different diameters, they can be used in different anatomic areas (Fig. 7-1). A thin Penrose drain may be used after scalene node dissection or evacuation of a vulvar hematoma, while those of large diameters would be used for a pelvic abscess or pelvic or subfascial hematoma. If much drainage is expected, an ostomy appliance may be placed over the drain for accurate fluid measurement (10). Small Penrose drains are usually removed within the first 24 hours, while the larger ones are advanced 3 to 5 cm/day when drainage has markedly diminished. The small Penrose drain is also ideal for exerting

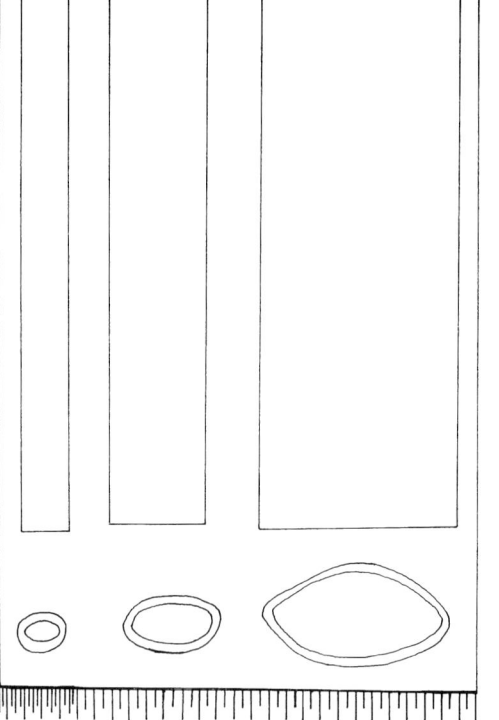

Fig. 7-1 Penrose drains are available in quarter-inch, half-inch, and 1 inch diameter.

gentle traction on the ureter during its dissection from the pelvic floor or from an adjacent retroperitoneal mass.

There is no role for Penrose drains in noninfected or clean wounds. Penrose drainage by gravity is difficult and inefficient, especially when compared with that of modern closed-suction drains. In addition, Penrose drains are two-way conduits that allow surface bacteria to colonize the drain tract quickly, and this can facilitate secondary infection.

Placing gauze inside a Penrose drain forms a cigarette drain. Although capillary action may be enhanced by the gauze, plugging can occur. We have found cigarette drains offer no advantage over standard Penrose drains.

Foley

Best known as the standard bladder drain, the inflatable balloon three-way Foley catheter was introduced in June 1935 by Frederic E. B. Foley to control hemorrhagic cystitis after transuretheral prostectomy (11,12). For gross hematuria from cystotomy or hemorrhagic cystitis, continuous bladder irrigation will help minimize blockage from clot formation.

A three-way Foley also provides excellent drainage for a pyometra. One can irrigate the uterine cavity continuously for 5 to 7 days, using a povidone-iodine solution, until the endometrial cavity is clear and the endocervical canal is sufficiently dilated to provide continuous spontaneous drainage. A No. 3-0 suture through the vestibule or vulva and around the catheter will help to stabilize it within the vaginal tube.

Foley catheters are also used for suprapubic bladder drainage and for decompression of the stomach following gastrostomy.

Malecot

The mushroom or wing-tipped Malecot catheter was introduced in France in 1892 by Achille-Etienne Malecot as a self-retaining urethral catheter or pleural drainage tube (13). It is commonly used for posterior colpotomy drainage of a pelvic abscess, or to drain the presacral space following posterior or total pelvic exenteration (14,15). Again, we suggest fixation to the vulva or perineal body for optimal stabilization.

Active drains

Open drains

Sump, or open, drains use two tubes with lumens of differing widths. The tube with the narrower lumen is placed within or adjacent to the tube with the wider lumen. Air enters the drained area through the narrower lumen to maintain patency of the wider one and to minimize the vacuum required (16). An important modification of the sump drain is the triple-lumen tube, which allows continuous irrigation through a third lumen. Drawbacks include possible entrance of airborne bacteria and rigidity of the drain (17). The addition of a filter to the vent lumen has reduced the amount of the particulate matter and the number of bacteria entering the smaller lumen. Sump drains are primarily used for closed-suction irrigation of wounds, enterocutaneous fistulas, and deep abscess cavities (1,18).

Closed drains

Closed suction drains are the most commonly used and are preferred to either open or passive drains for noninfected wounds and surgical spaces. Although all drains create a route for movement of bacteria to the drain site, there is much less movement of bacteria through closed drains. Examples of commonly used closed suction drain systems are the Blake or J-VAC (Fig. 7-2), Jackson-Pratt, and the T-tube. These drains are flat (7–10 mm) or round (10–19 Fr), soft, pliable, radiopaque, and multiperforated, and have ridged lumens to prevent collapse (19,20). They can be attached to a low-pressure (100-ml) or high-pressure (450-ml) reservoir. Although many of the drains come attached to a sharp trocar, we prefer insertion of the drain with a long Tonsil clamp to prevent inadvertent injury from the trocar. This is especially true if the drain is to be placed deep within the pelvis near great vessels, nerves, or the ureter.

Obstruction of closed-suction drains is usually due to small tissue fragments rather than clotted blood. Although Zacharski and associates have suggested sterile flushing to clear the drain (21), we agree with Moss that early suction should minimize this problem (3). With few exceptions, the low-pressure reservoirs should be used to minimize tissue damage and necrosis (22).

There is currently a trend toward decreased use of drains (1,2,23–28). Two important factors in this development are the routine use of prophylactic antibiotics (1,2,25) and minimal or no closure of the peritoneum (25,29,30). Nonclosure of the anterior parietal peritoneum eliminates the closed space between the anterior and posterior rectus sheath. Similarly, nonclosure of the posterior peritoneum eliminates a separate retroperitoneal space and allows absorption of lymph or serous fluid by the peritoneum. Suturing of the peritoneum can lead to ischemia of the edges, with potential loss of absorptive capacity and increased adhesion formation (30). Pelvic drains could likewise impair the reparative and absorptive capacities of the pelvic peritoneum, maintain lymphatic vessel patency, and therefore lead to prolonged, continuous, and unnecessary drainage (24).

In his survery of gynecologists and gynecologic specialists in the British Isles, Hilton (23) found very limited use of drains in cesarean sections and abdominal hysterectomy. Barton and associates. (24) compared vaginal T-tube to T-tube and two pelvic sidewall drains in radical hysterectomy and pelvic lymphadenectomy, and concluded that T-tube drainage should be sufficient. They also cited patient inconvenience and discomfort with the sidewall drains and a trend to a longer hospital stay. Jensen and colleagues (25) also evaluated the necessity of pelvic drainage following radical hysterectomy and pelvic lymphadenectomy. They found a higher morbidity in the drain group and concluded that prophylactic surgical drainage should not be used. Finally, data from the literature do not support the routine use of drains when large or small bowel has been repaired or resected (1,2,27).

The indications for prophylactic closed suction drainage are limited, but may include the prevention of hematoma or seroma formation, especially in large, deep incisions (31), the retropubic space following urologic surgery (23), and the subfascial space in Maylard incisions if the anterior peritoneum is closed (32), as well as obliteration of dead space and optimal apposition of flaps and skin, especially in the groin (1,2,23). This is the best indication for the high-pressure suction reservoir (23).

Complications of drains

Complications associated with surgical drains include the following:

1 Vessel laceration during insertion.
2 Infection and cellulitis of the drain site. Although abscess formation is unlikely, antibiotic therapy may be required (25).
3 Leakage around the drain due to obstruction of the drain or suboptimal suturing of the drain to the skin.
4 Pain.
5 Retention or breakage of the drain requiring subsequent surgical intervention.

Summary

Drains should be considered as foreign bodies and never be used as a substitute for hemostasis or meticulous surgical technique (17). Although therapeutic indications for prophylactic drainage are fairly clear, enthusiasm for its use in clean wounds and surgical spaces appears to be decreasing.

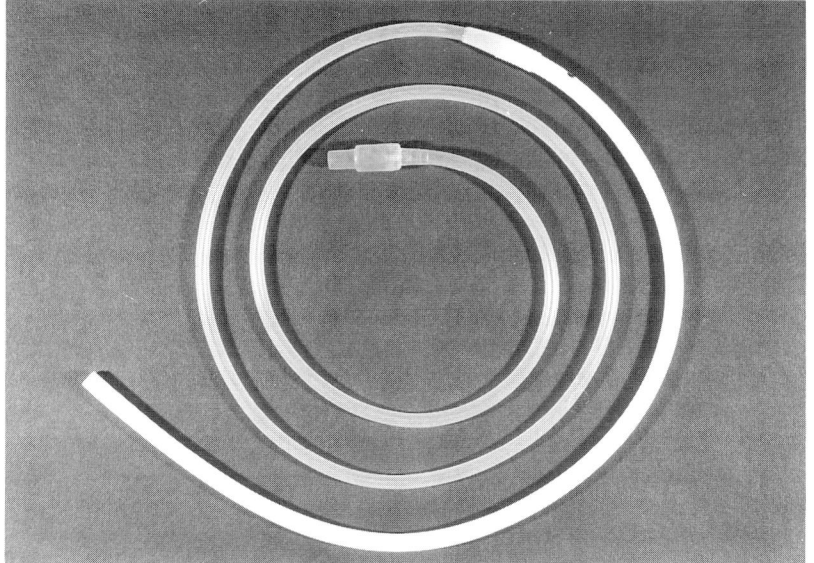

Fig. 7-2 A 19-Fr Blake silicone closed-suction drain.

Select the proper drain and adhere to strict surgical technique for insertion, management, and removal. Use soft, pliable drains with low-pressure reservoirs and remove them within 24 to 48 hours. This is especially important for drains adjacent to blood vessels, nerves, bowel, or the bladder.

There is little or no evidence to support the use of retroperitoneal drains. If the peritoneum is left unsutured, fluid collection or lymphocyst formation should be minimal (23–25).

Drains should never exit through the operative incision (1,7,20,23). This safeguard will significantly decrease the incidence of infection, wound disruption, and hernia formation.

By adhering to strict guidelines for the use of drains, patient care can only benefit. Hospital stay postoperatively will decrease, leading to substantial cost savings, and discomfort and complications associated with drains will be avoided.

References

1 Dougherty SH, Simmons RL. The biology and practice of surgical drains. I. Curr Probl Surg 1992;29:559.

2 Dougherty SH, Simmons RL. The biology and practice of surgical drains. II. Curr Probl Surg 1992;29:638.

3 Moss JP. Historical and current perspectives on surgical drainage. Surg Gynecol Obstet 1981;152:517.

4 Altemeier WA. Surgical infections: incisional wounds. In: Bennett JV, Brachman PS, eds. Hospital infection. Boston: Little, Brown, 1979;287.

5 McIlreth DC, Van Heerden HA, Edis AJ, et al. Closure of abdominal incisions with subcutaneous catheters. Surgery 1977;80:411.

6 Halstead WS. The treatment of wounds with especial reference to the value of the blood clot in the management of dead space. Johns Hopkins Hosp Rep 1891;2:255.

7 Cruse PJE, Foord R. A five-year prospective study of 23,469 surgical wounds. Arch Surg 1973;107:206.

8 Higson RH, Kettlewell MGW. Parietal wound drainage in abdominal surgery. Br J Surg 1978;65:326.

9 Abramson DJ. Charles Bingham Penrose and the Penrose drain. Surg Gynecol Obstet 1976;143:285.

10 Firlit CF, Canning JR. Surgical wound drainage: a simple device for collection. J Urol 1972;108:327.

11 Zorgniotti AW. Frederick E. B. Foley: early development of balloon catheter. Urology 1973;1:1.

12 Foley FEB. A self-retaining bag catheter for use as an indwelling catheter for constant drainage of the bladder. J Urol 1937;38:140.

13 Malecot A. Sonde se fixant d'elle-meme a demeure dans la vessie. Arch Tocologie Gynecologie 1892;19:321.

14 Rubenstein PR, Mishell DR Jr, Ledger WJ. Colpotomy drainage of pelvis abscess. Obstet Gynecol 1976;48:142.

15 Benigno BB. Medical and surgical management of the pelvic abscess. Clin Obstet Gynecol 1981;24:1187.

16 Dulthie HL. Drainage of the abdomen. N Engl J Med 1972;287:1081.

17 Magee C, Rodeheaver GT, Golden GT. Potentiation of wound infection by surgical drains. Am J Surg 1976;131:547.

18 Chaffin RC. Drainage. Am J Surg 1934;24:100.

19 Jackson FE, Fleming PN. Jackson-Pratt brain drain: use in general surgical conditions requiring drainage. Int Surg 1972;57:614.

20 Helmkamp BF, Krebs HB, Amstey MS. Correct use of surgical drains. Contemp Obstet Gynecol 1984;24:123.

21 Zacharski LR, Colt J, Mayor MB, et al. Mechanism of obstruction of closed wound suction tubing. Arch Surg 1979;114:614.

22 Cherry G, McClatchey K. Wound drainage: effects of negative pressure on healing. Infect Surg 1983;2:243.

23 Hilton P. Surgical wound drainage: a survey of practices among gynaecologists in the British Isles. Br J Obstet Gynaecol 1988;95:1063.

24 Barton DPJ, Cavanagh D, Roberts WS, et al. Radical hysterectomy for treatment of cervical cancer: a prospective study of two methods of closed suction drainage. Am J Obstet Gynecol 1992;166:533.

25 Jensen JK, DiSaia PJ, Lucci JA III, Manetta A, Berman ML. To drain or not to drain: a retrospective study of closed-suction drainage following radical hysterectomy with pelvic lymphadenectomy [abstract]. Presented at the 24th Annual Meeting of the Society of Gynecologic Oncologists, Palm Desert, Calif., February 7–10, 1993.

26 Cobb JP. Why use drains? J Bone Joint Surg 1990;72:993.

27 Johnson CD, Lamont PM, Orr N, Lennox M. Is a drain necessary after colonic anastomosis? J R Soc Med 1989;82:661.

28 Wihlborg O, Bergljung L, Martensson H. To drain or not to drain in thyroid surgery. A controlled clinical study. Arch Surg 1988;123:40.

29 Sutton GP. Splitting hairs about splitting muscles. Am J Obstet Gynecol 1991;164:1575.

30 Pietrantoni M, Parsons MT, O'Brien WF, et al. Peritoneal closure or non-closure at cesarean. Obstet Gynecol 1991;77:293.

31 Krebs HB, Helmkamp BF. Transverse periumbilical incision in the massively obese patient. Obstet Gynecol 1984;63:241.

32 Helmkamp BF, Krebs HB. The Maylard incision in gynecologic surgery. Am J Obstet Gynecol 1990;163:1554.

Chapter 8

Appendectomy

Stephen R. T. Evans, Richard V. Brenner,

and Thomas C. Lee

The gynecologist will encounter a variety of clinical situations in which appendectomy is warranted. There are patients with chronic recurrent abdominal or pelvic pain such as those with endometriosis in whom incidental appendectomy will clarify future presentations of abdominal pain. Other patients brought to the operating room with suspected gynecologic pain will have acute appendicitis. Mastery of open appendectomy is essential for all gynecologists. With more widespread application of both diagnostic and therapeutic laparoscopy, competency with laparoscopic appendectomy has become standard for gynecologists and general surgeons alike. The surgical approach using both of these procedures for acute appendicitis and incidental appendectomy will be described in this chapter.

Open appendectomy

Elective appendectomy

Incidental, elective appendectomy during an open gynecologic procedure should be performed in certain clinical situations. It does not significantly increase the length of the overall operation, risk of postoperative wound infection, or length of hospital stay. The rationale is that it obviates the future development of appendicitis and eliminates acute appendicitis in the differential diagnosis in patients with recurrent or chronic abdominal pain. This will be particularly beneficial in patients with recurrent episodic abdominal pain as it will eliminate appendicitis from the differential diagnosis. The gain may never be realized in an older patient who has lived beyond the period of maximal risk for developing appendicitis. Incidental appendectomy should not be performed when there is granulomatous disease, such as Crohn's, involving either the cecum or appendix.

The critical part of removing an appendix is making the organ accessible. The appendix is identified by following the anterior cecal taenia to the appendiceal base. Moist tapes are used to grasp and advance the cecum until the appendiceal base is reached. Occasionally, however, the cecum must be mobilized. The simplest way is by hooking the index finger behind the cecal taenia and slowly, repeatedly stretching the lateral peritoneal attachments (Fig. 8-1). If these do not give sufficiently, incising the avascular lateral peritoneal attachments with scissors or cautery will deliver the cecum into view.

When the cecum is delivered, the appendix usually follows, unless it is retrocecal or fixed by retrocecal adhesions. Then the appendix, too, must be mobilized. Keep in mind that any and all appendiceal antimesenteric adhesions are avascular, and that incising these tissues with scissors expedites rapid exposure. When the appendix is retrocecal, grasp the cecal taenia to its distal tip, then advance it into the wound (Fig. 8-2). There is no need to fear that this maneuver will tear the vascular supply and make it difficult to reach a torn appendiceal artery. The blood

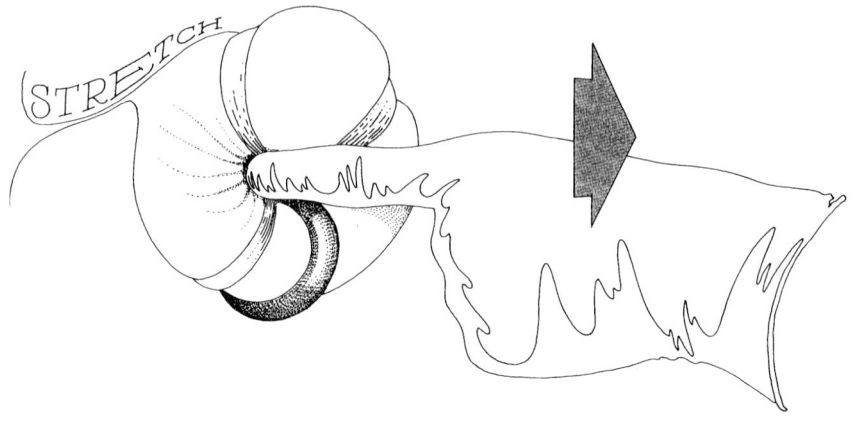

Fig. 8-1 To mobilize the cecum, hook the index finger behind the cecal taenia and pull medially (direction of arrow), stretching the lateral peritoneum.

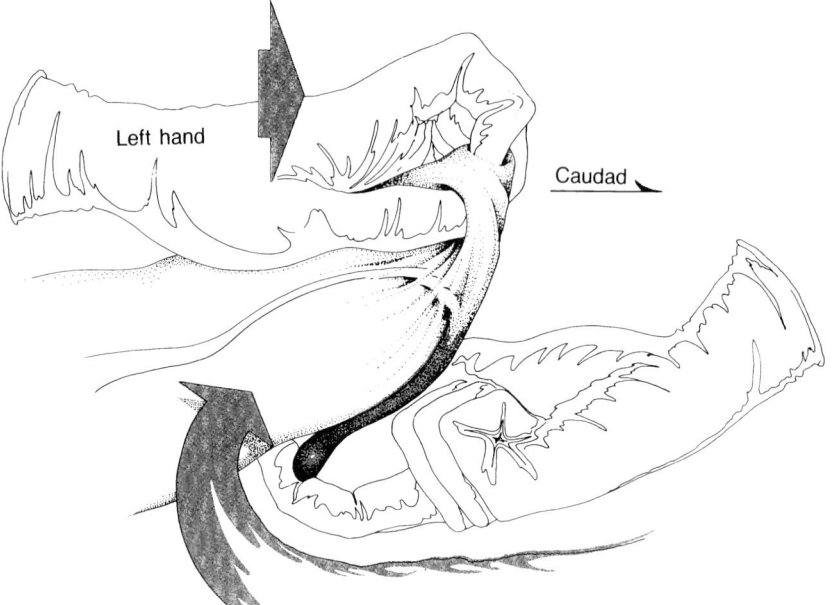

Fig. 8-2 Mobilizing the appendix. When the appendix is retrocecal, grasp the cecal taenia with a curved index finger. With the index finger of the other hand, palpate the appendix to its distal tip, then flip it into the wound.

supply is from the ileocecal artery and is always proximal to the tip, never distal.

If, as happens in less than 1% of cases, the appendiceal tip is not visible, consider retrograde appendectomy. Clamp the appendix at its base between two straight hemostats and transect the base. Then, using the clamp on the distal appendiceal side for leverage, slowly and progressively pull the full distal length and eventually the tip into view. Hemostasis of the divided mesoappendix is most easily achieved with medium or large surgical clips, but can also be accomplished with clamps and ligatures.

When the appendix is not inflamed, the mesoappendix is thin. Often, if the patient is not obese, the vascular supply is readily identified. A Babcock clamp is placed either on the distal tip of the appendix or on the mesoappendix near the appendiceal tip to elevate the entire structure from the wound. An assistant's hand or a second Babcock clamp is used to stretch the cecum caudad and at a right angle to the appendix. This maneuver tents the mesoappendix like a sail, with the appendix being the mast and the cecum the boat (Fig. 8-3).

Sharply stab a hemostat through the mesoappendix, spread it slightly, and withdraw and then replace it while clamping the vascular supply. A clamp is then placed on the appendiceal side as close to the appendix as possible. Use scissors to cut the mesoappendix along the clamp on the appendiceal side. This will ideally leave a 1-cm cuff, so the tie will not slip off when it is ligated. Use one to three pairs of hemostats to separate the mesosalpinx from the appendix. Care should be taken to secure the appendiceal artery at the base of the appendix. Ligate the clamped mesoappendix with resorbable suture material. We prefer 000 polyglactin (Vicryl).

The appendix is then doubly ligated at its junction with the cecum with heavy absorbable suture material. We prefer 0 Vicryl. One tie is placed exactly on top of the other

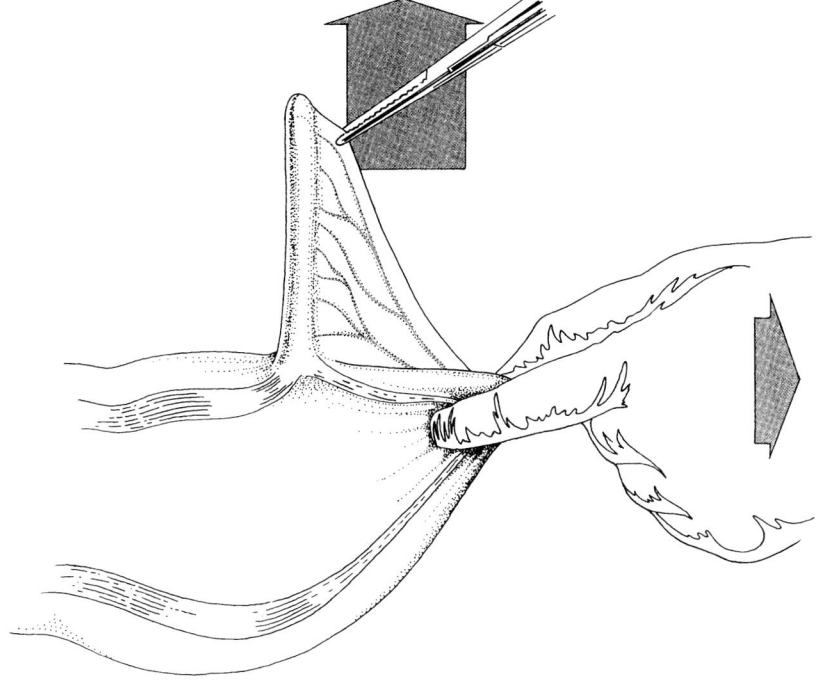

Fig. 8-3 Elevating the mesoappendix. Place a hemostat either on the distal tip of the appendix or on the mesoappendix near the appendiceal tip and elevate all of it from the wound. Use an assistant's hand or Babcock clamp to stretch the cecum caudad and at a right angle to the appendix (arrows indicate direction of traction).

rather than separating the ties by several millimeters. If a fecalith is present in this area, use a hemostat to milk it toward the appendiceal tip. Once the ligatures have been placed and cut, place a straight hemostat 5 mm distal to these ties. Use a scalpel to complete the appendectomy by cutting beneath the clamp.

The mucosa of the appendiceal stump may then be cauterized. A hemostat is used as a conduit for the Bovie current to avoid contamination of the Bovie tip. Dabbing the appendiceal stump tip with silver nitrate, phenol, alcohol, or povidone-iodine (Betadine) should not be done. It is unnecessary to suture the mesoappendix or omentum over the base of the cecum. Inversion of the base of the appendix should be considered when the base of the appendix is friable or inadequate for ligation. We prefer 000 silk for the purse-string stitch. The purse-string bites are seromuscular and do not traverse the full thickness of the bowel wall.

After the appendectomy is complete, the cecum is returned to its normal anatomic position without letting the appendiceal base touch the subcutaneous fat. Elective appendectomy should be done after the primary procedure, because bacteria may be spread to distant organs if the hands of the surgeon or the assistant have come in contact with the appendiceal stump. Another maneuver intended to minimize the risk of wound contamination is the placement of moist tapes around the wound edges. This should be done before manipulation of the cecum and appendix. Adherence to this procedure will allow for routine wound closure.

Ileus may be slightly prolonged because of manipulation and invasion of the intestines. Nasogastric suction is unnecessary, unless the patient has prolonged ileus accompanied by distention. Oral intake may begin with sips on the first postoperative day and is advanced to regular intake as tolerated. Warn patients to avoid enemas and suppositories other than glycerin for at least 2 weeks.

Acute appendicitis

The procedure just described also applies to the acutely inflamed appendix, with the following exceptions. Once it is certain that the disease is acute, it is wise to institute intraoperative antibiotic support immediately. Ideally, antibiotics should be given at least 30 minutes before surgery. Indeed, when acute appendicitis is within the differential diagnosis, coverage for this process should be instituted preoperatively.

Second-generation cephalosporins, such as Cefotan (Cefotetan, 2 g IV), are preferred for their better gram-negative rod, gram-positive cocci, and anaerobic coverage. This antibiotic coverage is continued for two doses postoperatively for focal or suppurative, nonperforated appendicitis.

The appendix is often thickened and tense and may appear ready to burst. If so, handle it gently. Intraoperative rupture is associated with increased morbidity and even mortality, thus cautious handling of the appendix is mandated. Intraoperative cultures are expensive and are of no value because they do not influence either the choice or duration of postoperative antibiotics.

Not uncommonly, the omentum has wrapped itself around the appendix, forming a mass. It usually can be freed by gentle finger dissection. It is during this maneuver that the appendix may perforate, as the omental fat may have sealed the perforation. If confronted with frank pus and contamination, use all efforts, including suction and occluding tapes, to localize it. Often the mesoappendix is more than 1-cm thick, so the vascular supply can no longer be seen. Under these circumstances, one of two approaches is possible. One can stab a hemostat blindly through both walls of the mesoappendix, spread it slightly, and have an assistant follow through with another 1-cm cuff. The problem with this is that the appendiceal artery, which is not visualized, may be stabbed. Certainly, this is not a disaster, but it necessitates quick hands to secure hemostasis. Because of this potential problem, an alternative method is preferred.

Stretch the thickened, opaque mesoappendix as much as possible to create a sail (Fig. 8-4). Gently snip the edge of the overlying peritoneum with dissection scissors. Continue incising the visceral peritoneum on both sides to the appendicocecal junction. The underlying mesoappendiceal edematous fat will bulge through. Then, with the thumb and index fingers on opposing sides of the mesoappendix, squeeze out edematous fluid. This maneuver will leave only the palpable and often visible appendiceal artery. Clamp, cut, and tie this vessel securely.

If acute inflammatory appendiceal process is beyond 1 cm from the appendicocecal junction, treat the base with an inverting purse-string stitch as described above. However, if the surrounding cecal tissue is necrotic, partial cecectomy will be necessary.

Perforated gangrenous appendicitis

Exercise even greater care when mobilizing a gangrenous appendix, to minimize distal contamination. Use suction freely along with sponges and tapes to keep the pus and contaminants as local as possible. If possible, the appendix should be removed at this time, not as a subsequent, staged operation. For all cases of perforation, copious irrigation is essential. When there is free perforation without abscess cavity formation, no drains are left within the peritoneal cavity. Drains are required only when distinct abscess cavities are present. All abscesses are drained with Jackson-Pratt drains brought through separate stab incisions.

Peritoneum and fascia are closed. A delayed primary closure of the skin is preferred. Excellent wound closure is achieved with the following method. First, 000 nylon mattress sutures are placed in the skin. They are left untied and are secured at their tips with either a hemostatic clip or a sterile strip to prevent them from pulling through. The open wound is packed with a betadine-soaked sponge. The packing is removed 48 hours postoperatively, and normal saline wet-to-dry dressing changes are instituted. On postoperative day 5, the margins are reapproximated in the delayed primary closure. This process minimizes risk of wound infection from approximately 30% to less than 5%.

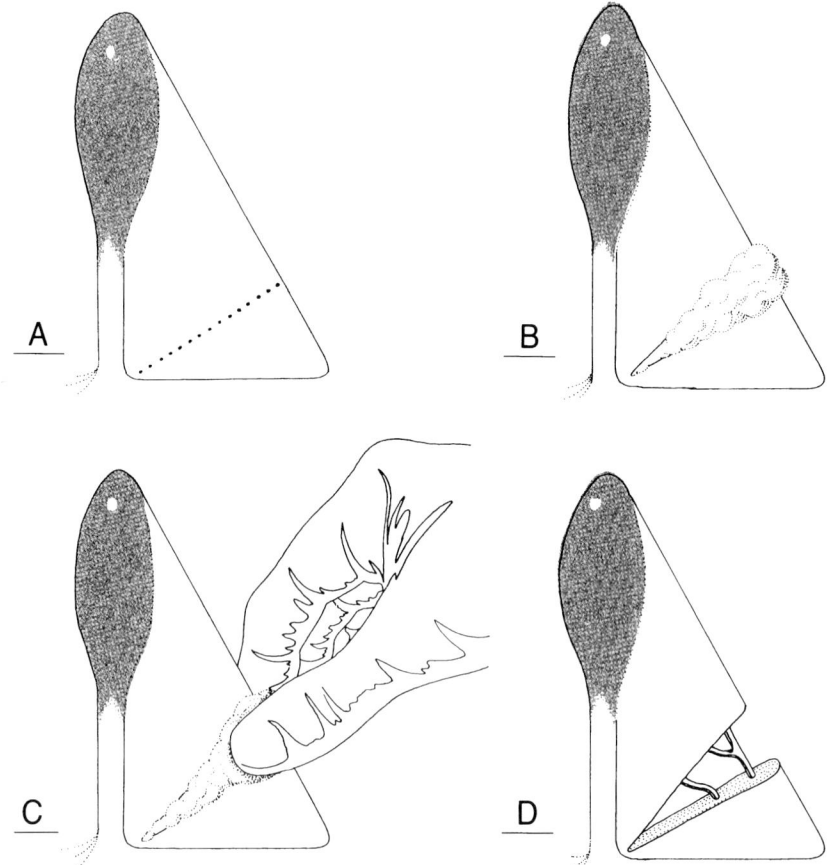

Fig. 8-4 Technique for localizing contamination. (A) Stretch the thickened, opaque mesoappendix as much as possible to create a sail. Gently snip the edge of the overlying peritoneum with dissection scissors. (B) Continue incising the covering on both sides to the appendicocecal junction. The underlying mesoappendiceal edematous fat will bulge through. (C) With the thumb and index fingers on opposing sides of the mesoappendix, squeeze out edematous fluid. (D) Clamp, cut, and tie the appendiceal artery.

Broad spectrum antibiotic coverage is continued for 10 to 14 days. A typical regimen includes ampicillin, gentamicin, and flagyl. A ruptured appendix is potentially life-threatening. Skin sutures may be removed on postoperative day 12. Oral feedings are withheld until flatus is manifested. Advancement of the diet is determined by the patient's temperature, bowel activity, and absence of abdominal distention.

Laparoscopic appendectomy

The emergence of diagnostic and operative laparoscopy as a viable option to laparotomy has led to new applications, including laparoscopic appendectomy. When performed by a skilled laparoscopist, incidental laparoscopic appendectomy is indicated in the same clinical situations as incidental open appendectomy. Several advancements in instrumentation have made the performance of this procedure easier. One of the most common settings in which incidental laparoscopic appendectomy is performed is in association with laparoscopy for endometriosis and pelvic adhesions. Again, the appendectomy is performed at the conclusion of the principal procedure. Laparoscopic appendectomy has less of a role in perforated appendicitis owing to the amounts of inflammation and contamination. Conversion to open appendectomy is more expeditious with a gangrenous, friable, or perforated appendix.

The 12-mm operating port is ideally located in the right upper quadrant, although this can be modified to the right lower quadrant if the port is already positioned there. The retractor port is suprapubic, and the videolaparoscope is positioned at the umbilical port. The cecum is lifted with an endo Babcock clamp to bring the appendix into view. The suprapubic grasper is then used to retract at the appendiceal tip. The mesoappendix is then isolated. The fastest,

albeit most expensive, way to transect the mesoappendix and appendix is with a multifire endo GIA (gastrointestinal anastomosis) 30 stapler. First, the measuring device is inserted to determine whether small (2.5-mm) or large (3.5-mm) staple cartridges will be used. Once this has been ascertained, the stapling device is inserted and fired across the appendix (Fig. 8-5). The measuring and firing process is repeated for the mesoappendix (Fig. 8-6). The staple line is then inspected for hemostasis. The free appendix is then grasped at its stapled end, brought up into the shaft of the port, and removed from the peritoneal cavity. An endoscopic retrieval bag is used to deliver the appendix if the appendix does not fit into the port.

An alternative to use of the endo GIA involves endo clips and endo loops. Hemostatic clips can be used to divide the mesoappendix. This step is often necessitated by a thickened or inflamed mesoappendix that cannot be hemostatically stapled and transected by the endo GIA. Two chromic endo loops are used to ligate the appendix. The appendix is then divided between the two loops, making sure to leave a sufficient length of appendiceal stump.

Meckel's diverticulectomy

Both the appendix and Meckel's diverticulum are true diverticula of the gastrointestinal tract because, unlike colonic diverticula, both contain a muscular layer. They differ mainly in the location and anatomy. While the appendix is always attached to the cecum, the Meckel's diverticulum may be anywhere from 3 to 500 cm from the ileocecal valve. The entire small bowel must be examined before ascertaining that there is no Meckel's diverticulum. In most cases, it will be 25 to 50 cm from the ileocecal valve.

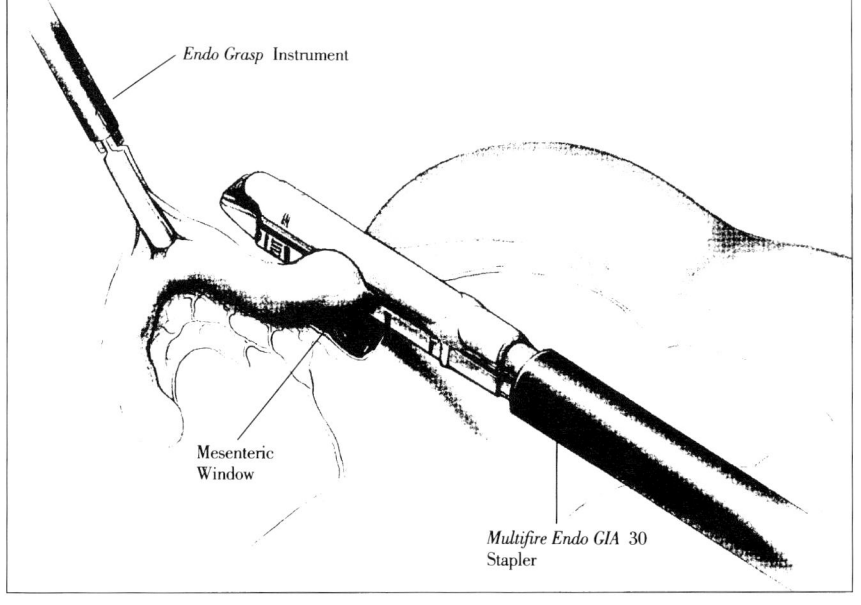

Fig. 8-5 Laparoscopic appendectomy. The appendix is grasped by its shaped base and retracted upward. After the tissue is measured with the Endo Gauge 30 instrument (which usually indicates a white vascular cartridge), the Multifire Endo GIA 30 stapler, now loaded with the proper-sized cartridge, is reinserted and closed around the mesoappendix. The instrument is fired, amputating the appendix from the gastrointestinal tract.

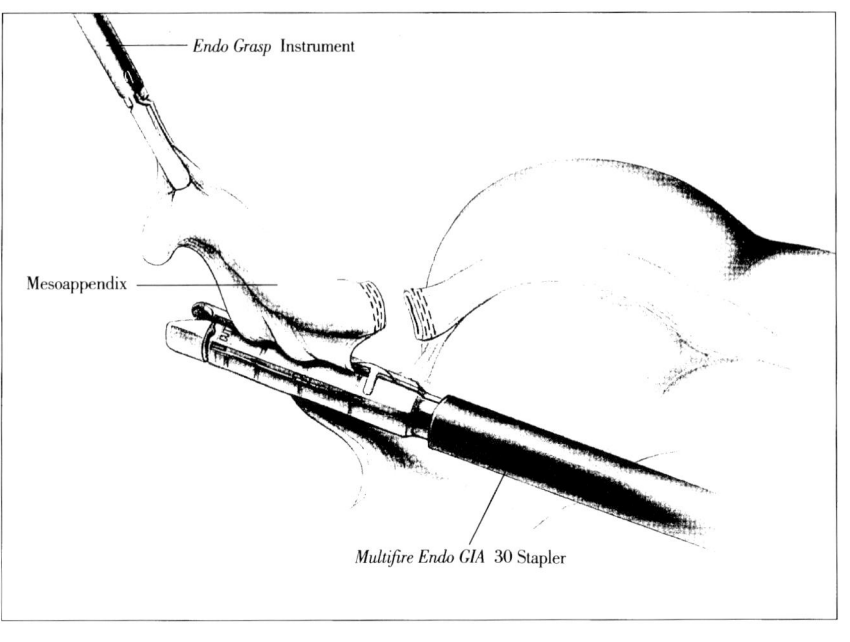

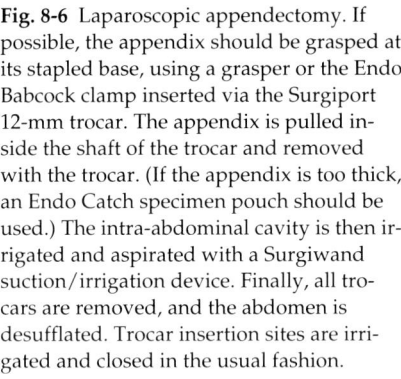

Fig. 8-6 Laparoscopic appendectomy. If possible, the appendix should be grasped at its stapled base, using a grasper or the Endo Babcock clamp inserted via the Surgiport 12-mm trocar. The appendix is pulled inside the shaft of the trocar and removed with the trocar. (If the appendix is too thick, an Endo Catch specimen pouch should be used.) The intra-abdominal cavity is then irrigated and aspirated with a Surgiwand suction/irrigation device. Finally, all trocars are removed, and the abdomen is desufflated. Trocar insertion sites are irrigated and closed in the usual fashion.

The other major difference between these two diverticula is in the size of their mouths. While the mouth of the appendix is small, the Meckel's usually has a broad opening to the small intestine and must be handled differently.

Most authorities agree that a Meckel's noted in a young patient should be excised, since a few will eventually bleed, obstruct, or perforate. This holds true especially for Meckel's with ectopic tissue and those with narrow mouths. It should not be removed in the setting of inflammatory bowel disease such as Crohn's. The diverticulum often has a mesentery of its own, called the mesenteriolum (Fig. 8-7), which connects to the small intestinal mesentery. Within this mesenteriolum is the vascular supply. Simply clamp, divide, and ligate it. Because of the large opening into the small intestine, be careful not to compromise the intestinal lumen in excising the diverticulum. Clamping, which must be done at right angles to the long axis of the small bowel, can be accomplished in one of several ways.

While an assistant stretches both ends of the proximal and distal adjacent intestine, elevate the Meckel's with a Babcock clamp, place a linear gastrointestinal stapler at right angles to the intestine, and fire it (Fig. 8-8). Place two Kocher clamps at the junction between the Meckel's and the intestine, again at right angles, clamp, and divide. With the intestinal-side Kocher in place, closure can be effected by a running, nonlocking, absorbable suture over the clamp, reinforced with interrupted 000 Prolene or Ethibond sutures; by a running, back-and-forth absorbable suture beneath the clamp, reinforced with Prolene or Ethibond; or by any one of many other accepted techniques for closing a rent in the intestinal lumen.

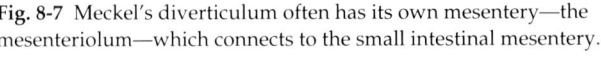

Fig. 8-7 Meckel's diverticulum often has its own mesentery—the mesenteriolum—which connects to the small intestinal mesentery.

For acute Meckel's diverticulitis, use the techniques just described, except in the following cases. Approximately 50% of Meckel's diverticula contain heterotropic tissue, usually gastric mucosa or pancreatic tissue. When there is gastric mucosal tissue, an ulcer may not only arise but bleed or perforate within the confines of the diverticulum. This is treated the same as a nonactive Meckel's. Gastric mucosa also may cause an ulcer in the opposite wall of the small intestine, perforating into the mesentery. If confronted with this situation, not only should the Meckel's be resected, but also a cuff of intestine, including the ulcerated area. A stapled side-to-side, functional end-to-end anastomosis is acceptable.

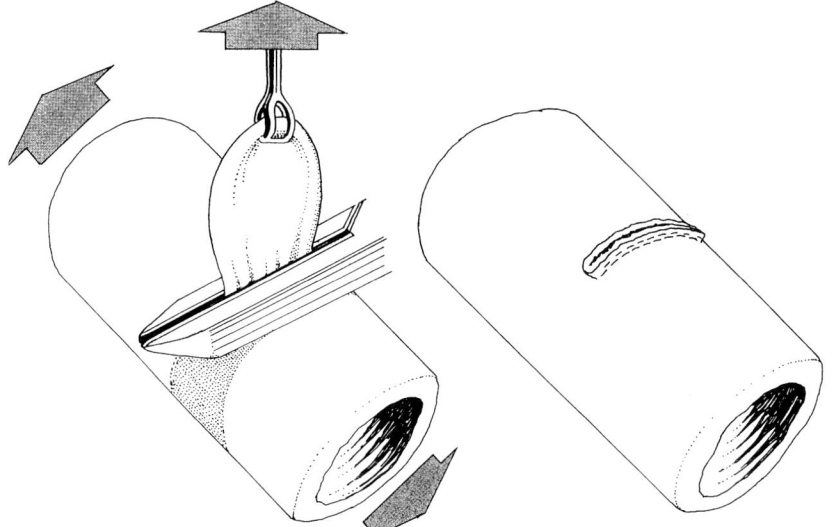

Fig. 8-8 Clamping Meckel's diverticulum. Arrows indicate the direction of traction as the stapling device is placed over Meckel's diverticulum. Note that the resulting staple line is at a right angle to the long axis of the intestine.

Chapter 9

Repair of incidental abdominal wall hernias

Stephen R. T. Evans, Richard V. Brenner,

and Thomas C. Lee

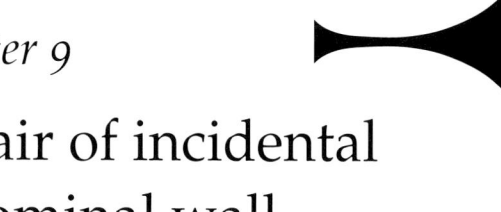

Abdominal wall hernias that will confront the gynecologist have two etiologies: congenital and iatrogenic. Congenital fascial weakness can cause umbilical and inguinofemoral hernias. Iatrogenic hernias are related to previous operation. Although the etiologies vary, the principles of incidental repair are similar. Fascial or ligamentous structures are secured to other fascial and ligamentous structures. Repair of any large or complex hernia or laparoscopic hernia should be done in conjunction with a general surgeon.

Diagnosis

A hernia can be defined as a facial defect in the abdominal wall through which a peritoneum-lined structure protrudes or may protrude (Fig. 9-1). Usually, it can be diagnosed by gliding the fingertips along the abdomen's smooth parietal peritoneal surfaces and searching for the defect.

In the umbilical area, which is usually explored first, small defects are occasionally palpable. Repair all defects, as even small defects can incarcerate.

Assess femoral hernias by following the course of the round ligaments through the internal inguinal ring. Again, all defects that are palpable must be repaired, as even small defects can incarcerate.

Incisional, or iatrogenic, hernias frequently have omentum or intestines incarcerated and adherent to the peritoneal sac. This involvement makes evaluation and repair more difficult.

Hernias should always be repaired unless the hernia is inaccessible, sepsis and shock coexist, or the primary procedure and contemplated herniorrhaphy are both complex. If the hernia is distant from the initial incision, the exposure may not be correct. Rather than extend the incision, it is best to abandon the attempt. Blind herniorrhaphies are to be condemned.

Adding a second procedure is unwise if its complications will negate the beneficial results of the primary one. Hence peritonitis and significant blood loss are considered contraindications. Similarly, a complex herniorrhaphy should not be attempted after a complex primary gynecologic procedure. However, a complex herniorrhaphy could follow a simple gynecologic procedure, and simple herniorrhaphy a complex gynecologic procedure. If there is any doubt, leave the herniorrhaphy for another time.

Umbilical herniorrhaphy

Hernias in this area are the result of a defect in the linea alba and usually vary from one to three fingerbreadths in diameter (Fig. 9-2a). Once the distinct fascial edge is palpated, it is grasped on each side with a sharp penetrating instrument such as an Allis, Adair, Lahey, Kocher, or towel clip (Fig. 9-2b). Then secure a No. 0 or 1 permanent suture, such as Prolene or Ethibond, just lateral to the tip of the clamp and also contralateral, but leave it untied (Fig. 9-2c).

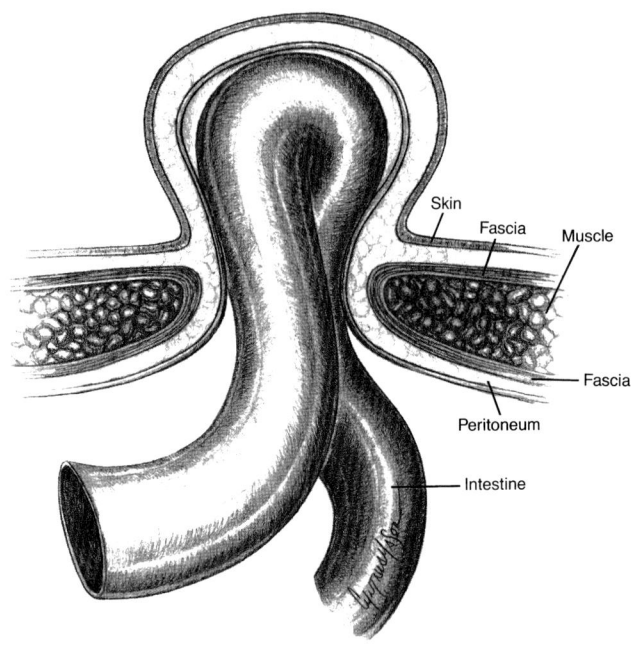

Fig. 9-1 A hernia is a viscus protruding through a fascial defect.

Once this initial suture is in place, remove the clamps and apply traction toward you to both sutures in order to bring the fascial edges closer to each other and to you (Fig. 9-2d). With this tension maintained, make a second placement of the same suture in the same plane, but more lateral than the initial suture, to buttress the defect (Fig. 9-2e). Then securely tie this second, lateral suture in a figure-of-eight fashion (Fig. 9-2f).

Place similar sutures at 1-cm distances. Therefore, if a defect is 3 cm, two or three such sutures will be needed; if 10 cm, nine or ten such sutures will be needed.

Occasionally, an umbilical defect will be incarcerated with omentum or, less often, with small intestine. If gentle traction cannot return these structures to their normal position, incising the fascial ring in the inferior midline will allow their release. This is usually done with heavy curved scissors by cutting between index and middle fingertips that have been forced into the hernial space (Fig. 9-2g). Once visceral reduction has taken place, repair is similar to that of any other umbilical hernia.

In the relatively young, resilient, and healthy patient, the umbilical skin will appear normal within several months.

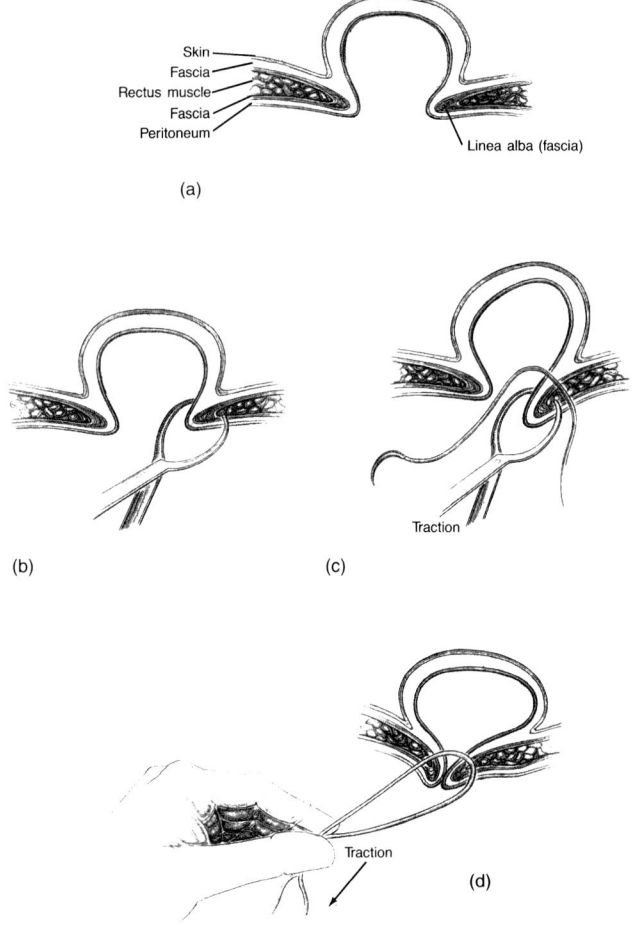

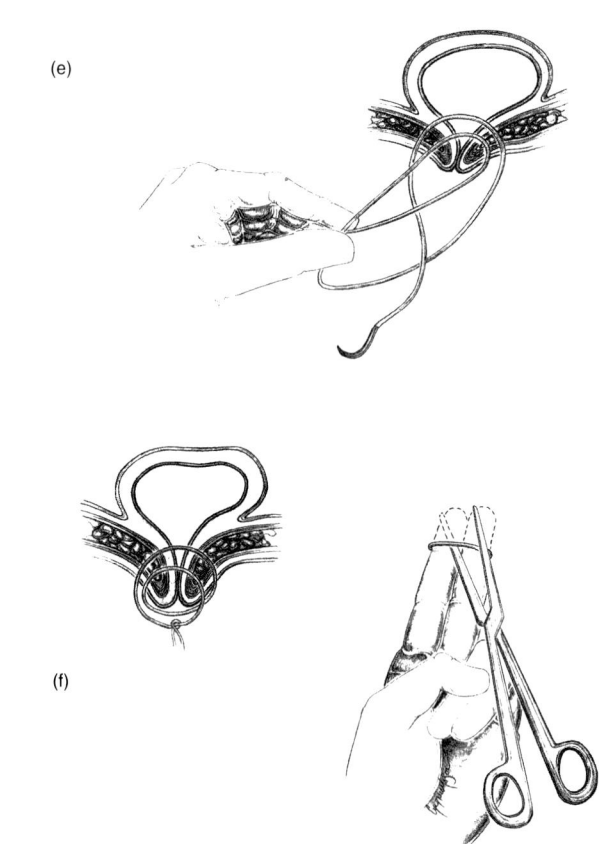

Fig. 9-2 Umbilical herniorrhaphy. (a) A linea alba defect is the cause. (b) Place a towel clip to grasp distinct edge. (c) Exert traction on towel clip and place first suture bite. (d) Apply traction on both sutures opposing defect. (e) A second throw completes the figure-of-eight into deeper tissues lateral to the first suture. (f) The suture is completed. (g) Incise the fascial ring to release incarcerated viscera.

On those rare occasions when redundancy persists, plastic procedures can easily restore a more attractive appearance.

Incisional herniorrhaphy

Repair of small incisional, or iatrogenic, hernias does not differ radically from that of umbilical hernias. However, a few distinctions are necessary. Repair is usually incorporated in the primary closure because, as a rule, it was the primary incision that caused the hernia. Therefore, repair should not substantially prolong the gynecologic procedure.

As noted earlier, omentum and intestinal viscera frequently adhere to the surrounding peritoneum. It is imperative to release these, not only along the projected site of repair but also for a distance of 3 to 4 cm laterally to allow the repairing sutures wide purchase.

Perhaps the best suture is one that uses a four-bite, near-far–far-near, Smead-Jones closure (Fig. 9-3). The first bite is near the wound edges and incorporates the fascia. The second bite is on the opposite side deep into the peritoneum, muscle, and fascia. The third bite recrosses to the first side, also going deep into muscle and fascia. The fourth and last bite, crossing once more to the opposite side, is similar to the first. This is a one-layer technique (not including skin) that disregards the value of or need for separate or incorporated peritoneal closure. Sutures should be 1 cm apart.

Femoral herniorrhaphy

This hernia is a triangular defect with no fascial plane on its lateral side. A mnemonic, NAVEL, is a convenient way to recall what lies between the inguinal (Poupart's) ligament and the ileal (Cooper's) ligament; from lateral to medial, N is the nerve, A the artery, V the vein, E the empty space (the fossa ovalis) through which the hernia extrudes, and L the lymphatic space (Fig. 9-4, top).

Frequently, a femoral hernia will contain incarcerated properitoneal fat. If it does, an incision must be made medially into the lacunar ligament to enlarge the opening and release the herniated structure, because cutting laterally would severely jeopardize the femoral vein. Once the herniated tissue, whether it is properitoneal fat, bladder, or small intestine, is reduced, the defect is readily palpated with one or two fingers.

Repair is straightforward so long as the fascial approximation is from Poupart's ligament to Cooper's ligament. Repair is never attempted in a medial-to-lateral plane as there is no lateral fascia, only vein. Thus herniorrhaphy is from fascia ligament to fascia ligament, white-to-white, employing figure-of-eight permanent sutures (Fig. 9-4, bottom).

Inguinal herniorrhaphy

Indirect inguinal herniorrhaphies are simpler in females than in males because there are neither vas deferens nor testicular vessels to preserve. Intraperitoneal repair is similar

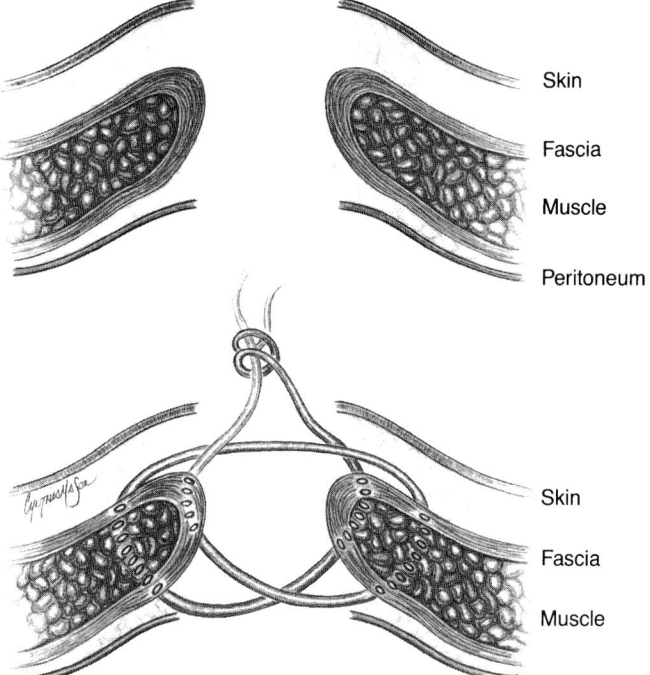

Fig. 9-3 The near-far–far-near closure. In the area to be repaired, sequence of suture placement is shown (top) for this one-layer technique. The suture is seen in place (bottom).

to that for umbilical hernia. Grasp the fascial edges of the deep internal ring with an instrument, and place and securely tie deep figure-of-eight sutures. Beware of the inferior epigastric vessels that lie just medial to the dilated internal inguinal ring. As with femoral herniorrhaphies, remember the location of the femoral vein. If a suture is inadvertently placed through the femoral vein, remove the suture and apply pressure for several minutes. Do not tie the suture, as this tends to make a larger opening in the vein.

Laparoscopic herniorrhaphy

Laparoscopic herniorrhaphy is a relatively new application of video laparoscopy that represents a new approach to an old problem: inguinofemoral hernias. To date, the only distinct advantage over traditional open approaches is an earlier return to physical activity postoperatively. No long-term follow-up data are available to prove superiority of this method over the extra-abdominal approach. Laparoscopic herniorrhaphy should not be attempted by anyone other than a general surgeon who has substantial experience in this field. The following description of laparoscopic herniorrhaphy will serve as a guide to the gynecologist, who will be asked to assist with the procedure when done in conjunction with a gynecologic operation. Review of the inguinofemoral anatomy as viewed via the laparoscope is essential for those assisting with a laparoscopic herniorrhaphy.

Three ports are needed for laparoscopic herniorrhaphy: the umbilical port for the camera, a 5-mm port for retrac-

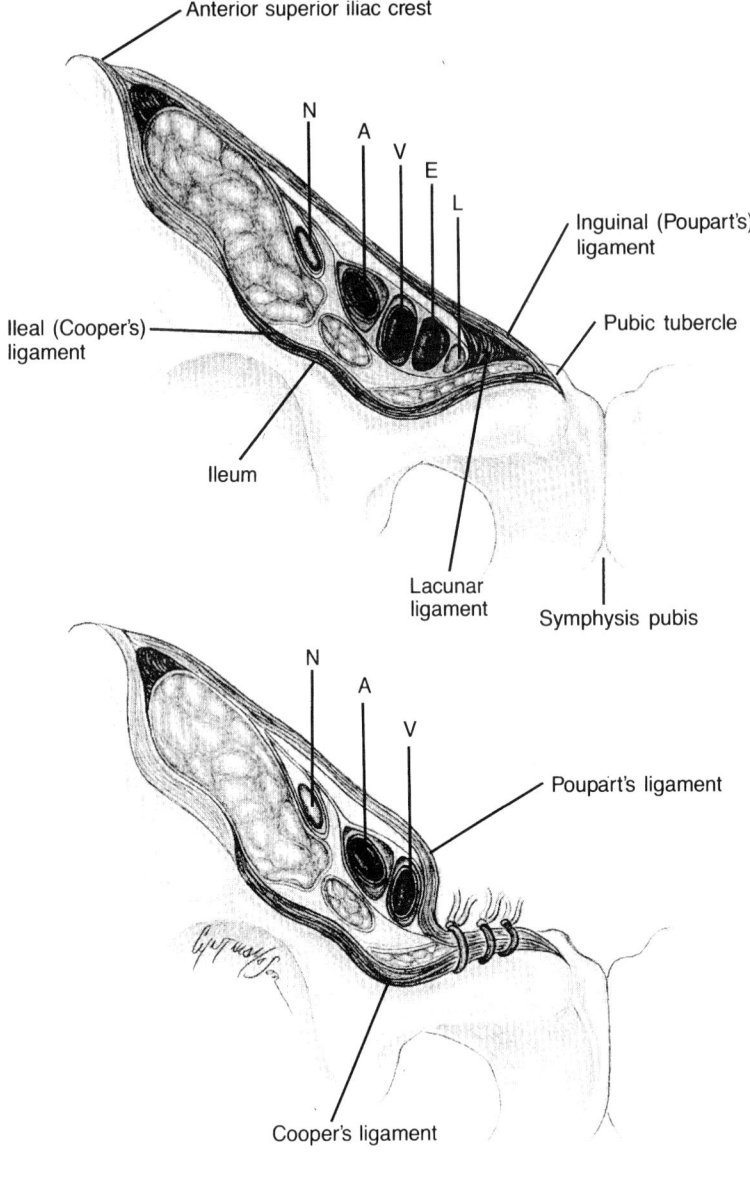

Fig. 9-4 Femoral herniorrhaphy. Schematic shows structure passing through the space between the inguinal and ileal ligament (top). Repair is approximation of the two ligamentous structures with figure-of-eight sutures (bottom). N, femoral nerve; A, femoral artery; V, femoral vein; E, empty space (fossa ovalis) through which hernia presents; L, lymphatics.

tion, and a 12-mm operating port. The working ports are placed at the level of the umbilicus at the lateral margins of the rectus abdominis. If bilateral hernias are present, two 12-mm ports are required. Initial recognition of the anatomy is challenging, as the peritoneum entirely covers all fascial and ligamentous landmarks. After identification of the hernia sac, epigastric vessels, and pubic tubercle, the sac contents are reduced. The peritoneal covering of the inguinal canal is opened, and upper and lower peritoneal flaps are developed. The hernia sac is pulled into the intra-abdominal cavity, and the peritoneum is inverted. Poupart's and Cooper's ligaments are identified as the anatomic landmarks. A 3-inch-by-5-inch piece of either Surgipro or Marlex mesh is fashioned to cover the entire inguinofemoral region with a cut made laterally to accommodate the round ligament. The mesh is then inserted and

stapled to the anatomic boundaries, using caution not to place a staple into the round ligament or the ileofemoral vessels. Direct, indirect, and femoral defects will be covered by the graft. Once the graft is secured in place, the edges of the peritoneal flaps are reapproximated. The abdomen is then desufflated, and the trocars are removed.

Postoperative care

The postoperative care of incidental herniorrhaphies is identical to that for other herniorrhaphies. Patients are instructed not to engage in heavy lifting for 4 to 6 weeks. An exception to this rule is made with laparoscopic herniorrhaphies, as there is no approximation of fascial edges.

Chapter 10

Evaluating a breast mass

William F. Feller

Carcinoma of the breast is the most common malignancy in women and is the second major cause of death from cancer. Breast cancer represents 32% of all cancers in women and is responsible for 18% of the cancer-related deaths in women. Approximately 182,000 women were diagnosed with breast cancer in the United States in 1993 (1). It is estimated that 46,000 women will die of this disease in 1993. In 1985 lung cancer surpassed breast cancer as the leading cause of cancer-related deaths in women. Of every 9 women, approximately one (11%) will develop breast cancer during her lifetime. The mortality is directly related to the stage of disease at diagnosis (i.e., the size and number of positive axillary lymph nodes).

A study by the Physician Insurers Association of America in 1990 found that failure to diagnose a breast cancer was the second most frequent reason for claims brought against physicians, and the most expensive. In most instances, diagnosis was delayed because the physical findings "failed to impress the physician," particularly when the mammogram was normal. Over two-thirds of the plaintiffs (69%) were young, premenopausal women (2).

Women frequently consult a gynecologist regarding a breast complaint or a breast mass found on self-examination. In addition, asymptomatic women often ask a gynecologist to perform a breast check and to order a screening mammogram to rule out the possible presence of a breast cancer. It is important for the gynecologist to be familiar with the proper procedures for an adequate breast evaluation. A few diagnostic tests can be very helpful, but their limitations must be understood. In general, four areas of investigation are required: history, including breast history and breast cancer risk status; physical examination of the breast; mammography; and invasive diagnostic tests including cyst aspiration, fine-needle and open breast biopsy. Table 10-1 summarizes diagnostic procedures used in the evaluation of a breast mass. About 75% of all breast cancers are detected by the patient, when she notices a new lump or thickening. Most patients who come to a physician with a breast complaint do not have cancer.

History

The purpose of a breast history is to elicit facts about the breast that the patient may have noted, such as a mass, breast pain, or nipple discharge, and to obtain information to establish the patient's breast cancer risk status. The four most important risk factors for developing breast cancer are age, family history, reproductive history, and biopsy-proved atypia, or carcinoma in situ (Table 10-2).

Breast history

The patient should be asked if she has noted a new mass or thickening in the breast, occurrence of breast pain, nipple

Table 10-1 Diagnostic evaluation procedures for breast mass

Procedure	Accuracy	Comment
Breast palpation	60%–70%	Always the first step.
Needle aspiration	99%	Should be done frequently. Diagnoses a cyst with 99% accuracy.
Mammography	85%	All women over 35. Single most accurate diagnostic test available.
Ultrasound	99%	Highly accurate for cysts. Low accuracy for cancer.
Fine-needle aspiration biopsy	98%	Need expert cytopathologist. Should correlate with mammography and physical findings.
Open breast biopsy	100%	Definitive diagnostic test.

Table 10-2 Risk factors for breast cancer

Age	*Incidence/100,000*
25	3
35–39	66
45–49	187
65–69	392

Family history	*Relative risk*
Premenopausal breast cancer, mother/sister	3
Bilateral breast cancer, mother/sister	5
Bilateral and premenopausal mother/sister	9

Parity	
First birth under age 18	0.6
First birth age 25	1.0
First birth over 35	1.5

Prior breast pathology	
Proliferative disease, no atypia	1.9
Proliferative disease, with atypia	5.3
Proliferative disease, atypia, family history	11

Postmenopausal estrogen	*Relative risk*
0.625 mg/d > 15 years	1.3–2.2
0.625 mg/d < 5 years	1.0
1.25 mg/d	2.0
0.625 mg/d, family history	3.4

discharge, or skin or nipple changes. If the patient has noted a mass or thickening, the physician should inquire how long it has been there, whether it changes in size with the menstrual period, and whether it is tender or painful. Cancers are generally painless, nontender, and do not change size with the menstrual cycle. A definite decrease in the size of a mass is strong evidence that it is not cancerous. However, some cancers can remain the same size for as long as one year. Historical information is helpful, but the clinician must always assess the patient's reliability. Is she an accurate and careful observer? Breast pain is hard to evaluate but usually is related to benign fibrocystic disease and is cyclic. Rarely, a cancer will be associated with breast pain. Skin dimpling or nipple inversion of recent origin is always suspicious for cancer and requires mammography and surgical consultation.

Nipple discharge is generally benign but may be a sign of early breast cancer. Two questions should be asked: Is the discharge spontaneous or is it produced by manipulation or stroking the breast? What color is the discharge? To be of clinical significance, a nipple discharge should be spontaneous, persistent, and nonlactational. A nipple discharge produced by breast manipulation or squeezing the nipple is almost never a sign of cancer. The clinician should try to reproduce the discharge by gentle finger pressure on the areola. The color and the consistency of the discharge can be observed. The discharge can be checked for blood on a hemoccult slide. Milky, multicolored and sticky, and purulent discharges are not related to cancer and can be managed medically except for the need of an incision of an abscess related to a purulent discharge. Four types of nipple discharge require a biopsy of the involved duct to establish a diagnosis: watery, yellow or serous, pink or serosanguinous, or bloody. Cancer is found in 15% of women with spontaneous and persistent nipple discharges of these four types. Leis (3) reported that 33% of women with clear, watery nipple discharge had invasive cancer, and 27% of women with bloody discharge had cancer.

Breast cancer risk status

The following information should be obtained from the patient to establish a risk profile.

Age

Because the incidence of breast cancer is age specific, this is the most important risk question. Cancer of the breast is rare in women under the age of 25. At age 25 the incidence of breast cancer is estimated to be 3/100,000, at age 35 it is 66/100,000, at age 45 it is 187/100,000, and at age 65 it is 392/100,000.

Family history

Breast cancer is a genetic disease. It can be caused by an inherited or an acquired gene defect. A strong family history of breast cancer is a clue to the possible presence of an inherited breast cancer gene. It is now believed that an inherited defective breast cancer gene is probably responsible for 5% of all breast cancers. One woman in 200 carries this defective gene, and those who do face an 80% to 90% risk of developing breast cancer (4). Epidemiologic studies have shown that the greatest risk of breast cancer is for a woman under the age of 50 whose sister and mother both had breast cancer. If first-degree relatives (mother or sister) had bilateral breast cancer, that women has a breast cancer risk about five times that of the general population (i.e., a 50% lifetime risk). If the relative had bilateral premenopausal breast cancer, that patient has a risk of breast cancer nine times that of the general population and probably carries the defective breast cancer gene. Commercially available tests to detect the presence of this gene should be available in early 1994. Three questions to ask: Whether mother or sister had breast cancer, age of onset of their cancer, and was it bilateral?

Reproductive history

Two factors increase risk of breast cancer: nulliparity and late first pregnancy. Women who have their first full-term pregnancy at 18 years or younger have a risk one-third that of women who are nulliparous or have their first child after 35.

Hormone replacement therapy

Prolonged use of estrogens for menopausal symptoms has been cited as a risk factor for breast cancer. The issue is controversial. Many studies have found no relationship between postmenopausal estrogen replacement therapy and cancer, while others have found that these hormones elevate breast cancer risk in some subgroups of patients. A recent meta-analysis of 16 case control studies of estrogen replacement therapy strongly supports the view of a small but statistically significant increase in breast cancer risk due to long-term estrogen use (5). This increased risk of breast cancer was demonstrated for estrogen users who had experienced a natural menopause or who had undergone a bilateral oophorectomy. After 15 years of estrogen use, this meta-analysis found a 30% increase in risk of developing breast cancer (relative risk 1.3). This risk did not appear to increase before 5 years of estrogen use. This analysis also showed that those case-control studies including premenopausal women or women using estradiol had a higher relative risk (i.e., 3.2). The highest risk (i.e., 3.4), was among estrogen users with a family history of breast cancer.

Another meta-analysis of 28 case-control studies reported by Dupont and Page (6) arrived at different conclusions. These authors showed that women who took 0.625 mg/day or less of conjugated estrogen had a risk of breast cancer that was 1.08 times that of women who did not receive this therapy. On the other hand, women who took 1.25 mg/day or more of conjugated estrogens had a breast cancer relative risk of 2.0 or slightly less in all studies. The relative risk of breast cancer associated with estrogen replacement therapy among women with a history of benign breast disease was 1.16. In summary, this meta-analysis suggested there is considerable and consistent evidence

that a daily dosage of 0.625 mg of conjugated estrogen for several years does not appreciably increase the risk of breast cancer. It is now accepted that estrogen replacement therapy reduces the risk of ischemic heart disease in women and also of osteoporosis. As the age-adjusted mortality due to ischemic heart disease is about four times that due to endometrial and breast cancer, there is likely to be an increase in the use of postmenopausal estrogen. The use of estrogen therapy for menopausal symptoms is contraindicated following breast cancer treatment. There is minimal evidence that contraceptive estrogen increases the risk of breast cancer except for a subgroup of women under age 45 who have used contraceptives for a long period of time beginning at an early age.

Benign breast disease

The patient should be asked if she has had a previous breast biopsy, and if so, the type of pathology should be ascertained. A classic study by Dupont and Page (7) showed that the risk of breast cancer for women with atypical hyperplasia (atypia) was 5.3 times that of women with nonproliferative lesions. They also showed that for women who had atypia and a family history of breast cancer, the risk of breast cancer was 11 times that of women without atypia or a family history of breast cancer. Table 10-2 summarizes risk factors.

Risk status summary

On the basis of the risk factors presented here—age, family history, reproductive history, postmenopausal estrogen use, and presence of atypical benign breast disease—a woman can be classified into one of four risk classes:

1 Normal risk, 11% lifetime risk
2 High risk, 20% to 25% lifetime risk
3 Very high risk, 50% lifetime risk
4 Extremely high risk, 80% to 90% lifetime risk

The patient should be informed about her risk status and if it is high, very high, or extremely high, should be advised to have breast examinations and high-quality mammograms yearly. Women with very high or extremely high risk status may be candidates for treatment with tamoxifen. Prophylactic mastectomy may also be considered. If the breast cancer gene test becomes commercially available in 1994, it should be carried out on women whose family history suggests very high or extremely high risk status.

Physical examination of the breast

The physical examination of the breast consists of visualization and manual palpation of the breast, axillae, and supraclavicular node areas. Breast visualization can reveal nipple retraction, nipple ulceration or crusting, skin dimpling, or localized skin edema (peau d'orange). Occasionally a breast mass or tumor causes a "localized fullness" that can be seen. The breasts are visualized both with the arms at the patient's sides and with the arms extended over her head. Skin dimpling is accentuated with the arms extended over the patient's head. Palpation is carried out with the patient in the sitting position with arms at her sides and also with her arms fully extended above her head. Palpation is done with the flat of the fingers in each of the four breast quadrants. Also with the patient in the sitting position, the axillae and supraclavicular areas are examined by palpation. The patient is then placed in the supine position, and one arm is extended above her head. The breast on that side is then examined. Sometimes the patient is rotated so that the breast falls medially to facilitate lateral palpation. After both breasts are examined carefully, the nipple and subareolar tissue is examined by gentle, single-finger palpation.

The exact location of a breast mass or breast thickening should be noted in the patient's record. Often it is impossible to distinguish a definite mass from a thickening, or fibrocystic area. A mass generally has an "edging effect." A fibrocystic area can be described as a "localized hard or firm area." Fibrocystic areas typically occur over a larger segment of breast tissue. The physician who is not certain should note "questionable mass." Four descriptive terms can be used to describe physical findings: definite mass, breast cyst, questionable mass, and fibrocystic area. A physician who records feeling a definite mass is "obligated" to rule out cancer by mammography, fine-needle aspiration, or surgical consultation. Likewise, a designation of breast cyst must be proved by ultrasonography or a cyst aspiration procedure.

The accuracy of palpation to evaluate a breast mass is limited. Cysts cannot be distinguished reliably from solid masses. One study found that physical examination correctly identified only 58% of 66 palpable cysts (8). A study by Boyd et al. (9) showed a significant lack of agreement between experienced surgeons about physical findings. Four surgeons independently agreed on the need for a biopsy of only 73% of 15 women subsequently proved to have had a malignant breast mass. If a breast cancer is larger than 2.0 cm, its chance of being identified by palpation is probably 85%; however, less than half of cancers smaller than 1.0 cm in size can be identified by breast palpation.

Mammography

Mammography is the single most important noninvasive diagnostic test in breast assessment. Its accuracy in detecting early breast cancer is clearly recognized. Several large screening studies have shown that mammography alone can detect 40% of all cancers picked up by a combined physical examination and mammography screening technology. When data from the studies of the American Cancer Society Breast Cancer Detection Demonstration Project (10) were

analyzed for detection of early or minimal breast cancers (less than 1 cm in diameter), mammography's record was outstanding. Of 1153 minimal cancers detected in this project, 656 (or 57%) were detected by mammography alone; only 6% were detected by physical examination alone.

All women over the age of 35 with a breast complaint or a breast mass should have a diagnostic mammogram. Failure to obtain a mammogram at the time of initial breast evaluation for a breast complaint has resulted in several malpractice suits in cases in which a breast cancer occurred at a later date.

Currently, both appropriate breast palpation and high-quality mammography are required to properly assess a breast complaint. There are a few exceptions to this rule. In women under 35 (certainly under 30) there is concern about the hazard of breast irradiation from a mammogram. Furthermore, mammography in women under 30 is not very accurate. Likewise, mammography in a pregnant woman is generally avoided to protect the fetus, and again, the accuracy of mammography in breasts of pregnant women is low. Mammography is safe in breasts of lactating women, but the diagnostic results are highly inaccurate.

Concern over the hazard of inducing breast cancer by radiation from mammography has been generally overemphasized. Extensive analysis, using data from three large series of studies on breast irradiation, has shown that relatively low doses of radiation (10 to 25 rad) do slightly increase the risk of breast cancer. All the data suggest that there is a linear dose response to x-ray and that any exposure could be harmful in some women. These studies have also shown that breast tissue of adolescents and women under age 25 is much more sensitive to cancer inducement by radiation than is the breast tissue of women age 40 or older. With current technology, the likelihood that a woman over age 35 will develop a radiation-induced breast cancer is extremely small. Radiation scientists have calculated that a one-rad exposure of the breast could add six or seven excess breast cancers to the 2000 that occur per million women each year.

Over the past 10 years, several studies on the accuracy of mammography have been carried out. In general, an 85% accuracy can be achieved in most large teaching centers. Three studies from very high-volume cancer centers have achieved 90% accuracy or better. Community-based hospitals should achieve an accuracy rate of approximately 80%. A study of 1385 cases of breast cancer found that mammograms were erroneously interpreted as benign in 8.2% of cases; when they were interpreted as showing cancer, the error rate was 16.1% (11). This same study reported that when both palpation and mammography suggested a mass was benign, the error rate was 3.7%, and when both suggested that it was cancerous, the error rate was 3.6%.

In younger women, mammography is less accurate. Several studies have shown that accuracy falls to 60% to 70% in women age 35 to 50. In a series at Georgetown University

Hospital, we achieved an overall accuracy of 87%, but when we studied 24 women under 50 who had breast cancer, our accuracy fell to 71% (W. F. Feller and O. J. Cigtay, unpublished data). Kalisher analyzed 52 women who had false-negative mammograms and showed that 50% fell into the unvisualized category—those having dense breasts or tumors outside the field (12). He concluded that the small, dense breast characteristic of the young nullipara was the most difficult to evaluate radiologically.

In general, mammography is a highly accurate diagnostic tool, particularly in women over 50. However, a negative mammogram should not be used to rule out breast cancer. Be particularly cautious about interpreting the results of mammography in women under age 50 and in those with radiologically dense breasts. Mammography should probably not be used in women under age 30 or in pregnant women. Rather, consider other imaging modalities.

Other imaging modalities

Ultrasonography is not sensitive in detecting breast cancer. Ultrasonography is widely used to differentiate breast cysts from solid tumors and for this purpose is generally considered very accurate. Breast thermography is not clinically useful because of a low sensitivity in detecting early cancers. Diaphonography (concentrated visible light) is not helpful, as it does not detect deeper-lying tumors. Magnetic resonance imaging of the breast is still in a research phase of development.

Mammographic screening of asymptomatic women

For several years, the American Cancer Society and the American College of Radiology have recommended screening mammograms in asymptomatic women beginning at age 40 (Table 10-3). These guidelines suggest a screening mammogram every one or two years between the ages of 40 and 50, and a yearly mammogram over age 50. Women of higher breast cancer risk status may have yearly mammograms beginning at age 40. All health organizations that have reviewed the subject of the value of screening mammograms for women over 50 agree that mammography for older women is definitely beneficial in terms of saving lives.

Table 10-3 American Cancer Society mammography guidelines for asymptomatic women

Age	Recommendation
40	Baseline mammogram
40–49	Mammogram every year or two
50 and over	Mammogram every year

Guidelines as of February 1993.

Recently, there has been controversy on the value of screening mammograms to reduce breast cancer mortality in women under age 50. A large Canadian study reported in late 1992 that women under age 50 do not benefit, as shown by a lower breast cancer mortality from yearly mammographic screening (13). In February 1993, the American Cancer Society reviewed several studies that had examined this question and concluded that the present guidelines for mammographic screening of women between the ages of 40 and 49 should stand. It cited three large studies that showed a mortality benefit from mammographic screening for younger women.

Invasive diagnostic tests

Breast cyst aspiration

About 20% of solitary breast lumps in patients between ages 25 and 50 are cysts; thus a properly done needle aspiration can achieve a diagnostic accuracy of 99%. Any solitary breast tumor that is round, soft, and movable in surrounding tissue is probably a cyst, and aspiration should be attempted. Explain to the patient that aspiration is a diagnostic test and a biopsy need not be done if fluid is obtained.

Aspirate the cyst with a No. 22 needle and 10-ml disposable syringe. Very small (1-cm) cysts can be aspirated with a No. 23 or No. 25 needle. Manipulating the needle into a small cyst is much easier without the syringe attached. Once the fluid is withdrawn, the tumor should disappear. Most often the fluid is clear; the color may be green, brown, or yellow. Most surgeons do not send clear fluid for cytology. Ciatto et al. (14) found no malignant cells in specimens from 6747 cysts with nonbloody fluids. If the fluid is turbid, opaque, or bloody, it should be sent for study. Blood cyst fluid always raises the suspicion of an intracystic type of carcinoma, although this kind of malignant lesion is rare. Most often, the bloody fluid contains no cancer cells, and the blood results from injury to a vessel by the aspirating needle.

After needle aspiration, apply firm pressure over the needle hole to prevent bleeding. Subcutaneous or internal bleeding severe enough to cause ecchymosis is rare, but does occur. Although bruising or ecchymosis is distressing to the patient, it usually requires only reassurance. Less than 20% of simple cysts will refill.

Most solitary breast lumps should be aspirated for fluid. Fluid should be clear or nonbloody, and the tumor mass should disappear completely following aspiration. Bloody fluid, incomplete disappearance of the mass, or failure to obtain fluid mandate further study and probably open breast biopsy.

Fine-needle aspiration biopsy

Fine-needle aspiration (FNA) biopsy of a solid breast tumor is finding increasing acceptance in the surgical world;

however, most gynecologists do not feel comfortable in carrying out this procedure and refer patients to a general surgeon or cytopathologist for this diagnostic test. It has been practiced in Sweden since 1968 and is very popular in Britain. It removes cells from a breast tumor via a No. 20 or No. 22 needle and fairly strong vacuum pressure. The vacuum is achieved with a glass syringe and a special holder or, often, an ordinary plastic syringe. The cells removed are put on a glass slide and viewed by an experienced cytopathologist. The technique is simple to perform, and there are almost no complications. The major problem is reliability; the needle may miss the tumor, or the cytopathologist may misinterpret the specimen. In highly experienced hands, overall accuracies of 99% have been attained. False-positive results are below 2%. All studies show that it is critical to have highly experienced surgical pathologists interpreting the aspirates.

Several studies have compared the accuracy of combining physical examination, mammography, and FNA cytology as a triple approach to evaluation of a breast mass. The combination of physical examination, mammography, and FNA is highly accurate when all the tests give the same results. In a large review study by Layfield et al. (11), cancer was found in only 3 of 457 cases (0.7%) in which all three evaluations indicated that a mass was benign. Many reports have shown no false-positive errors. Women with inadequate aspirates should have an open biopsy. In one study, 17% of the inadequate aspirates (few or no cells) were malignant. One report (15) indicated that a negative FNA result in very expert hands can be used to defer open biopsy. Patients in this study followed for 3 years showed a 1.9% false-negative rate. In the present malpractice climate, many surgeons would not accept this very low risk.

Open breast biopsy

An open breast biopsy carried out by a trained surgeon is the definitive diagnostic step in a breast workup. In competent hands it has achieved 100% accuracy. Before 1975, a one-step, biopsy-mastectomy procedure, based on a positive frozen section, was the standard approach. The main drawback to this routine was the immense psychological stress on all patients undergoing biopsy. Most surgeons now use a two-step approach: an outpatient open breast biopsy under local anesthesia and a definitive surgical procedure (i.e., mastectomy or tumor excision and axillary dissection) under general anesthesia one to two weeks after a positive breast biopsy. With this approach the patient with a positive cancer diagnosis has a week or two to discuss treatment options with her surgeon or primary physician. She may also seek a second opinion.

Indications

There are two main indications for an open breast biopsy: a definite or questionable mass in women over 25 unless ul-

trasonography or needle aspiration has clearly shown that the mass is a cyst, and an abnormal mammographic finding when no mass can be palpated. This would include abnormal radiographic densities and small clustered areas of microcalcification.

Pathology

The pathologic findings following a breast biopsy include benign fibrocystic disease, fibroadenoma, cancer, cyst, and lipoma. The most common breast pathology is fibrocystic disease, which is found in about 50% to 60% of biopsy specimens. About 10% to 20% of biopsy specimens yield cancer, depending on the age of the patient and the indication. Age is a major determinant of pathology. Less than 5% of biopsy specimens from those under age 35 reveal cancer, whereas close to 75% of biopsy specimens from those over age 70 show malignancy. About 25% to 30% of women biopsied for a mammographic microcalcification cluster yield a diagnosis of cancer.

Once breast palpation reveals a solitary mass, the physician must rule out carcinoma. Several nonsurgical diagnostic tests are available, and most of these have relatively high diagnostic accuracies. However, an open breast biopsy is 100% accurate and should probably be used as a diagnostic step in women over age 25 with a breast mass unless other tests show the mass is a cyst.

Treatment of breast cancer

The diagnosis of a primary or localized breast cancer requires surgical treatment. The extent of the local surgery is controversial, but two alternative surgical approaches are widely accepted for most early breast cancers: either modified radical mastectomy or tumor excision, breast irradiation, and axillary dissection. Preoperatively the extent of the disease—staging—is determined. In addition to breast and axillary palpation, a chest x-ray, mammogram, and bone scan are obtained. A patient with locally advanced disease or metastatic breast cancer requires combined treatment modalities (i.e., chemotherapy, breast irradiation, and limited surgery).

Discussion of treatment alternatives with the patient

After a definite biopsy-proved diagnosis of stage I or II breast cancer is made, treatment alternatives are discussed with the patient. Women with large primary tumors (greater than 4 cm) or multiple primary cancers in the same breast, and those whose cancer contains extensive intraductal disease, are advised that the results of a breast-conserving operation may not be as good as those of a mastectomy. Women with small, early, single-focus lesions (2 to 3 cm) with minimal intraductal components are ideal candidates for local excision and breast irradiation. Some surgeons may express a personal preference for mastectomy, but most will discuss the treatment alternatives fairly with the patient and explain that the clinical results of the two alternatives are equal. Breast irradiation should be carried out at a medical center by a radiation therapist skilled in this type of procedure. There is some concern about the long-term effects of intensive irradiation to the breast and chest wall, which may occur after 15 or 20 years. Some reports have suggested that complications, such as breast fibrosis, skin changes, fractured ribs, local pleuritis, or local pericarditis, may occur at a later date. However, such problems are uncommon if the irradiation is carried out by an experienced radiation physician.

Surgical strategies

Local tumor excision and axillary dissection

Tumor excision and axillary dissection are carried out under general anesthesia. Many surgeons routinely reexcise the biopsy site unless there is direct or first-hand knowledge that all of the gross tumor was removed at the time of the diagnostic biopsy. Extensive surgical excision of healthy breast tissue is usually avoided because it produces poor cosmetic results. The axillary dissection is usually done through a separate oblique or transverse incision low in the axillae. The extent of the axillary dissection is controversial. Most surgeons remove all the axillary lymph nodes in level I and II of the axillae. This includes dissection of the axillary contents extending from the tail of the breast inferiorly, the latissimus dorsi muscle laterally, and the axillary vein superiorly, and generally involves removing the axillary tissue beneath the pectoralis minor. This limited technique avoids dissecting level III or the high axillary area. High or total axillary dissection produces more significant arm disabilities and, if not properly done, can damage the blood supply or innervation to the pectoralis major muscle. Debilitating arm edema is rare with limited axillary dissection.

Modified radical mastectomy

The surgical strategy for a modified radical mastectomy is well known. In many centers, an immediate breast reconstruction is performed at the time of the mastectomy using a two-team approach. In this procedure, a general surgeon performs a standard modified radical mastectomy, and a plastic surgeon performs a breast reconstructive procedure.

Before 1991, most plastic surgeons used a silicone gel implant as a prosthetic device in breast reconstructive procedures. When it was used by experienced plastic surgeons, the cosmetic results were very good. In July 1991, the Food and Drug Administration raised concerns about the long-term safety of silicone gel implants, and in 1992 it removed silicone implants from the market except for breast reconstructive procedures following mastectomy for cancer. The safety concern grew out of several anecdotal reports of se-

rious autoimmune disease such as scleroderma in women whose implants leaked silicone gel into the surrounding breast tissue. It is now believed that 5% of implants will leak over a period of 5 years. Magnetic resonance imaging can depict the normal morphologic features of silicone gel breast implants and is probably the best imaging method to detect leakage. The actual number of women who may have adverse effects from the silicone gel implants appears likely to be very small (i.e., one in 500). The saline-filled breast implants appear to be safer than those filled with silicone gel and may be an acceptable alternative. To avoid plastic prosthesis implants altogether, some plastic surgeons are using autologous tissue from the abdomen. The transabdominal myocutaneous (TRAM) flap using the rectus abdominis muscle is gaining in popularity as a breast reconstructive procedure. Cosmetic results of TRAM flaps are generally excellent.

Nonsurgical therapy

Breast irradiation

For women who have chosen a breast-conserving option, breast irradiation is usually started one to two weeks after tumor excision and axillary dissection. It is given to the breast and chest wall in a tangential manner over 5 weeks. The total x-ray dose is between 5000 and 6000 rad. Some centers use a supplemental boost of x-ray to the biopsy site by an external electron beam or an interstitial iridium implant, which is left in place for 2 days. If the axilla has been surgically dissected, it is generally not irradiated. It is believed that both axillary surgery and axillary irradiation are not necessary for cancer control and that the two treatment modalities applied to the axilla can cause significant arm edema in many women. The immediate side effects of breast irradiation are minimal.

Adjuvant chemotherapy

In general, it is standard practice to use adjuvant chemotherapy in women with positive axillary lymph nodes. All node-positive premenopausal women should receive chemotherapy. Tamoxifen treatment may be added after chemotherapy for women with estrogen-receptor (ER) positive cancers. For postmenopausal women with such tumors, tamoxifen is the accepted treatment. Some data suggest additional benefit from chemotherapy. For postmenopausal women with ER negative tumors, adjuvant chemotherapy is strongly recommended.

It is likely that 50% of women with node-negative breast cancer will benefit from systemic adjuvant therapy. Although some medical oncologists recommend adjuvant chemotherapy for almost all node-negative women, most oncologists use adjuvant therapy in a subset of women with poor prognosis. The most reliable prognostic factors for selecting women for adjuvant therapy appear to be tumor size, histologic grade, and estrogen receptor status. Node-negative women with tumors larger than 2.0 cm, or of poor histologic grade (grade III), or with a negative estrogen receptor status should probably receive adjuvant chemotherapy.

Breast cancer treatment results

A study by Bloom and coworkers (16) of old hospital records in England showed that women with untreated breast cancer and coworkers had a 5-year survival of 18% and a 10-year survival of 3.6% Currently, more than 80% of stage I breast cancer patients will be alive and free of disease 10 years after modern surgical treatment alone. In addition, 91% of women with stage I disease and tumors less than 1.0 cm in size will be disease-free after 10 years. Survival can be accurately predicted when the stage of the disease, the actual number of positive axillary lymph nodes, the tumor size, and the histologic grade are known at the time of diagnosis. The single best prognostic indicator of disease-free survival is the actual number of axillary nodes involved with cancer. A study by Carter and colleagues (17; Fig. 10-1) on the relation of tumor size, lymph node status, and survival also illustrates the impact of positive node number on survival. Figure 10-1A shows the 7-year survival of women with breast cancer divided into three axillary node groups. The 7-year survival of node-negative women is 90%, whereas women with four or more positive nodes have a survival rate of 43%. These figures are independent of tumor size.

Tumor size is the second best prognostic indicator of survival and also can be used independent of axillary node status to predict survival. Again from the Carter study, Fig. 10-1B illustrates the prognostic value of tumor size. At 7

years, women whose tumors were less than 2 cm in diameter have a 90% survival rate while women whose tumors were larger than 5.0 cm have a survival rate of less than 50%. Histologic grade has also been shown to have a dramatic effect on prognosis, independent of stage or within any stage category. Two of the major prognostic factors, number of positive axillary lymph nodes and size of the tumor, are related to early diagnosis. If all women with breast cancer were diagnosed in the early stage of the disease with negative nodes and tumor size of 1.0 cm or less, the present overall 10-year mortality of 30% could be reduced to 10%.

Breast cancer in pregnancy

Breast cancer is the most likely cancer to be found during pregnancy. Delay in diagnosis is a serious problem with pregnant patients, who usually present with a more advanced stage than nonpregnant women. Ribeiro and associates. (18) reported that 89% of pregnant women who have breast cancer have positive axillary lymph nodes at the time of surgery. Any mass in the breast of a pregnant or lactating woman should be evaluated promptly. Mammography is generally ineffective owing to the increased density of the breast. Needle aspiration or open biopsy should be carried out for any persisting mass in the breast of a pregnant woman. In biopsy-proved cases, staging should be limited to routine chest x-rays that are done with proper abdominal and pelvic shielding. A modified mastectomy should be performed in all patients with stage I and II operable breast cancer. This procedure allows the pregnancy to continue normally with minimal risk to the mother or to the fetus. The use of breast conservation and irradiation as a primary treatment modality should be postponed until after delivery, because the dose of x-ray scattered to the fetus is unac-

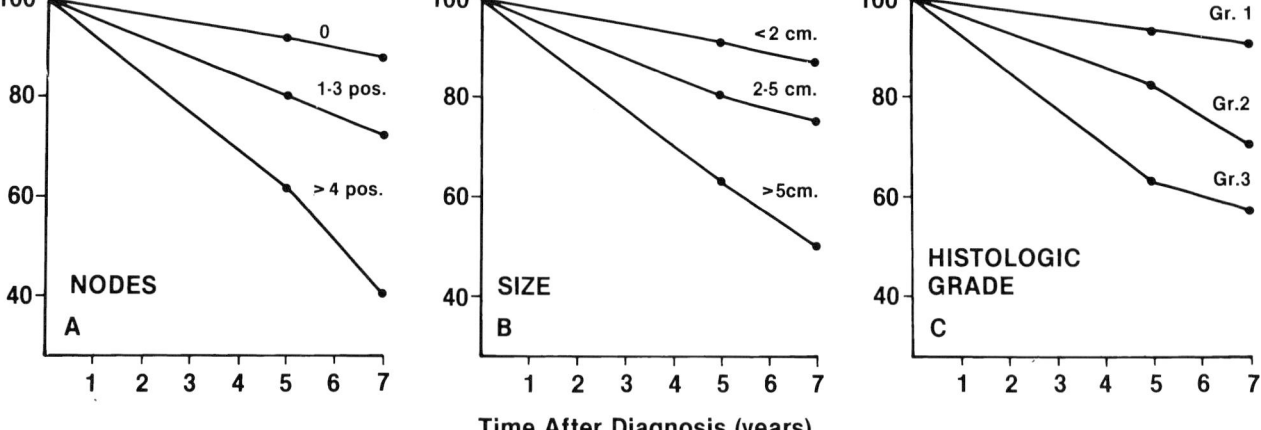

Fig. 10-1 Seven-year survival curves of breast cancer patients in three different prognostic groups. The curves represent the percentage of patients actually surviving at the specified times in years. (A) Patients separated according to the number of positive axillary nodes. (B) Patients separated according to tumor size. (C) Patients separated according to the histologic grade of the cancer. (Adapted with permission from Carter CL, Allen C, Henson DE. Relation of tumor size, lymph node status, and survival in 24,740 breast cancer cases. Cancer 1989;63:181–187.)

ceptably high. The use of any chemotherapeutic agent during the first trimester of pregnancy is not considered safe. Chemotherapy probably induces few, if any, abnormalities during the second or third trimester, and can be given if necessary. The drugs usually chosen are cyclophosphamide and doxorubicin. Pregnant patients who are diagnosed early with negative axillary lymph nodes have an expected outcome similar to that of nonpregnant women. For women of childbearing age who have had breast cancer, most surgeons recommend a delay of 3 years following mastectomy before childbearing is considered. This policy is not because a risk of recurrence is necessarily increased but because the use of chemotherapy, if a recurrence should occur, would complicate the pregnancy.

References

1 Cancer facts & figures—1993. Atlanta, American Cancer Society, 1993.

2 Breast cancer study. Pennington, NJ, Physicians Insurers Association of America, 1990.

3 Leis HP. Management of nipple discharge. World J Surg 1989;13:736–742.

4 Roberts L. Zeroing in on a breast cancer susceptibility gene. Science 1993;259:622–625.

5 Steinberg KK, Thacker SB, Smith SJ, et al. A meta-analysis of the effect of estrogen replacement therapy on the risk of breast cancer. JAMA 1991;265:1985–1990.

6 Dupont WD, Page DL. Menopausal estrogen replacement therapy and breast cancer. Arch Intern Med. 1991;151:67–72.

7 Dupont WD, Page DL. Risk factors for breast cancer in women with proliferative breast disease. N Engl J Med 1985;312:146–151.

8 Rosner D, Blaird D. What ultrasonography can tell in breast masses that mammography and physical examination cannot. J Surg Oncol 1985;28:308–313.

9 Boyd NF, Sutherland HJ, Fish EB, Hiraki GY, Lickley HLA, Maurer VE. Prospective evaluation of physician examination of the breast. Am J Surg 1981;142:331–334.

10 Seidman H, Gelb SK, Silverberg E, et al. Survival experience in the Breast Cancer Detection Demonstration Project. CA Cancer J Clin 1987;37:258–289.

11 Layfield LJ, Glasgow BJ, Cramer H. Fine-needle aspiration in the management of breast masses. Pathol Annu 1989;24:23–62.

12 Kalisher L. Factors influencing false negative rates in xeromammography. Radiology 1979;133:297.

13 Miller AB, Baines CJ, To T, Wall C. Canadian National Breast Screening Study. I. Breast cancer detection and death rates among women aged 40 to 49 years.

14 Ciatto S, Cariaggi P, Bulgaresi P. The value of routine cytologic examination of breast cyst fluids. Acta Cytol 1987;31:301–304.

15 Goodson WH, Mailmon R, Miller TR. Three year follow-up of benign fine-needle aspiration biopsies of the breast. Am J Surg 1987;154:58–64.

16 Bloom HJ, Richardson WW, Harres EJ. Natural history of untreated breast cancer (1803–1933): comparison of untreated and treated cases according to histological grade of malignancy. Br Med J 1962;213:5299.

17 Carter CL, Allen C, Henson DE. Relation of tumor size, lymph node status, and survival in 24,740 breast cancer cases. Cancer 1989;63:181–187.

18 Ribeiro G, Jones DA, Jones M. Carcinoma of the breast associated with pregnancy. Br J Surg. 1986;73:706–709.

Chapter 11

Stapling techniques for abdominal hysterectomy

Joseph A. Riggs and John C. Riggs

History

The use of metal staples in abdominal surgery (gastrectomies) was introduced in Budapest, Hungary, in 1908 as developed by Hültl (1). The Russians further pioneered the use of stapling devices during the 1950s (2). The use of metal staples in abdominal surgery began in the United States in the late 1960s, and over the next two decades use of various models of stapling instruments was reported by general, thoracic, and vascular surgeons. The use of metal staples in gynecology for closure of the vaginal cuff was first reported in 1968 by Kahn, who stressed speed, safety, and good hemostasis (3). A follow-up study by Albert in 1974 noted excellent healing with the use of metal staples (4). In 1987, Barter and Sanz suggested that surgery with staples was neater, faster, and more accurate than suturing in gynecologic surgery (5). Finally, in 1990, Riggs noted that absorbable staples offer many advantages for patients, surgeons, and operating room personnel (6).

Over the years, metal stapling procedures for intra-abdominal use became obsolete for various reasons. Some possible disadvantages were noted after unusual complications following an abdominal hysterectomy (7). Two significant problems with metal stapling procedures were realized at that time. First, the metal instruments were difficult to assemble and clean and were cumbersome to use because they contained many parts. Second, the use of stainless steel staples produced dyspareunia and urinary urgency in 6% of patients (8,9). Consequently, most gynecologists became reluctant to place permanent stainless steel staples near the vaginal cuff, fearing migration, extrusion, urinary problems, and dyspareunia.

In 1984, Beresford (9) reported on the use of absorbable stapling techniques in abdominal hysterectomy. The development of an absorbable staple, the Polysorb 55, made the techniques suitable not only for vaginal cuff closure but also for adnexal surgery. The Polysorb 55 absorbable staple combined all the benefits of surgical stapling: minimal inflammation during healing, reduced tissue trauma, decreased blood loss, and reduced operative time. These features were combined with the advantages of the staples being absorbable, radiolucent, and easy to apply. Thus, the postoperative disadvantages of metal staples were virtually eliminated.

Introduced in 1984, Polysorb absorbable staples opened up a whole new world of gynecologic stapling applications. Modern internal staplers rely on the principle of placing B-shaped staples of titanium or absorbable polymer material in double staggered rows. The B-shaped staple allows micro vessels to pass through, ensuring tissue viability. The staples are 4.4 mm in width and fit exactly into a retainer plate that measures 6.6 mm. Once locked into the retainer plate, the staples cannot come apart until absorption takes place (Fig. 11-1).

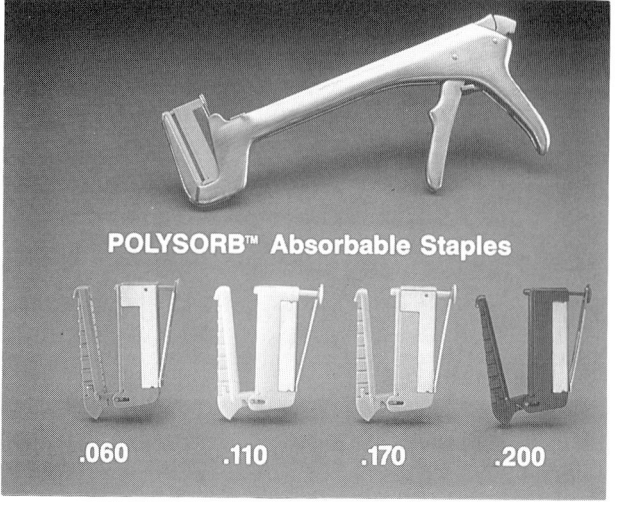

Fig. 11-1 Polysorb 55 absorbable staples.

Polysorb absorbable staples

Polysorb 55 absorbable staples are made of a lactomer absorbable copolymer, a blend of polyglactic and polyglycolic acid similar to the polyglycolic suture material currently used to made absorbable sutures (Fig. 11-2). The staples maintain tensile strength during the critical first few postoperative weeks. Thereafter, they begin to crumble and absorb rapidly. The staples are completely absorbed by 6 to 8 weeks postoperatively; breakdown time of the staples can vary from patient to patient. The advantages of total absorption and radiotransparency make Polysorb 55 the material of choice when staples are used in abdominal hysterectomy.

Instruments

All staple sizes are available in colored cartridges that can be loaded into a reusable stapling instrument. There are several different types of stapling instruments that can be used during abdominal hysterectomy. The thoracoabdominal (TA) Premium 55 instrument is a one piece stainless steel unibody applicator that is easy to clean and handle by operating room personnel (Fig. 11-3). When the adnexa are being preserved, the TA 55 instrument, using a 0.060 (aqua) cartridge, is used to staple ovarian and broad ligaments solely or combined with the round ligament. When the adnexa are being removed, the same cartridge can be used across the infundibulopelvic ligament. However, when the adnexal vessels are large and tortuous, it may be best to apply a TA 30 Premium (white) instrument, which contains a smaller cartridge that applies a triple layer of titanium permanent staples across the infundibulopelvic ligament.

The aqua cartridge with shorter absorbable staples is used for relatively thin tissue; it should not be used on the vaginal cuff, which contains thicker tissue. The aqua cartridge leaves a row of absorbable staples across the adnexal tissues on the patient's side, necessitating cutting the proximal edge with a knife or electrocautery.

A recently developed device, the Polysorb 75 (Fig. 11-4), can be used on the adnexa whether or not ovarian preservation is desired. The Polysorb 75 places two rows of absorbable staples on each side and divides the staples up the middle with a blade at the same time. This instrument is faster because it places staples on the patient and specimen sides of the adnexa, thus eliminating the need for clamps to control backbleeding.

For the vaginal cuff, either one of two instruments may be used. The TA Premium 55 instrument is the nondisposable applicator with no removable parts. It accommodates either one of two cartridges for the vaginal cuff. The 0.170 (light brown) cartridge contains shorter staples to be used in postmenopausal women who have a thinner atrophic vagina. The 0.200 (dark brown) cartridge has longer staples and is used in younger patients who possess a thicker vaginal mucosa.

The 0.170 and 0.200 staples can be used in a modified TA instrument called a Roticulator 55 Poly stapler. The Roticulator 55 Poly stapler is very useful because it has an adjustable, flexible swivel head allowing for easier access to the vaginal cuff (Fig. 11-5). It is disposable and is used most often in patients with a deep pelvis in whom accessibility to the cuff is more difficult. Because it is easier to apply, the Roticulator 55 is also recommended for neophyte surgeons who are still learning how to use this new technology.

Technique

There has been significant development and use of staples in gynecology since 1984 with the introduction of polysorb absorbable staples (PAS). These staples can be applied for ligating and dividing the adnexa and vaginal cuff closure during abdominal hysterectomy. However, the technique

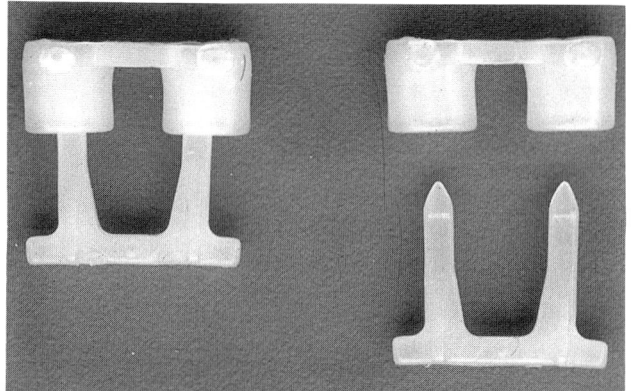

Fig. 11-2 Absorbable staples begin to break down after the first 2 postoperative weeks and are completely absorbed by 6 to 8 weeks.

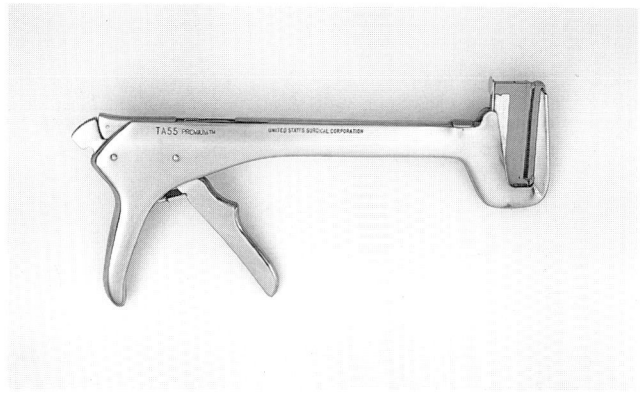

Fig. 11-3 The TA 55 Premium instrument can be used to staple the ovarian and round ligaments and the vaginal cuff.

of abdominal hysterectomy completed with the use of staples is not much different from that completed with sutures. After entrance into the abdominal cavity, an O'Sullivan-O'Connor retractor is placed. The lower retractor blade is used to displace the anterior peritoneum inferiorly. The upper blade is used to displace the bowel superiorly after approximately three lap pads are placed. The uterus is then grasped with a double-toothed tenaculum. A decision is made either to leave or to remove the ovaries. Large Kelly clamps are used to grasp bilaterally the utero-ovarian ligament, round ligament, and fallopian tubes adjacent to the uterus. The bladder flap is then sharply dissected from the midline to the proximal one-third of the round ligaments on each side. It is important to push the bladder flap downward to approximately 2 cm below the cervical-vaginal junction anteriorly. This will allow for later placement of an absorbable stapler across the vaginal cuff.

Lateral to the fundus and just below the round ligament, the surgeon's index finger dissects through the avascular space of the broad ligament, just above and away from the uterine vessels. This opening accommodates placement of the retaining pin of the stapling instrument. A large Kelly clamp is placed adjacent to the fundus to control reverse bleeding from the specimen.

If the ovaries are to be preserved, a 0.060 (aqua) cartridge is applied anteriorly over the utero-ovarian ligament, fallopian tube, and round ligament by placing the distal end of the stapler through the "window" in the broad ligament (Color Plate 1). After the stapler is set in the appropriate position, with the retaining pin fitting into the anvil, the cartridge is closed, the safety is locked, and the instrument is fired. The safety is then reset. The tissue is cut with a scalpel immediately adjacent to the cartridge. Any tissue that extends past the cartridge is electrocoagulated. Lateral to the stapler, the round ligament is grasped with a small Kelly clamp so that the pedicle can be held after stapling is completed. The cartridge is released, and the TA 55 Premium instrument is removed. The pedicle is held up by the small

Kelly clamp, allowing for careful inspection of the edges of the pedicle along the staple line. If necessary, electrocoagulation is used to cauterize any minor oozing along the staple line. The divided utero-ovarian tissue is nicely sealed with a double row of staples. There is little or no tissue distal to the staple line and no bunching up of adnexal pedicles (Color Plate 2). The small Kelly clamp is released, allowing the pedicle to lie flat along the lateral pelvic wall.

If the adnexa, including tubes and ovaries, are to be removed, a Babcock clamp is used to hold these organs medially. The same cartridge can be placed across the infundibulopelvic ligament and the round ligament, with care to avoid proximity to the ureter, which has been previously identified as lying more lateral and inferior to the application. The cartridge is closed, and the safety is released. The instrument is fired using the same technique as described above.

The tissues adjacent to the uterine vessels are skeletonized, and minor bleeders may be coagulated or suture ligated, or Polysurgiclips may be applied. Again, the ureter is identified before the uterine vessels are clamped with a Heaney clamp. The uterine vessels are cut and doubly ligated using absorbable sutures.

The cardinal and uterosacral ligaments are suture ligated close to the cervix. At this point, it is often beneficial to take an extra bite of tissue on each side of the vaginal cuff, taking care not to enter the vagina. This allows for easier application of the stapler to the vaginal cuff. The bladder flap must be approximately 2 cm below the anterior cervicovaginal junction prior to placement of the PAS. The cervix and vagina are now adequately prepared for application of the stapler (Color Plate 3).

A single-toothed tenaculum is used to grasp the middle portion of the cervix anteriorly, while keeping traction on the cervix during stapler application. Either the TA 55 Premium reusable instrument or the disposable Roticulator 55 Poly stapler is placed across the vaginal cuff below the cervix at the vaginal junction. Either instrument allows for placement of the 0.170 (light brown) cartridge for a thin postmenopausal vaginal cuff or a 0.200 (dark brown) car-

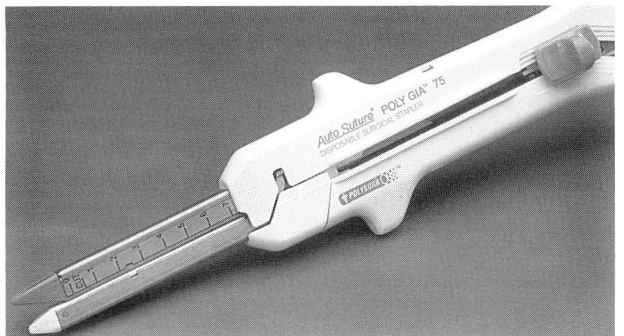

Fig. 11-4 The Polysorb 75 instrument places two rows of absorbable staples on each side and divides the staples with a blade up the middle.

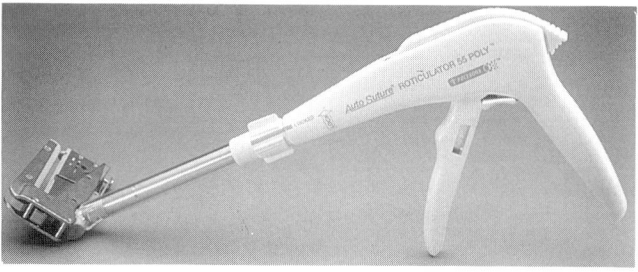

Fig. 11-5 The Roticulator 55 Poly is a disposable stapler with an adjustable swivel head for use in patients with a deep pelvis.

tridge for a thicker premenopausal cuff. The Roticulator, with a rotating swivel head, is often used in a deep pelvis because this allows for better visualization and easier placement. Care must be taken to avoid the previously sutured pedicles, the bladder, and the bowel before closing the cartridge. The stapling instrument is held with one hand, and the index and middle fingers of the opposite hand are placed behind the cervix to guide the head of the instrument posteriorly. With this method, the wide open cartridge will easily slip into place. Again, the retaining pin must be set into the anvil as the cartridge is closed (Color Plate 4). The safety is unlocked, and the instrument is fired. A scalpel on a long handle is used to cut adjacent to the cartridge as the entire specimen is removed (Color Plate 5). The cartridge is opened, and the instrument is removed. On rare occasions electrocoagulation or a small suture is used to control oozing and remove any excess tissue along the staple line.

A double row of Polysorb absorbable staples closes the vaginal vault uniformly and hemostaticly without crushing the vaginal mucosa (Color Plate 6). There is virtually no blood loss or spillage of vaginal fluid into the peritoneal cavity. This may prevent contamination from vaginal organisms because entrance into the vagina does not occur. This could possibly lead to less pelvic infection in the postoperative period. However, if drainage of the pelvis is desired, a T-tube or vacuum drain may be inserted easily through a stab wound in the posterior vaginal wall just below the staple line. The uterine specimen, as sent to pathology, shows a minimal rim of vaginal tissue around the cervix. This preserves as much vaginal tissue as possible while causing no shortening of the vagina.

The pelvis is irrigated with 200 cc of sterile water to check for any mild bleeding. If necessary, electrocoagulation, a Polysurgiclip, or sutures may be applied as indicated. Closure of the retroperitoneal space is not necessary as there is little chance for adhesions along the fine, flat hemostatic pedicles. After removal of the retractors and lap pads, the anterior peritoneum is closed inferiorly to superiorly in normal fashion. The fascia is closed from each lateral edge with a running suture to the midline. The skin is approximated with metal skin staples, a subcuticular

stitch, or the newly introduced stapler using absorbable skin staples.

Discussion

The problems of staple migration from the vaginal cuff, causing urinary discomfort and dyspareunia after the use of metal staples, have been alleviated by the use of absorbable staples. Beresford's success with Polysorb absorbable staples through the 1980s changed the general attitude of gynecologists and allowed for an alternative method for abdominal hysterectomy (9). Currently, gynecologists, after proper training, use Polysorb absorbable staples as an appropriate standard of care.

Over the past decade, many studies have compared Polysorb absorbable staples with traditional suturing techniques, relating advantages and disadvantages for abdominal hysterectomy. In 1982 in France, Brun and associates compared 170 patients in whom Polysorb absorbable staples were used for vaginal cuff closure with 231 patients in whom polyglycolic absorbable sutures were used during abdominal hysterectomy. They found a reduction in hospital stay, lack of granulation tissue, and a lower infection rate in the absorbable staple group (10). Other studies have reported a reduction in operating time of 14 to 30 minutes (11,12). Riggs, in 1990 (6), compared over a 3-year period of time a group of patients undergoing total abdominal hysterectomy in whom an interrupted absorbable sutured cuff closure was used with a similar group of patients in whom an absorbable staple cuff closure was used. The most important difference noted in the stapled group 6 weeks postoperatively was a significant decrease of granulation tissue in the majority of patients. Nearly half of the patients in the suture group had a slight to moderate degree of granulation tissue, whereas only 11% in the stapled group exhibited only minimal granulation tissue. In most cases, healing in stapled patients was complete at the time of the 6-week postoperative examination, with only a fine line present across the vaginal apex (Color Plate 7).

Advantages

There are many advantages with the use of absorbable staples in abdominal hysterectomy (Table 11-1). When Polysorb absorbable staples are applied to the adnexa, the advantages include flat, unbundled pedicles, possibly leading to little or no tissue necrosis and no need for reperitonealization.

There are many advantages when absorbable staples are applied to the vaginal cuff. Closure is easier, and there is much less tissue manipulation, traction, and trauma. There is less or no blood loss with absorbable staples. Tissue strangulation and bunching are eliminated. Closure of the vaginal cuff is achieved before resection of the uterus, reducing

Table 11-1 Advantages of Polysorb absorbable sutures

Advantages for adnexa

Flat, unbunched pedicles

Little or no tissue necrosis

Peritonealization not needed

Simple to apply

Advantages for vaginal cuff

Better healing

Easier to close

Less blood loss

Less contamination

Less granulation tissue

Quicker to close (< one minute)

the potential for contamination of the peritoneal cavity and possibly leading to less postoperative infection and cuff induration (11). Once the procedure has been mastered, up to 15 minutes of operating time can be saved (12,13).

Contraindications and complications

Polysorb absorbable staples should not be used on tissue that is too thick or too thin for the staple size. This rarely occurs in the adnexal area but occasionally may occur in the vaginal cuff area in a multiparous patient with a very thick cervix. Likewise, the absorbable staples should not be placed over an existing line of stainless steel staples and vice versa. In either case, the staples may not close or approximate the tissue edges properly.

If staples are used with care, complications are rare. However, possible complications that theoretically can occur with the use of stapling devices include ureteral obstruction, bladder fistulas, bowel trauma, and pelvic abscess. Whether or not complications occur may depend on the experience of the operating surgeon. For the neophyte, practice on experimental animals or tissues is encouraged. It is recommended that the beginner operate with a surgeon well experienced in the use of absorbable staples until a level of comfort is obtained with this technology.

Summary

Standard basics have to be followed with stapling techniques just as they are with any surgical procedure. Knowledge of anatomy, vascular supply, and tissue approximation is always essential. Applying the stapling instruments properly will minimize tissue trauma, and it is understood that good surgical judgment is necessary at all times. For difficult

situations, such as those presented by a deep, narrow pelvis, multiple adhesions, extensive endometriosis, large pelvic masses, or widespread malignancy, Polysorb absorbable staples may not be applicable.

The TA 30 Premium permanent nonabsorbable staples are marketed for use on the infundibulopelvic ligament, especially with large, tortuous adnexal vessels. Although the Polysorb absorbable staples are not recommended by the manufacturer for placement across the infundibulopelvic ligament, they can be placed safely with or without the round ligament, using the 0.060 (aqua) cartridge, without difficulty and with good hemostasis (6).

Greater costs associated with the use of Polysorb absorbable staples were anticipated. However, it has been shown (6) that the increased cost of absorbable staples compared with sutures can readily be counterbalanced by the savings allowed by the shorter operating room time and fewer anesthesia units required. Moreover, there is no doubt that the patient benefits considerably by having a shorter operation and receiving less anesthesia.

When staples were first used in gynecology, they were made of stainless steel, and occasional migration and extrusion caused patient discomfort and dyspareunia. Thus, most gynecologists felt reluctant to place steel staples in the vaginal cuff for a hysterectomy, and the procedure did not gain popularity. Since their introduction in 1984, the use of Polysorb absorbable staples has been found to be as safe, accurate, and reliable as the conventional suture method. In the majority of cases, they can add neatness, precision, speed, and superior healing to the adnexal and vaginal cuff areas. No studies have shown that traditional suturing techniques provide better results than stapling devices. Further data and more long-term follow-up are needed to confirm these impressions. Recent experience with the Polysorb absorbable staples has been encouraging, and it is recommended that these techniques be used more extensively in gynecologic teaching programs and in private practice in appropriate cases.

References

1 Hültl H. Il Kongress der Ungareschen Geseheschaft fur Chirurgie, Budapest, May 1908. Pester Med Cin Presse 1909;45:108–110, 121–122.

2 Babkin SE, Astofev GV, Kolimina TV. Contemporary equipment for operation on the intestines. New surgical apparatus and instruments and experience in their use. Moscow: Ministry of Health USSR, 1957.

3 Kahn E. Auto suture in abdominal hysterectomy. Obstet Gynecol 1868;31:852–854.

4 Albert RO. Use of automatic staplers in vaginal hysterectomy, etc. Tex Med J 1974;70:66–76.

5 Barter J, Sanz L. Staplers for gyn surgery—what's available? Contemp Obstet Gynecol 1987;87–97.

6 Riggs J. Absorbable stapler value after hysterectomy. Contemp Obstet Gynecol 1990;105–120.

7 Zerner J, Miller B, Nelson B. Unusual complications following abdominal hysterectomy, etc. J Me Med Assoc 1980;71:169–170.
8 Messitt J. Dyspareunia from auto staples. Obstet Gynecol
   1977;49:369–370.
9 Beresford J. Automatic stapler techniques in abdominal hysterectomy. Surg Clin North Am 1984;64:609–617.
10 Brun G, Spaultz F, Girard P, et al. Mechanical vaginal sutures after
   hysterectomy. Rev Fr Gynecol Obstet 1982;77:773–776.

11 Buka N. Absorbable staples in abdominal hysterectomy.
   1988;166:175–176.
12 McTammany JR. Vaginal cuff closure during abdominal hysterectomy using absorbable staples. Berk's County Med Rec 1986;
   77:35–36.
13 Beresford J. Using automatic staplers in gyn surgery. Contemp Obstet Gynecol 1987;147–153.

Chapter 12

Anesthesia for gynecologic procedures

Young K. Shin

Gynecologic procedures such as pelvic examination may be simple and brief. On the other hand, radical pelvic surgery may require invasive monitoring and careful fluid management for optimal care. Women undergoing such surgical procedures may be elderly and may have concurrent systemic disease. Thereby, the anesthetic management of women undergoing gynecologic surgical procedures should not differ from that of general surgical patients.

This chapter attempts to focus on new developments in the anesthesia field such as comprehensive preanesthetic evaluation, improved intraoperative monitoring techniques, new anesthetics and muscle relaxants, and new techniques of postoperative pain management, as well as anesthetic considerations in specific gynecologic procedures, especially for physicians untrained in anesthesia.

Preanesthetic evaluation and preparation

The main objective of preoperative evaluation and preparation is to maximize the patient's physical status for the surgical procedure; therefore, it is to reduce intraoperative complications and postoperative morbidity. It is also to acquaint a patient with anesthetic procedures and to dispel misconceptions or fear about the anesthesia.

An increasing number of patients are admitted to the hospital on their day of surgery. A preanesthetic evaluation by an anesthesiologist should be arranged before admission. The preanesthetic visit will focus on a review of previous anesthetic experiences, adverse effects of anesthetics, familial problems with anesthetics, concurrent systemic disease, and medication history. A patient with a history of familial malignant hyperthermia, for example, requires special preparation for anesthetic management. Upon physical examination, upper airway assessment is essential to predict difficult endotracheal intubation. A short thyromental distance and invisibility of the posterior pharyngeal wall may be predictors of difficult tracheal intubation (1).

Cardiovascular and pulmonary disease have been the two major risk factors in the perioperative period. The patient with hypertension, coronary artery disease, or chronic pulmonary disease may require preoperative medical consultation. The objective of the medical consultation is to determine whether the patient needs further therapeutic intervention to optimize cardiac and pulmonary functions, thereby minimizing development of intraoperative and postoperative complications. At an increased risk of cardiac mortality and morbidity in the perioperative period are patients older than 70 years of age, and those with a history of recent myocardial infarction, evidence of heart failure, aortic stenosis, and frequent atrial or ventricular arrhythmias (2). Patients with hypertension to diastolic pressure of 110 torr or higher may also have increased cardiac complications (3). Patients with a history of heavy smoking, obesity, or pulmonary disease, or over 70 years of age are candidates for preoperative evaluation of pulmonary function (4).

Antihypertensive medications such as methyldopa (Aldomet) or beta-blockers should continue until the time of surgery. Rebound hypertension can develop after discontinuation of clonidine (5). Monoamine oxidase inhibitors, however, may be discontinued 2 weeks before surgery because of the hemodynamic instability under anesthesia.

Another area deserving mention is discussion of blood transfusion. Because of risks of hepatitis and human immunodeficiency virus infection with banked blood, many patients are interested in autologous blood transfusion, which can be readily arranged by a hospital blood bank.

Choice of anesthesia

The decision about anesthetic techniques is based on surgical requirement, physical status of the patient, the patient's desire, and the anesthesiologist's skill.

Most gynecologic surgery is performed under general anesthesia; however, in patients with respiratory disease, avoidance of general anesthesia will reduce the associated respiratory depression. In patients with ischemic or congestive cardiac disease, less hemodynamic instability is noted with the use of regional anesthesia. Regional anesthesia (epidural or spinal) may also be preferred in patients with a full stomach or when difficult tracheal intubation is anticipated. However, regional anesthesia is contraindicated in patients with coagulopathy or on anticoagulants for fear of space-occupying hematoma in the epidural or subarachnoid space. Regional anesthesia may also be avoided in patients with a fixed cardiac output. Sympathetic blockade accompanying regional anesthesia can lead to hypotension and sudden cardiac decompensation in a patient with aortic stenosis.

Combined regional anesthesia (continuous epidural technique is most frequently used) with general anesthesia can provide anesthesia and postoperative analgesia in the form of epidural or intrathecal narcotic therapy. Moreover, fewer cardiopulmonary complications have been reported in high-risk patients who had combined epidural anesthesia with general anesthesia (6).

Physical status and risk

The anesthesiologist uses a classification of the surgical patient's physical status (adopted by the American Society of Anesthesiologists) to assess or predict operative risk under anesthesia and the outcome of the surgery.

Class 1 patients in good general health
Class 2 patients with mild or moderate systemic disease
Class 3 patients with severe systemic disease such as limiting organic heart disease
Class 4 patients with life-threatening systemic disease such as organic heart disease with cardiac insufficiency
Class 5 moribund patients

Patients with poor physical status such as class 3 or 4 are not candidates for outpatient surgery.

Premedication

Almost all patients have some degree of preoperative anxiety or apprehension. Relief of anxiety can be achieved by adequate preparation of the patient, by mere reassurance and an informative discussion. However, premedication with a variety of narcotics, sedatives, tranquilizers, and anticholinergics may be given depending on the patient's emotional status and magnitude of the surgical procedure.

Laboratory tests

Although there is no routine laboratory screening test for preanesthetic evaluation, hematocrit and urinalysis are usually required. Further studies including electrocardiogram (ECG), chest x-ray, or determination of electrolytes are based on concurrent systemic diseases or medications.

Patient monitoring

With great advances in technology, more sensitive or easily applicable monitorings are readily available in the perioperative period.

Electrocardiogram

The ECG remains the standard monitor used intraoperatively to assess cardiac function. In a patient with coronary artery disease, V5 and V4 are the most sensitive leads to detect the myocardial ischemia. However, transesophageal echocardiography is a better instrument to diagnose intraoperative myocardial ischemia (7).

Pulse oximetry

Pulse oximetry can provide a means of noninvasive assessment of arterial blood oxygenation. With light-emitting diodes (LED) as the light source and a photocell to detect wavelengths of light, a pulse oximeter estimates continuously arterial hemoglobin saturation. The main application in anesthesia is detection of hypoxemia in the perioperative period (8). Pulse oximetry has become a standard for basic intraoperative monitoring (adopted by the American Society of Anesthesiologists). Its use in anesthesia is included during the patient's transport and in the recovery room.

Capnography

The capnograph is an instrument that measures respiratory CO_2 by an infrared analyzer or a mass spectrometer system. Its primary use in anesthesia is to confirm the correct placement of an endotracheal tube by identifying CO_2 (end-tidal) in the expired gas (9). Maintenance of normocarbia under general anesthesia is readily achieved by capnography, avoiding physiologic consequences of hypocarbia or hypercarbia. Absence of CO_2 in the expired gas may be indicative of esophageal intubation, disconnection of mechanical ventilation, or apnea. From an abnormal capnogram, obstruction to gas flow or malfunction of an inspiratory valve can be suspected.

Anesthetics

Intravenous anesthetics

Although thiopental remains an intravenous induction agent, new intravenous agents such as etomidate, midazolam, and propofol have been available for induction as well as for maintenance of anesthesia by continuous infusion technique.

Thiopental

Thiopental (Pentothal), a barbiturate, was introduced as the first intravenous induction drug in the practice of anesthesia in 1934. Upon intravenous injection, the drug concentration rises rapidly in the highly vascular organs such as the brain. Through redistribution to muscle and fat, the action on the brain is terminated so that the patient awakens within 5 to 10 minutes of injection.

Thiopental has potent respiratory and circulatory depressant effects. Minor pharyngeal stimulation with an artificial airway or secretion often precipitates cough or laryngeal spasm. But thiopental may be beneficial in patients with an increased intracranial pressure because of its property to reduce cerebral blood flow and cerebral metabolism.

Recovery is gradual, depending on the total dose of the drug given, and will be slow with repeated doses because of the slow release of the drug stored in fat.

Ketamine

Ketamine provides not only unconsciousness but also analgesia. Characteristics of ketamine anesthesia include normal maintenance of the airway with retention of pharyngeal and laryngeal reflexes, bronchodilation, and circulatory stimulation by endogenous release of catecholamines. Therefore, it is often selected as an induction agent in high-risk patients. However, delirium or unpleasant dreams during awakening or in the postoperative period have been associated with the use of ketamine (10).

Etomidate

Etomidate results in less respiratory and cardiovascular depression than thiopental does. But etomidate suppresses the adrenocortical response to surgical stress for 5 to 8 hours (11). Excitement phenomena during induction and recovery often negate the advantages of this drug.

Midazolam

Midazolam hydrochloride (Versed), a benzodiazepine derivative, is used as a premedicant, sedative, and anesthetic induction as well as maintenance drug (12). It also has an amnestic property. The onset of action and recovery are slower than those of thiopental, but its cardiorespiratory depression is less than that of thiopental. Midazolam causes less venous irritation and has higher metabolic clearance than diazepam. Despite minimal respiratory depression when used alone, the combination with narcotics may produce a significant respiratory depression. A specific benzodiazepine antagonist, flumazenil, became available to reverse the depressive actions of this drug (13).

Propofol

Propofol (Diprivan) is a short-acting intravenous anesthetic agent for induction and maintenance of general anesthesia as well as sedation during local and regional anesthesia. Its rapid distribution and elimination makes recovery significantly faster than with the use of thiopental (14). Rapid recovery on termination even with a prolonged infusion is usual. Its cardiorespiratory depression is similar to that produced by thiopental, but postoperative nausea and vomiting are less common than with the use of thiopental. The preparation is formulated in an emulsion of soy bean oil and egg yolk lecithin, and pain on injection can be reduced with lidocaine pretreatment.

Synthetic opioids

Several synthetic agonist opioids (fentanyl, sufentanil, and alfentanil) and agonist-antagonist opioids (butorphanol and nalbuphine) are currently used in anesthetic practice in the form of parenteral as well as intraspinal injection. All these synthetic opioids produce a dose-dependent respiratory depression with relative stability of cardiovascular function. The fentanyl derivatives have a shorter duration of action and higher potency than morphine. Sufentanil is the most potent opioid, being 5 to 10 times more potent than fentanyl. Alfentanil, which has a shorter elimination half-life than fentanyl or sufentanil, seems more suitable for infusion techniques in outpatient procedures (15). Nalbuphine produces analgesic effects at κ receptors equipotent to those of morphine, but has a moderate antagonism at μ receptors with fewer psychomimetic side effects than with the use of butorphanol.

Inhalation anesthetic gases

Desirable elements to be considered in choosing an inhaled anesthetic gas include rapid onset of action, smooth mask induction, minimum organ toxicity from biodegradation, and rapid emergence.

Halothane, enflurane, and isoflurane depress cardiorespiratory function in a dose-related manner. These inhaled gases produce cerebral vasodilatation and an increase in cerebrospinal fluid pressure. They have a muscle-relaxant property, potentiating the action of muscle relaxants and also causing relaxation of the uterine muscle.

Hepatic dysfunction has been reported with halothane. It is thought that products of reductive metabolism of halothane cause hepatic damage. Although enflurane or isoflurane is much less associated with hepatic injury, metabolism of enflurane to inorganic fluoride may impair urine concentrating ability. They all induce malignant hyperthermia in a susceptible patient.

Sevoflurane and desflurane are new inhaled anesthetic gases whose solubility in blood is less than that of isoflurane (16,17); therefore, a more rapid emergence appears to be a potential advantage over halothane, enflurane, and isoflurane. Airway problems including breath holding, coughing, and excessive secretion, however, are common on induction with desflurane. No clinical cases of nephrotoxicity or hepatotoxicity have been reported.

Local anesthetics

Local anesthetics commonly used for infiltration, peripheral nerve block, and central neural block for gynecologic procedures may be classified based on their clinical properties as follows (18):

1 Low potency with short duration: procaine, 2-chloroprocaine
2 Moderate potency and duration: lidocaine, mepivacaine
3 High potency and long duration: bupivacaine, etidocaine (Table 12-1).

Large nerve fibers such as motor and proprioceptive fibers require higher concentrations of local anesthetics. Lower concentration is necessary for local infiltration. With rapid clearance of procaine and 2-chloroprocaine, the potential for systemic toxicity of ester-local anesthetics is low, but short duration of action limits its clinical utility. Epinephrine 1:200,000 (5 μg/ml), when added to local anesthetic, prolongs the duration of anesthesia, reduces peak blood levels of local anesthetics, and increases the intensity of neural blockade. The alkalinization of local anesthetic solutions (e.g., addition of 1 mEq of sodium bicarbonate to each 10 ml of lidocaine solution) produces a faster onset of anesthesia. Although systemic toxicity can result from administration of an excessive dose of local anesthetic, its central nervous system toxicity and profound cardiac toxicity are largely due to an inadvertent intravascular injection. A toxic dose of bupivacaine and etidocaine can produce serious cardiac arrhythmias and asystole. The current recommended technique to avoid such severe systemic toxicity is

Table 12-1 Recommended maximum single dose for infiltration of local anesthetics

Drugs	Concentration (%)	Duration (min)	Maximum dose (mg)
Procaine	1.0	30–60	1000 (100 ml)
Chloroprocaine (Nesacaine)	1.0	30–60	800 (80 ml)
			1000 + epinephrine (100 ml)
Lidocaine (Xylocaine)	0.5	60–120	300 (60 ml)
	1.0		300 (30 ml)
			500 + epinephrine (0.5% 100 ml)
			(1.0% 50 ml)
Mepivacaine (Carbocaine, Polocaine)	0.5	90–180	400 (80 ml)
	1.0		400 (40 ml)
			500 + epinephrine (0.5% 100 ml)
			(1.0% 50 ml)
Bupivacaine (Marcaine, Sensorcaine)	0.25	120–360	175 (70 ml)
			225 + epinephrine (90 ml)

Epinephrine = 1:200,000
(Reproduced with permission from Covino BG. Clinical pharmacology of local anesthetic agents. In: Cousins MJ, Bridenbaugh PO, eds. Neural blockade, ed. 2. Philadelphia: JB Lippincott, 1988: 112–113.)

to use local anesthetic solution at divided doses with frequent aspirations of the syringe. Treatment of the systemic toxicity includes oxygen administration and drug therapy with succinylcholine and with diazepam or a barbiturate. Allergic reactions to amide local anesthetic are rare, but such solutions may contain a preservative, methylparaben, and an antioxidant, metabisulfite, which can produce allergic reactions. There are local anesthetic preparations free from methylparaben (Xylocaine-MPF) or free from methylparaben and bisulfite (Nesacaine-MPF).

Ropivacaine is a new amide local anesthetic undergoing clinical trials. It is structurally similar to bupivacaine but has fewer cardiotoxic properties (19).

There are a few neural blockades, by local anesthetics, suitable for gynecologic procedures: paracervical block may be suitable for dilatation and curettage, or the uterine sound for laparoscopy. Its potential risks include intravascular injections of local anesthetic and paracervical hematoma; pudendal nerve block provides anesthesia for the lower part of the vagina and perineum, but anesthesia for the anterior one-third of the labia requires local infiltration for genitofemoral and ilioinguinal nerve block. Lidocaine 1% with epinephrine 1:200,000 can be used for these blocks. A total of 20 to 25 ml in volume should be sufficient, with a maximum volume of 50 ml (500 mg).

Muscle relaxants

Desirable properties of muscle relaxants are rapid onset of action, good relaxation for tracheal intubation, minimum side effects, easy antagonism of residual blockade, and elimination without cumulative effect.

Succinylcholine is the choice of a relaxant for endotracheal intubation for its rapid onset of action. However, its side effects include bradycardia and arrhythmias due to stimulation of autonomic ganglia and muscarinic receptors in the heart. Succinylcholine is contraindicated in patients with burns, massive trauma, and neurologic disease for fear of development of hyperkalemia. Postanesthetic myalgia is also noted.

d-Tubocurarine and pancuronium are long-acting muscle relaxants. d-Tubocurarine is a potent histamine releaser and a ganglionic blocker, resulting in arterial hypotension. Pancuronium has a vagolytic effect that may increase heart rate. Their duration of action may be prolonged in patients with renal or hepatic dysfunction because of their elimination by the hepatic and renal system.

Atracurium and vecuronium are intermediate-acting muscle relaxants. Atracurium is a choice of muscle relaxant in patients with renal failure because of its spontaneous degradation independent of kidney function (20). Vecuronium, despite a structural analog of pancuronium, has no vagolytic effect.

Mivacurium is a short-acting, nondepolarizing ester relaxant. As a result, it is hydrolyzed by plasma cholinesterase. The clinical duration of action varies between 14 and 25 minutes (21). Therefore, it is suitable for short procedures or for maintenance of relaxation for longer procedures by infusion.

Doxacurium is a new long-acting muscle relaxant with few cardiovascular effects. Because of renal elimination, however, there is potential for prolongation of the duration of action in patients with renal failure (22).

The action of muscle relaxants may be potentiated by inhaled anesthetic gases, aminoglycoside antibiotics, verapamil, lithium, and potassium-depleting diuretics. In addition to clinical signs, the depth of neuromuscular blockade should be monitored by a peripheral nerve stimulator. The train-of-four is the most useful method. Residual neuromuscular blockade may be antagonized by acetylcholinesterase inhibitors (neostigmine, or pyridostigmine with anticholinergic drugs), and recovery from the blockade should be assessed by complete recovery of the train-of-four, a sustained tetanus, and head lift.

Postoperative pain management

Adequate pain relief not only reduces the patient's suffering but also improves the ability to ambulate, thereby reducing postoperative complications. With a variety of treatment modalities, it is appropriate to address a plan for postoperative pain management on preanesthetic evaluation.

Conventional intermittent intramuscular injection and intravenous injection of opioids have been the most frequently used methods of pain control in the postoperative period. They are simple and effective in most circumstances. However, because steady-state drug levels in blood can readily be produced by continuous infusion, a more constant degree of analgesia can be achieved by the continuous infusion of opioids.

Patient-controlled analgesia

Patient-controlled analgesia devices allow the patient to self-administer small bolus doses of opioids within lockout intervals. This management of postoperative pain is routine in most gynecologic surgical procedures. Patient-controlled analgesia with intravenous morphine provides satisfactory pain relief after abdominal hysterectomy (23). The patient initiates a bolus of morphine of 0.5 to 2 mg with lockout intervals of 5 to 20 minutes.

Intraspinal opioids

Intrathecal or epidural injection of opioids acts on opioid receptors in the substantia gelatinosa of the dorsal horn of the spinal cord, producing selective analgesia without motor or sympathetic blockade. The major clinical application is in the area of postoperative pain management and in obstetrics. A variety of opioids have been administered intrathecally or epidurally by intermittent injection, continuous infusion, or patient-controlled technique. An intrathecal single dose of preservative-free morphine (Astramorph, Duramorph) of 0.5 to 1 mg or an epidural dose of morphine of 3 to 5 mg appears to be effective for postoperative pain for up to 24 hours (24). Continuous epidural infusion of morphine also provides good postoperative analgesia after hysterectomy (25). Epidural meperidine in doses of 50 to 100 mg produces analgesia up to 6 hours. Intrathecal meperidine in doses of 50 to 80 mg provides surgical anesthesia as the sole anesthetic for postpartum tubal ligation and provides excellent postoperative analgesia, in part attributable to its local anesthetic properties (26). Epidural fentanyl produces a more rapid onset of action than morphine. The use of patient-controlled analgesia epidurally for fentanyl administration can be set with a maintenance dose of 20 μg with a lockout interval of as short as 6 minutes (27). The major side effects of intraspinal opioids are nausea, vomiting, pruritus, and urinary retention. Respiratory depression, usually at 6 to 10 hours postinjection with morphine, was reported with an incidence of 0.2% (24). Although these side effects can be antagonized by naloxone, small doses of an antiemetic such as droperidol (0.625 mg IV) or transdermal scopolamine patches containing 1.5 mg of scopolamine (Transderm Scop) are effective in treating nausea and vomiting. The transdermal scopolamine placed on the skin behind the ear before surgery can also reduce the incidence of postoperative nausea (28). Diphenhydramine (Benadryl) at 25 to 50 mg may relieve pruritus, although the pruritus is not related to histamine release. Frequent assessments of the patient's level of sedation and respiratory rate are necessary to minimize serious ventilatory depression.

Transdermal fentanyl

A rate-controlled transdermal patch of fentanyl (at a rate of 75 μg/hour) can reduce supplemental analgesics for postoperative pain. However, the long latency, difficulty in adjusting dose, and high incidence of nausea appear to be limiting factors to its use (29).

Local infiltration

Infiltration of local anesthetic at the operative site may provide analgesia for postoperative pain. Incisional infiltration with bupivacaine 0.25% at the end of abdominal surgery can reduce postoperative opioid requirements.

Ketorolac

Ketorolac tromethamine (Toradol) is a new nonsteroidal analgesic drug with anti-inflammatory properties (30). It is administered by intramuscular injection or orally. Its single-dose efficacy is greater than that of morphine and meperidine in postoperative pain. Unlike opioids, it does not cause respiratory depression; therefore, it may be a useful alternative to opioids. A 30-mg intramuscular dose seems effective for moderate postoperative pain; the dose may be repeated every 5 to 6 hours. Oral dosages range from 10 to 20 mg four times daily. Side effects include somnolence, headache, nausea, gastrointestinal pain, and gastric ulceration and bleeding. It inhibits platelet aggregation and may prolong bleeding time. The systemic dose should be reduced in patients with renal impairment because of its dependency on renal elimination.

Specific procedures

Vaginal and pelvic floor surgery

These surgical procedures may require a steep Trendelenburg position in addition to lithotomy. In the lithotomy position, the legs should not be placed against stirrups to avoid

peroneal nerve palsy, and the arms should not be overstretched to protect from bracheal plexus injury. Although minute ventilation and gas exchange are not compromised by the Trendelenburg position in patients breathing spontaneously under anesthesia (31), the potential effect of the steep Trendelenburg position on respiratory function is cause for concern among anesthesiologists because it decreases total lung volume and functional residual volume as a result of pressure by the abdominal contents upon the diaphragm. In addition, the altered lung mechanics under general anesthesia may interfere with pulmonary gas exchanges.

Although major vaginal surgery can be associated with substantial blood loss and it is sometimes difficult to estimate the blood loss with accuracy, the use of epidural anesthesia can reduce blood loss (32).

Laparoscopy

Laparoscopic examinations require pneumoperitoneum of carbon dioxide or nitrous oxide and the use of a steep Trendelenburg position. Although a rise in $PaCO_2$ from absorption of carbon dioxide from the peritoneal cavity and mechanical impairment of ventilation by the pneumoperitoneum and Trendelenburg position has been implicated as a cause of cardiac arrhythmias, the rise of $PaCO_2$ is clinically insignificant (33) when peritoneal insufflating pressure is less than 25 cm H_2O. End-tidal CO_2 monitoring is essential in this respect. Another danger of the excessive intra-abdominal pressure greater than 25 cm H_2O is the potential for interfering with venous return to the heart.

The majority of laparoscopic examinations are performed under general anesthesia with controlled ventilation. However, epidural anesthesia has been used safely without the rise in $PaCO_2$ (34). Local anesthesia consisting of a periumbilical field block may also be used in combination with narcotics in patients undergoing diagnostic laparoscopy and tubal ligation (35).

Significant vagal reflex with bradycardia and hypotension can be observed during uterine manipulation. Cessation of the uterine manipulation and atropine (0.4–0.6 mg) can reverse the reflex.

Gynecologic cancer surgery

The anesthetic considerations in patients who have previously received chemotherapy involve effects of the chemotherapy on organ systems and its potential interaction with anesthetics.

Doxorubicin (Adriamycin) can produce cardiac arrhythmias and cardiomyopathy (36). Furthermore, a patient treated with doxorubicin may have left ventricular dysfunction without clinically evident congestive heart failure. Pulmonary artery catheter pressure monitoring may be indicated (37). Cyclophosphamide (Cytoxan) has also been associated with myocarditis resulting in heart failure. Concomitant use of cyclophosphamide and halothane can be detrimental to myocardial function.

Patients treated with bleomycin are at risk of developing the postoperative respiratory failure. Careful monitoring of fluid replacement and minimal fractional concentration of inspired oxygen ($FiO_2 < 0.3$) during operation may reduce postoperative pulmonary complications (38).

Cis-platinum may increase serum creatinine and blood urea nitrogen, and causes hypomagnesemia, hypocalcemia, and hypokalemia. Cis-platinum causes peripheral neuropathy. If regional anesthetic technique is to be used, preexisting neurologic deficits should be documented.

Laser surgery

A laser does not interfere with the patient's monitoring equipment. The illumination of the operating room may not be sufficient to observe the color of the patient; a pulse oximeter and end-tidal CO_2 monitoring are essential. Operating room personnel should wear protective eyeglasses, and the patient's eyes should be taped closed under general anesthesia.

Hysteroscopy

Hysteroscopy is a diagnostic procedure, but it is also used therapeutically, using a laser to remove submucosal myomas and for endometrial ablation for intractable uterine bleeding. Insufflation with carbon dioxide or instillation of a liquid medium such as saline, water, or dextran (Hyskon) is necessary as an aid in distending the uterine cavity for optimal visualization of its surface. As a result, gas embolism ascribed to carbon dioxide insufflation, disseminated intravascular coagulation, and pulmonary edema from rapid intravascular absorption of the visualizing medium have been reported (39). In addition to the recommendation that the lowest dose of the irrigating solution with a minimum injection pressure and duration of the injection be used, patients undergoing operative hysteroscopy should be closely observed for signs of fluid overload.

Postpartum hemorrhage

When pharmacologic intervention with oxytocin, ergometrine, and prostaglandins in postpartum hemorrhage fails, surgical measures such as hypogastric artery ligation and hysterectomy may become necessary.

Careful assessment of blood loss, fluid administration, urine output, and vital signs is essential. Volume resuscitation with crystalloid fluids and blood is the main measure. Establishment of two large-bore intravenous lines and an intra-arterial catheter for arterial pressure monitoring are recommended.

The patient should receive antacid, 30 ml of sodium citrate, preoperatively. General anesthesia can be induced with thiopental or ketamine using a rapid sequence induction. Although a low concentration of inhaled anesthetic gases may not increase uterine bleeding, all potent inhaled anesthetic gases relax uterine muscles.

In those patients with an epidural catheter in place for labor and delivery, extension of the block may provide anesthesia for the surgery. However, one should be aware that sympathetic blockade accompanying epidural block causes vasodilatation resulting in hypotension.

Elderly patients

Preexisting disease and decline in organ system function due to the aging process may increase perioperative risks in elderly patients. Moreover, anesthetic requirements for geriatric patients are reduced, and drug elimination may be prolonged.

The incidence of perioperative hypothermia in the elderly is common and may cause an increased demand on cardiopulmonary work. Every measure should be taken to maintain a thermo-neutral environment, including the use of the patient's warming device.

Significant impairment of mental function up to 3 days postoperatively following general anesthesia is not uncommon in the elderly. Studies have shown that the maintenance of mental function is better following spinal anesthesia without sedation (40).

Summary

A thorough preoperative preparation of the patient's physical status to its maximum can lead to a better outcome of surgery. Intraoperative monitoring of oxygenation and ventilation has been much improved by the use of pulse oximetry and end-tidal CO_2 monitoring. The newer anesthetics such as propofol, midazolam, desflurane, and mivacurium have shorter duration of action, which allows better control over their effects. Thereby, rapid and complete recovery from anesthesia can be achieved. Although no particular anesthetic technique has been shown to be superior for any given patient, the use of epidural anesthesia alone or in combination with light general anesthesia may have multiple beneficial effects, including postoperative pain management with epidural opioids, in most gynecologic surgical procedures. Patient-controlled analgesia is the choice of technique in postoperative pain management. Patients undergoing laparoscopy, major vaginal surgery, or operative hysteroscopy and patients treated with anticancer drugs may deserve specific anesthetic considerations.

References

1 Frerk CM. Predicting difficult intubation. Anaesthesia 1991; 46:1005.

2 Goldman L, Caldera DL, Nussbaum SR, et al. Multifactorial index of cardiac risk in noncardiac surgical procedures. N Engl J Med 1977;297:845.

3 Tisi GM. Preoperative evaluation of pulmonary function, validity, indications and benefits. Am Rev Respir Dis 1979;199:293.

4 Goldman L, Caldera D. Risks of general anesthesia and elective operation in the hypertensive patient. Anesthesiology 1979;50:285.

5 Houston MC. Abrupt cessation of treatment in hypertension: consideration of clinical features, mechanisms, prevention and management of the discontinuation syndrome. Am Heart J 1981; 102:415.

6 Yeager MP, Glass DD, Neff RK, Brinck-Johnsen T. Epidural anesthesia and analgesia in high-risk surgery patients. Anesthesiology 1987;66:729.

7 Smith JS, Cahalan MK, Benefiel DJ, et al. Intraoperative detection of myocardial ischemia in high-risk patients: electrocardiography versus two-dimensional transesophageal echocardiography. Circulation 1985;72:1015.

8 Severinghaus JW, Kelleher JF. Recent developments in pulse oximetry. Anesthesiology 1992;76:1018.

9 Coté CJ, Liu LMP, Szyfelbein SK, et al. Intraoperative events diagnosed by expired carbon dioxide monitoring in children. Can Anaesth Soc J 1986;33:315.

10 White PF, Way WL, Trevor AJ. Ketamine—its pharmacology and therapeutic uses. Anesthesiology 1982;56:119.

11 Fragen RJ, Shanks CA, Molteni A, et al. Effects of etomidate on hormonal response to surgical stress. Anesthesiology 1984;61:652.

12 Reves JG, Fragen RJ, Vinik HR, Greenblatt DJ. Midazolam: pharmacology and uses. Anesthesiology 1985;62:310.

13 Philip BK, Simpson TH, Hauch MA, Mallampati SR. Flumazenil reverses sedation after midazolam-induced general anesthesia in ambulatory surgery patients. Anesth Analg 1990;71:371.

14 Sebel PS, Lowdon JD. Propofol: a new intravenous anesthetic. Anesthesiology 1989;71:260.

15 White PF, Coe V, Shafer A, Sung ML. Comparison of alfentanil with fentanyl for outpatient anesthesia. Anesthesiology 1986;64;99–100.

16 Fink EJ, Malan TP, Atlas M, et al. Clinical comparison of sevoflurane and isoflurane in healthy patients. Anesth Analg 1992;74:241.

17 Smiley RM. An overview of induction and emergence characteristics of desflurane in pediatric, adult, and geriatric patients. Anesth Analg 1992;75:S38.

18 Covino BG. Clinical pharmacology of local anesthetic agents. In: Cousins MJ, Bridenbaugh PO, eds. Neural blockade, ed 2. Philadelphia: JB Lippincott, 1988.

19 Feldman HS, Arthur GR, Pitkanen M, et al. Treatment of acute systemic toxicity after the rapid intravenous injection of ropivacaine and bupivacaine in the conscious dog. Anesth Analg 1991;73:373.

20 Miller RD, Rupp SM, Fisher DM, et al. Clinical pharmacology of vecuronium and atracurium. Anesthesiology 1984;61:444.

21 Savarese JJ, Ali HH, Basta SJ, et al. The clinical neuromuscular pharmacology of mivacurium chloride (BW B109OU). Anesthesiology 1988;68:723.

22 Basta SJ, Savarese JJ, Ali HH, et al. Clinical pharmacology of doxacurium chloride. Anesthesiology 1988;69:478.

23 Parker RK, Holtmann B, White PF. Effects of a nighttime opioid infusion with PCA therapy on patient comfort and analgesic requirements after abdominal hysterectomy. Anesthesiology 1992;76:362.

24 Ready LB, Loper KA, Nessly M, Wild L. Postoperative epidural morphine is safe on surgical wards. Anesthesiology 1991;75:452.

25 Asantila R, Eklund P, Rosenberg PH. Continuous epidural infusion of bupivacaine and morphine for postoperative analgesia after hysterectomy. Acta Anaesthesiol Scand 1991;35:513.

26 Curran C, Dickerson SE, Bailey SL. Efficacy of intrathecal meperidine as the sole anesthetic for postpartum tubal ligation [Abstract]. Anesthesiology 1992;77:A1004.

27 Glass PSA, Estok P, Ginsberg B, Goldberg JS, Sladen RN. Use of patient-controlled analgesia to compare the efficacy of epidural to intravenous fentanyl administration. Anesth Analg 1992;74:345.

28 Bailey PB, Streisand JB, Pace NL, et al. Transdermal scopolamine reduces nausea and vomiting after outpatient laparoscopy. Anesthesiology 1990;72:977.

29 Caplan RA, Ready LB, Oden RV, et al. Transdermal fentanyl for postoperative pain management. A double-blind placebo study. JAMA 1989;261:1036.

30 Buckley MMT, Brogden RN. Ketorolac: a review of its pharmacodynamic and pharmacokinetic properties, and therapeutic potential. Drugs 1990;39:86.

31 Scott DB, Slawson KB. Respiratory effects of prolonged Trendelenburg position. Br J Anaesth 1968;40:103.

32 Moir DD. Blood loss during major vaginal surgery. A statistical study of the influence of general anesthesia and epidural analgesia. Br J Anaesth 1968;40:233.

33 De Sousa H, Tyler IL. Can absorption of the insufflating gas during laparoscopy be hazardous? [Abstract]. Anesthesiology 1987;67:A476.

34 Ciofolo MJ, Clergue F, Seebacher J, Lefebvre G, Viars P. Ventilatory effects of laparoscopy under epidural anesthesia. Anesth Analg 1990;70:357.

35 Brown DR, Fishburne JI, Roberson VO, Hulka JF. Ventilatory and blood gas changes during laparoscopy with local anesthetic. Am J Obstet Gynecol 1976;124:741.

36 Lewis KP. Anesthetic implications in the patient receiving cancer chemotherapy. Part II. Anesth Rev 1988;15(3):45.

37 Powell L, Garfield JM. Anesthetic considerations for gynecologic cancer surgery. Semin Surg Oncol 1990;6:194.

38 Goldiner PL, Carlon GC, Cvitkovic E, Schweizer O, Howland WS. Factors influencing postoperative morbidity and mortality in patients treated with bleomycin. Br Med J 1978;1:1664.

39 Jedeikin R, Olsfanger D, Kessler I. Disseminated intravascular coagulopathy and adult respiratory distress syndrome: life-threatening complications of hysteroscopy. Am J Obstet Gynecol 1990; 162:44.

40 Chung F, Meier R, Lautenschlager E, et al. General or spinal anesthesia: which is better in the elderly? Anesthesiology 1987;67:422.

Part 2

Vaginal Surgery

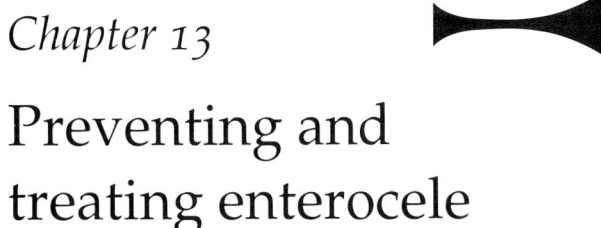

Chapter 13

Preventing and treating enterocele

David H. Nichols

An enterocele or pudendal hernia is a sac, generally filled with small intestine and omentum, that has separated between the posterior wall of the vagina and the anterior wall of the rectum. Not uncommon, the condition usually is progressive. If the sac extends all the way to the perineal body, it may cause a wide separation between the vagina and the rectum.

The bottom of the cul-de-sac of Douglas may extend behind and below the uterine cervix or vaginal vault even as far as the perineal body but should always be obliterated at surgery to lessen the chance of future enterocele. This deep cul-de-sac may or may not be filled with loops of small intestine. For the latter to be present there must be coincident pathologic elongation (beyond the usual 15 cm) in the length of the small bowel mesentery. The weight of a food-laden small intestine with pathologically long mesentery lying upon the site of the freshly obliterated cul-de-sac invites recurrence of enterocele by disrupting the integrity of the scar. This incidence of recurrent enterocele may be reduced by strengthening the scar at the neck of the sac through the use of a nonabsorbable suture material and by closing the peritoneal sac with more than one layer of suture.

The four main types of enterocele—congenital, pulsion, traction, and iatrogenic—each have a different cause, location, and treatment (1–3). To be successful, the surgical procedure must correlate with a particular enterocele's etiology.

Types of enterocele

Congenital enterocele results when the fetal sac of peritoneum between rectum and vagina fails to fuse or reopens because of pathology. This sac is located posterior to the vagina, and there is no associated cystocele or rectocele. The sac represents a split layer of the peritoneal fusion fascia of Denonvilliers (the rectovaginal septum) (Fig. 13-1A).

In the pulsion type of enterocele (Fig. 13-1B), increased intra-abdominal pressure creates the hernial sac and often pushes the vaginal vault down along with the peritoneal sac. As the vault drops, it drags the anterior vaginal wall with it, producing a displacement cystocele. Often there is no rectocele. Because the enterocele is truly a sliding hernia, the uterus, cervix, and anterior vaginal wall slide along the anterior surface of the rectum. Should these structures be firmly attached and remain in place, the anterior rectal wall may move along the posterior surfaces of the vagina and cause a rectal prolapse or intussusception (4).

Traction enterocele (Fig. 13-1C) results when both a large cystocele and a rectocele pull on the vaginal vault. In due course, the downward pull of gravity gradually accentuates this condition.

When an enterocele occurs anterior to the vagina, it looks like a cystocele, although it is, in fact, a peritoneal sac separating the bladder from the anterior vaginal wall (Fig. 13-1D). This variant generally results when excess anterior peritoneum is not resected at the time of hysterectomy and

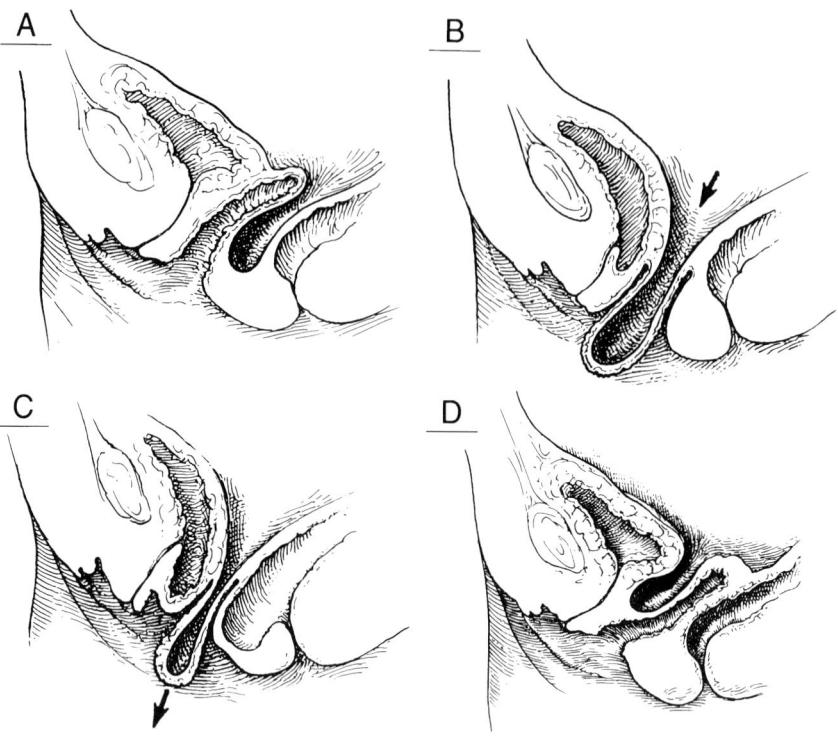

Fig. 13-1 The four types of enterocele:
(A) posterior, (B) pulsion, (C) traction,
(D) iatrogenic.

the abdomen subsquently reperitonealizes. This is likely to occur at vaginal hysterectomy when there was difficulty identifying the anterior vesicouterine peritoneal fold, and the peritoneal cavity was finally entered cranial to the bladder and close to the fundus of the uterus.

The most common type of iatrogenic enterocele results from a surgically produced change in the normal vaginal axis. Figure 13-2 shows the upper vagina almost horizontal and the rectum lying on and parallel to the levator plate.

Both the Marshall-Marchetti-Krantz operation and the Burch suprapubic vesicourethral suspension displace the vagina anteriorly (5). These procedures leave the cul-de-sac

of Douglas exposed, unprotected, and vulnerable to damage from the full range of increases in intra-abdominal pressure that occur during a normal day.

A rare type of enterocele follows sudden, short, but massive increases in intra-abdominal pressure. A rupture of the pelvic diaphragm ensues, often lateral to the vagina, and the hernial sac lies along a lateral vaginal wall, sometimes extending all the way to the vulva (Fig. 13-3). Because the neck of this lateral sac is small, intestinal obstruction may follow. Should the local bowel become caught within this sac, this situation may produce the presenting symptoms. The hernial defect in the pelvic floor becomes apparent dur-

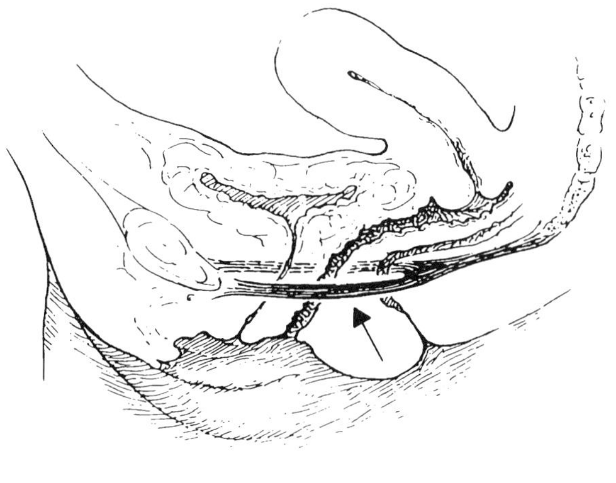

Fig. 13-2 The normal vaginal axis. The pubococcy-geal muscles (arrow) are normally fused posterior to the rectum as shown.

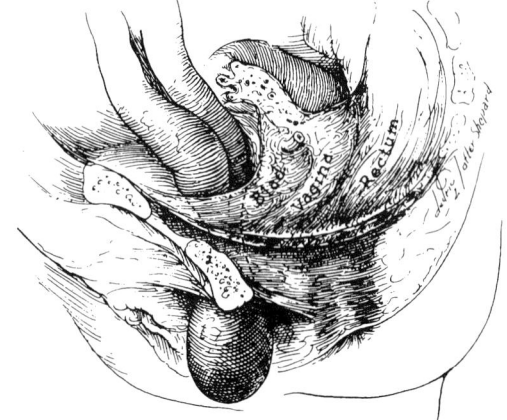

Fig. 13-3 Lateral pudendal enterocele.

ing surgery, when the bowel is traced to its disappearance in the sac, within the pelvic floor. Gentle traction brings it back into the peritoneal cavity.

Mixtures of several of these events may be at work in a particular enterocele. To lessen the chance of recurrence, determine each of these influences preoperatively, so specific remedies can be incorporated into the surgical procedure. The location of the enterocele correlates with the cause, which, in turn, determines the optimal treatment, as noted in Table 13-1.

Ventral suspension or ventrofixation of the uterus or vagina may render an unprotected cul-de-sac vulnerable to subsequent enterocele (Fig. 13-4). To avoid this hazard, fix the vagina to the promontory of the sacrum by a retroperitoneal bridge.

Making the diagnosis

Enterocele and high rectocele often coexist, but it is important to distinguish both conditions. Suspect an enterocele when a fullness can be felt in the vaginal vault of a patient in the lithotomy position. However, diagnosis is most accurate when the patient is examined in the standing position. The effect of gravity helps maximize the filling of the enterocele cavity with bowel and omentum (Fig. 13-5). A thumb gently introduced into the vagina will clearly establish whether there is a prolapse of the vault or cystocele. Gently elevate the vaginal vault with the thumb and insert an index finger through the anus to palpate the perineal body and posterior vaginal wall. This makes it possible to detect any weakness and note the full extent and location of a rectocele, be it low, middle, or high in the vagina, or all three. Then ask the patient to bear down as in a Valsalva maneuver and gently press the tips of the index finger and the thumb against each other. A hernial sac and its contents will generally be evident. Carefully note the presence or absence of a normal, horizontally inclined upper vaginal axis.

Table 13-1 Enterocele correlation

Type and cause	Location	Treatment
Congenital	Posterior to vagina	Excision of the sac with high ligation of its neck.
Pulsion (pushed)	With eversion of vaginal vault	Restore vault depth by transvaginal sacrospinous fixation, or transabdominal sacropexy if cardinal and uterosacral strength is poor, or culdeplasty if strong. Coincident hysterectomy often desirable.
Traction (pulled)	Lower vaginal eversion (cystocele and rectocele) pulling vault into descent and upper vaginal eversion	Same as above, plus anterior and posterior colporrhaphy.
Iatrogenic	Anterior to vagina, or posterior from change in vaginal axis	Excise or obliterate sac and and restore normal vaginal axis, if defective.

The patient's discomfort generally is caused by one or more of these symptoms:
• Backache produced by traction to the pathologically long small intestine mesentery coincident with the pull of gravity acting against the supports of the vaginal vault in the standing patient. This type of backache is characteristically minimal in the morning, worsens as the day goes on, and peaks by evening. Lying down relieves it.
• A sense of fullness in the pelvis, the result of the filling of the enterocele sac by omentum or small bowel with traction on the mesentery.
• Pressure from a pelvic or vaginal mass, worse when the patient stands. A sufficiently large mass may cause dyspareunia.

Preventive steps or surgery

Enterocele often can be prevented by resecting redundant or excess peritoneum at the time of hysterectomy (7). It is important to recognize a potential enterocele (deep cul-de-sac) or an existing one by carefully exploring the cul-de-sac with the bent finger (Fig. 13-6). Packing a suspected sac with a gauze sponge makes it easier to confirm and identify the excess peritoneum.

Using both sharp and blunt dissection, separate the enterocele sac from the surrounding connective tissue down to a point where the excision of excess peritoneum extends across the anterior surface of the rectum. Any fat belongs on the rectal side of the dissection. The characteristic condensations of fat or the longitudinal muscle fibers of the outer layer of the rectal wall indicate one has reached the rectum. Inspect the anterior peritoneum and excise the redundant

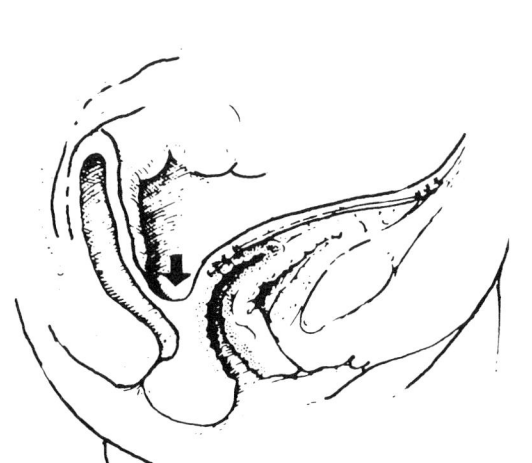

Fig. 13-4 The unprotected cul-de-sac (arrow), which resulted after ventral fixation of vagina.

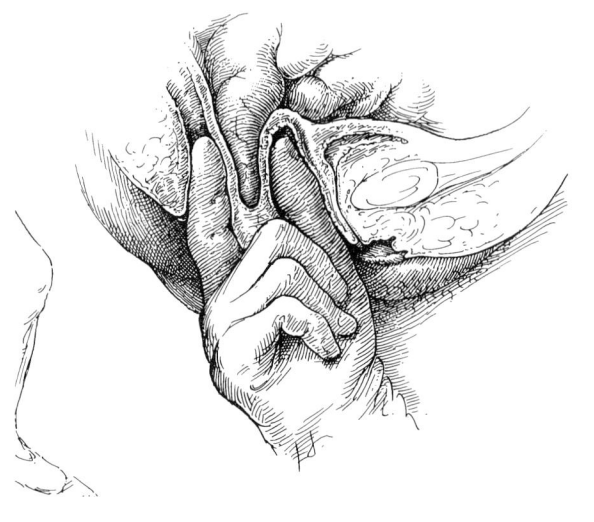

Fig. 13-5 Examination for enterocele. With the patient upright, place the thumb in the vagina and the index finger in the rectum. When the patient strains, palpation of a bowel-filled sac dissecting the rectovaginal septum indicates enterocele. (Reproduced with permission from Nichols DH. Repair of enterocele and prolapse of the vaginal-vault. In: Barber H, ed. Goldsmith's practice of surgery. Philadelphia: JB Lippincott, 1981:1–16, and Nichols DH, Randall CL. Vaginal surgery, ed 2. Baltimore: Williams & Wilkins, 1989:313–327.)

peritoneum anteriorly before accomplishing high peritonealization (Fig. 13-7).

If a marking suture has been placed, and it is difficult to locate the anterior peritoneum, catheterize the patient and lightly grasp the tissue of the bladder wall below the anterior peritoneum and with successive gentle bites on an unlocked hemostat, "walk up," until one recognizes the cut edge of peritoneum and can grasp it with forceps.

Use a full length of absorbable 0 or 2-0 suture, held in a light hemostat for later identification. Sutures usually are of the delayed absorption variety, such as polyglycolic (Dexon) or polyglactin (Vicryl).

Uterosacral ligaments may be shortened and sewn to one another following hysterectomy, and a pathologically wide vaginal vault may be narrowed by excising an appropriate wedge of tissue from the posterior wall of the vagina (4). If the uterosacral ligaments are both long and strong, they may be incorporated in a New Orleans or McCall-type culdeplasty, which not only brings them together in the midline, but also fixes them at a point cranial to that at which the peritoneum will be closed.

Surgical procedures on the birth canal should restore to normal a defective vaginal axis, particularly when the abnormality is in the upper vagina (8).

Operations that change the normal vaginal axis include ventrosuspension, ventrofixation, and suprapubic vesicourethral pin-up operations. In all such procedures, it is advisable to obliterate the cul-de-sac deliberately, often plicating the uterosacral ligaments as well. At the time of vaginal hysterectomy and repair for uterine prolapse, it is advisable to shorten pathologically elongated uterosacral ligaments, then attach them to the vaginal vault (4).

Surgical treatment may be either transvaginal or transabdominal. For transvaginal procedures, I recommend excising the sac with high ligation of its neck, along with any colporrhaphy that may be necessary, permitting restoration of a normal vaginal depth and axis (4). Transabdominal procedures include reducing the width of the vaginal vault by excising a wedge of tissue to narrow the vault, (4,9) and obliterating the sac by concentric purse-string Moschcowitz-type stitches (10) or, better yet, sagittally placed Halban-type stitches (6,11), as the latter do not interfere with the ureter.

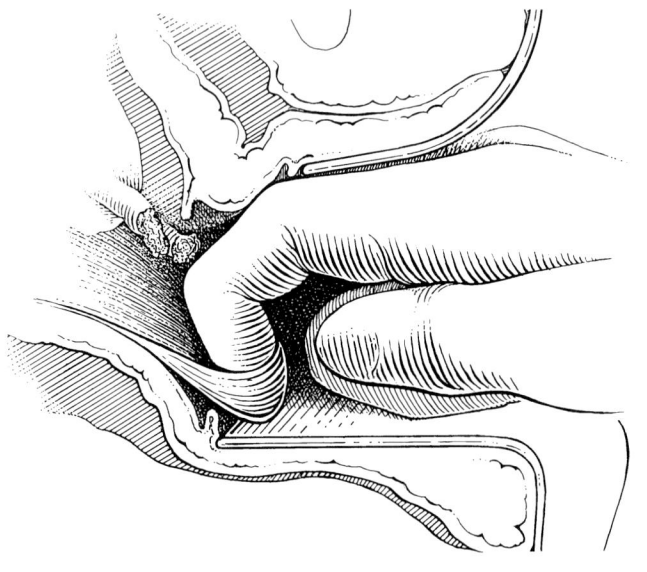

Fig. 13-6 Exploring cul-de-sac for enterocele. At surgery, explore cul-de-sac for enterocele, as shown in this sagittal section. (Reproduced with permission from Nichols DH. Repair of enterocele and prolapse of the vaginal vault. In: Barber H, ed. Goldsmith's practice of surgery. Philadelphia: JB Lippincott, 1981:1–16, and Nichols DH, Randall CL. Vaginal surgery, ed. 2. Baltimore: Williams & Wilkins, 1989:313–327.)

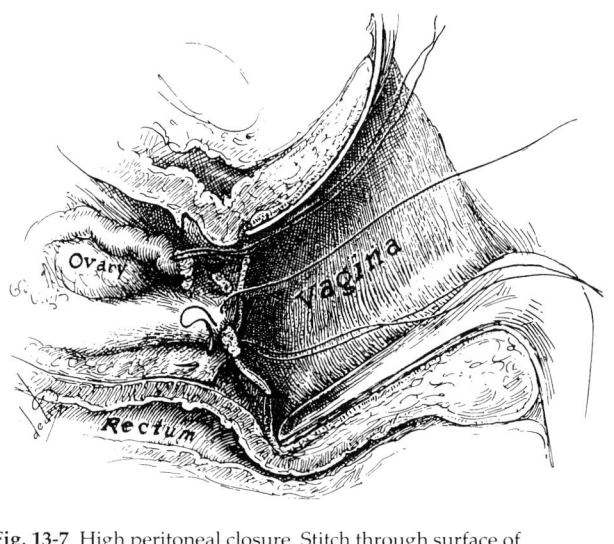

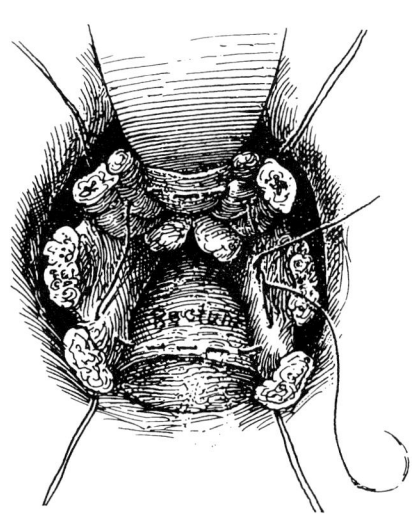

Fig. 13-7 High peritoneal closure. Stitch through surface of uterosacral ligament above posterior cut edge of peritoneum. Reef posterior peritoneum, then do opposite uterosacral ligament, round ligament, anterior peritoneum, and other round ligament. (Reproduced with permission from Nichols DH. Repair of enterocele and prolapse of the vaginal vault. In: Barber H, ed. Goldsmith's practice of surgery. Philadelphia: JB Lippincott, 1981:1–16, and Nichols DH, Randall CL. Vaginal surgery, ed 2. Baltimore: Williams and Wilkins, 1989: 313–327.)

Fig. 13-8 Closing the cavity. Place one purse-string suture to incorporate the uterosacral and round ligaments. Reinforce with a second suture 1 cm distal to the first. (Reproduced with permission from Nichols DH, Randall CL. Vaginal surgery, ed 2. Baltimore: William & Wilkins, 1989:313–327.)

When an enterocele sac has been excised transvaginally, close the neck of the sac by two purse-string sutures (Fig. 13-8), the upper one being a nonabsorbable monofilament material such as size 0 Novafil or Prolene. The double closure will increase the thickness of the scar, and the extra suture line will take some of the pull from the first suture and its knot.

Treat coincident eversion of the vaginal vault by appropriate colpopexy (12–16; Fig. 13-9). In postmenopausal patients, estrogenic hormone therapy may help restore pelvic elasticity and vascularity.

Certain preventive steps—no heavy lifting, or tight, constricting girdles or corsets—may minimize progression of the lesion. Treat chronic respiratory disease such as asthma, emphysema, and bronchitis. Impress on the patient the importance of discontinuing smoking. Following surgical repair of any enterocele, the patient should also take these precautions to minimize the chance of recurrence.

When surgery is contraindicated, these changes in lifestyle and avoidance of heavy lifting may afford some relief. A well-fitting vaginal pessary, doughnut, or inflatable balloon may displace the enterocele. A ring-type or Gellhorn pessary may be used if the uterus has dropped.

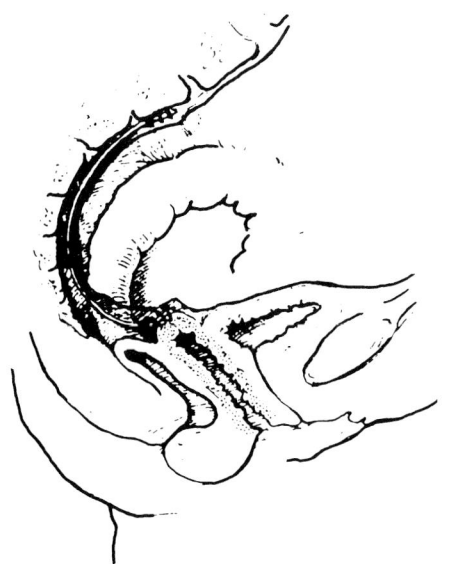

Fig. 13-9 Transabdominal sacral colpopexy. After the vagina has been fixed to the promontory of the sacrum, cul-de-sac is no longer vulnerable. (Reproduced with permission from Nichols DH. Repair of enterocele and prolapse of the vaginal vault. In: Barber H, ed. Goldsmith's practice of surgery. Philadelphia: JB Lippincott, 1981:1–16.)

Summary

There are at least four types of enterocele, each with a different etiology, each identifiable by its location within the pelvis. Successful surgery requires choosing a procedure that takes into account the cause of the hernia. Carefully weigh and judge possible contributing medical factors and recommend changes in lifestyle.

References

1 Weed JC, Tyrone C. Enterocele. Am J Obstet Gynecol 1950;60:324.

2 Read CD. Enterocele. Am J Obstet Gynecol 1951;62:743.

3 Nichols DH. Types of enterocele and principles underlying the choice of operation for repair. Obstet Gynecol 1972;40:257.

4 Nichols DH, Randall CL. Vaginal surgery, 3rd ed. Baltimore: Williams & Wilkins, 1989:313–327.

5 Burch JD. Urethrovaginal fixation to Cooper's ligament for correction of stress incontinence, cystocele, and prolapse. Am J Obstet Gynecol 1961;81:281.

6 Nichols DH. Repair of enterocele and prolapse of the vaginal vault. In: Barber H, ed. Goldsmith's practice of surgery. Philadelphia: JB Lippincott, 1981: 1–16.

7 Litschgi M, Kaser O. The problem of enterocele. Geburtshilfe Frauenheilkd 1978;38:915.

8 Nichols DH, Milley PS, Randall CL. Significance of restoration of normal vaginal depth and axis. Obstet Gynecol 1970;36:251.

9 Torpin R. Excision of the cul-de-sac of Douglas for the surgical cure of hernias through the female caudal wall: including prolapse of the uterus. J Med Assoc Ga 1947;36:396.

10 Moschcowitz AV. The pathogenesis, anatomy and cure of prolapse of the rectum. Surg Gynecol Obstet 1912;15:721.

11 Halban J. Gynakologische operationslehre. Berlin-Vienna: Urban and Schwarzenberg, 1932:171–172.

12 Randall CL, Nichols DH. Massive eversion of the vagina. Obstet Gynecol 1971;38:330.

13 Nichols DH. Gynecologic and obstetric surgery. St. Louis: Mosby-Yearbook, 1993:420–430.

14 Nichols DH. Effects of pelvic relaxation on gynecologic urologic problems. Clin Obstet Gynecol 1978;21:770.

15 Nichols DH. Sacrospinous fixation for massive eversion of the vagina. Am J Obstet Gynecol 1982;142:901.

16 Nichols DH, Milley PS. Clinical anatomy of the vulva, vagina, lower pelvis, and perineum. In Sciarra J, ed. Gynecology and obstetrics. New York: Harper & Row, 1993.

Chapter 14

Repair of total uterovaginal prolapse

Luis E. Sanz

Uterovaginal prolapse can be caused by obstetric trauma, a weakening of the tissues produced by postural strain, or congenitally attenuated fascia. This involves elongation of the levator ani muscles, especially the pubococcygeus and puborectalis muscles. Treatment encompasses a variety of nonsurgical and surgical techniques, including colpocleisis, vaginal hysterectomy with anterior and posterior colporrhaphy, abdomino sacrocolpopexy (1), the Le Forte procedure (2), sacrospinous colpopexy (3,4), and the use of pessaries. Choice of appropriate therapy depends on individual assessment of the patient.

The pelvic diaphragm, which supports the pelvic organs, consists of pelvic floor muscles, ligaments, and fascia. In patients with strong cardinal and uterosacral ligaments, vaginal hysterectomy with repair of anterior and posterior vaginal wall relaxation is a good way to correct a mild genital prolapse.

Many etiologic factors are involved in vaginal relaxation: congenitally weak tissues (5), obstetric trauma, heavy occupational lifting, obesity, chronic cough, chronic constipation, and the menopause with its atrophy and weakening of vaginal tissues and ligaments.

Proper selection of patients and techniques includes the mobility, size, and position of the uterus, gross pelvic pathology, and previous pelvic surgery, such as a large inflammatory adnexal mass or ovarian tumor, which is a contraindication (6). However, with the advent of laparoscopic surgery, laparoscopic-assisted vaginal hysterectomy (LAVH) could be easily performed in selected patients.

A uterus up to a size compatible with a 12-week gestation can be removed vaginally, using a morcellation technique. If the increase in size is secondary to fibroids, reduce it with the use of gonadotropin analogs (Lupron Depot). To repair a total vaginal prolapse without compromising sexual function, I recommend a modified surgical approach to the anterior colporrhaphy as part of the total vaginal hysterectomy and posterior colporrhaphy. Instead of starting with the hysterectomy, begin by dissecting the anterior vaginal mucosa, using the uterus for traction. This allows for better identification of the pubovesical fascia and its separation from the anterior vaginal mucosa. A trapezoidal incision on the anterior vaginal mucosa makes it easier to identify the bladder base and pillars (Fig. 14-1).

This approach allows one to visualize the bladder base and pillars before dissecting the bladder base from the cervix and lower uterine segment. Because this method avoids blind blunt dissection, it should result in less bladder trauma and bleeding. It also permits better access to the pubovesical fascia before the Kelly plication or paravaginal repair. The enterocele repair stresses the importance of high ligation of the hernial sac and obliteration of the posterior cul-de-sac, McCall coldoplasty, in an attempt to minimize any recurrence (7).

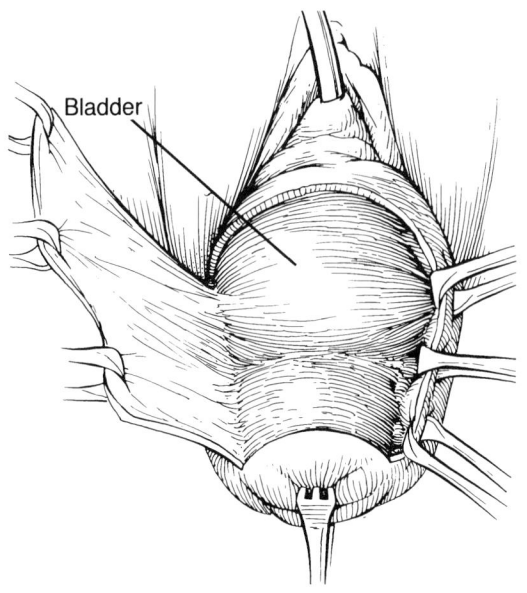

Fig. 14-1 Remove anterior mucosa. Using the uterus for traction, remove only the anterior vaginal mucosa. Leave pubovesical fascia attached to bladder.

Preoperative evaluation

Because a patient with marked pelvic prolapse may remain asymptomatic, preoperative evaluation is critical. Usually, however, such patients experience pelvic fullness, pelvic pain, annoying protrusion of pelvic organs, or a need to apply digital pressure to the posterior vaginal wall to achieve rectal evacuation. They may have recurrent urinary tract infections caused by large postvoid residuals, or symptoms of overflow urinary incontinence.

The preoperative evaluation should include careful examination of the introitus to estimate vaginal dimensions. Examine the anterior and posterior vaginal walls and ask the patient to cough or strain to delineate the degree of pelvic relaxation. If she gives a history of urinary stress incontinence, urine may be observed to spurt from the urethral meatus when she bears down.

To differentiate an enterocele from a high rectocele, it is helpful to inspect the posterior vaginal wall by rectal digital examination in conjunction with the Valsalva maneuver. Depress the rectum by placing a finger on the patient's posterior vaginal wall, and ask her to strain. If the posterior vaginal wall bulges forth, then an enterocele is present. One can delineate the degree of uterine relaxation by placing a single-tooth tenaculum on the anterior cervical lip and applying gentle traction. The magnitude of the prolapse is best evaluated by having the patient stand up and bear down. Do a thorough pelvic examination to determine the site, position, and motility of the uterus and rule out adnexal pathology. If there is massive procidentia, one must try to replace the uterus and vagina in place with estrogen cream packing to reduce swelling and improve the vaginal tissue.

If needed, the preoperative evaluation may include cervical cytology, endometrial biopsy, and an intravenous pyelogram (IVP) to reveal any significant ureteral displacement or hydronephrosis. As a research tool magnetic resonance imaging can give a great deal of information about the pelvic floor (8). In menopausal patients, an estrogen vaginal cream helps restore structural integrity to the atrophic vaginal mucosa and the supporting structures. Urodynamic studies (urethroscopy and cystometrics) are sometimes needed to determine the degree of rotational descent of the urethra, if any, and to rule out urinary stress incontinence. A mechanical bowel preparation with GoLytely the day before the operation may be required if the patient has a history of constipation; otherwise, a laxative (e.g., Colace) may be enough to clear the distal colon. An enema, on the day of the procedure is helpful during the surgery. Prophylactic antibiotics (cephalosporins, ampicillin, or doxycycline) are given one hour before the surgery to reduce infection morbidity.

Technique

Begin general or epidural anesthesia and then place the patient in the dorsolithotomy position using Allen stirrups. I place most of my patients under epidural anesthesia, which minimizes the postoperative complications especially in older patients. I also infiltrate the surgical area, especially the perineum, with bupivacaine (Marcaine) 0.25%, which markedly reduces the use of postoperative analgesics. Be careful not to inject bupivacaine intravascularly, as it is cardiotoxic. The main advantage of bupivacaine is that it is a long-acting anesthetic, lasting up to 12 to 16 hours, especially bupivacaine with epinephrine. Empty the bladder with a Foley catheter and then instill 150 cc of a solution of normal saline and methylene blue to reveal any bladder perforation during the dissection or the suturing. Reassess the anesthetized patient for uterine size, mobility, and degree of relaxation. Grasp the cervix with a single-tooth tenaculum or a Lahey clamp.

If the patient is to continue sexual activity, then the vagina must be reconstructed. If not, a partial vaginectomy is faster and will give much better results. If the vagina is going to be reconstructed, try to replace the uterus in its correct anatomic position by pushing the Lahey clamp in a cephalad direction. Place two Allis clamps on the anterior vaginal wall and draw them together to estimate the amount of vaginal mucosa to be removed. The redundant portion of the midanterior vaginal mucosa between the drawn clamps will be excised. It is important that one not remove too much of the anterior vaginal wall, as this will shorten the vagina and will produce dyspareunia. One must leave between 8 and 10 cm of vaginal depth (9).

The patient in Color Plate 8 has a total uterovaginal prolapse. The dotted lines represent the initial incisions on the cervix and the anterior vaginal wall. Infiltrate the anterior vaginal mucosa with bupivacaine with epinephrine 0.25% to separate the vaginal mucosa from the perivesical fascia and also to anesthetize the area and decrease bleeding. Then, make a 180-degree incision of the anterior cervical mucosa at the level of the cervicovaginal junction. Next, incise the anterior vaginal wall mucosa in a trapezoidal fashion with the apex no closer than 2 cm from the urethral meatus.

Figure 14-2 shows partial removal of the anterior vaginal wall mucosa. With this step, excise only vaginal wall mucosa and leave the perivesical fascia intact.

Figure 14-3 illustrates full visualization of the bladder base and pillars as well as the reflection of the anterior peri-

toneum. Dissecting the bladder base from the cervix under direct visualization allows for better control of bleeding and minimizes the possibility of bladder injury. This procedure affords easy identification and isolation of both the periurethral and perivesical fascia, for subsequent Kelly plication or (my preference) a Cullen-Richardson type of paravaginal repair. Sometimes one may have to perform both procedures. This depends on the area of weakness around the bladder (Color Plate 9). Continue dissecting the bladder base until the anterior peritoneal reflection can be identified, which permits one to enter the anterior cul-de-sac under direct visualization (Fig. 14-4). The bladder prolapses because of separation from the arcus tendineus fasciae pelvis laterally and central perivesical tears (10; Fig. 14-5). Therefore, to do a good physiologic repair, the best approach is a combination of a Kelly plication, without reducing bladder capacity, and approximation of the torn lateral perivesical fascia to the arcus tendineus under the symphysis pubis. One should use a continuous suture of 3-0 polydioxanone (PDS) or polyglyconate (Maxon) for the Kelly plication and 2-0 PDS or Maxon for the paravaginal repair. One must be very careful not to perforate the bladder, ureter, or urethra during this procedure. Make sure to preserve a good posterior urethrovesical angle to avoid overcorrection and incontinence (11,12). At this point, drain the bladder by opening the Foley catheter. Otherwise, the full bladder will make the hysterectomy very difficult.

Extend the cervical incision and with Metzenbaum scissors, and then dissect the posterior vaginal mucosa until the posterior peritoneal reflection is identified. A transverse in-

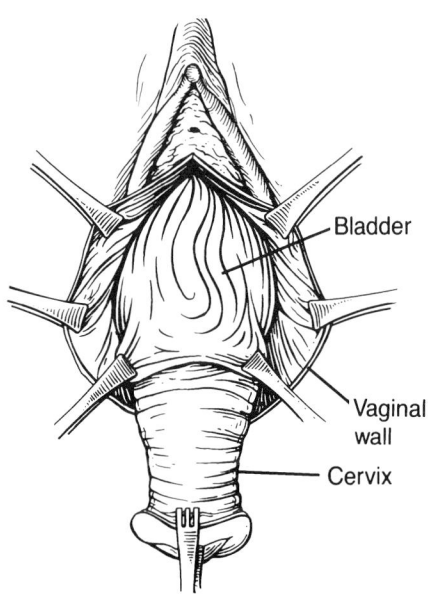

Fig. 14-2 Separate bladder. To separate the bladder from the cervix easily, first identify the bladder base and pillars.

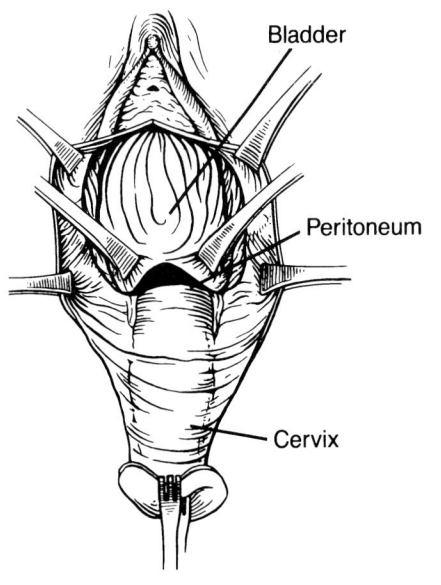

Fig. 14-3 Identify anterior peritoneum. Dissect the bladder base up to the anterior peritoneal reflection, so the anterior cul-de-sac is visible.

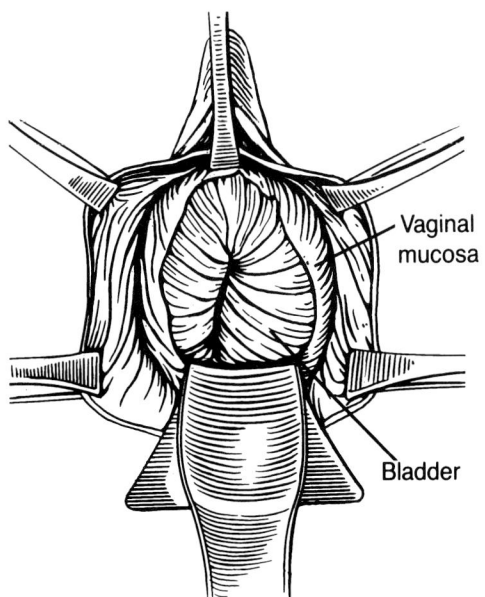

Fig. 14-4 Locate perivesical fascia. Before undertaking the anterior repair, locate the perivesical fascia, which must be identified to do an appropriate Kelly plication.

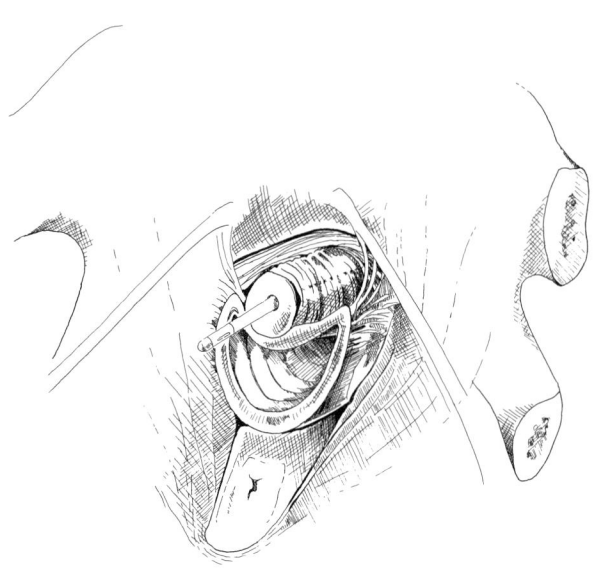

Fig. 14-5 The urethra (U), vagina (V), and rectum (R) are transected at the level of the arcus tendineus fasciae pelvis (ATFP). PD, pelvic diaphragm; PS, pubic symphysis; SFPD, superior fascia of the pelvic diaphragm.

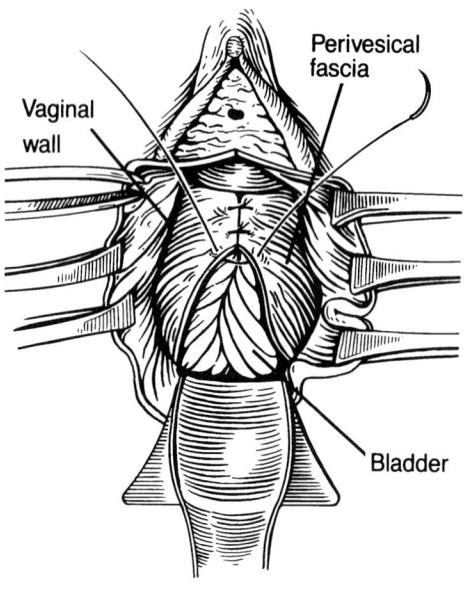

Fig. 14-6 Approximate anterior vaginal mucosa. Keep sutures away from proximal urethra. Approximate anterior vaginal mucosa with continuous sutures.

cision through the peritoneum allows access into the posterior cul-de-sac (13). Perform a digital examination through the anterior and posterior pelvic peritoneum, to identify any adhesions or other pathology.

In a very few patients in whom there is only a second-degree prolapse of the uterus, and the woman is young and wants more children, I will leave the uterus in place. However, one must find the cardinal ligaments and cross them anteriorly and then find the uterosacral ligaments and tie them posteriorly. This suspends the uterus away from the introitus. I have performed three such procedures with good results up to 5 years. Most of the time it is better to wait for childbearing to end and then do the hysterectomy for better results.

Now perform the hysterectomy in the usual fashion (Fig. 14-6). Always try to palpate the ureters laterally and above the cardinal ligaments. Ascertain the strength of the cardinal ligament and the uterosacral ligaments. If they are weak and elongated, do a sacrospinous ligament suspension.

To prevent central vaginal cuff prolapse or enterocele, it is important to attach the cardinal ligaments to the ipsilateral side of the vaginal mucosa and to plicate the uterosacral ligaments with a McCall colpoplasty. Close the pelvic peritoneum using a purse-string suture with 2-0 poliglecaprone (Monocryl) or 2-0 polyglactin (Vicryl).

Take care to place the suture high posteriorly to prevent an enterocele (Fig. 14-7). However, if there is an enterocele, repair this first while the peritoneum is open to prevent injury to the sigmoid colon (14,15). After peritoneal closure, if needed, finish the reconstruction of the posterior aspect of the bladder. After completing the anterior colporrhaphy,

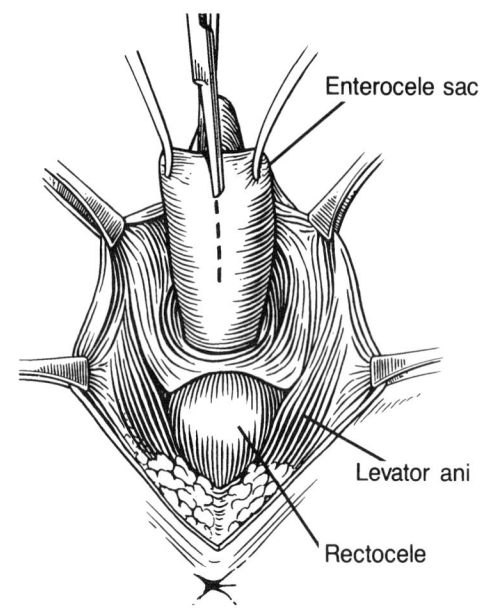

Fig. 14-7 Combined rectocele and enterocele. A band of perirectal fascia separates rectocele and enterocele. Pull it forward by placing a finger in the rectum.

begin to repair the rectocele. Figure 14-8 shows a combined enterocele and rectocele.

The rectocele is usually combined with a perineoplasty to prevent recurrence of the rectocele. First inject 10 or 15 cc of Marcaine 0.25% into the perineal body and perirectal fascia to diminish postoperative pain. Then make a diamond-shaped incision on the perineovaginal junction and resect it

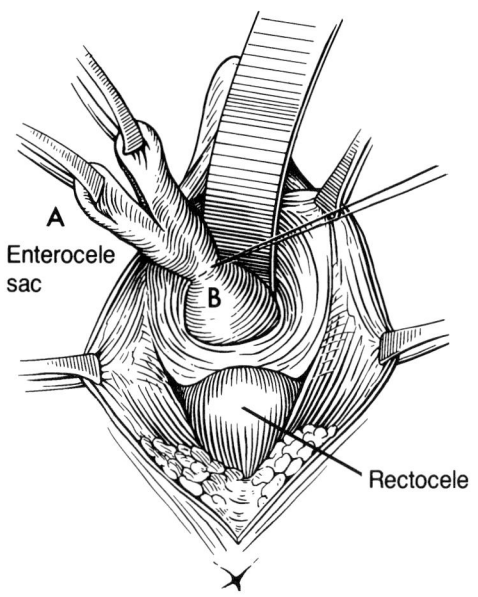

Fig. 14-8 High ligation of hernial sac. Notice open enterocele sac (A). High ligation (B) of hernial sac is essential to prevent recurrence.

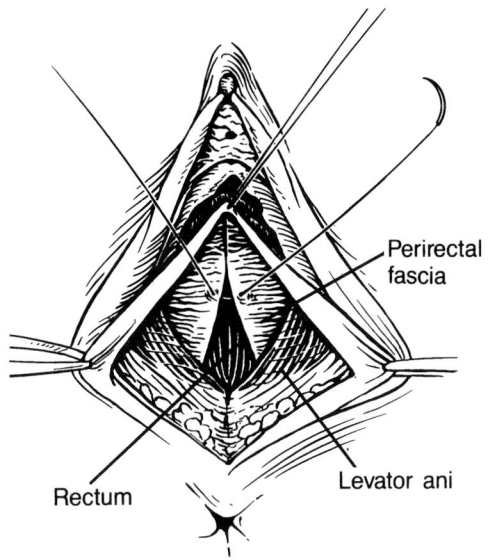

Fig. 14-9 Close perirectal fascia. Close the perirectal fascia from the vaginal vault to the level of the levator axis with interrupted sutures of 3-0 Maxon or PDS.

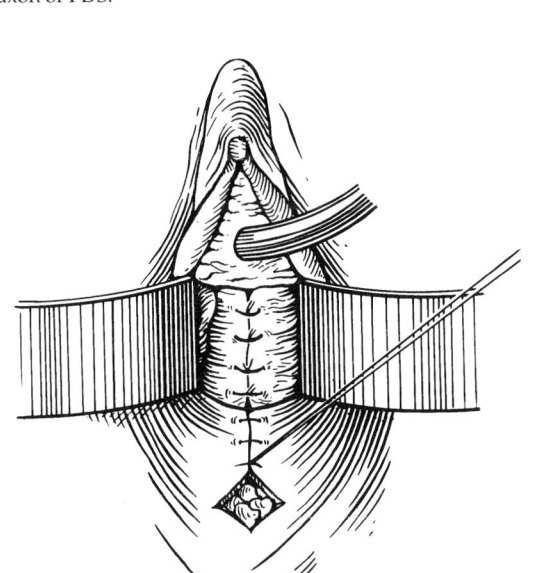

Fig. 14-10 Completed procedure. After perineoplasty, the operation is complete. Place a Foley catheter and leave it there for 3 to 5 days.

from the underlying fascia. Take a midline vertical incision through the posterior vaginal mucosa to the level of the enterocele. If the enterocele has not been repaired, then isolate it from the vaginal mucosa as high as possible with Metzenbaum scissors. It is critical to reduce the hernia and ligate the hernial sac as high as possible. Place a purse-string closure, including the uterosacral ligaments if possible to obliterate the cul-de-sac. These two steps are crucial in preventing a recurrence of the enterocele.

Correct the rectocele by dissecting the perirectal fascia from the vaginal mucosa and then approximating it with a continuous suture of 3-0 PDS (Fig. 14-9; Color Plate 10). With the advent of longer-lasting and stronger monofilament sutures, it is better to run the sutures to prevent multiple areas of devascularization and weakness as seen with interrupted sutures. Also there is a greater chance of granuloma formation around the area of the knot. At this point one may decide to perform a sacrospinous ligament fixation (Nichol's procedure) (3,4,9). Care must be taken to avoid injuring the rectum, the pudendal vessels and nerve, or the sciatic nerve. Try to place a suture of 0 Prolene on the superior medial aspect of the sacrospinous ligament on the left side to avoid the sigmoid colon. For the sacrospinous ligament suspension I use the Shult suture punch developed by Dr. Caspari for knee surgery. I use the 4mm tip. The advantage of the Caspari suture punch is that it is much easier to place the suture. Essentially it is a safer and faster method (Fig. 14-11). Following excision of excess vaginal mucosa, reapproximate the edges by a running suture of 3-0 Monocryl. Leave the tails of the suture inside the vaginal mucosa so as to avoid injury to the penis during intercourse. Monocryl is a new monofilament synthetic material with

great tensile strength, but it is absorbed within 2 to 3 weeks. To preserve adequate sexual function, close the introitus so as to allow easy introduction of two to three fingers. Now perform a perineoplasty to change the axis of the inferior aspect of the vagina (16–18). Figure 14-10 and Color Plate 11 illustrate the complete procedure. Place a vaginal packing of MetroGel vaginal impregnated Kerlix and remove it the next day. Monitor the hematocrit on the evening of the surgery and the next morning. The Foley catheter is left in place for one or two days. If work around the bladder was extensive, do a cystoscopy in the operating room to make sure that there are no sutures into the bladder and to see the elevation of the trigone.

In an older patient who is not sexually active, do a partial vaginectomy. This will maximize a successful operation and decrease the failure rate. It also makes for a much faster operation, because vaginal reconstruction takes a long time. The Le Forte procedure is done only in patients who are very sick and restricted to bed.

The management of the postoperative period includes vaginal packing soaked with Sultrin cream or MetroGel for 24 hours, Foley catheter, ice pack to the perineum, stool softener, sitz bath on day 2, and ketorolac tromethamine (Toradol) or acetaminophen (Tylenol No. 3) for pain. If the patient has diarrhea, then Lomotil is given as needed.

Complications

Many of the complications to this procedure can be serious, so care must be taken in identifying important anatomic landmarks. The complications of this surgery are as follows: perforation of the bladder, cutting or tying the ureters, bleeding, infection, damage to the sciatic or pudendal nerve or vessels, and perforation of the rectum. Late complications are as follows: urge incontinence that tends to improve with time, vesicovaginal fistula, urinary stress incontinence, rectovaginal fistula, shortening of the vagina, tight introitus, and recurrence (16).

Results

In a series of 152 cases of repair of total uterovaginal prolapse at Georgetown University, there was a 4% failure rate. The failures were recurrence of the cystocele or the vaginal cuff or both. For the first 6 to 10 weeks, 20% to 25% of the patients complained of irritable bladder and some urge incontinence. Only 1% maintained the symptoms after 10 weeks. The Foley catheter is usually removed on the second or third day after the surgery. About 15% of the patients have to go home with the Foley catheter, and then it is removed 7 days later in the office. Three patients had the catheter longer than 8 days. One had the catheter for 3 weeks. This problem with urinary retention is secondary to denervation of the bladder during surgery, swelling, and the elevation of the bladder. The patients are usually very satisfied with the results of the surgery to repair their prolapses. The only restrictions after 6 weeks are to avoid heavy lifting, to empty the bladder regularly, and to do Kegel's exercises.

Summary

Cystourethrocele and symptomatic rectocele may occur in conjunction with uterine prolapse. Total vaginal hysterectomy with anterior and posterior colporrhaphy is required to treat these patients successfully. A sacrospinous ligation will be needed in a case of vaginal prolapse. Remember that proper selection of patients is critical. The surgical tech-

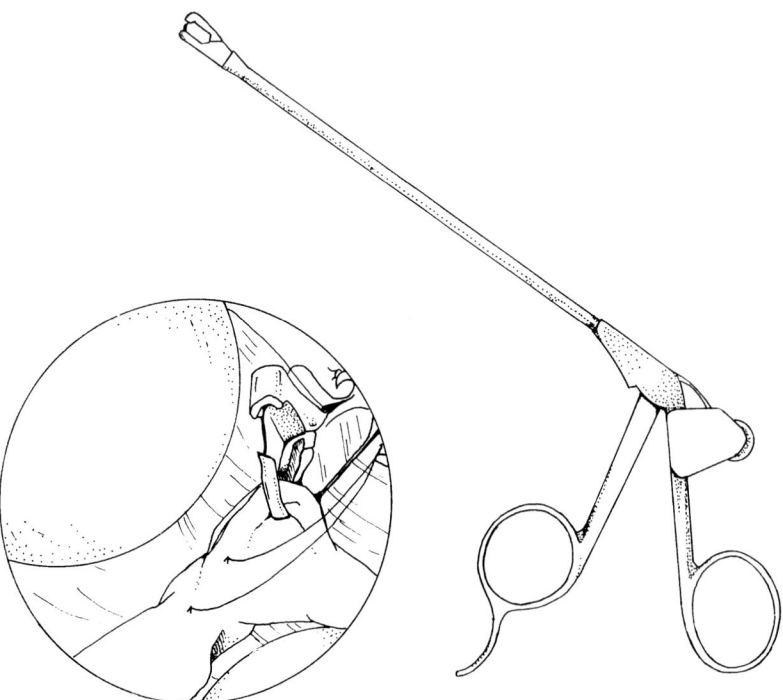

Fig. 14-11 Caspari suture punch. The advantage of Caspari suture punch is that it is much easier to pass the needle through the sacrospinous ligament. A monofilament suture has to be used. A 0 prolene suture makes the procedure safer and faster.

nique described here represents an alternative to the repair of uterine and vaginal prolapse. This technique will minimize bladder trauma, reduce blood loss, and allow for easier identification of periurethral and perivesical fascia. This procedure will eliminate symptoms by restoring normal anatomy and will maintain proper sexual function.

References

1 Timmons M, Addison A, et al. Abdominal sacral colpopexy in 163 women with posthysterectomy vaginal vault prolapse and enterocele. J Reprod Med 1992;37:323.

2 Ahranjani M, et al. Neugebauer–Le Forte operation for vaginal prolapse. J Reprod Med 1992;37:959.

3 Nichols D. Sacrospinous fixation for massive eversion of the vagina. Am J Obstet Gynecol 1982;142:901.

4 Nichols D. Effects of pelvic relaxation on gynecologic urologic problems. Clin Obstet Gynecol 1987;21:759.

5 DeLancey J. Pelvic floor dysfunction: causes and prevention. Contemp Obstet Gynecol 1993;37:68.

6 Sanz L, Holden R, Bourque D. How to repair a vaginal prolapse. Contemp Obstet Gynecol 1984; Special Issue.

7 McCall M. Posterior culdeplasty: surgical correction of enterocele during vaginal hysterectomy. Obstet Gynecol 1957;10:595.

8 Aronson M, Lee R, Berquist T. Anatomy of anal sphincters and related structures in continent women studied with magnetic resonance imaging. Obstet Gynecol 1990;76:846.

9 Morley G, DeLancey J. Sacrospinous ligament fixation for eversion of the vagina. Am J Obstet Gynecol 1988;158:872.

10 DeLancey J. Structural aspects of the extrinsic continence mechanism. Obstet Gynecol 1988;72:296.

11 Symmonds R, Jordan L. Iatrogenic stress incontinence of urine. Am J Obstet Gynecol 1964;82:1231.

12 Mills A. The management of genital prolapse. Ur J Hosp Med 1978;20:586.

13 Telinde R. Prolapse of the uterus and allied conditions. Am J Obstet Gynecol 1966;52:444.

14 Immon W. Pelvic relaxation and repair including prolapse of vagina following hysterectomy. South Med J 1963;56:577.

15 Ranney B. Enterocele, vaginal prolapse, pelvic hernia: recognition and treatment. Am J Obstet Gynecol 1981;34:53.

16 Grody T. The postoperative dysfunctional vagina. Clin Pract Sexuality 1990;7:8.

17 Fuut M, Thompson J, Birch H. Normal vaginal axis. South Med J 1978;71:1534.

18 Nichols D, Randall C. Vaginal surgery, ed 3. Baltimore: Williams & Wilkins, 1989:1.

Chapter 15

Transvaginal sacrospinous colpopexy after prolapse of the vaginal vault

David H. Nichols

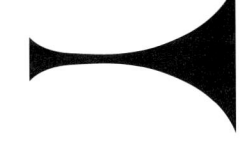

Massive eversion of the vagina and vaginal vault is generally associated with cystocele and rectocele. Enterocele is present 60% of the time, and the uterus may or may not be present. It is important to remember that a dropped uterus is the *result*, not the cause, of vaginal prolapse. Therefore, although coincident vaginal hysterectomy is desirable, the key to treating massive vaginal prolapse is the appropriate repair.

When the cardinal and uterosacral ligaments are evidently strong although considerably elongated, shortening them, attaching them to the vaginal vault, and performing appropriate culdeplasty may afford adequate support. This, combined with appropriate colporrhaphy, may restore the vaginal vault to its normal position near the hollow of the sacrum and reconstitute the normal, horizontally inclined upper vaginal axis.

Indications for transvaginal sacrospinous colpopexy

If the cardinal and uterosacral ligaments have atrophied and cannot adequately support the vaginal vault, as following hysterectomy, the vagina can be sewn to one or both sacrospinous ligaments. This colpopexy with coincident colporrhaphy will provide firm, permanent, and adequate support, will restore vaginal depth and axis, and will ensure sexual function (1; Fig. 15-1).

It is sometimes possible to predict with reasonable accuracy the patient with uterine procidentia who will require coincident sacrospinous colpopexy. This can be achieved by identifying the primary site of weakness as either in the upper or in the lower vaginal supports, with the patient in the lithotomy position on the examining table (as suggested by Victor Bonney). The gynecologist should replace the prolapse within the pelvis and have the patient bear down and observe to see which organs appear first. If the cervix and uterus appear first followed by the rest of the vagina and some cystocele and rectocele, the patient has massive damage to the upper supports of the vagina, particularly the cardinal and uterosacral ligaments, and will probably require hysterectomy *and* colpopexy as part of the primary procedure.

If, on the other hand, the cystocele and rectocele appear first followed by the cervix, the primary damage in all likelihood is concentrated on the supports of the lower pelvis, particularly the pelvic and urogenital diaphragms, and the patient will probably be best treated by a skillful vaginal hysterectomy with colporrhaphy and will not require planning for a probable coincident sacrospinous colpopexy.

Such a procedure is distinctly preferable to total or partial colpocleisis, which results in permanent loss of vaginal coital function. It is also preferable to transabdominal colpopexy, because the latter does not repair coincident cystocele and rectocele, which must then often be corrected by a subsequent secondary procedure.

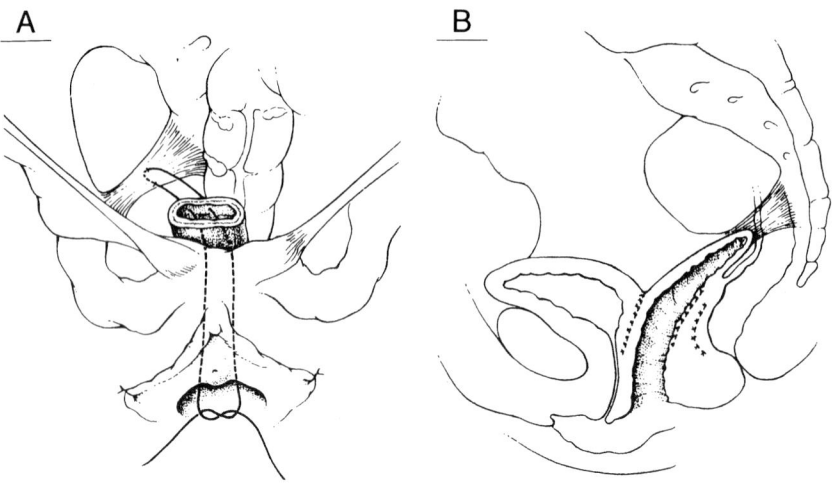

Fig. 15-1 Favorable results of sacrospinous colpopexy. The everted vagina has been sewn to the right sacrospinous ligament one-and-a-half fingerbreadths medial to the ischial spine seen in frontal view (A) and sagittal view (B). Note the restoration of normal vaginal depth and axis. (Reproduced with permission from Randall CL, Nichols DH. Surgical treatment of vaginal inversion. Obstet Gynecol 1971;38:327.)

Transabdominal attachment of an intermediate bridge of plastic mesh such as Mersilene from the vagina to the sacral promontory poses certain risks: damage to the veins of the sacral foramina with troublesome hemorrhage, and erosion into adjacent sigmoid diverticula with subsequent infection and abscess formation necessitating removal of the mesh (2).

Preoperative steps

History

Keep a number of points in mind while reviewing the patient's history. First, massive eversion of the vagina may result when insufficient attention has been paid to supporting the vaginal vault at hysterectomy. Failure to excise an enterocele or peritoneum of a redundant cul-de-sac that may not have been recognized at the time of either abdominal or vaginal hysterectomy may also be a cause of prolapse; so, too, may be clinically increased intra-abdominal pressure related to heavy lifting occasioned by the patient's occupation or work habits. Severity of such pressure may intensify postmenopausally, once hormone support has been withdrawn from estrogen-dependent tissues supporting the vagina.

Although most patients with massive vaginal eversion are multiparous, suggesting an element of obstetric damage, some are nulliparous. There will often be a family history of the disorder, indicating congenital weaknesses. The presence of many abdominal wall striae suggests an inherited connective tissue weakness.

Physical examination

It is important to establish preoperatively all sites of damage to pelvic support so that each may be repaired during surgery. Because gravity intensifies displacement, examine the patient who is awake and standing. The examining surgeon should manually replace the vaginal vault in its normal position and reobserve the findings on pelvic examination noting any cystocele, rectocele, or enterocele. Even if these are minor, they should be repaired coincident with colpopexy, both to improve the end result and to decrease necessity for a separate, secondary procedure. The surgeon should give particular attention to restoring support to the vesicourethral junction (see Chapter 24, Treating Incontinence Transvaginally) as part of anterior colporrhaphy in order to forestall any postoperative urinary stress incontinence.

Anatomic orientation

The sacrospinous ligament, located deep within the coccygeal muscle, connects the ischial spine to the sacrum (3; Fig. 15-2). Locate it by careful palpation of the ischial spine and identify it as a firm ridge running posteromedially toward the lower sacrum.

Although the ligament of both the right and the left sides can be used for colpopexy, bilateral colpopexy does not seem to offer any particular advantage. The right-handed operator will generally find that it is easier to use the patient's right sacrospinous ligament. There are four reasons that one may choose to use one side rather than two:
1 Unilateral colpopexy works anatomically and physiologically—and without dyspareunia.
2 Using one side rather than two decreases the risk of perforation or obstruction to the bowel.
3 Narrowing the vaginal vault at the time of surgery decreases the risk of postoperative enterocele.
4 If the patient has undergone a previous operation, including some resection of the vagina, the residual vaginal vault must be wide enough to be suspended to each sacrospinous ligament, requiring that the vault be wide enough to reach from one side of the pelvis to the other.
To ensure safety, it is generally best to approach the ligament by direct entry first into the rectovaginal potential

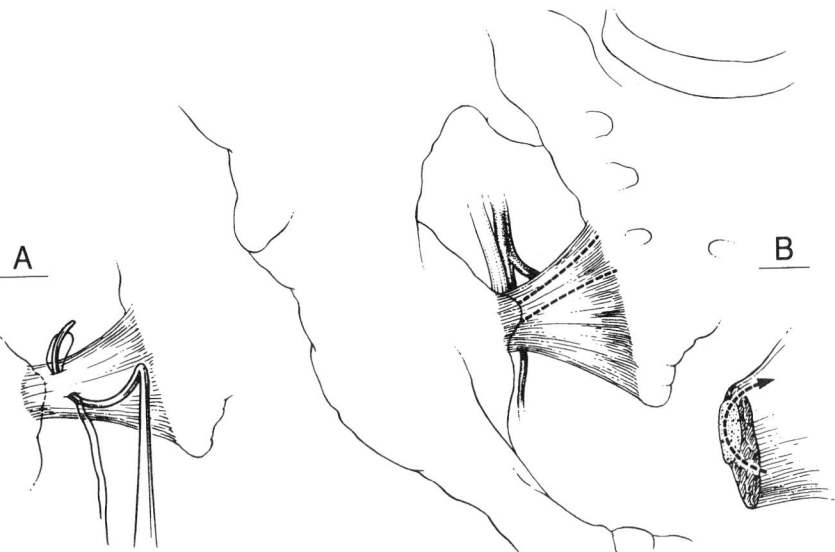

Fig. 15-2 Location of sacrospinous ligament. The dotted line shows the sacrospinous ligament deep within the substance of the coccygeal muscle. To avoid the pudendal vessels and nerves and sciatic nerve, penetration of the muscle and ligament is made one-and-a-half fingerbreadths medial to the ischial spine (A). Also shown is the path of the ligature through the muscle and ligament (B). (Reproduced with permission from Nichols DH. Effects of pelvic relaxation on gynecologic urologic problems. Clin Obstet Gynecol 1978;21:759.)

space, then by penetration and fenestration through the rectal pillar opening into the pararectal space.

To avoid the pudendal nerve and vessels beneath the ischial spine, one must penetrate the coccygeus muscle and sacrospinous ligament at a site one-half to two fingerbreadths medial to the ischial spine, with penetration in a direction perpendicular to those of the fibers of both muscle and ligament, and thus entrance and exit of the needle or ligature carrier are equidistant from the ischial spine.

Operative procedures

Initial exploration

First, incise the perineum and enter the rectovaginal space. Carry dissection the full length of the posterior vaginal wall. Remove a dropped uterus, if present, by vaginal hysterectomy, and carefully note the size and strength of the uterosacral ligaments. If these appear inadequate to support the vaginal vault surgically, excise any enterocele or redundant cul-de-sac and close the peritoneal cavity.

Reaching the ligament

Next, anteriorly displace the cardinal ligament containing the ureter by a suitable retractor. Then displace the rectum to the patient's contralateral side using a straight, long retractor. Identify the ischial spine by palpation and penetrate the overlying rectal pillar, either by blunt dissection or, to overcome resistance, by the tip of a curved Mayo scissors or a sharp-pointed hemostat. The window thus created will expose the right ischial spine and coccygeus muscle.

Expose the surface of the coccygeus muscle, and at a point one-half to two fingerbreadths medial to the ischial spine,

penetrate the muscle and the sacrospinous ligament from below upward with the blunt point of a long-handled Deschamps ligature carrier holding polyglycolic acid (No. 2 Dexon) and a nonabsorbable monofilament suture such as polybutester (0 Novafil) or polypropylene (Prolene).

There should be some resistance to the passage of the ligature carrier. Absence of resistance indicates either that the ligament has not been penetrated at all or, equally undesirable, that both the ligament and the surrounding muscle have been pierced completely and that the ligature carrier has penetrated underlying structures.

Making the ligature

If exposure is adequate, one may grasp the muscle and ligament with a long-handled Babcock clamp and apply gentle traction, which will facilitate penetration by the Deschamps ligature carrier. If visibility is poor because of extensive scarring from previous surgery, first make sure the rectum has been safely displaced to the opposite side.

One may place a second or even third suture through the ligament provided each is always medial to the first, that is, still farther away from the pudendal nerve and vessels. Sew one end of each suture to the undersurface of the vaginal vault at the point chosen for anchoring it to the ligament, but do not tie them yet. If the vaginal wall is thin, one pair of absorbable Dexon stitches may be placed *through* the vagina at the vault. The knot of the absorbable suture will be tied within the vaginal lumen later in the procedure.

Now look at the anterior vaginal wall, and correct any cystocele and rotational descent of the bladder neck by appropriate anterior colporrhaphy (see Chapter 24). When this is done, begin posterior colporrhaphy, starting at the vaginal vault. After closing the vault for its upper 1.5 to 2 inches, tie the

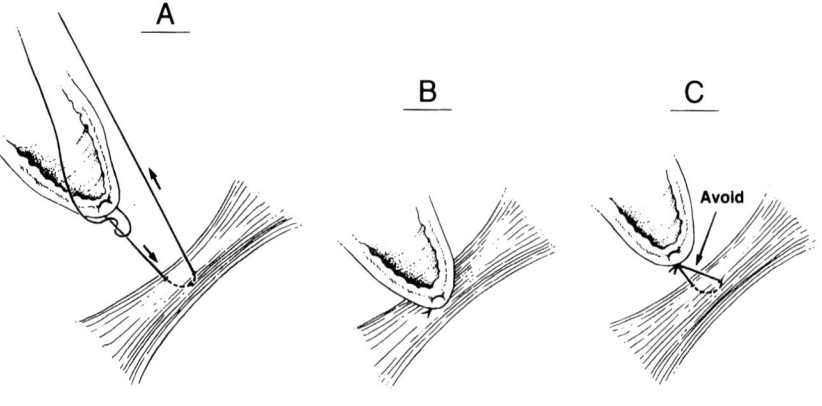

Fig. 15-3 Placing the suture. (A) A suture passed through the sacrospinous ligament is fixed to the vaginal wall by a single half stitch. (B) The movable wall has been brought into direct contact with the ligament and a conventional knot tied. (C) Avoid a suture bridge, as shown. (Reproduced with permission from Randall CL, Nichols DH. Surgical treatment of vaginal inversion. Obstet Gynecol 1971;38:327.)

sacrospinous fixation stitches, bringing the vault to the surface of the coccygeal muscle and sacrospinous ligament (Fig. 15-3). The tissues should clearly be in direct contact with one another, with no intervening suture bridge. Tie all sacrospinous colpopexy stitches, cut the remaining suture ends, and finish the posterior colporrhaphy and perineorrhaphy.

Finally, confirm the integrity of the rectum with rectal examination and, if desired, insert an iodoform gauze pack in the vagina to be left in for 24 hours, but packing is usually unnecessary.

Postoperative considerations

Care following transvaginal sacrospinous colpopexy is the same as for other vaginal reconstructions. The day after surgery, get the patient up and stimulate normal bowel activity by a stool softener and laxative. Duration of hospitalization is generally 5 days.

The principal, though rare, complication, which must be identified promptly, is trauma or ligation of the sciatic or pudendal nerve. In my experience of more than 800 procedures performed since 1968, this has occurred twice early in the series. It is obvious postoperatively when the patient has severe pain down the back of the homolateral leg.

In such an instance, return the patient promptly to surgery and replace the sutures in a safer position. This complication can be avoided by placing stitches precisely in the substance of the ligament and muscle one-and-a-half to two fingerbreadths medial to the ischial spine. To date I have encountered neither hemorrhage nor infection following this procedure.

References

1 Randall CL, Nichols DH. Surgical treatment of vaginal inversion. Obstet Gynecol 1971;38:327.
2 Timmons MC, Addison WA. Pelvic relaxation involving the middle compartment. Curr Opin Obstet Gynecol 1993;5:452–457.
3 Nichols DH. Effects of pelvic relaxation on gynecologic urologic problems. Clin Obstet Gynecol 1978;21:759.

Suggested readings

Bonney V. The principles that should underlie all operations for prolapse. J Obstet Gynecol Br Emp 1934;41:669–683.

Nichols DH. Gynecologic and obstetric surgery. St. Louis: Mosby-Yearbook, 1993:431–464.

Nichols DH, Milley PS, Randall CL. Significance of restoration of normal vaginal depth and axis. Obstet Gynecol 1970;36:251.

Nichols DH, Randall CL. Vaginal surgery, ed 3. Baltimore: Williams & Wilkins, 1989:328–357.

Parsons L, Ulfelder H. An atlas of pelvic operations, ed 2. Philadelphia: WB Saunders, 1968:280.

Richter K. Die operative Behandlung des prolabierten Scheidengrundes nach Uterus-exstirpation, ein Beitrag zur Vaginaefixatio sacrotuberalis nach Amreich. Geburtshilfe Frauenheilkd 1967;27:941.

Symmonds RE, Jordan LT. Iatrogenic stress incontinence of urine. Am J Obstet Gynecol 1961;82:231.

Chapter 16

The Martius graft technique for repair of rectovaginal fistula

Luis E. Sanz and Kenneth Blank

Rectovaginal fistula is a condition of multiple etiology. For the patient, it is a distressing and shameful condition. Its repair, always a surgical challenge, may call for one of many operative techniques. Choice of appropriate method depends on the surgeon's assessment of the size and location of the opening. The specific repair technique we describe is applicable to a wide variety of rectovaginal fistulas.

Uses of Martius graft

Techniques for repairing rectovaginal fistulas include approximation and grafting. In 1932, Martius described a graft involving the bulbocavernosus muscle and overlying fat pad. We prefer this flap for closing fistulas located midway in the vagina when the rectovaginal septum is very thin or markedly scarred.

One advantage of this closure is that it interposes a vascularized pedicle between the vagina and rectum. This buffer prevents direct apposition of suture lines in different tissues. When the procedure is properly executed, risk of recurrence is slight. For a low or midpoint rectovaginal fistula, one must use a vaginal approach, handle tissue gently, mobilize it adequately, excise the fistulous tract thoroughly, and reapproximate accurately and without tension.

Essential anatomy

The bulbocavernosus muscle is one of three paired muscles in the superficial perineal space. It arises from the central tendon of the perineum. Its fibers blend with the sphincter externus of the anus, pass ventrally on either side of the vagina, and are inserted into the corpus cavernosus of the clitoris. The fatty tissues of the labia majora overlie the muscle, which contains the vestibular glands.

The terminal branches of the internal pudendal artery provide the muscle's blood supply. One of these, the dorsal artery of the clitoris, anastomoses with branches of the superficial external pudendal artery in the superior aspect of the labia majora.

Description

Rectovaginal fistulas are classified both by location and by size. Any point along the 10-cm-long rectovaginal septum may be involved.

A fistula's position is important both for determining the repair method and for deciding whether to use an abdominal or vaginal approach. Daniels, as cited by Rothenberg and Goldberg, describes rectovaginal fistulas as low when located on or immediately below the dentate line, with the vaginal opening just inside the fourchette; as high when the vaginal opening is behind or near the cervix; and as mid when the opening is neither high nor low (1).

Daniels calls a fistula small if it is less than 0.5 cm in diameter, medium if it is between 0.5 and 2.5 cm, and large if it is more than 2.5 cm. Most rectovaginal fistulas are less than 2 cm in diameter. Finally, rectovaginal fistulas may be either simple, involving only the vagina and rectum, or compound, involving the bladder, ureter, or bowel as well.

Etiology

Rectovaginal fistulas may be congenital or acquired (Table 16-1). Obstetric trauma from episiotomy, especially a fourth-degree perineal tear, is a frequent cause. Necrosis arising from pressure on the rectovaginal septum during prolonged labor is another source. A foreign body, such as a pessary or a sponge left after surgery, may also erode the rectovaginal septum to produce a fistula.

Fistulas can result, too, from ulcerative colitis and even more commonly from Crohn's disease. Spontaneous development of a rectovaginal fistula should raise the suspicion of Crohn's disease, even when all the other signs of this condition are clinically absent. Any infection involving the septum, especially one originating in the anal or vaginal canal, can produce a rectovaginal fistula. Examples are Bartholin's or cul-de-sac abscess, diverticular disease, tubercular perirectal abscess, and lymphogranuloma venereum.

Incidence of rectovaginal fistula after irradiation for cervical cancer has been reported as between 1% and 10% by White and coworkers (2) and by Rothenberg and Goldberg (1). Most such fistulas develop between 6 months and 2 years after treatment. If one occurs during radiotherapy, a more likely cause is tumor penetrating the rectal and vaginal mucosa. Primary, recurrent, or metastatic cancers causing rectovaginal fistulas are usually colorectal, cervical, vaginal, or uterine.

Finally, leukemia, aplastic anemia, agranulocytosis, endometriosis, and even condylomata have been reported occasionally to produce fistulas, which can lead to septal breakdown from ulceration in the vagina and rectum.

Table 16-1 Types of rectovaginal fistula

Congenital

Acquired

 Traumatic

 Obstetric

  Caused by foreign body

  Operative

  Violence-induced

 Inflammatory

  Bowel disease

  Infectious

 Irradiation-induced

  Neoplastic

  Miscellaneous

Diagnosis

If the fistula is small, the patient may fail to notice flatus from the vagina or a tiny amount of feces in a vaginal discharge. With a slightly larger fistula, complaints of gas leakage or of fecal odor in a discharge are more likely. Passage of the entire bowel contents through the vagina may occur if the fistula diameter is greater than 2.5 cm.

Usually, a low fistula may be noted by spreading the labia. Viewing a higher fistula may require a speculum. Look for feces in the vagina or the dark red rectal mucosa at the fistula's opening.

Identification of a small fistula may prove difficult. In such cases, one may carefully use a small lacrimal probe to define the fistulous tract and permit visualization of both ends. Care must be taken not to perforate the rectal mucosa and create another fistula. Another option is to insert a tampon into the vagina, and a tampon soaked with methylene blue dye into the rectum. If the tampon is unstained after 20 minutes, a fistula is unlikely.

Dye may also aid proctoscopic visualization of the rectal opening. To rule out a fistula to another bowel portion, fistulograms, vaginograms, barium enemas, intravenous pyelograms, or endoscopy may be useful.

Preoperative considerations

Surgical repair is not always needed. Removing a foreign body or successfully treating an infection may allow the fistula to heal spontaneously. Mattingly and Thompson state that 50% of small rectovaginal fistulas heal by themselves (3). They recommend waiting 6 months before attempting surgical repair of one caused by obstetric trauma. However, new information in the literature indicates that with the advent of new antibiotics and better synthetic sutures early repairs can be performed as long as there is no evidence of infection.

When an operation is deemed necessary, first be sure the patient is in optimal physical condition and that any underlying disease has been treated aggressively. Local tissue should be as near normal as possible, with inflammation resolved and the septum returned to its normal soft, pliable state. We advise a wait of 3 months after acute inflammation resolves before undertaking surgery for small fistulas, because they can heal on their own or by placing the patient NPO (nothing per oral) and with hyperalimentation.

We also recommend prophylactic antibiotics, enemas, GoLytely, and vaginal douching (Table 16-2). Give the last enema the night before surgery to avoid the expulsion of fecal matter into the operative field. Place the patient on a clear liquid diet the day before surgery, and give nothing by mouth after 6 P.M. GoLytely should be given the day before the surgery to empty the colon. Proper mechanical bowel preparation is critical to avoid defecation after surgery.

Opinions vary widely about the need for a temporary diverting colostomy. Russell and Gallagher hold it unnecessary in most cases (4), whereas Graham routinely performs

Table 16-2 Preoperative preparation

GoLytely and enema day before surgery

Antibiotics

  Cefotetan, 1 g IV, one hour before the surgery

Diet

  Low residue 7 days before surgery

  Full liquids 2 days before surgery

  Clear liquids one day before surgery

  Nothing by mouth from 6 P.M. on evening before surgery

it (5). We believe a diverting colostomy is not necessary for repair of most simple rectovaginal fistulas. If there is inflammation, perform the colostomy first and defer fistula repair until local tissues are more normal. When inflammation is absent, both procedures can be done at the same time.

Posterior or lateral sphincterotomy is no longer done. It was formerly used by some to prevent a buildup of rectal pressure that was thought to increase risk of recurrence. However, external sphincter muscle repair to halt rectal fecal incontinence may be needed in conjunction with the rectovaginal fistula repair.

Intravenous hyperalimentation or an elemental diet may also be necessary. However, these options are often reserved for the second repair attempt. Central hyperalimentation, which provides mechanical and secretory rest to the bowel, sometimes permits spontaneous closure of small fistulas.

Selection of procedure

The specific method of operative repair will depend on an evaluation of many factors: etiology, location, and size of the fistula, number and type of previous repairs, associated abnormalities, the patient's operative risk, and the surgeon's experience. Regardless of the procedure, good surgical principles with proper preoperative and postoperative management are essential for a successful outcome.

Operative technique

First place the patient in the dorsal lithotomy position. Inject the perineum and the rectovaginal septum with bupivacaine (Marcaine 0.25%) regardless of the anesthesia used for the surgery. This is done to alleviate postoperative pain. Identify the fistula by placing one finger in the rectum and positioning right-angle vaginal retractors laterally (Fig. 16-1; Color Plate 12). Search carefully for any other occult fistulas. Undermine the vaginal mucosa around the fistulous tract for 1 cm (Fig. 16-2). Carefully ligate all bleeding vessels with fine sutures or with electrocoagulation if the bleeding is from small vessels. Then trim all devitalized tissue from the fistulous tract's circumference with Metzenbaum scissors (Color Plate 13).

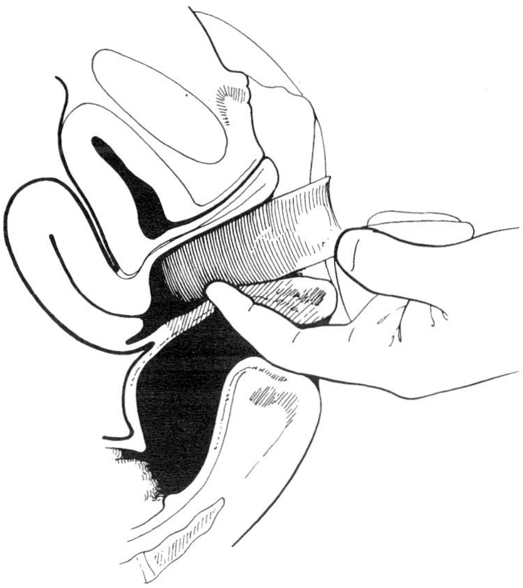

Fig. 16-1 Identify the fistula by viewing vaginally a finger placed in the rectum.

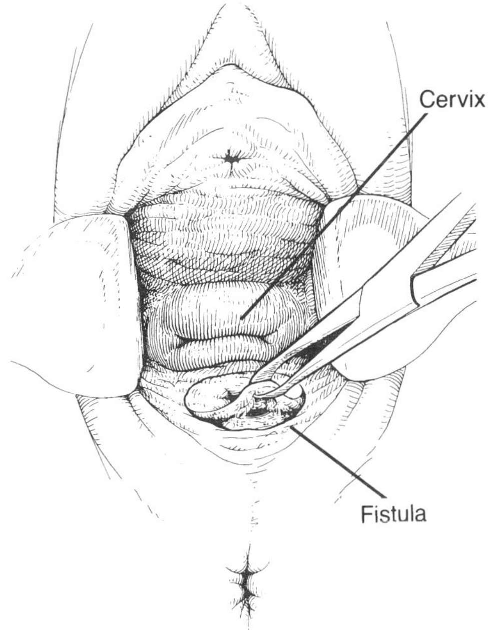

Fig. 16-2 Undermine vaginal mucosa by making an incision around the fistula for a distance of 1 cm. Remove the doughnutlike fistulous tract.

Identify, dissect, and mobilize the rectal mucosa, perirectal fascia, and vaginal mucosa beyond the fistulous tract (Fig. 16-3). Undermine this portion of the vaginal mucosa and separate it from the rectal mucosa with Metzenbaum scissors.

Repair the rectum horizontally with running continuous sutures of 3-0 poliglecaprone 25 (Monocryl) or polyglactin (Vicryl). Do not enter the mucosa. If the fistula is small, one may use a purse-string suture. Approximate the perirectal

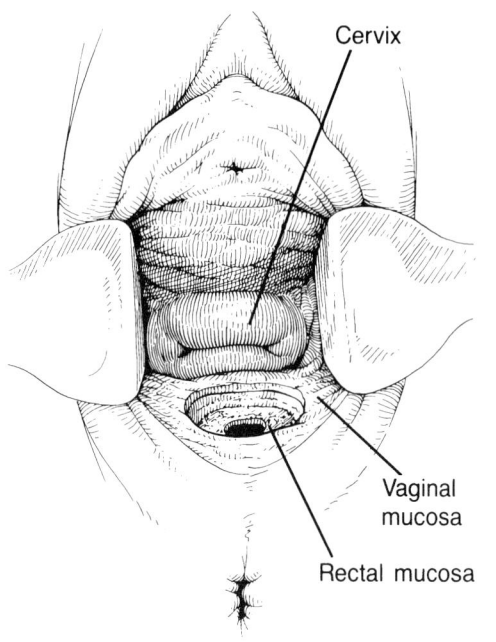

Fig. 16-3 The vagina after excision of the fistulous tract.

fascia with simple interrupted sutures of No. 3-0 polyglyconate (Maxon), or polydioxanone (PDS). If the rectovaginal fistula is small and there is good healthy tissue, then there is no need to do a Martius graft.

Next extend an incision from the vaginal mucosa up toward the labia majora to perform the Martius graft technique. Incise the fat pad and underlying bulbocavernosus muscle, and dissect them free from the skin and underlying fascia (Color Plate 14). Begin superiorly and continue inferiorly to maintain the pedicle's blood supply from the internal pudendal artery, which enters posteriorly (Fig. 16-4). Ligate small perforating branches from the external pudendal artery superiorly, using free ties of No. 3-0 polyglycolic acid (Dexon or Dexon-S) or Vicryl.

Next bring the bulbocavernosus muscle with its overlying fat pad down through the subcutaneous tunnel created. Place it over the excised fistula. The tunnel's diameter should be wide enough to avoid compressing the pedicle. This may compromise its blood supply (Fig. 16-5). Secure the pedicle between the vagina and perirectal fascia with interrupted sutures using No. 3-0 polyglyconate.

Make sure not to place any tension on the fat pad and underlying muscle. Close the vaginal mucosa over the pedicle down to the introitus with a continuous suture of No. 3-0 Monocryl. Then irrigate the labia majora with dilute povidone-iodine (Betadine) and check for hemostasis.

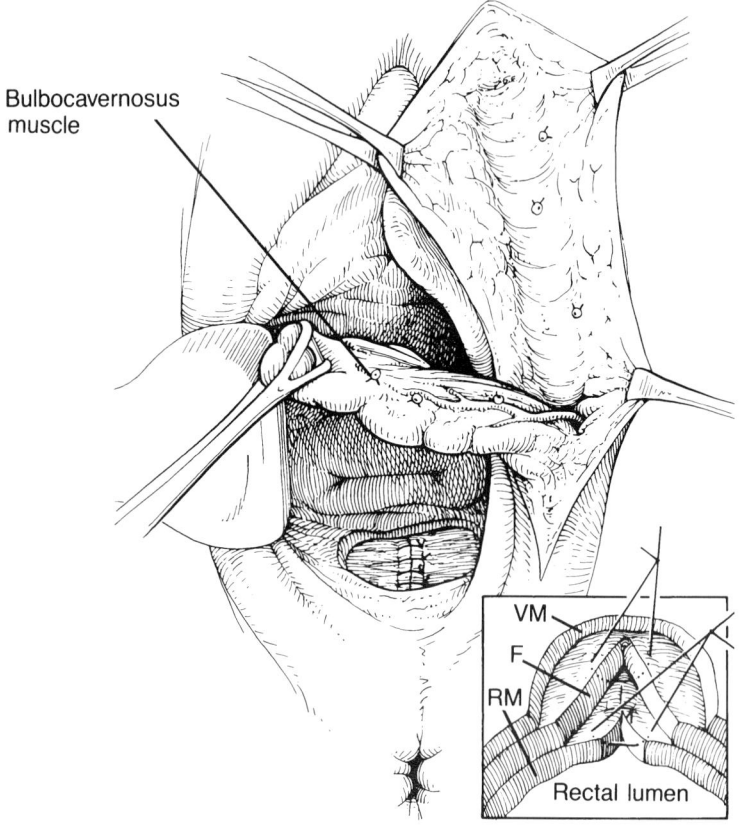

Fig. 16-4 Close the rectal mucosa. Free the bulbocavernosus muscle, taking care to preserve the blood supply. Ligate the branches of the external pudendal artery with free ties. VM, vaginal mucosa; F, fascia; RM, rectal mucosa.

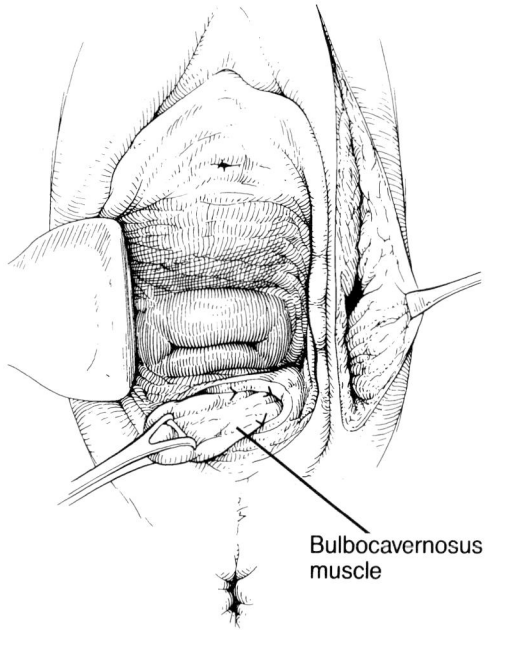

Fig. 16-5 Place the bulbocavernosus muscle over the excised fistula, leaving a tunnel wide enough to avoid compressing the pedicle.

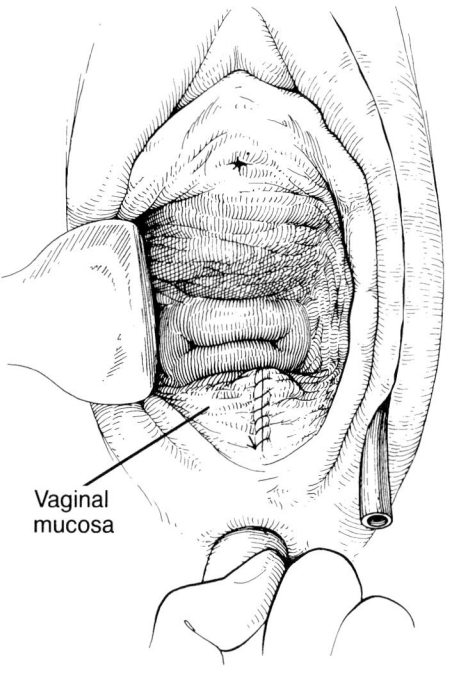

Fig. 16-6 Close the labial skin with a running subcuticular suture. At this point, a finger inserted in the rectum is no longer visible vaginally.

The next step is inserting a drain into the dead space of the labia majora, allowing it to exit from their lower third. Then close the labial skin with a running subcuticular suture of No. 5-0 polyglycolic acid (Fig. 16-6). Finally, one should carefully place one finger in the rectum and one in the vagina to check completion of repair. Avoid connecting the fistula with the perineum by making a cut through the perineum and the anal canal, because a breakdown will result in a case of total incontinence. This is done only in cases of small superficial rectovaginal fistulas close to the introitus.

Postoperative management

Apply an ice pack to the area for the first 12 hours to decrease inflammation. Maintain the patient on clear liquids for 3 days and then place the patient on a caloric diet with Ensure or Sustecal. Prevent constipation by allowing early ambulation and administering a stool softener and mineral oil to soften the stools. The regimen should be tailored to avoid diarrhea and constipation. If the patient has diarrhea, prescribe Diphenoxylate with atropine (Lomotil), 1 tab q.i.d. for 5 to 10 days. Ketorolac tromethamine (Toradol) or codeine can be used for relief of pain in the immediate postoperative period. Start sitz baths on the second day. Remove the drain on the first or second day.

Complications

The most common complications of this surgery are as follows: early and late infections, bleeding and hematoma,

wound breakdown, fistula formation, granuloma formation, and dyspareunia. Infection must be treated aggressively with antibiotics and sitz baths. The patients should be seen on a weekly basis to detect late infection, which is common in this type of repair unlike other types of gynecologic surgery. If there is evidence of abscess formation, one must incise and drain it as soon as possible to prevent breakdown of the repair. If bleeding occurs, one must make a small incision in the vagina to allow it to drain. Granulomas are the result of chronic inflammation around knots. As a rule, these patients should be followed very closely to avoid complications.

Summary

A rectovaginal fistula may result from many causes. Diagnosis may be elusive, and choice of reparative techniques is challenging. Careful evaluation of the problem and proper patient selection are critical. The Martius graft is an easy, safe, and successful means of managing some rectovaginal fistulas. When its use is combined with good surgical technique, the expected recurrence rate will be low.

References

1 Rothenberg DA, Goldberg SM. The management of rectovaginal fistulae. Surg Clin North Am 1983;63:61.
2 White AJ, Buchsbaum HJ, Blythe JG, et al. Use of the bulbocavernosus muscle (Martius procedure) for repair of radiation-induced rectovaginal fistulas. Obstet Gynecol 1982;60:114.

3 Mattingly RF, Thompson JD. TeLinde's operative gynecology. Philadelphia: JB Lippincott, 1985.
4 Russell TR, Gallagher DM. Low rectovaginal fistulas, approach and treatment. Am J Surg 1977;134:13.
5 Graham JB. Vaginal fistulas following radiotherapy. Surg Gynecol Obstet 1965;120:1019.

Suggested readings

Greenwald JC, Hoexter LB. Repair of rectovaginal fistulas. Surg Gynecol Obstet 1978;146:443.

Hibbard CT. Surgical management of rectovaginal fistulas and completer perineal tears. Am J Obstet Gynecol 1978;130:139.

Hodgkins WJ, Park RC, Long R, et al. Repair of urinary tract fistulas with bulbocavernosus myocutaneous flap. Obstet Gynecol 1984;63:588.

Hodgkinson CP. Rectovaginal fistula repair—succeeding on the second try. Contemp Obstet Gynecol 1984;23:93.

Leuchter RS. Management of postexenteration perineal hernias by myocutaneous axial flaps. Gynecol Oncol 1982;14:15.

McCall ML, Bolter KA. Martius gynecological operations with emphasis on topographic anatomy. Boston: Little, Brown, 1956.

Piraka H, Parsa MH, Jahanmir F. Rectovaginal fistula: management by intravenous feeding and surgical repair. Int J Gynaecol Obstet 1978;16:103.

Rock JA, Woodruff JD. Surgical correction of a rectovaginal fistula. Int J Gynaecol Obstet 1982;20:413.

Rosenshein NB, Genandry RR, Woodruff JD. An anatomic classification of rectovaginal septal defects. Am J Obstet Gynecol 1980;137:439.

Zacharon RF. Grafting as a principle in the surgical management of vesicovaginal and rectovaginal fistulae. Aust N Z J Obstet Gynecol 1980;20:10.

In studying the surgical anatomy of the ureter during vaginal hysterectomies, we found that the uterine artery is not the primary factor drawing the ureter closer to the uterus. Traction on the cardinal ligament is the chief factor affecting movement of the ureter; this action protects the ureter. Added protection by the cardinal ligament occurs with bladder retraction and cutting of the uterosacral-cardinal ligament complex, with the ureter displacing to a lateral and superior position. A technique for dissecting the ureter during vaginal hysterectomy is narratively and pictorially described.

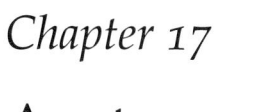

Chapter 17

Anatomy of the ureter during vaginal hysterectomy

Stephen H. Cruikshank and

S. Robert Kovac

Introduction

The relationship of the ureter to the uterine artery during hysterectomy has always been of major concern to the operating gynecologist. The percentage of all ureteral injuries associated with gynecologic procedures has been as low as 0.25% to 3.0% and as high as 30% (1–3). Up to one third of these injuries occur during vaginal (as opposed to abdominal) operations (2,3). Nichols (4) has suggested that the risk of ureter injury during a vaginal procedure is greater because the ureters may be pulled down to the uterus by the uterine artery. This might easily occur if the vesicovaginal space has not been developed adequately. However, Hofmeister and Wolfgran (5) and Kamina (6) have suggested that there is a margin of ureteral safety during each step of a vaginal hysterectomy.

To help avoid ureteral injury, operators performing abdominal procedures attempt to identify the ureters during surgery (7,8). This practice should be incorporated into vaginal procedures. Bilateral vaginal ureteral dissection can be attempted during vaginal hysterectomy (9). Little additional time is necessary, morbidity is minimal, and there have been no deaths.

Clinical observations

Two observations were made suggesting that the ureter is protected during vaginal hysterectomy by mechanisms not previously described. Two patients were evaluated with computed axial tomography (CAT) scans before their hysterectomy for uterovaginal prolapse. These patients were premenopausal and had significant symptoms of uterovaginal prolapse with an attenuated but palpable uterosacral and cardinal ligament complex. CAT scan films were obtained with a tenaculum placed on the cervix in a resting state and under traction. When traction was applied to the cervix, the ureter's position was displaced downward and lateral to the position of the ureter at rest. This movement allowed us to determine radiographically that the ureters were displaced further lateral from the cervix, to a position of surgical safety. We also observed during surgical identifications of the ureter, at the time of vaginal hysterectomy (9), that once the uterosacral-cardinal ligament complex was cut, the ureter actually moved out of harm's way. If the ureters had not been dissected before the cutting of the uterosacral-cardinal ligament complex, it was quite difficult to dissect and visualize them vaginally.

We wondered what brought about the change in the angles of the ureteral catheters noted by Hofmeister and Wolf-gran (5) in the area of the parametrial tissue. The degree of angulation was increased further once the bladder was dissected free, lifting the ureters (to the extent possible) away from danger. To investigate this mechanism more carefully, we investigated the relationship of the ureter to the operative field during vaginal hysterectomy.

General precautions during surgery

We have always considered it preferable for the gynecologic surgeon to see and palpate the ureter during a pelvic operation. Therefore, we ask residents performing such procedures abdominally to open the retroperitoneal space, identify the ureter and vascular structures, and perform a "mock" hypogastric ligation (8). In addition, for vaginal surgery, we have devised a specific technique for dissecting the ureters vaginally.

Vaginal surgery involves the ureters' lower third, which is close to the upper vagina, uterus, and adnexa. Those parts of the ureters near the uterus are especially exposed to injury during surgery (Figs. 17-1 and 17-2).

Symmonds reported that more than 75% of ureteral fistulas resulted from gynecologic operations (10). Of these,

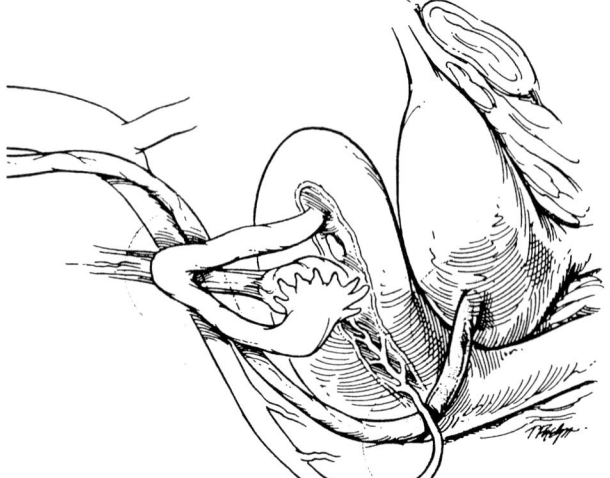

Fig. 17-2 Common sites of ureteral injury are shown in lateral view.

more than 50% were from abdominal hysterectomies. He reported, too, that most genitourinary tract injuries were from straightforward gynecologic surgery rather than complicated procedures.

To help prevent injury during vaginal hysterectomy, observe the following general precautions:
• Avoid blind clamping and suturing.
• Identify the ureters at the time of pelvic surgery and keep them in view (already almost axiomatic in abdominal surgery and appropriate for vaginal surgery as well).
• If necessary, insert ureteral catheters intraoperatively to identify the ureters.
• Obtain an intravenous pyelogram before a difficult pelvic operation.

Ureteral dissection technique

When this method of vaginal ureteral dissection was first attempted, it was performed successfully without complications in 37 of 40 patients (9). Subsequently, we have been successful with the same technique, bilaterally or unilaterally, in more than 300 patients.

However, over the past 4 years it has become more obvious that the ureter moves with cervical traction and is somewhat dependent on the patient's degree of uterovaginal prolapse.

All patients underwent standard vaginal hysterectomy. We began by entering the anterior and posterior cul-de-sacs, thus penetrating the abdominal cavity. Placing a retractor under the bladder to elevate it out of the operative field helped as well to elevate and displace the ureters (Fig. 17-3).

We then explored the abdominal cavity, and also palpated the pelvic sidewalls by inserting one or more fingers through the anterior colpotomy incision. We noted the

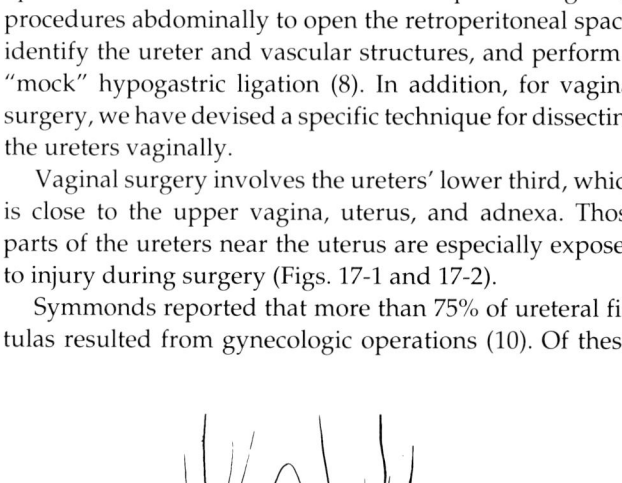
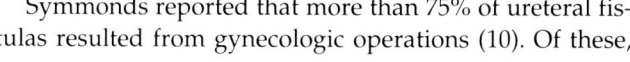
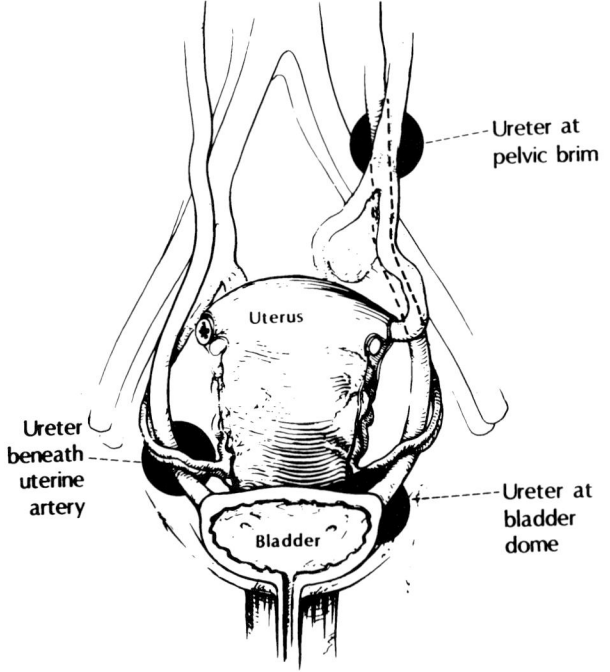

Fig. 17-1 The ureters' lower third, near the uterus and bladder, is especially vulnerable during vaginal hysterectomy.

Ureter at pelvic brim

Uterus

Ureter beneath uterine artery

Bladder

Ureter at bladder dome

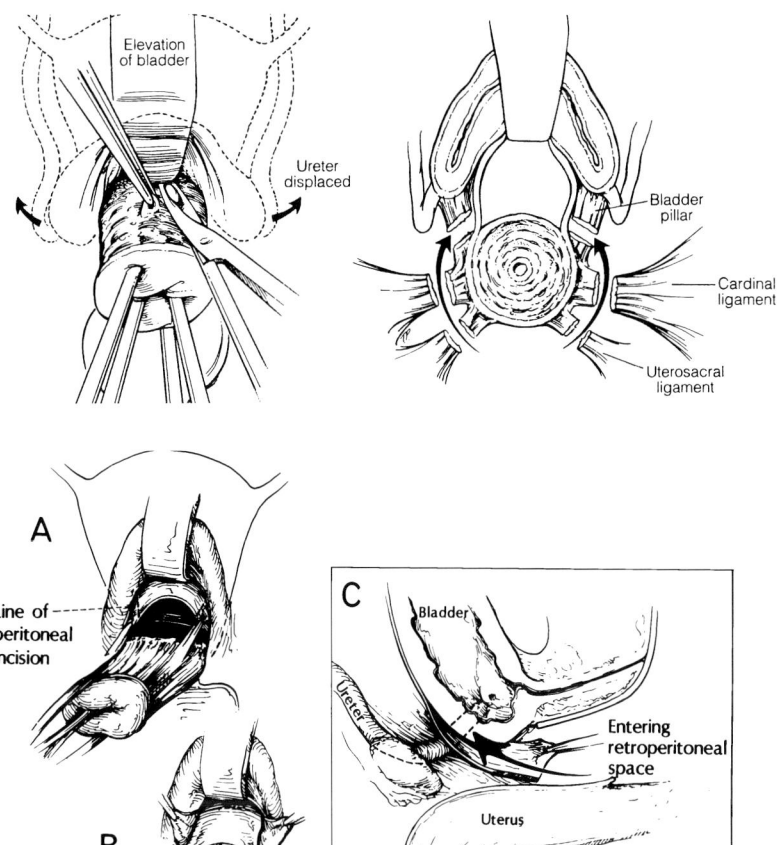

Fig. 17-3 Elevating the bladder out of the operative field with a retractor also helps elevate and displace the uterus.

Fig. 17-4 When approaching the ureters vaginally, pulling the peritoneum toward the surgeon (A) and incising it cephalad (B) permits access to the retroperitoneal space (C).

bladder pillars and identified the infundibulopelvic ligament and its pulsating ovarian artery. Below is another pulsatile structure, the hypogastric artery. Between the two, one can palpate the ureter directly through the peritoneum.

Next, the peritoneum on either bladder pillar was pulled toward the surgeon, undermined with long Metzenbaum scissors, and incised for approximately 5 cm cephalad (Fig. 17-4). In this manner, we gained access to the retroperitoneal space through the vagina.

In performing this step, be sure the scissor tips always point away from the pelvic sidewall to avoid damaging such retroperitoneal structures as the obturator nerve, ureter, and hypogastric arteries and veins. By holding the scissors against the peritoneum while undermining it, and by constantly watching the retroperitoneal space during blunt dissection, one can avoid causing bleeding from vaginal, uterine, middle hemorrhoidal, and vesical veins near the pelvic ureter.

Next place an index finger in the retroperitoneal space to dissect the areolar tissue bluntly. If lateral vaginal retrac-

tion is adequate, one will be able to see the ureters as they enter the bladder base or infundibulopelvic ligament, and cephalad for 3 to 4 cm (Fig. 17-5).

At times, one must perform vaginal hysterectomy without initially entering the anterior cul-de-sac. If so, enter the retroperitoneal space postoperatively and dissect the ureters to confirm absence of damage or make immediate repairs.

We succeeded in identifying the bladder pillars in all patients and in accomplishing retroperitoneal ureteral dissection in more than 90% of cases. Difficulty in seeing the ureters was most common in obese patients, in whom the ureters were concealed by soft tissue dystocia and fat.

Incidences of morbidity and complications were quite low. More than 90% of patients remained afebrile postoperatively. Reasons for fever in the remainder included bladder infection and vaginal cuff cellulitis. Average blood loss with bilateral ureteral dissection was approximately 200 ml, and average operating time was 75 minutes. Figure 17-6 shows lateral views of the ureteral anatomy during abdominal and vaginal hysterectomies.

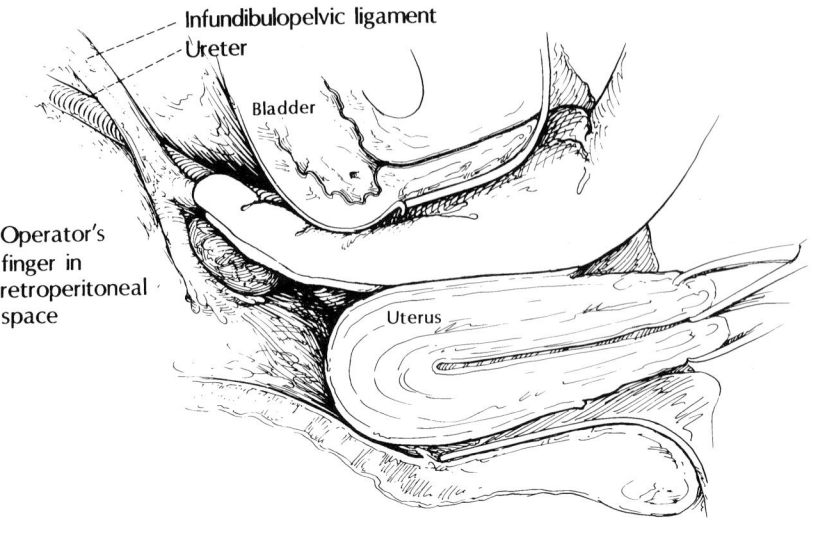

Fig. 17-5 Place an index finger in the retroperitoneal space to dissect the areolar tissue bluntly.

Newer anatomic findings

We studied another group of patients undergoing vaginal hysterectomy for benign disease with varying degrees of uterovaginal prolapse, too. Patients with either moderate or severe uterovaginal prolapse or procidentia were selected. Moderate prolapse was defined as the extension of the cervix to the midvagina or to the introitus with Valsalva's maneuver; severe prolapse was defined as protrusion of the cervix past the introitus with or without Valsalva's maneuver (excluding an elongated cervix) (11). Procidentia was defined as complete prolapse. Forty patients had moderate to severe uterovaginal prolapse and ranged in age from 29 to 65 years. The remaining 20 patients had procidentia and ranged in age from 32 to 77 years.

In patients with moderate to severe uterovaginal prolapse, the ureters were identified by direct vision or palpa-

tion prior to clamping of the uterosacral-cardinal ligament complex. The ureter's position was identified after traction was applied and after each ligament was cut. In the patients with procidentia, the ureters were easily palpated and dissected free because of the procidentia. All ureters were visualized surgically, and their position, as well as the effect of the uterine artery on the ureter, was noted after traction and the cutting of each ligament.

In the first 40 patients, when forceful traction was applied to the cervixuteri and there was no upward retraction on the bladder, the ureter did not move significantly. When the bladder was retracted upward and forceful traction on the uterus was applied, the ureter was displaced cephalad to the pelvis. This finding is consistent with Hofmeister and Wolfgran's observations (5). Once the uterosacral-cardinal ligament complex near the cervix was cut, with upward bladder retraction and forceful traction on the uterus, the

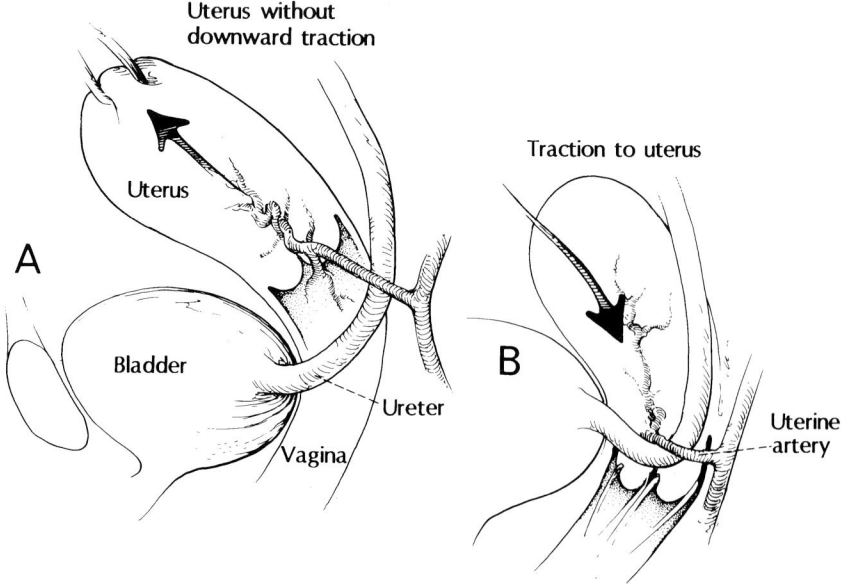

Fig. 17-6 Upward traction in abdominal hysterectomy allows the ureter to escape the operative field (A); downward traction in vaginal hysterectomy (B) makes it more vulnerable in certain circumstances unrelated to the uterine artery.

ureter was pulled away from the operative field and could not be visualized or palpated (Figs. 17-7 and 17-8).

The same operative steps were followed in the patients with procidentia. When forceful traction was applied to the uterus with no retraction of the bladder, the ureter was pulled medially in all 20 patients. The uterine artery was ruled out as the cause of this pulling; the size of the uterine artery was markedly diminished owing to atrophy or arteriosclerotic change and demonstrated no ability to kink the ureter. Rather, the marked attenuation of the uterosacral-cardinal ligament complex and marked absence of ligamentous tissue surrounding the ureter appeared to be the factors that allowed the ureter to be displaced. When bladder retraction was used with forceful traction on the uterus, this effect became less pronounced. When the uterosacral ligaments were cut, the ureter was still visualized or palpable, but once the cardinal ligaments were incised, the ureter was again pulled out of the operative field.

Summary

The uterosacral-cardinal ligament complex supplies blood vessels and nerves and holds the cervix and upper third of the vagina in place over the levator plate. The ureter passes through the cardinal ligament and beneath the uterine artery and vein approximately 1.5 to 2.0 cm lateral to the internal cervical os (1,4). It continues medially for about 2.0 cm, where it crosses the anterior fornix to enter the base of the bladder in the trigone.

We postulate that the uterosacral-cardinal ligament complex plays the major role in determining the ureter's position during vaginal hysterectomy. Range and Woodburne (12) suggest that as traction is applied to the uterosacral-cardinal ligament complex, the loosely arranged connective tissue (including the ureter) within these structures is stretched in the direction of the force applied. Because of the histology of

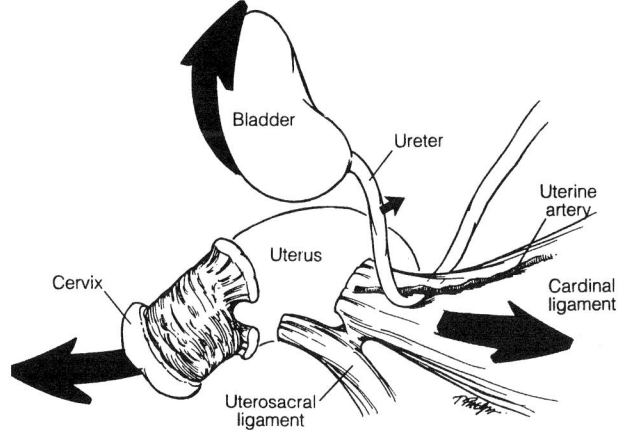

Fig. 17-8 Lateral view. This view shows that the position of the ureter is determined by the uterosacral-cardinal ligament complex, not the uterine artery.

these ligaments and the effect of traction on this tissue, we believe that it is the cardinal ligament that causes angulation of the ureter during vaginal hysterectomy. Once these ligaments are cut, the connective tissue returns to its pretraction state, pulling the ureter out of the operative field.

The precise effect of traction on these ligaments will depend on the consistency of the connective tissue. In our experience, there is considerable individual variation in both the thickness and the length of these ligaments. Uterine size and width will also affect the amount of movement. We believe that the wider uterus will further displace the cardinal ligaments laterally, pushing the ureters in the same direction.

Our observations explain the greater ureteral safety margin that exists with vaginal hysterectomy. Anatomic changes in position due to traction on the uterus, retraction of the bladder, and cutting of the uterosacral-cardinal ligament complex account for this safety margin. The angulation of the ureters noted by Hofmeister and Wolfgran (5) is probably the result of a release-and-elevation phenomenon produced when the uterosacral-cardinal ligament complex retracts toward its origin, the pelvic sidewall.

References

1 Mattingly RF, Thompson JD. Operative injuries of the ureter. In: Mattingly RF, Thompson JD, eds. Telinde's operative gynecology, ed 6. Philadelphia: JB Lippincott, 1985: 325.

2 St Martin EC. Ureteral injury in gynecologic surgery. J Urol 1953;70:51.

3 Thompson JD, Benigno BB. Vaginal repair of ureteral injuries. Am J Obstet Gynecol 1971;3:601.

4 Nichols DH. Vaginal hysterectomy. In: Nichols DH, Randall CL, eds. Vaginal surgery, ed 3. Baltimore: Williams & Wilkins, 1989:182.

5 Hofmeister FJ, Wolfgran RC. Methods of demonstrating measurement relationships between vaginal hysterectomy ligatures and the ureters. Am J Obstet Gynecol 1962;83:938.

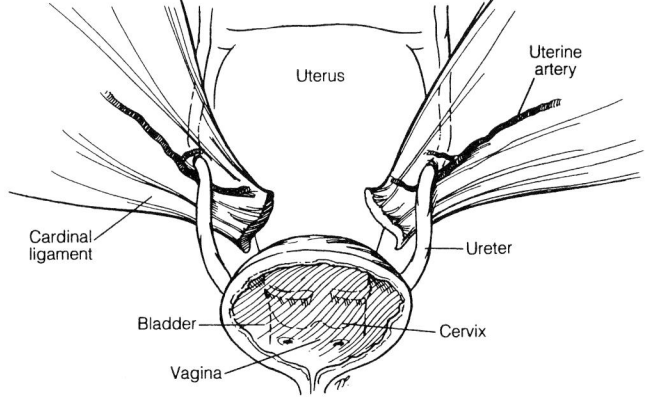

Fig. 17-7 Frontal view. The uterosacral-cardinal ligament complex is cut, and the ureter is displaced lateral and cephalad to the pelvic sidewall. After this complex is dissected, it pulls the ureter away from the operative field, thus protecting it.

6 Kamina P. De l'anatomie a la technique de l'hysterectomie vaginale. Rev Fr Gynecol Obstet 1990;85:435.

7 Thompson JD. In: Nichols DH, ed. Clinical problems, injuries and complications of gynecologic surgery. Baltimore: Williams & Wilkins, 1983:8–10.

8 Cruikshank SH. Retroperitoneal dissection in gynecologic surgery for benign disease. South Med J 1987;80:296.

9 Cruikshank SH. Surgical method of identifying the ureters during total vaginal hysterectomy. Obstet Gynecol 1986;67:277.

10 Symmonds RE Jr. Urological injuries: ureter. In: Schaefer G, Graher EA, eds. Complication in obstetrics and gynecologic surgery. Hagerstown, Md: Harper & Row, 1981:412.

11 Cruikshank SH, Cox DW. Sacrospinous fixation at the time of transvaginal hysterectomy. Am J Obstet Gynecol 1990;162:1611.

12 Range RL, Woodburne RT. The gross and microscopic anatomy of the transverse cervical ligament. Am J Obstet Gynecol 1964;90:460.

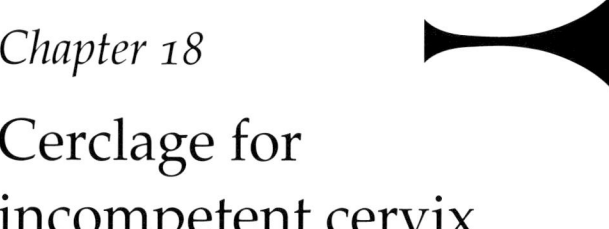

Chapter 18

Cerclage for incompetent cervix

Miles J. Novy

In cervical cerclage, the narrow neck of the uterus is encircled with a nonabsorbable material to prevent midtrimester abortion or premature delivery due to cervical or isthmic incompetence. It usually is done transvaginally. However, patients whose cervices are extremely short, scarred, deeply lacerated, or markedly effaced will benefit more from a transabdominal approach.

Which women are candidates?

Success depends on selecting patients who have a history of painless cervical dilation associated with second-trimester loss, excluding factors other than incompetence, and placing the cerclage early (1,2). There is no evidence that cerclage prolongs gestation or improves fetal survival if it is applied randomly to patients at risk for preterm delivery (3,4). Patients who have had even one second-trimester abortion should postpone pregnancy until thorough clinical examination and a hysterosalpingogram (HSG) have ruled out a müllerian duct anomaly or other intrauterine abnormality.

A diagnosis of cervical insufficiency is strengthened if between pregnancies the cervix is patulous and easily admits passage of a No. 8 or larger Hegar dilator during the luteal phase. In such cases, the HSG may show a uterine isthmic diameter larger than 8 mm.

About two thirds of women exposed to diethylstilbestrol (DES) in utero have abnormal HSGs—commonly showing T-shaped, constricted, irregular, or boxy uterine cavities. But it is still too early to know how many of these women will manifest signs and symptoms of cervical incompetence. Therefore, it is necessary to perform frequent cervical examinations of all pregnant DES daughters and to be alert for incompetence. The application of ultrasonography to diagnose premature cervical effacement and protrusion or "beaking" of the membranes into the internal os has been an encouraging recent development (5). Often these early signs can be detected before cervical changes are palpable by vaginal examination.

Question any patient who has had previous midtrimester losses about upper vaginal or pelvic heaviness or pressure and bloody or watery discharge. These could signal the occurrence of early cervical changes or premature distention of the lower uterine segment.

At our institution, we obtain a cervical culture for aerobic and anaerobic bacteria and *Ureaplasma urealyticum.* Anaerobes are commonly pathogens in chorioamnionitis and *Ureaplasma* are involved in some cases of second-trimester abortion (6).

Also, before contemplating cerclage, exclude syphilis, isoimmunization, abnormal placentation, endocrine disorders, and immunogenetic abnormalities as causes of midtrimester abortion. Use preoperative ultrasound to establish fetal viability and gestational age and to help rule out congenital anomalies. Offer genetic amniocentesis or chorionic villus biopsy as an option for older women and those who have a history of fetal anomalies.

Cervical injury accounts for most incompetence. Extensive conization or amputation of the cervix are other causes. Incompetence may also be congenital, without history of DES exposure, since some patients without history of trauma manifest it in their first pregnancy. Finally, some may be due to premature release of cervical prostaglandins, which seem to promote effacement and dilation of the cervix, or to a lower than normal cervical collagen content (7).

Elevated basal levels of circulating metabolites herald a high level of prostaglandin release after cerclage and help to identify the patient who is at risk for early postoperative complications or premature delivery (8). When the cervix is markedly effaced or dilated, preoperative determination of plasma PGFM and PGFM-II levels may be a useful adjunct to the usual clinical criteria for identifying those patients who are not optimal candidates for cervical cerclage.

Cervical incompetence may coexist with congenital defects of the uterine fundus. Some have recommended cerclage to prevent abortion or premature delivery in the woman with a septate or bicornuate uterus (9). However, in these cases most U.S. gynecologists prefer a Tompkins metroplasty or hysteroscopic resection as the primary procedure, with cerclage as a possible adjunct.

Operative techniques

In 1950, Raoul Palmer in Paris and Abraham Lash in Chicago advocated correcting cervical incompetence in nonpregnant patients by excising a wedge of tissue at the cervicouterine junction and suturing the excised defect. Results, compared with those of current procedures, were unsatisfactory, primarily because of a high incidence of secondary infertility.

Subsequently, the late V. N. Shirodkar of Bombay, India, advocated encircling the incompetent cervix during pregnancy with fascia lata (10). Since then many have attempted to find more suitable permanent ligature material. Barter and associates used a Dacron mesh, and Easterday and Reid a stainless steel wire encased in 26-gauge polyethylene tubing (11,12). Most widely used today is the 5-mm polyester (Mersilene) tape Ethicon RS-21.

Shirodkar method

Common to this method and its modifications is transverse incision of the vaginal mucosa at the anterior and posterior cervical vaginal junctions. The operation is usually performed between 12 and 26 weeks' gestation under halothane or conduction anesthesia, but it may have to be done earlier if the cervix is widely patulous and the patient's history is characterized by early abortions of normal embryos.

Begin by injecting a 1:1000 solution of epinephrine in 20 ml of saline in the anterior vaginal fornix and posteriorly at the level of the uterosacral ligaments. Then make a transverse incision at the cervicovaginal junction and extend it

laterally about 1.5 cm on either side (Fig. 18-1A). Separate the areolar tissue bluntly by spreading the scissors until the glistening vesicouterine fascia can be identified. Then advance the bladder a short distance and retract it, and similarly incise the posterior vaginal wall, taking special care not to enter into the cul-de-sac.

Next use Allis forceps to compress the lateral paracervical tissue containing the blood supply. Grasp the anterior and posterior edges of the cut vaginal mucosa (Fig. 18-1B). This maneuver facilitates the next step—passing a 5-mm Mersilene tape swaged to double-armed tapered needles between the blood vessels laterally and the fibromuscular substance of the cervix (Figs. 18-1B and 18-1C). Tighten this suture as firmly as possible. If the cervix is patulous or dilated, place a finger in the cervical canal to help guide the needle and avoid perforating the cervix or membranes. Verify closure of the cervical canal digitally, taking care that the tape is flat and will not cut through the cervix.

Place a high suture through the cervical fascia and secure it to the tape to prevent the cerclage from sliding downward. If deemed necessary for cerclage, place a second tape above the first one.

Tie the knot anteriorly or posteriorly (Fig. 18-1D). A posterior knot, although easily identified, is hard to secure tightly and may erode through the vaginal mucosa. Let a tail of tape protrude anteriorly from the incision to ease removal before vaginal delivery. Close the anterior and posterior vaginal incisions with interrupted chromic catgut or polyglycolic acid sutures. Neither vaginal packing nor an indwelling catheter is necessary.

McDonald method

First, place a purse-string suture around the cervix without incising the mucosa or advancing the bladder (13). Although McDonald used No. 4 Mersilene, I recommend 5-mm Mersilene tape to reduce cutting through tissue. Then, using an atraumatic needle, insert the suture as high as possible at the cervicovaginal junction while avoiding the edge of the bladder. Take four or five bites with the needle through the mucosa and into the fibromuscular substance of the cervix without entering the cervical canal (Fig. 18-2).

Be especially careful to undermine the blood vessels laterally and to insert the suture deeply on the cervix's posterior aspect, as it is most likely to pull out in this location. Cervical ischemia is not a problem if the lateral blood supply is external to the ligature.

An alternative approach that avoids incisions (*Wurm procedure*) is to place mattress sutures at right angles to each other—at the 12 o'clock and 6 o'clock and 3 o'clock and 9 o'clock positions.

Emergency cerclage

Cervical dilation or herniation of the membranes into the vagina is associated with a poor prognosis; therefore incompetence is best treated prophylactically before the

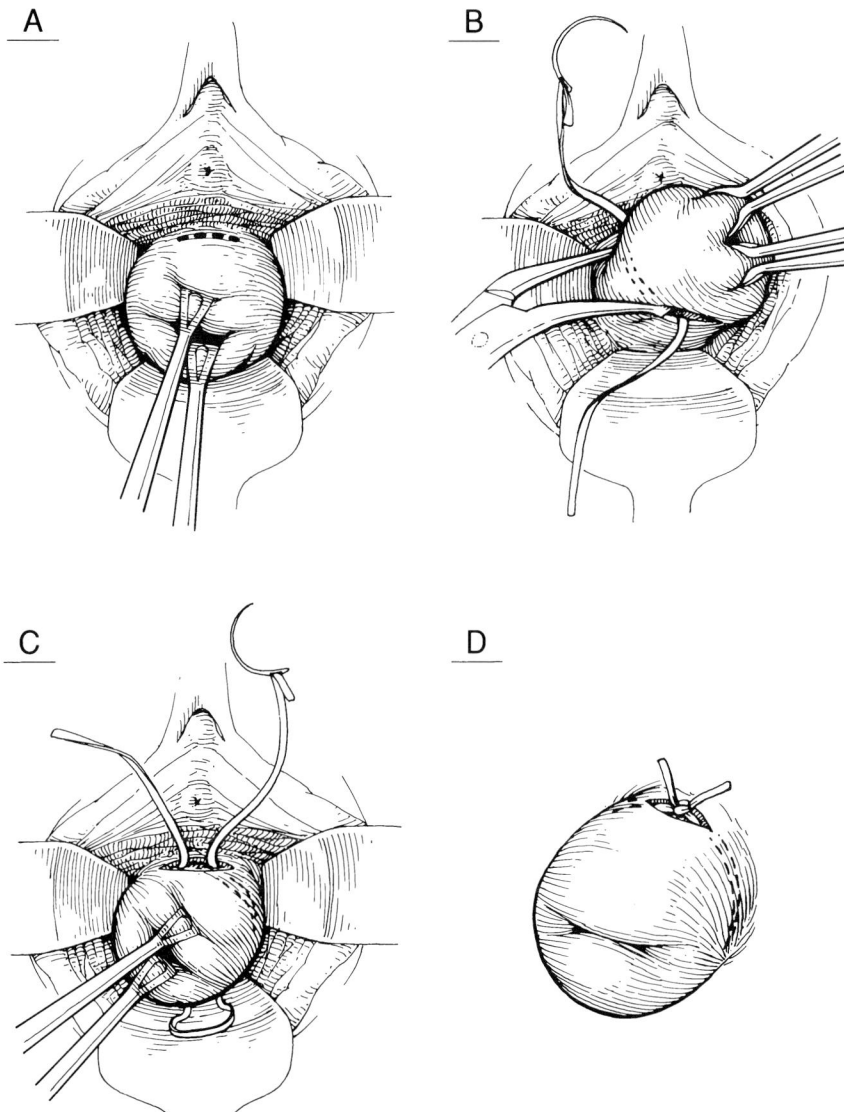

Fig. 18-1 Shirodkar method. Make an incision anteriorly at the cervicovaginal junction (A) and then posteriorly. Next compress the cervical tissue with curved Allis clamps, insert the suture, and bring it out (B, C). Tie the knot either anteriorly or posteriorly (D).

cervix is markedly dilated or effaced (13). However, should emergency cerclage be necessary, one may attempt a modified Shirodkar or McDonald procedure if membranes are still intact, if there is no fetal anomaly, premature labor, vaginal bleeding, or clinical infection, and if dilation is determined to be not more than 4 cm.

Hospitalize the patient at bed rest in the Trendelenburg position and delay surgery until as many of the above conditions as possible are met. Since fetal survival at 28 weeks exceeds 50% in most U.S. tertiary neonatal intensive care units, cerclage is usually contraindicated after 26 weeks.

Put the patient under deep general anesthesia (or after subarachnoid block) in steep Trendelenburg position. The choice of anesthetic is less important than the manner in which it is carried out. Expert care must be given to prevent a Valsalva maneuver during the surgical procedure. Nausea and vomiting or difficulties with intubation and extubation will increase abdominal pressure and promote

prolapse of the membranes. Maintain a full urinary bladder, as it has been shown that distention of the bladder promotes replacement of prolapsed fetal membranes (14).

Prepare the vulva as usual, but because membranes are exposed, simply irrigate the vagina with an antiseptic solution (Fig. 18-3A). If the membranes are not prolapsed, it is preferable to perform a cerclage by the Shirodkar technique. Because the thin cervical edges are friable and tear easily, it is advisable to apply traction to the cervix with Babcock forceps placed at the cervicovaginal junction. Insertion of the Mersilene band in the lateral paracervical tissue by the Shirodkar method reduces the risk of accidental perforation of the membranes. Additional support and elongation of the cervix can be achieved by placing a second higher Shirodkar stitch after each initial one is tied and used as a marker and traction device. The risk of membrane perforation or suture erosion into the cervical canal is greater when the cervix is markedly effaced, regardless of

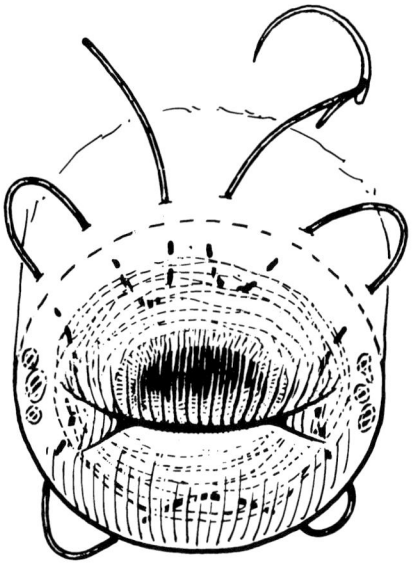

Fig. 18-2 McDonald method. Insert the suture or Mersilene band into the substance of the cervix without entering the canal and beneath the blood vessels laterally.

the cerclage method used. However, the McDonald technique is somewhat riskier under these conditions because it requires multiple entries into the cervical substance.

If the membranes are completely prolapsed and the Shirodkar method is not technically feasible, then attach six to eight cervical stay sutures of No. 0 Mersilene (or similar material) to the margins of the effaced cervix with a free needle "Saskatchewan" procedure (Fig. 18-3B) (15).

Exert traction on the stay sutures to move protruding membranes back into the uterine cavity or push them back gently with a sponge-holding forceps covered by a condom or a finger cot (Fig. 18-3B). If membranes are not completely prolapsed, one may push them higher into the uterus by inserting a deflated 30-ml Foley balloon catheter through the external os and slowly filling the balloon with water to displace the forewaters above the level of the internal os. After placing cerclage with the catheter in situ, deflate the balloon and withdraw the catheter.

When all else fails to reduce herniated membranes, insert an amniocentesis needle suprapubically or under ultrasonic guidance and withdraw several hundred cubic centimeters of amniotic fluid (16). Ensure uterine relaxation either by deep halothane anesthesia or with tocolytic agents, such as 0.25 mg of terbutaline sulfate administered subcutaneously.

With membranes displaced upward and protected from accidental perforation, place two rows of No. 1 Mersilene or similar encircling purse-string sutures as high as possible into the substance of the effaced cervix (Fig. 18-3C). Tighten these sutures and tie the knot anteriorly. Remove half the stay sutures and tie the others across the external os to close the cervix effectively (Fig. 18-3D).

Transabdominal cervicoisthmic approach

Indications include a congenitally short, surgically amputated, markedly scarred, deeply notched, or multiply defective cervix, unhealed penetrating forniceal lacerations, subacute cervicitis, extensive conization, a previous failed vaginal approach, or effacement precluding high placement of cerclage vaginally (17,18).

Pfannenstiel entry into the peritoneal cavity provides adequate exposure for cerclage placement at 12 to 15 weeks' gestation. However, a vertical incision is advisable thereafter. Divide the peritoneal reflection transversely and advance the bladder.

Identify the space between the ascending and descending branches of the uterine arteries lateral to the cervicouterine junction. Develop it carefully by blunt dissection medially to the uterine arteries and veins and laterally to the connective tissue of the uterine isthmus. Long right-angle forceps with tapered jaws are ideal for this step. Have an assistant provide firm upward traction on the uterine fundus to expose the internal os and tense the vessels.

After developing a 1- to 2-cm tunnel in the avascular space, puncture the broad ligament's posterior leaf with right-angle forceps. Pass a 15-cm segment of 0.5-cm Mersilene tape through the aperture under direct vision to prevent slippage of the forceps or inclusion of tissue with ribbon and consequent laceration of thin-walled veins. Perform the identical procedure on the contralateral side.

Next pass the Mersilene band around the uterine isthmus and over the posterior peritoneum at the level of the uterosacral ligament insertions. Make sure the band lies flat, fits snugly, and compresses intervening tissue. Secure it anteriorly with a single knot, fix the cut ends to the band with nonabsorbable sutures, and close the peritoneum and abdomen.

To perform the modification of this technique described by Mahran, elevate the uterus from the abdominal cavity (19). Then palpate the uterine vessels and pull them laterally away from the isthmus.

Pass the needle and tape around the isthmus, keeping as close to the uterine wall as possible. Then puncture the broad ligament's posterior leaf just medial to the uterosacral ligament attachment on both sides, draw the tape tightly, and tie it either posteriorly or anteriorly. Palpation of the cerclage and its position relative to cervical length is easier during vaginal examinations on subsequent prenatal visits if the knot is placed anteriorly; erosion of the bladder wall by the knot has not been observed in the author's experience. Place a moist laparotomy sponge in the posterior pelvis to protect the bowel and surrounding major vessels from injury by the needle or retractors.

The Mahran approach has been used successfully by the author in six consecutive patients between 11 and 13 weeks' gestation without significant blood loss.

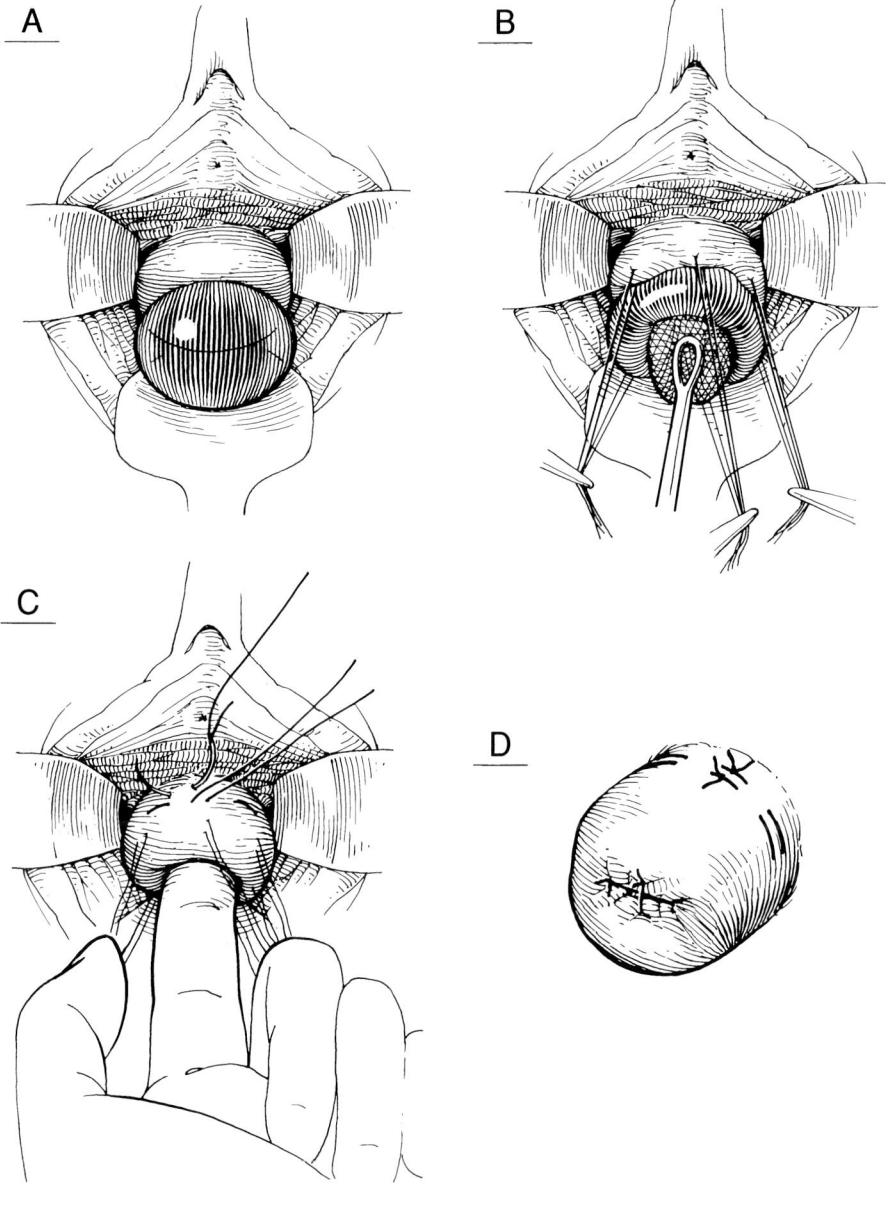

Fig. 18-3 Emergency cerclage. Membranes are shown herniating through an effaced and partially dilated cervix (A). Insert stay sutures, exert traction to move the bulging membranes back into the uterus (B), and place two rows of encircling sutures (C). Remove half of the stay sutures and tie the remaining ones across the external ones to close the cervix (D). (Adapted with permission from Olatunbosun OA, Dyck F. Cervical cerclage operation for a dilated cervix. Obstet Gynecol 1981;57:166.)

Postoperative care

Monitor for evidence of uterine irritability. This is uncommon unless there has been marked effacement or dilation of the cervix.

Do not routinely give prophylactic hormones, uterine relaxants, or antibiotics. Allow the patient's history, gestational age, and degree of uterine activity to dictate whether to use tocolytic agents. Routine administration of prostaglandin inhibitors is not indicated for transvaginal or transabdominal cervicoisthmic cerclage since circulating prostaglandin metabolite levels subside rapidly after surgery and the magnitude of the increase does not correlate with gestational age, with mild to moderate cervical changes, or with fetal survival (8). Conversely, the patient with advanced premature cervical dilation or effacement who demonstrates an elevation in circulating prostaglandin (PG) metabolites might benefit from PG inhibition if a minimal risk-to-benefit ratio has been established (20).

The patient can get up to go to the toilet, but should otherwise lie supine for 24 hours. If the cervix was significantly dilated, insert an indwelling urinary catheter and extend bedrest. Follow bedrest with in-hospital ambulation before discharge.

If the postoperative course is smooth, do not limit physical activity but discourage strenuous exercise. It is unknown whether intercourse or orgasm involve risks, but it is prudent to advise patients to abstain from intercourse. Do weekly cervical examinations and periodic ultrasound scans, and tell the patient to immediately report any signs of premature labor.

Complications

More frequent after emergency than after elective cerclage, complications include hemorrhage, rupture of membranes, chorioamnionitis, suture erosion, premature labor and delivery, and cervical dystocia after the band has been removed (2). Incidence of premature rupture of membranes, chorioamnionitis, and intrauterine infection increases three-fold for cerclage performed after the 20th week, and prophylactic antibiotics are recommended when it is done after the 18th week (21). However, incidence of sepsis does not differ between the Shirodkar and McDonald techniques (22).

A potential complication of the transabdominal approach is blood loss extensive enough to require transfusion. Use hemostatic clips and suture ligatures to achieve hemostasis following laceration of thin-walled parametrial veins.

Premature labor and delivery remain major complications with all techniques. Rare complications are uterine rupture, maternal septicemia, and vesicovaginal fistulas. One can prevent or treat all of them but should always balance management exigencies against the patient's desire to have a mature live baby.

Although a higher cesarean section rate has been reported after the Shirodkar procedure, most patients can have a normal vaginal delivery after transvaginal cerclage (1). However, after transabdominal cervicoisthmic cerclage, the usual delivery method has been elective cesarean section near term. Leave the tape in place, as bleeding will follow forceful attempts to remove it.

Moreover, the patient may desire future pregnancies. If premature labor unresponsive to therapy occurs shortly after transabdominal cerclage, visualize and cut the band by performing posterior colpotomy.

Success rate of cervical cerclage

Although the broad consensus is that cervical cerclage has been successful when patients are properly selected, a few obstetricians remain skeptical. In most reported series, fetal survival ratios before cerclage are 20% to 30% and afterwards are 70% to 90% (Table 18-1).

In 1984, Rush and coworkers. (23) from South Africa reported a prospective randomized trial of cervical cerclage in 194 women at risk for preterm delivery. There was no significant difference in perinatal outcome between the two groups; the cervical cerclage group experienced a higher rate of hospitalization and tocolytic therapy. Lazar and colleagues. (24) from France also presented a randomized, prospective study of 506 patients at risk for preterm delivery with similar results. Both studies are flawed in several important respects. First, they excluded patients who had "obvious cervical incompetence" by history or anatomic abnormalities. Second, they had a variable time of registration of their patients. In one study, patients were admitted up to 28 weeks' gestation, and the results were

not clearly separated according to the trimester in which the cerclage was applied. It was not clear whether the decision to intervene surgically was based on preexisting factors or on evolving cervical changes. A tendency for selection bias was noted in that patients allocated to the cerclage groups had had more previous abortions or adverse pregnancy outcomes. If the results of these two studies are accepted at face value, one might conclude that cerclage is a relatively safe procedure and does not predispose to preterm delivery even when applied to patients who are not in all respects ideal candidates.

Harger reported that, regardless of technique, fetal survival was better after elective than after emergency cerclage (1). Once dilation has begun and the membranes protrude, one can anticipate a success rate of less than 50% (9).

Most studies (all retrospective) show no significant difference in fetal survival following McDonald's as opposed to Shirodkar's procedure. However, evidence suggests the rate of premature births is lower after an elective Shirodkar than after an elective McDonald purse-string cerclage (1).

I recommend the Shirodkar procedure when technically feasible because it provides a stronger circumferential support of the internal os by higher placement of the encircling suture. Also, sutures are less likely to erode into the cervical canal. The McDonald procedure, which is easier to perform, may be used when there is significant cervical effacement.

The combined series shows excellent results for transabdominal cervicoisthmic cerclage (Table 18-1). One reason may be that all patients had an anatomically well-defined syndrome and a history of multiple late fetal loss. In several patients who had had normal deliveries earlier but experienced repeated loss after a traumatic event, such as cervical amputation, successful pregnancy followed the performance of this procedure (18).

A more basic reason for the success of transabdominal cervicoisthmic cerclage may be that it provides the stronger circumferential support of the isthmus. Decreased slippage of the band is achieved abdominally by placing the ribbon above the cardinal and uterosacral ligaments. Substantiating this view is the observation that 50% of the patients in the combined series experienced pregnancy failure after a transvaginal procedure, while none did after the transabdominal one (18).

A successful cerclage holds a distensible cervix closed, but does not prevent the ripening process. To partially restore resistance normally provided by the intact collagenous cervix, place a band at the cervicouterine junction.

It is evident that patients who undergo cerclage represent a heterogeneous group. Epidemiologic data have linked several genitourinary pathogens (e.g., *Ureaplasma urealyticum, Chlamydia trachomatis,* Group B streptocci, *Gardnerella vaginalis,* and associated anaerobic bacteria), with premature uterine contractions, cervical ripening, and rupture of the fetal membranes (25). Many of these microor-

Table 18-1 Treatment results

	Fetal survival before treatment		Fetal survival after treatment		
	No. of pregnancies	*Survivors (%)*	*No. of pregnancies*	*Survivors (%)*	*Fetal salvage ratio**
Transabdominal cervicoisthmic cerclage					
Benson and					
Durfee, (17) 1965†	47	11	11	82	7.45
Watkins, 1972	9	44	2	100	2.27
Novy, 1981	55	24	22	95	3.96
Transvaginal uterosacral-cardinal ligament cerclage					
Ritter, 1978†	134	22	54	98	4.45
Shirodkar method					
Cousins, (7) 1980†	1957	22‡	898	82‡	3.78
McDonald purse-string method					
Cousins, 1980†	751	27‡	272	74‡	2.71

*Percentage of survivors after treatment divided by percentage of survivors before treatment.
†First-trimester abortions not uniformly excluded.
‡Average results based on review of the literature.

ganisms are able to produce phospolipase A_2, an enzyme capable of initiating prostaglandin synthesis by cleaving arachidonic acid from phospholipids (26). According to this hypothesis either the presence of phospholipase-containing organisms in the decidua or fetal membranes directly produces prostaglandins, or the prostaglandins are released secondarily as a result of the local inflammation.

A combined approach of antibiotic prophylaxis or treatment and cerclage to prevent increasing ascending infection may be an appropriate treatment for a subgroup of patients. This idea requires testing in a prospective clinical trial. Application of new imaging techniques together with bacteriologic screening and possibly prostaglandin metabolite measurements should result in more specific and objective criteria for performing cervical cerclage.

References

1 Harger JH. Comparison of success and morbidity in cervical cerclage procedures. Obstet Gynecol 1980;56:543.

2 Thomason JL, Sampson MB, Beckman CR, et al. The incompetent cervix. J Reprod Med 1982;27:187.

3 Lazar P, Gueguen S, Dreyfus J, et al. Multicentered controlled trial of cervical cerclage in women at moderate risk of preterm delivery. Br J Obstet Gynaecol 1984;91:731.

4 Rush RW, Isaacs S, McPherson K, et al. A randomized controlled trial of cervical cerclage in women at high risk of spontaneous preterm delivery. Br J Obstet Gynaecol 1984;9:724.

5 Michaels WH, Montgomery C, Karo J, et al. Ultrasound differentiation of the competent from the incompetent cervix: prevention of preterm delivery. Am J Obstet Gynecol 1986;154:537.

6 Knudsin RB, Driscoll SG. Mycoplasmas and human reproductive failure. Surg Gynecol Obstet 1970;131:89.

7 Cousins L. Cervical incompetence, 1980: a time for reappraisal. Clin Obstet Gynaecol 1980;23:467.

8 Novy MJ, Ducsay CA, Stanczyk FZ. Plasma concentrations of prostaglandin $F_{2\alpha}$ and prostaglandin E_2 metabolites after transabdominal and transvaginal cervical cerclage. Am J Obstet Gynecol 1987;156:1543.

9 Abramovici H, Faktor JH, Pascal B, et al. Congenital uterine malformations as indication for cervical suture (cerclage) in habitual abortion and premature delivery. Int J Fertil 1983;28:161.

10 Shirodkar VN. A new method of operative treatment for habitual abortions in the second trimester of pregnancy. Antiseptic 1955;52:299.

11 Barter RH, Dusbabek JA, Tyndal CM, et al. Further experiences with the Shirodkar operation. Am J Obstet Gynecol 1963;85:792.

12 Easterday CL, Reid DE. The incompetent cervix in repetitive abortion and premature labor. N Engl J Med 1959;260:687.

13 McDonald IA. Cervical cerclage. Clin Obstet Gynaecol 1980;7:161.

14 Scheerer LJ, Lam F, Katz M. A new technique for cervical cerclage in the presence of prolapsed fetal membranes [abstract 144]. Proceedings from the 7th Annual Meeting of the Society of Perinatal Obstetricians, February 5–7, 1987, Lake Buena Vista, Florida.

15 Olatunbosun OA, Dyck F. Cervical cerclage operation for a dilated cervix. Obstet Gynecol 1981;57:166.

16 Goodlin RC. Cervical incompetence, hour-glass membranes and amniocentesis. Obstet Gynecol 1979;54:748.

17 Benson RC, Durfee RB. Transabdominal cervicouterine cerclage during pregnancy for the treatment of cervical incompetency. Obstet Gynecol 1965;25:145.

18 Novy MJ. Transabdominal cervicoisthmic cerclage for the management of repetitive abortion and premature delivery. Am J Obstet Gynecol 1982;143:44.

19 Mahran M. Transabdominal cervical cerclage during pregnancy. Obstet Gynecol 1978;52:502.

20 Repke JT, Niebyl JR. Role of prostaglandin synthetase inhibitors in the treatment of preterm labor. Semin Reprod Endocrinol 1985;3:259.

21 Charles D, Edwards WR. Infectious complications of cervical cerclage. Am J Obstet Gynecol 1981;141:1065.

22 Kuhn RJP, Pepperell RJ. Cervical ligation: a review of 242 pregnancies. Aust N Z J Obstet Gynaecol 1979;17:79.

23 Rush RW, Isaacs S, McPherson K, et al. A randomized controlled trial of cervical cerclage in women at high risk of spontaneous preterm delivery. Br J Obstet Gynaecol 1984;91:724.

24 Lazar P, Guegen S, Dreyfus J, et al. Multicentered controlled trial of cervical cerclage in women at moderate risk of preterm delivery. Br J Obstet Gynaecol 1984;91:731.

25 Gravett MG, Hummel D, Eschenbach DA, et al. Preterm labor associated with subclinical amniotic fluid infection and with bacterial vaginosis. Obstet Gynecol 1986;67:229.

26 Bejar R, Curbelo V, Davis C, et al. Premature labor. II. Bacterial sources of phospholipase. Obstet Gynecol 1981;57:479.

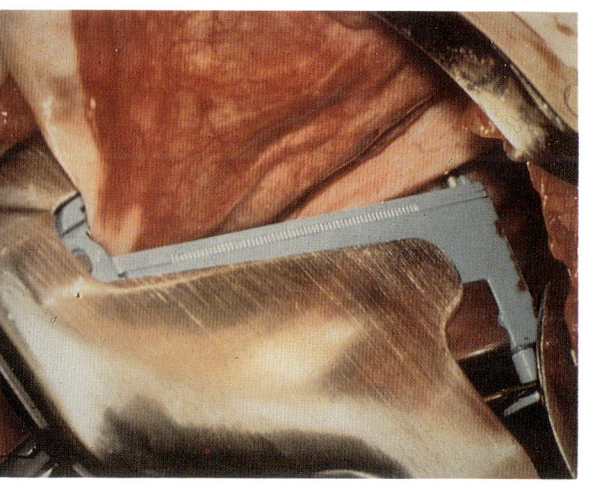

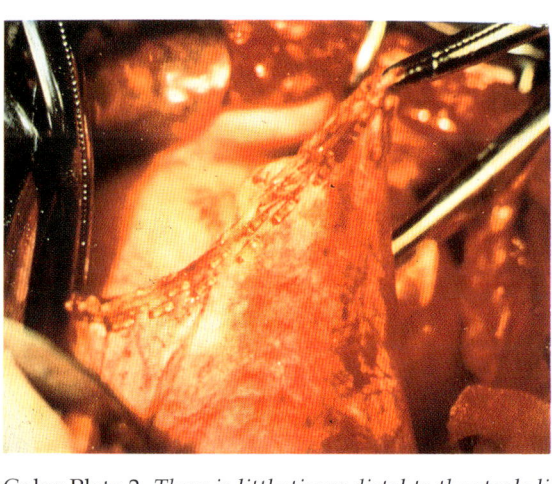

Color Plate 1 *The stapler is applied over the uterosacral ligament, the broad ligament and the round ligament.*

Color Plate 2 *There is little tissue distal to the staple line and no bunching up of pedicles.*

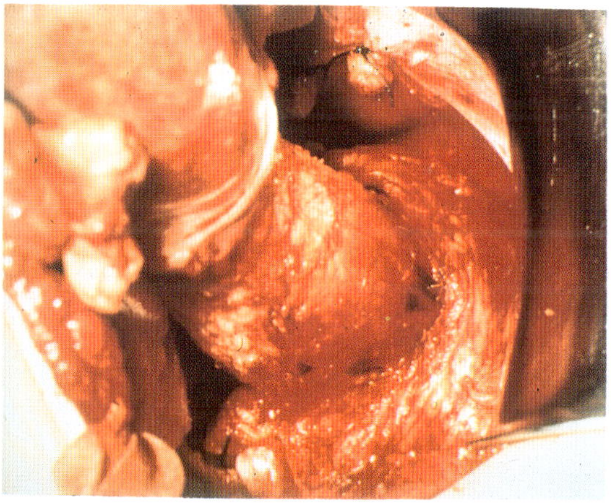

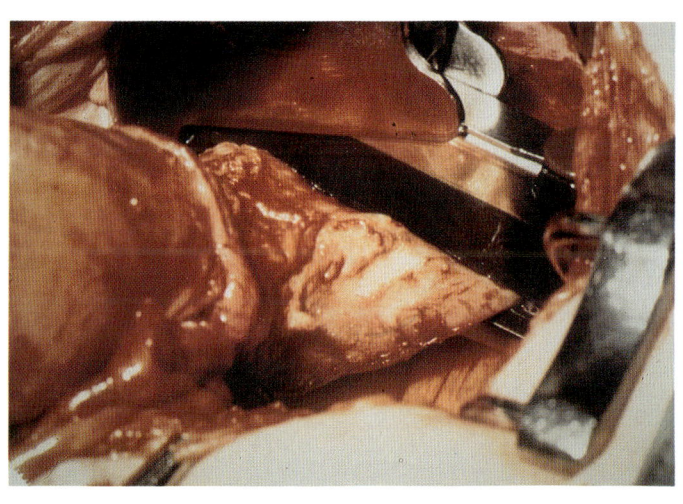

Color Plate 3 *The cervix and upper vagina are now prepared for application of the TA 55 premium instrument with PAS.*

Color Plate 4 *The cartridge is in place before firing.*

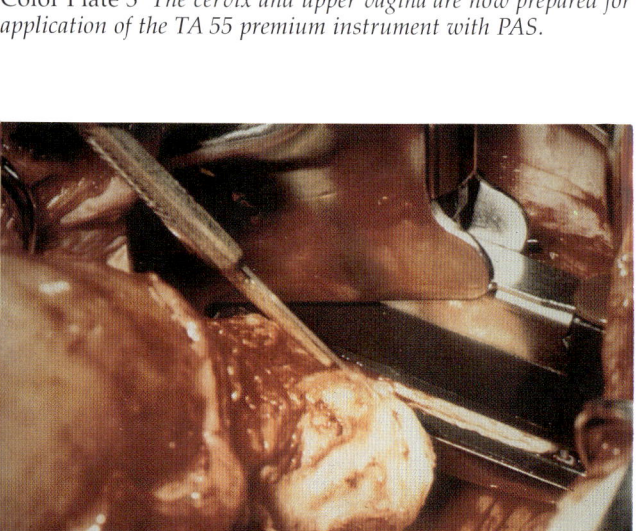

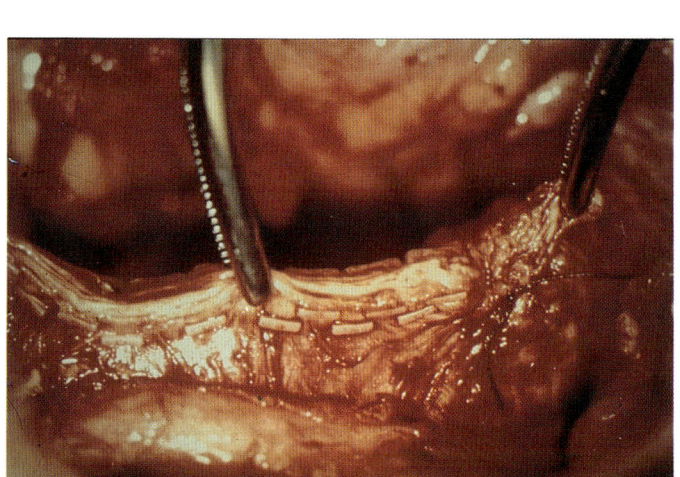

Color Plate 5 *A scalpel is used to divide the vaginal vault close to the cartridge edge.*

Color Plate 6 *A double row of PAS closes the vaginal vault uniformly and hemostatically.*

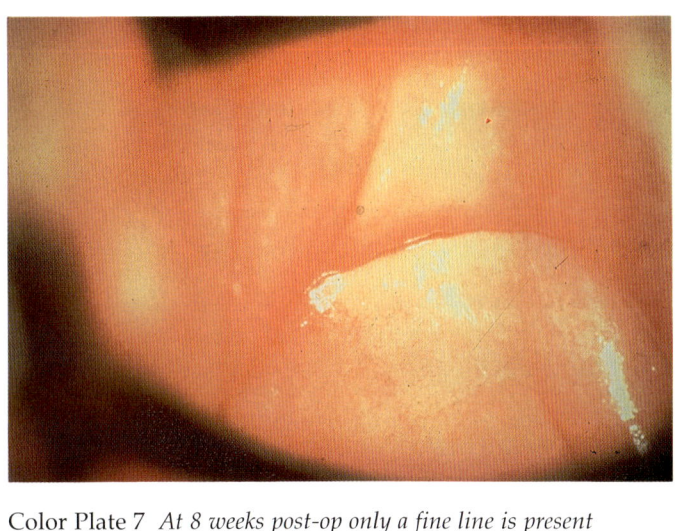

Color Plate 7 *At 8 weeks post-op only a fine line is present showing lack of granulation tissue.*

VAGINAL PROLAPSE

Color Plate 8 (right) *In this total uterovaginal prolapse, the dotted line indicates the initial trapezoidal incision of the anterior vaginal mucosa. The cystocele is dissected first.*

Color Plate 9 (below, left) *The cystocele is dissected from the anterior vaginal wall.*

Color Plate 10 (below, middle) *Rectocele. The finger is in the rectum for the dissection from the posterior vaginal wall. This is done to avoid injury to the rectum.*

Color Plate 11 (below, right) *This slide shows the perineum after the surgery.*

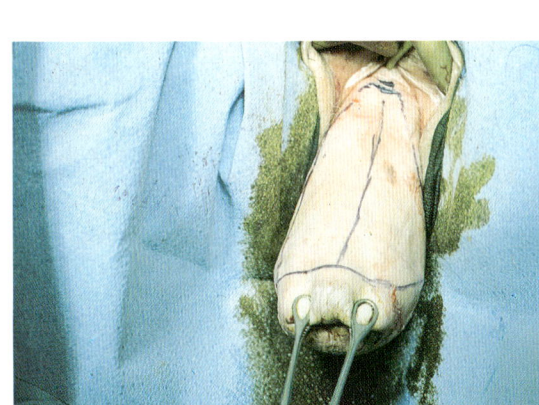

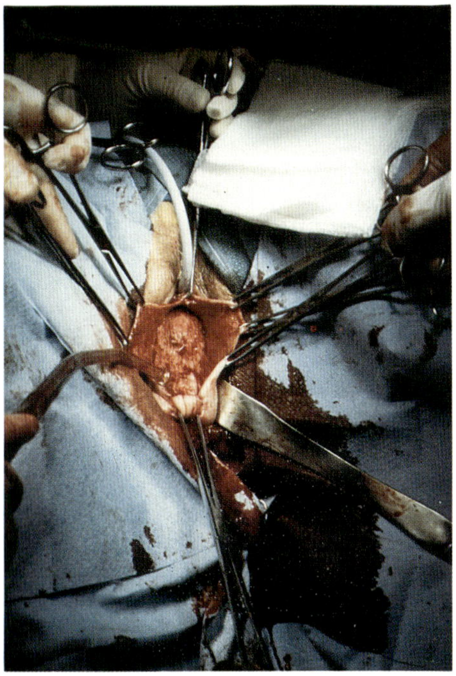

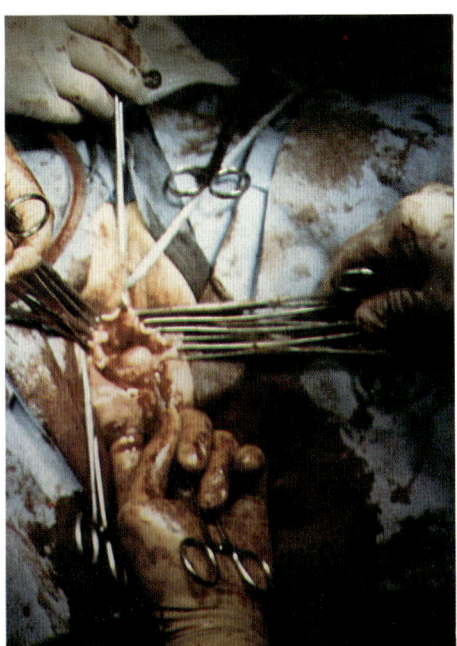

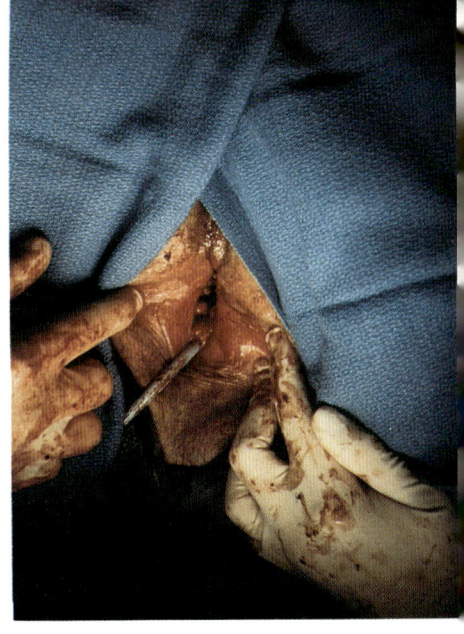

RECTOVAGINAL FISTULA

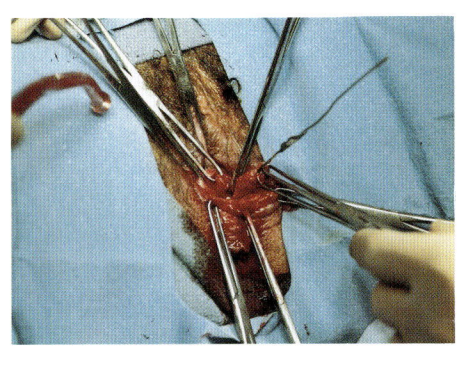 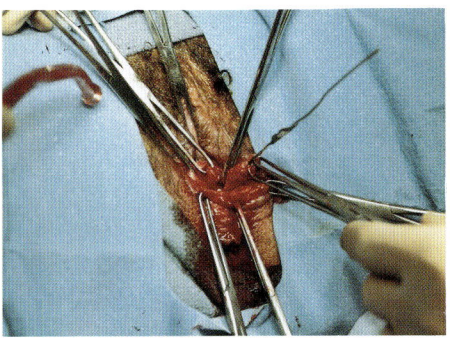 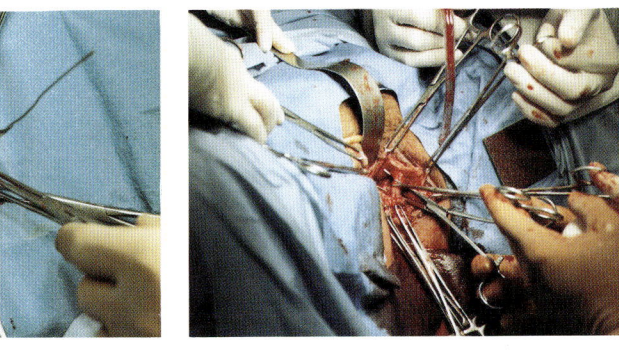

Color Plate 12 *Notice probe marking the vaginal opening of the rectovaginal fistula. Care must be taken not to make a new opening.*

Color Plate 13 *This slide shows the circumferential excision of the rectovaginal fistula.*

Color Plate 14 *The left bulbocavernous muscle is dissected free to perform a Martius graft.*

ANAL INCONTINENCE

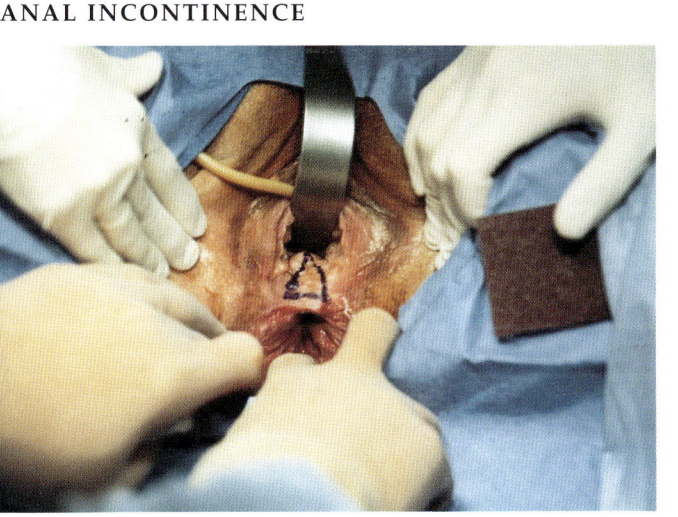

Color Plate 15 *Notice the loss of the external sphincter and the perineal body. The rectovaginal septum is very thin. There is no sphincter tone present. Notice the pen markings for the incision.*

VAGINAL HYSTERECTOMY

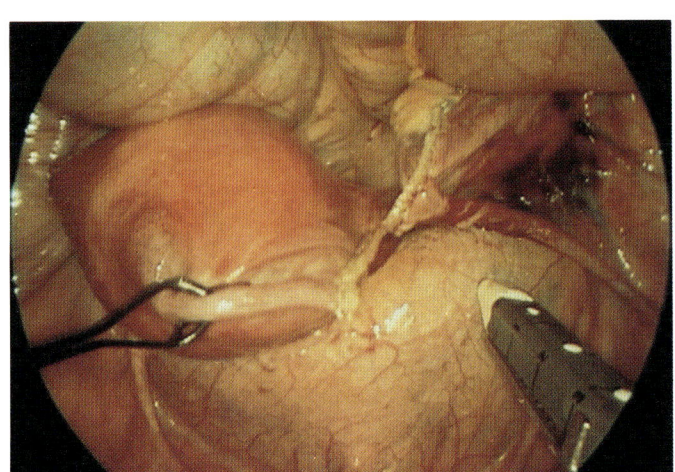

Color Plate 16 *Holding vesicouterine fold.*

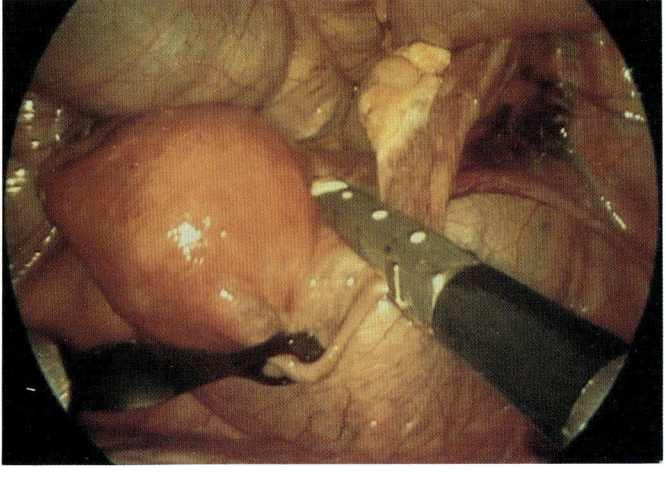

Color Plate 17 *Multifire endo GIA* 30 applied to round ligament and utero-ovarian pedicle.*

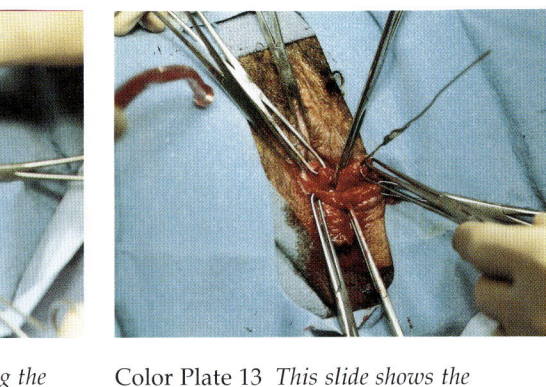

Color Plate 18 *After stapling the ligaments.*

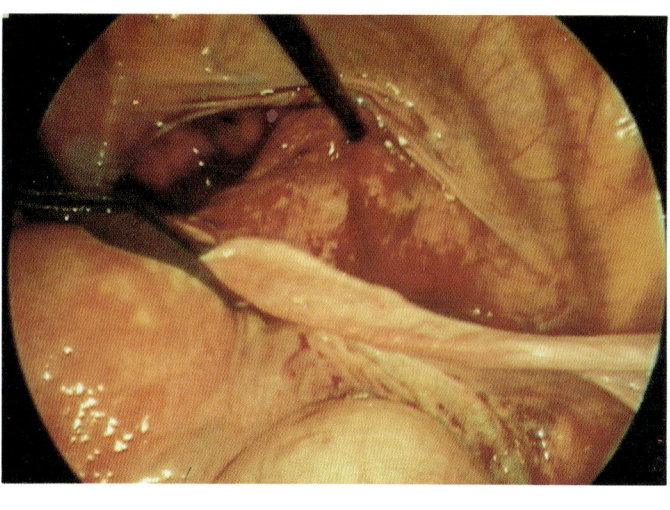

Color Plate 19 *Uterine vessels and dissected bladder.*

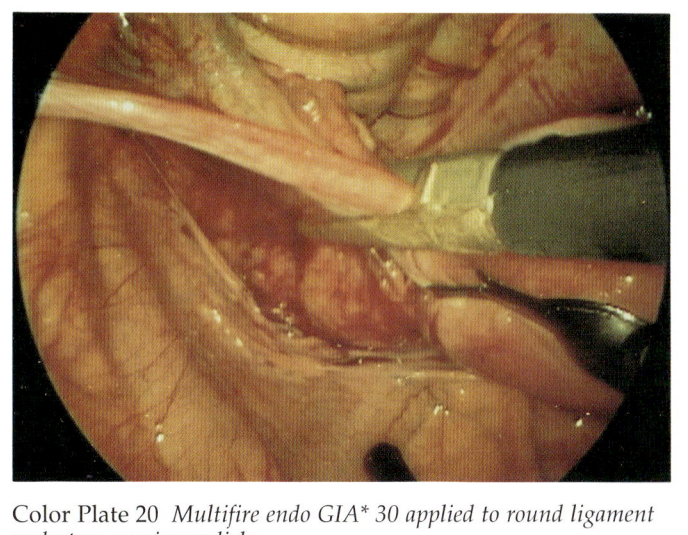

Color Plate 20 *Multifire endo GIA* 30 applied to round ligament and utero-ovarian pedicle.*

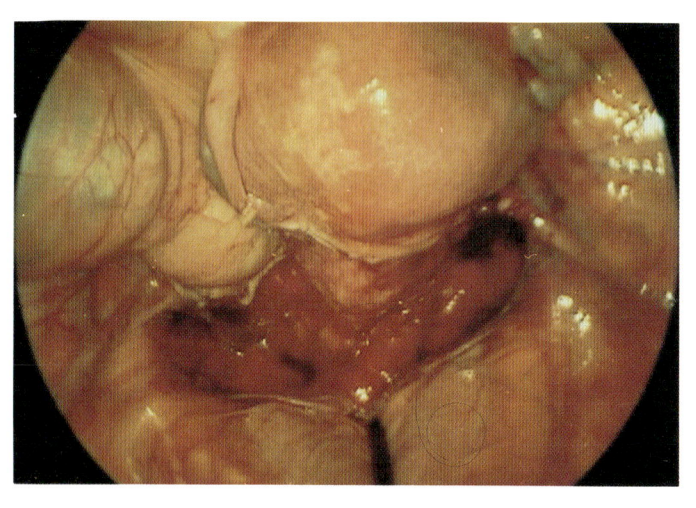

Color Plate 21 *Anterior view of the uterus after transection of the ligaments.*

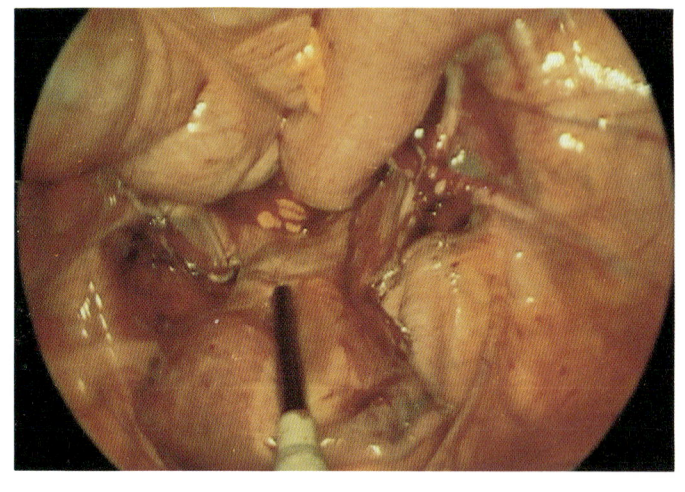

Color Plate 22 *Posterior view of the uterus after transection.*

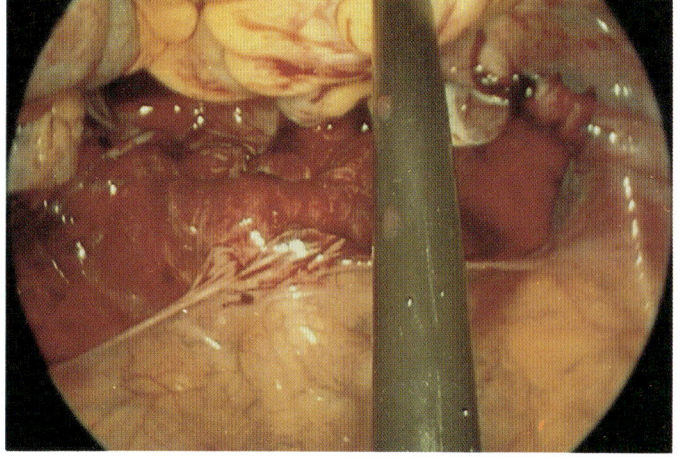

Color Plate 23 *End of LAVH. Notice closed vaginal cuff.*

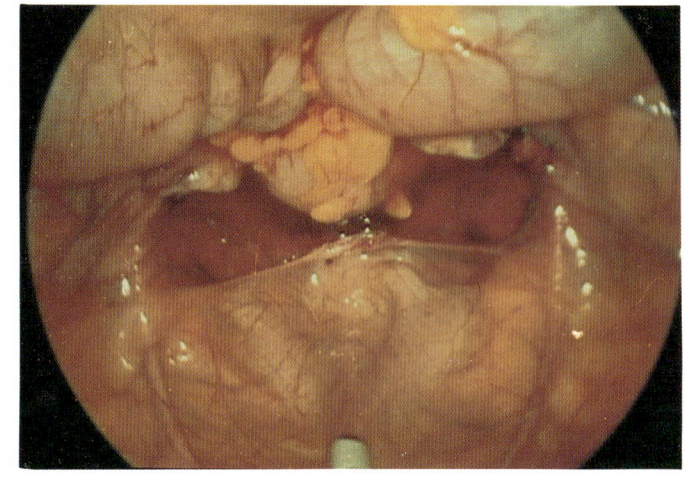

Color Plate 24 *End of procedure.*

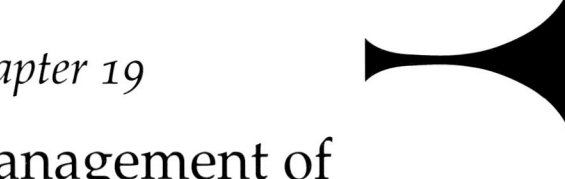

Chapter 19

Management of episiotomies

Brendan Burke and Luis E. Sanz

Episiotomy comes from the Greek and translates as incision of the pudenda. Although perineotomy may be more accurate, episiotomy is defined as a surgical incision into the perineum and vagina to prevent traumatic tearing during delivery (1). The most comprehensive literature review of episiotomy by Thacker and Banta recorded an incidence of 62.5%, yet in some centers, incidences of up to 80% in nulliparous women have been reported (2,3).

Prophylactic episiotomy, first popularized in the 1920s, has become a routine part of obstetrics since 1945. The incidence of episiotomies varies from country to country. In the Netherlands it is as low as 7%. Despite its common practice, performance of episiotomy is decreasing in the United States. Traditional indications for the use of episiotomy have come under question. As more studies are completed, routine or liberal performance can no longer be justified, especially in multiparous women. The importance of antepartum perineal massage and the positioning of women during delivery are rapidly gaining recognition in an attempt to reduce the need for episiotomy. Despite these trends, several indications do remain; therefore proper evaluation, performance, and repair are necessary.

Benefits and risks

Commonly quoted benefits of episiotomy are protection against uterine prolapse and pelvic relaxation in later years; decreased fetal head compression, thereby reducing birth asphyxia; and the provision of two clean wound edges that can be more easily repaired, thereby producing better healing (4). A reduction in perineal lacerations has also been reported as an indication for episiotomy; however, if we consider the episiotomy as a second-degree laceration, the number of patients with lacerations is higher in the episiotomy group (5). Also of concern is the increased number of third- and fourth-degree lacerations in those patients undergoing episiotomy.

Despite the decreasing evidence to substantiate the use of episiotomy for some of the traditional indications as well as evidence to suggest greater trauma in patients undergoing episiotomy, several indications still exist. Situations requiring expeditious delivery, the need for operative vaginal delivery, maximization of the vaginal outlet when dystocia is encountered or anticipated, vaginal breech delivery, or concern for possible clitoral, urethral, or labial tears continue to justify the use of episiotomy to reduce fetal and maternal morbidity.

Nomenclature

Lacerations are reported in degrees between one and four. A first-degree laceration involves the perineal skin or the vaginal mucosa or both. A second-degree laceration involves the vaginal mucosa and submucosa, the perineal skin, and the underlying perineal muscles. A third-degree laceration involves the external anal sphincter. A partial third-degree laceration does not involve all the fibers of the external anal sphincter. Total transection of the muscle is a complete third-degree laceration. A fourth-degree laceration involves any break in the rectal mucosa.

As an episiotomy involves incision of the vaginal mucosa, the perineal skin, and into the perineal muscles, it is thereby anatomically equivalent to a second-degree laceration. If there is involvement of the external anal sphincter or the rectal mucosa, this should be described as an episiotomy with a third-degree or fourth-degree extension, respectively.

Procedure and repair, midline episiotomy

Proper timing of an episiotomy is important, as a premature incision can result in a greater blood loss and delaying too long can result in damage that one is ultimately trying to avoid. The incision should be made when the presenting part is continuously distending the perineum. After adequate anesthesia is documented, a Mayo scissors is used to make an incision along the median raphe of the perineum, extending 2 to 4 cm into the vagina. Transection of the vaginal mucosa, perineal skin, perineal body (fusion of the bulbocavernosus muscles), and superficial transverse perineal muscle is carried out in one motion.

After the delivery of the baby and the placenta, the cervix, vagina, and perineum are inspected closely for any other lacerations. Proper hemostasis to avoid hematoma formation is extremely important. The apex of the vaginal incision is then identified. Beginning just above the apex, the vaginal mucosa is closed using a running locking suture of 3-0 poliglecaprone 25 (Monocryl, Ethicon) or 2-0 chromic catgut with attention that opposite sides are properly aligned (Fig. 19-1). This is carried down to the hymenal ring. The suture needle is then placed perpendicular to the suture plane and is driven into the space beneath the vaginal mucosa. Using a separate suture of 2-0 polyglactin 910 (Vicryl, Ethicon) or 2-0 poliglecaprone 25, a single interrupted "crown stitch" can then be placed to reapproximate the bulbocavernosus muscle (Fig. 19-2). Two or three more single interrupted sutures are then used to reapproximate the fascia and fibers of the superficial transverse perineal muscle (Fig. 19-3). Loose approximation of these tissues to prevent devascularization thereby improves healing and decreases pain. The continuous suture is then used to reapproximate the superficial fascia down to the most inferior point of the perineal incision (Fig. 19-4). Continuing back toward the vagina, the perineal skin edges are reapproximated using a subcuticular technique (Fig. 19-5). The suture is carried upward and behind the hymenal ring, where the suture is tied, thereby avoiding a knot in the perineal area. The use of continuous sutures minimizes the number of knots that have to be placed in the healing wound, therefore decreasing the chances of granuloma formation and swelling.

Upon completion, the suture line should be inspected for any bleeding areas. A bimanual examination should be performed to remove any excess blood clot or sponges remaining in the vagina. Finally, a rectal examination should be performed to ensure a fistula has not gone undetected as well as to document that no suture has been placed through the rectal mucosa.

Procedure and repair, mediolateral episiotomy

The mediolateral episiotomy was first described by DeLee in 1920 and gained initial acceptance in its adjunctive use with forcep deliveries (6). Still commonly used outside of

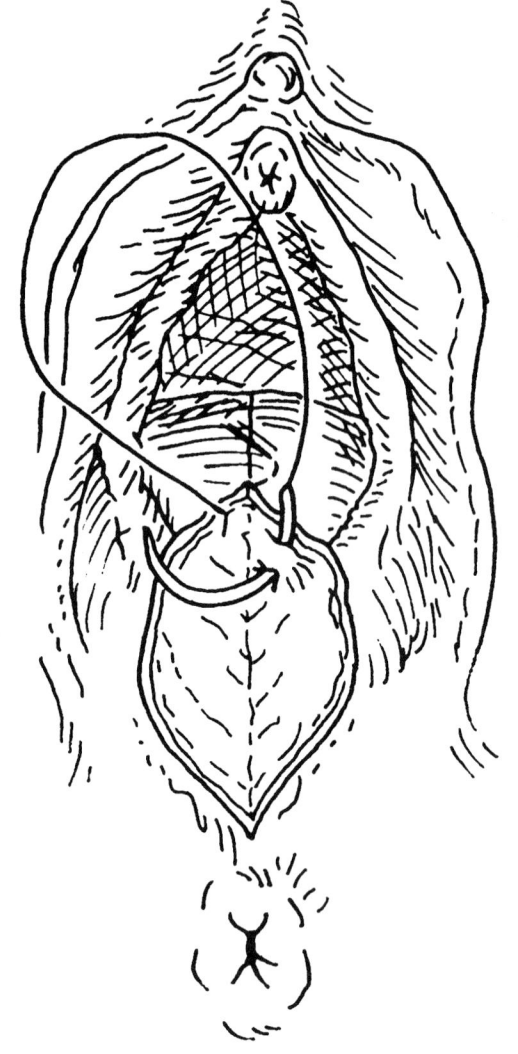

Fig. 19-1 The midline episiotomy is repaired by a continuous suture on the vaginal incision, starting at its very top. The suture is carried down to the hymenal margin.

the United States, its use has fallen from routine practice secondary to increased blood loss expectancy and more pain in both the short and long term. However, situations such as a short perineum or previous rectal surgery or those requiring maximization of the vaginal outlet still justify its use.

The initial incision is made in the midline of the posterior fourchette to the area immediately inside the hymenal ring. The blades of the Mayo scissors are then directed laterally, and the bulbocavernosus, superficial transverse perineal, and part of the levator ani muscles are transected. Depending on the degree of extension, fat within the ischiorectal fossa can be identified.

If immediate delivery of the placenta is not anticipated, repair should commence in an effort to reduce blood loss. The apex of the vaginal mucosa is identified. Beginning just above the apex the vaginal mucosa is closed using a running locking suture of 3-0 poliglecaprone 25 or 2-0 chromic catgut. This is carried down to the hymenal ring with attention to proper alignment of the mucosal edges. The bulbocavernosus muscle is then reapproximated to restore normal anatomy (Fig. 19-6). The muscle and fascia of the superficial transverse perineal and levator ani muscles are then reapproximated using interrupted sutures of 2-0

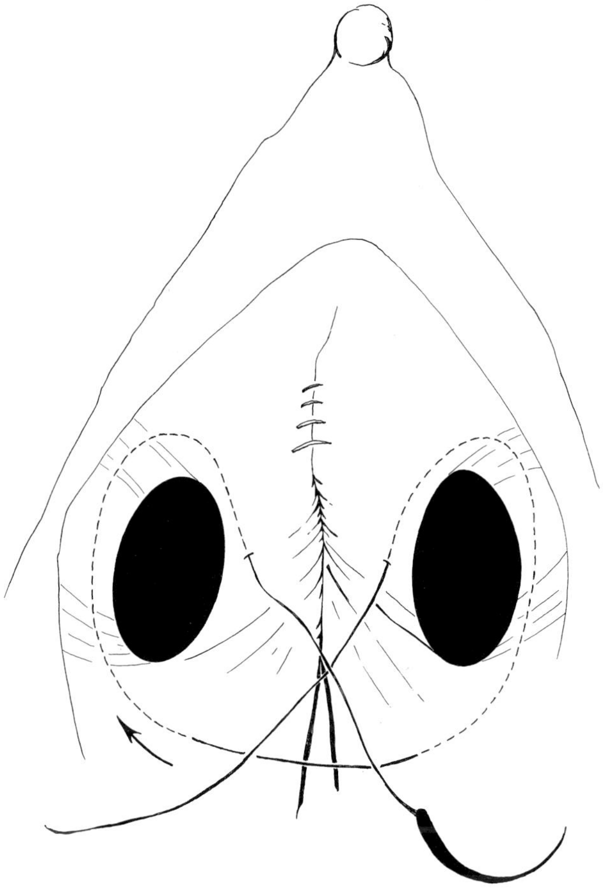

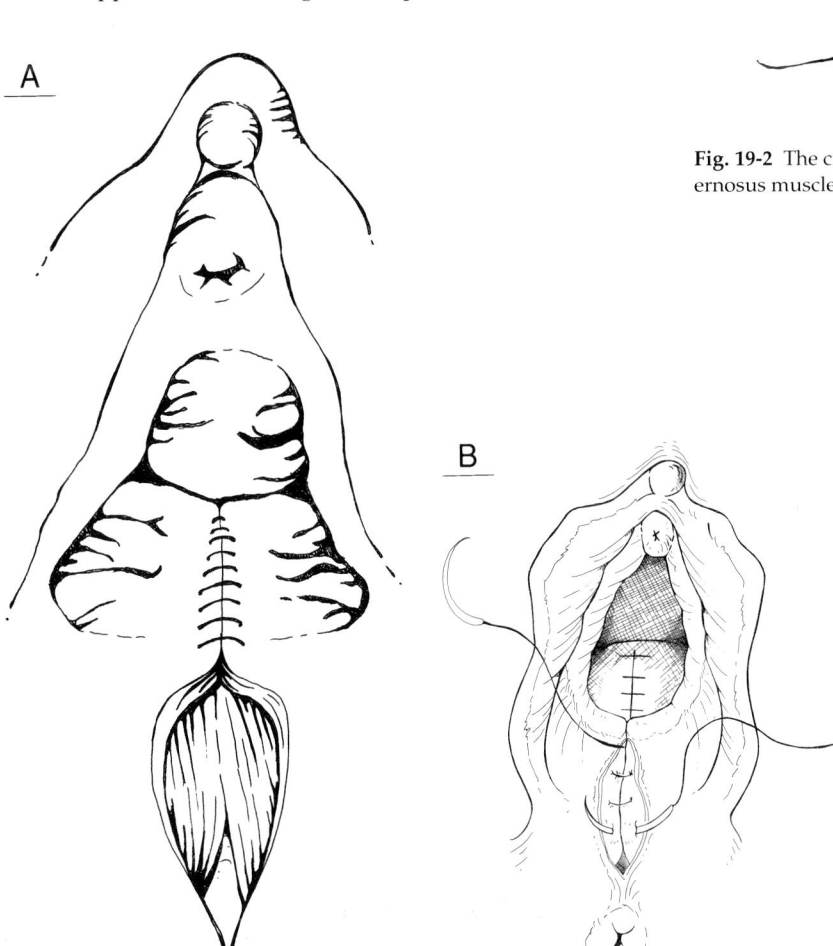

Fig. 19-2 The crown suture, reuniting the divided bulbocavernosus muscle.

A

B

Fig. 19-3 (A) Drawing together the perineal muscles and fascia with interrupted sutures; (B) after the interrupted sutures are tied, the vaginal suture is continued downward.

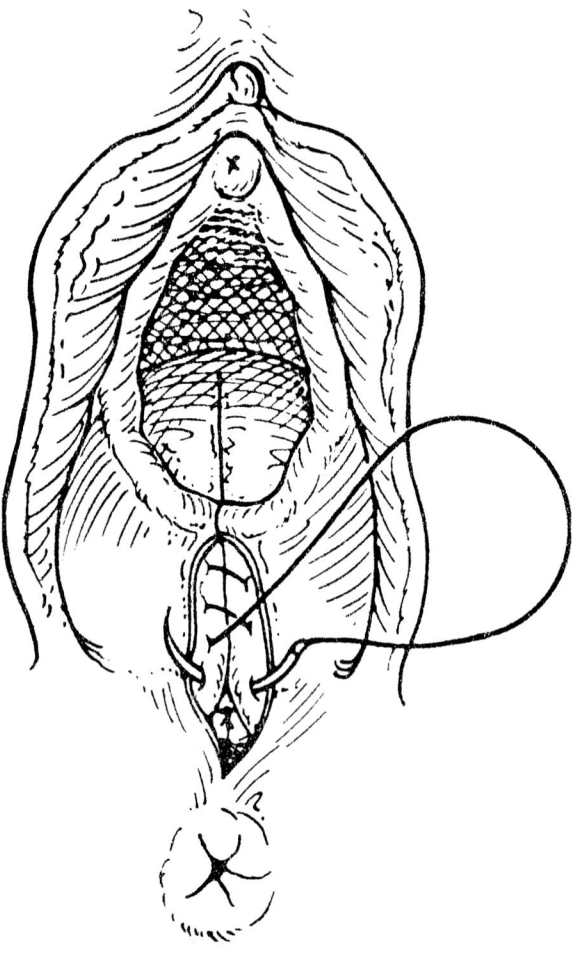

Fig. 19-4 If desired, the vaginal suture may be continued as a running layer to reunite the sides of the perineal body.

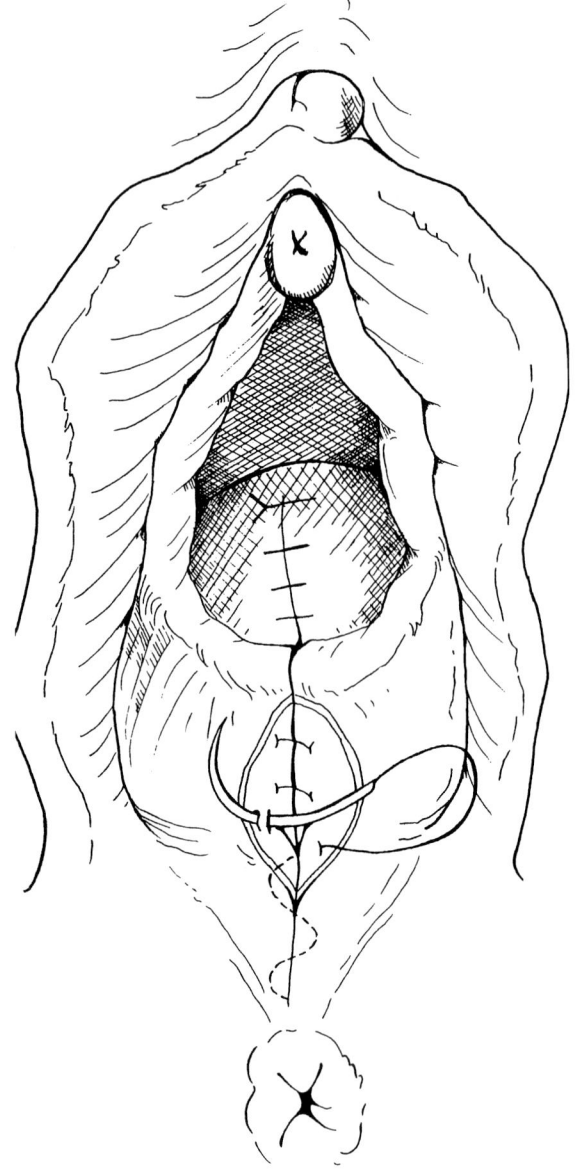

Fig. 19-5 Subcuticular closure of perineal skin.

polyglactin 910 or 2-0 poliglecaprone 25 (Fig. 19-7). Beginning at the most inferior aspect of the incision, the skin edges are reapproximated using a subcuticular suture of 3-0 poliglecaprone 25 or 2-0 chromic catgut. This should be carried past the hymenal ring to avoid a knot on the perineum (Fig. 19-8).

Upon completion the suture line should be inspected and a bimanual examination performed. A thorough rectal examination to document anal sphincter integrity and the absence of suture material into the rectal mucosa should complete the repair.

Third- and fourth-degree extensions

Various degrees of laceration of the external anal sphincter can occur. The capsule of the external anal sphincter must be inspected, and if there is a break of any degree, the capsule should be reapproximated using interrupted sutures of 2-0 poliglecaprone 25 or 2-0 polyglycolic acid placed .05 cm apart (Fig. 19-9).

If there is a defect in the rectal mucosa, the edges must first be identified. Beginning at the apex a continuous su-

ture of 4-0 poliglecaprone 25 (Monocryl) or 3-0 chromic catgut is placed 0.5 cm from the edge through the serosa and extending to, but not through, the mucosa (Fig. 19-10). This is carried out until the entrance of the anus is reapproximated. A second layer of interrupted or continuous 3-0 poliglecaprone or polyglycolic sutures reapproximating the rectovaginal fascia is then placed. The external anal sphincter is repaired by placing a figure-of-eight suture of 2-0 poliglecaprone 25 or 2-0 polyglycolic acid and approximating the edges loosely (Fig. 19-11). Recent evidence suggests that attention to the restoration of the broad band structure of the external anal sphincter, as opposed to the traditional small bundle of muscle fibers view, plays a role in subsequent continence of gas or liquid stool (7). The re-

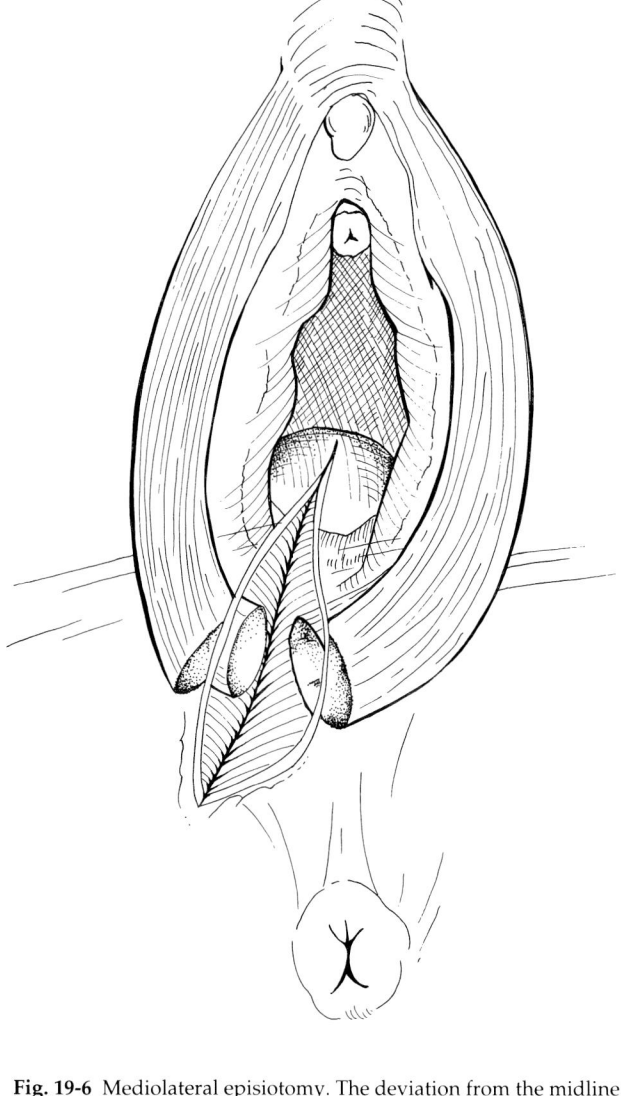

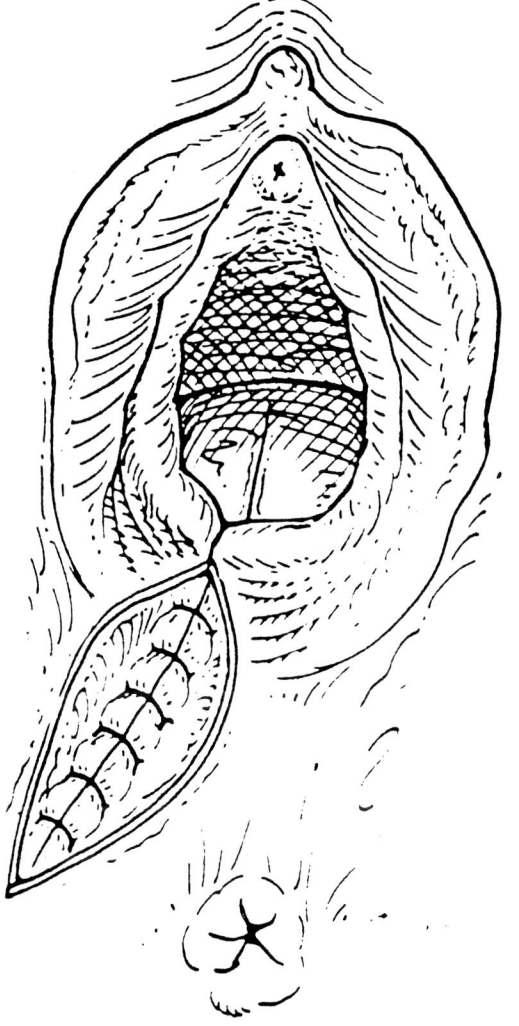

Fig. 19-6 Mediolateral episiotomy. The deviation from the midline will depend on the "handedness" of the operator.

Fig. 19-7 When the deeper tissues have been reunited, as shown, the subcutaneous layer is closed by a running subcuticular suture.

mainder of the episiotomy is repaired in both situations as described above.

Suture material

A 2-0 or 3-0 caliber suture is usually used throughout the repair except when reapproximating the rectal mucosa, when a 3-0 or 4-0 suture is more appropriate. Although the derivatives of polyglycolic acid were associated with less pain in a 4-week follow-up period when compared with chromic catgut, long-term superiority of the former suture material has not been as clear (8,9).

A promising new suture material, poliglecaprone 25 (Monocryl, Ethicon), is a monofilament, rapidly-absorbed suture that may prove superior to the materials currently used. Polydioxanone (PDS, Ethicon) should be avoided because of its slower resorption. Finally, in tying any suture material, attention must be focused on the proper number

of knots as well as on keeping these knots flat in an attempt to maximize strength and facilitate proper resorption.

Anesthesia

With any operative procedure, there is always concern that the patient be given the best anesthesia during and after its performance. Epidural and pudendal blockade provide excellent relief for patients undergoing episiotomy, yet there appears to be a higher incidence of episiotomy in patients receiving this anesthesia. This may be attributed to the possibility that it is easier to perform an episiotomy when the perineal region is anesthetized (10).

When only local anesthesia is used, infiltration of 1% lidocaine or 1% 2-chloroprocaine into the perineum is done prior to incision. The latter anesthesia is preferred by some investigators because very little, if any, unchanged 2-chloroprocaine reaches the fetus (11). Patients not undergoing episiotomy who have lacerations requiring suturing

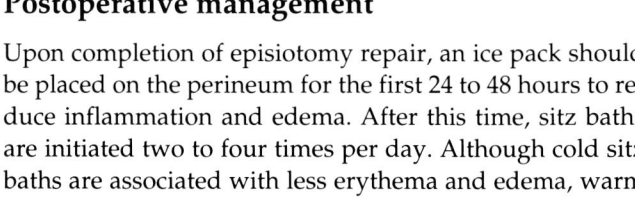

Fig. 19-8 Increased blood loss may be expected with deviation from the midline. Timely repair may need to be initiated before a completed third stage of labor.

are anesthetized best by infiltration of a local anesthetic prior to repair if no regional anesthesia is being used.

Postoperative management

Upon completion of episiotomy repair, an ice pack should be placed on the perineum for the first 24 to 48 hours to reduce inflammation and edema. After this time, sitz baths are initiated two to four times per day. Although cold sitz baths are associated with less erythema and edema, warm sitz baths are generally better tolerated by the patient (12).

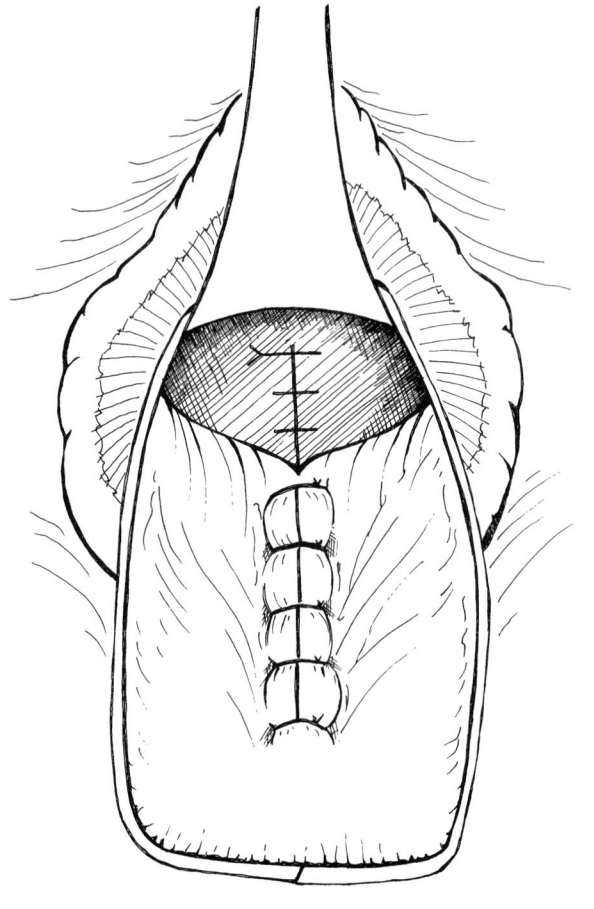

Fig. 19-9 Transected ends of anal sphincter are reapproximated in the midline.

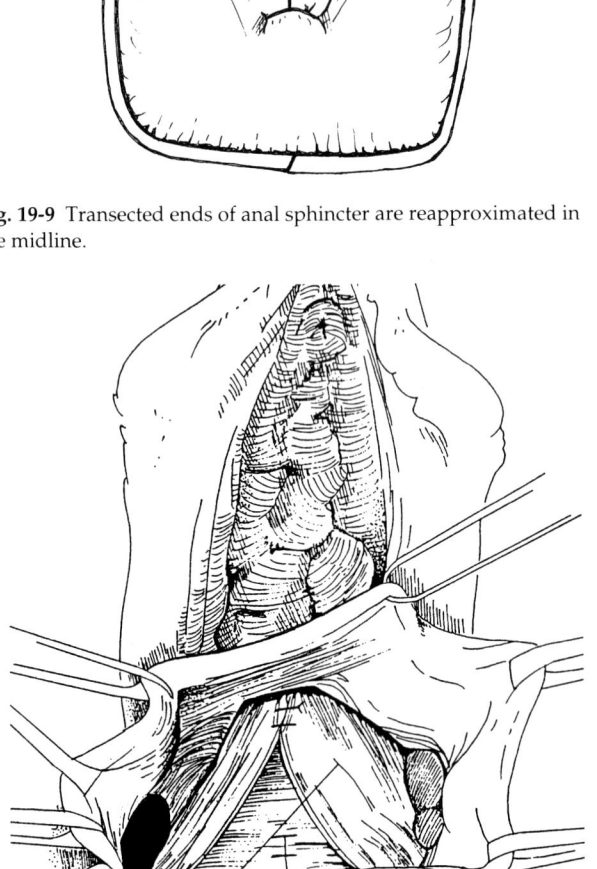

Fig. 19-10 Repair of fourth-degree extension. Minimal tension should be placed on the repaired edges of rectal mucosa and perirectal fascia.

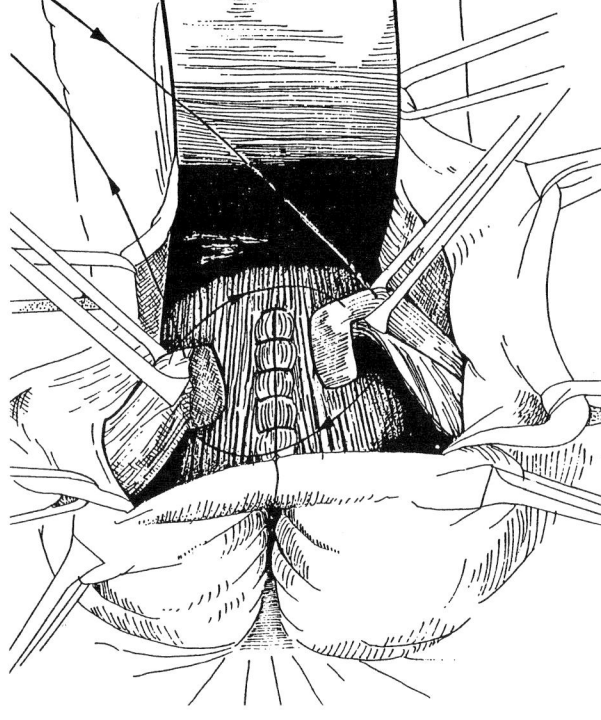

Fig. 19-11 Repair the third-degree extension. The transected ends of the anal sphincter should be brought to the midline and reapproximated incorporating the fascia.

Meticulous care including use of stool softeners, avoidance of rectal examination, and use of sitz baths in patients with fourth-degree tears is necessary to reduce the chance of breakdown.

When analgesics are necessary, ibuprofen, acetaminophen, or a combination of acetaminophen with either codeine or oxycodone are all effective and safe. Ketorolac tromethamine (Toradol) offers excellent analgesia, but its safety with breast-feeding has not been established. Some investigators have advocated infiltration of the episiotomy site with lidocaine after delivery under epidural anesthesia in an effort to reduce analgesic requirements in this patient group (13).

The episiotomy site should be inspected in 24 hours for any evidence of excessive edema, infection, separation, or bleeding. Local perineal care instruction should be reviewed with the patient before discharge. The site is then inspected 4 to 6 weeks postpartum or earlier if complications arise. Poor healing should be observed closely in those patients with a history of human papillomavirus infection and in those who smoke (14).

Should any nodule appear in the previous episiotomy site at any point in the patient's lifetime, the area should be biopsied to rule out the presence of endometriosis or carcinoma (15,16).

Complications

Even with excellent care, obstetrical lacerations and episiotomies do not always heal well. As with any complica-

tion, timely identification can often prevent further difficulties. Breakdown of an episiotomy has been reported with an incidence as high as 3.0% (17). Minimally separated vaginal mucosa or perineal skin usually granulates together without need for surgical intervention. Dehiscence of the external anal sphincter or rectal mucosa requires more aggressive management. Traditionally, repair was delayed to await a decrease in inflammation and formation of granulation tissue to facilitate repair. One group of investigators successfully managed early repair when a dehiscence was identified in an attempt to avoid the definite disability encountered with delayed repair (18).

The formation of a rectovaginal or rectoperineal fistula is often less readily identified than a complete breakdown. Suspicion should arise if the patient reports passage of flatus or stool from either the vagina or perineum. These may close spontaneously if small; however, larger defects usually require surgical intervention. Unabsorbed suture material should be removed, and any underlying infection should be treated before any surgery is considered. Infection has been reported in up to 3.0% of women having an episiotomy (2). Complications can range from a simple wound infection to *Clostridium myonecrosis*. Simple wound infection can be treated with opening of the episiotomy site with drainage and does not require antibiotic treatment unless a cellulitis is present. Sitz baths to facilitate irrigation of the area should be performed. The wound should be allowed to heal by granulation or by placing externally two loosely tied sutures of 3-0 polypropylene (Prolene). They will have to be removed in 5 or 6 days.

An uncommon yet often fatal infection of the superficial fascia and subcutaneous tissue is necrotizing fasciitis. Usually occurring in patients with compromised vascularity, necrotizing fasciitis has a demonstrated mortality incidence of 60% (18). Any patient with an apparently infected episiotomy site associated with hypoesthesia and massive edema should be treated aggressively. Wide debridement and use of broad spectrum antibiotics is mandatory. Hemodynamic status should be monitored closely. Less life-threatening complications include pain and short-term dyspareunia. In those patients in whom pain or dyspareunia persists, epithelial inclusion cysts or suture granuloma should be sought and removed. New studies have shown that as many as one third of patients having a third- and fourth-degree laceration have some degree of gas or fecal incontinence later in life, despite primary repair (7). This can be documented now with sophisticated magnetic resonance imaging analysis of the perineal muscles dealing with continence.

Summary

Although there is a decreasing trend in the use of episiotomy, proper technique is necessary. One must try to prevent the use of episiotomy unless indicated, especially in multiparous patients. The goal should be to continue to reduce tissue damage, maximize healing, and minimize postoperative pain and discomfort, in both the short and the long term. If an episiotomy is performed or a laceration occurs involving the sphincter, proper repair is essential to prevent incontinence later in life.

References

1 Dorland's illustrated medical dictionary. Philadelphia: Harcourt Brace Jovanovich, 1988.

2 Thacker SB, Banta HD. Benefits and risks of episiotomy: an interpretative review of the English literature, 1860–1980. Obstet Gynecol Surv 1983;36:322–338.

3 Thorp JM Jr, Bowes WA Jr. Episiotomy: can its routine use be defended? Am J Obstet Gynecol 1989;160:1027–1030.

4 Shiono P, Klebanoff MA, Carey JC. Midline episiotomies: more harm than good? Obstet Gynecol 1990;75:765–770.

5 Gass MS, Dunn C, Stys SJ. Effect of episiotomy on the frequency of vaginal outlet lacerations. J Reprod Med 1986;31:240–244.

6 DeLee JB. The prophylactic forceps operation. Am J Obstet Gynecol 1920;1:34–44.

7 Aronson MP, Lee RA, Berquist TH. Anatomy of anal sphincters and related structures in continent women studied with magnetic resonance imaging. Obstet Gynecol 1990;76:846–851.

8 Grant A. The choice of suture materials and techniques for repair of perineal trauma: an overview of the evidence from controlled trials. Br J Obstet Gynaecol 1989;96:1281–1289.

9 Grant A. Repair of episiotomies and perineal tears. Br J Obstet Gynaecol 1986;93:417–419.

10 Larsson PG, Platz-Christensen JJ, Bergman B, Wallstersson G. Advantage or disadvantage of episiotomy compared with spontaneous perineal laceration. Gynecol Obstet Invest 1991;31:213–216.

11 Philipson EH, Kuhnert BR, Syracuse BS. 2-Chloroprocaine for local perineal infiltration. Am J Obstet Gynecol 1987;157:1275–1288.

12 Lafoy J, Geden EA. Postepisiotomy pain: warm versus cold sitz bath. J Obstet Gynecol Neonatal Nurs 1989;18:399–403.

13 Khan GQ, Lilford RJ. Wound pain may be reduced by prior infiltration of the episiotomy site after delivery under epidural anesthesia. Br J Obstet Gynaecol 1987;94:341–344.

14 Snyder RR, Hammond TL, Hankins GD. Human papillomavirus associated with poor healing of episiotomy repairs. Obstet Gynecol 1990;76:664–667.

15 Sayfan J, Benosh L, Segal M, Orda R. Endometriosis in episiotomy scar with anal sphincter involvement. Dis Colon Rectum 1991; 34:713–716.

16 Burgess SP, Waymont B. Implantation of a cervical carcinoma in an episiotomy site. Case report. Br J Obstet Gynaecol 1948;41:814–882.

17 Kaltreider DF, Dixon DM. A study of 710 complete lacerations following central episiotomy. South Med J 1948;41:814–882.

18 Hauth JC, Gilstrap JC, Ward SC, Hankins GDV. Early repair of an external sphincter ani muscle and rectal mucosa dehiscence. Obstet Gynecol 1986;67:806–809.

19 Sutton GP, Smirz LR, Clark DH, Bennett JE. Group B streptococcal necrotizing fasciitis arising from an episiotomy. Obstet Gynecol 1985;66:733–736.

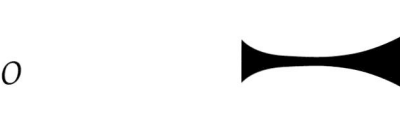

Chapter 20

Surgical management of anal incontinence and episiotomy dehiscence

Luis E. Sanz

Anal incontinence is a debilitating social problem defined as the inability to control the passage of feces or flatus. The degree of incontinence may vary from occasional inability to control flatus to complete inability to prevent the passage of feces.

Physiology of continence

Continence of stool and flatus is dependent upon intact neurologic and muscular function. Consistency of stool also plays an important role in the maintenance of continence. Liquid feces may be difficult to control despite adequate sphincter tone, while an incompetent sphincter may retain normal stool without a problem.

Neurogenic continence is the result of a highly integrated physiologic process. When stool reaches the rectum, mechanoreceptors respond to the distention, and the involuntary internal sphincter relaxes. Central nervous system inhibition overrides furthering of the process until the time to defecate is deemed appropriate. At the "designated" time, stool arrives in the anal canal, and the voluntary, external sphincter relaxes. Increased intra-abdominal pressure and descent of the pelvic floor musculature force the walls of the anal canal apart, allowing defecation to be completed (1).

Neurogenic incontinence may be detected by atony of the pelvic musculature, with laxity of the anal canal, insensibility to tactile stimulation, inability to voluntarily contract musculature, or absence of anal reflexes.

In traumatic or postoperative causes of incontinence, the circumference of the anorectal ring is disrupted. This defect may be felt during digital rectal examination. In addition, loss of the normal perianal corrugation and wrinkling provide visual aid in the diagnosis of the problem.

Etiology

Causes of fecal incontinence are numerous and include mechanical disruption of the anal sphincter, factors that decrease stool bulk (inflammatory bowel disease, gastroenteritis, mucus-secreting colorectal tumors), altered sensation in the rectum, and nervous system defects. The pudendal nerve (S2, S3, S4) innervates the levator ani and external sphincter musculature. Thus, any damage to this portion of the nervous system will affect anal continence (2).

Damage and impairment of the anorectal musculature are frequent causes of incontinence. Division of the external or the internal anal sphincter during childbirth, episiotomy, or surgical correction of complicated anal fissures may damage this musculature. Even appropriately performed episiotomy repairs may break down, resulting in damage to the anorectal muscles.

Dr. Lee (personal communication) from the Mayo Clinic has found that if one asks questions related to anal incontinence, the incidence of mild anal incontinence is significantly greater than it is reported in the literature. Therefore, proper repair of episiotomies with good perineoplasty is extremely important. Also, many women with this problem will benefit from a perineoplasty.

Other abnormalities leading to anal incontinence that can be repaired surgically are congenital anomalies, rectal prolapse, hemorrhoidal prolapse, and rectal trauma associated with sphincter injury. Causes of medical incontinence requiring only medical treatment are those related to the aging process, chronic diarrhea, laxative abuse, and radiation proctitis.

Anatomy

The levator ani muscles (sphincter vaginate, puborectalis, pubococcygeus, and ileococcygeus) and the coccygeus muscle with their respective fascial coverings make up the pelvic diaphragm (3). The levator ani forms a broad sling of musculature that originates from the posterior surface of the ischial spines, and from the obturator fascia in between (Fig. 20-1). These muscles surround the vagina and the rectum, and occupy a median raphe between the vagina and rectum, and a raphe below the rectum, and into the coccyx.

The urogenital diaphragm lies external to the pelvic diaphragm in the triangle between the symphysis pubis and the ischial tuberosities. It is composed of the deep transverse perineal muscles, the urethra constrictor muscle, and the internal and external fascial coverings.

The anal canal is surrounded by an inner and outer muscular tube. The inner muscular tube, or internal anal sphincter, is a thickened continuation of the circular smooth muscle of the rectum. The external anal sphincter is divided into three parts: the subcutaneous, the superficial, and the deep. The deep portion of the external sphincter blends with the puborectalis portion of the levator ani muscles.

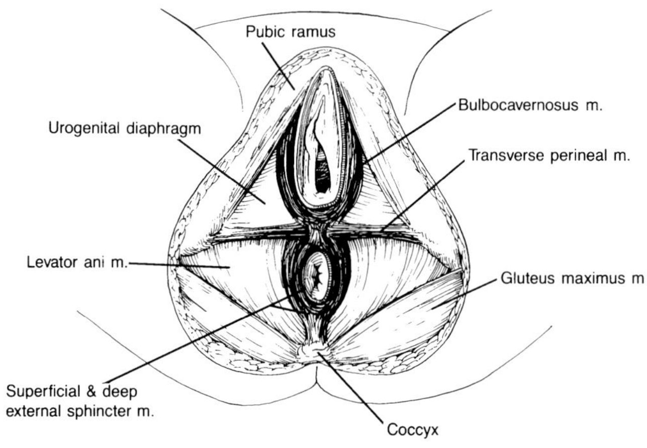

Fig. 20-1 Anatomy of the perineum. Notice the close relationship among the bulbocavernosus muscle, the transverse perineal muscle, and the external sphincter muscle. It is important to restore this anatomy during the surgical repair to maintain continence.

The perineal body is composed of fibers of the levator ani that unite in a median raphe between the vagina and rectum. This is reinforced by the central perineal tendons, which are composed of fibers from the bulbocavernosus muscle, the deep transverse perineal muscles, and the external anal sphincter. These structures are often lacerated during vaginal delivery (4).

Preoperative evaluation and preparation

The diagnosis and etiology of anal incontinence can often be determined by taking a thorough history. Physical examination, including digital rectal examination, is imperative to complete understanding of the problem (5).

Treatment options depend on the etiology and severity of symptoms. Minor incontinence can often be treated conservatively with diet modification (i.e., such as the addition of bulk additives), exercises to increase sphincter tone (Kegel's) and biofeedback. The timing of the repair is either within 10 days of or 3 months after an episiotomy breakdown (6). Incontinence caused by laceration of the anorectal musculature is often corrected by surgical repair. The patient should be in optimal physical condition at the time of surgery. Prophylactic antibiotics, enemas, and vaginal douching are part of the preoperative regimen (7; Table 20-1). The last enema should be given the night before surgery to avoid expulsion of fecal matter into the operative field during surgery. The patient should be placed on a clear liquid diet the day before surgery and have nothing by mouth after 6 P.M. GoLytely should be given the day before the surgery as a mechanical bowel preparation.

Operative technique

With the patient in the dorsal lithotomy position, a thorough pelvic examination should be performed under general anesthesia to better evaluate the relative position of the different perineal muscles (Fig. 20-2). Bupivacaine (Marcaine) 0.25% with epinephrine is injected throughout the perineal area as extra anesthetic for the postoperative period. Most procedures can be performed under epidural

Table 20-1 Preoperative preparation

Laxative and enema
Antibiotics
Cefotetan, 1 g IV, one hour before the surgery and 12 hours after the surgery
Diet
Low-residue diet 7 days before surgery
Full liquids 2 days before surgery
Nothing by mouth from 6 P.M. on evening before surgery

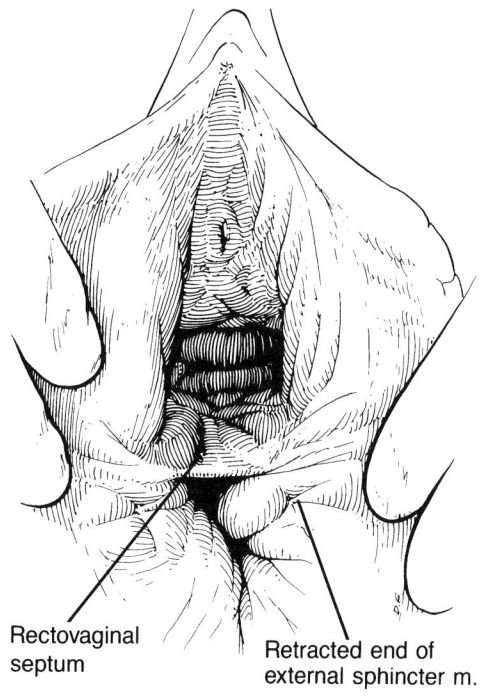

Rectovaginal
septum

Retracted end of
external sphincter m.

Fig. 20-2 Position of perineal muscles. Retracted external sphincters and their rectovaginal septum typical of patients with anal incontinence.

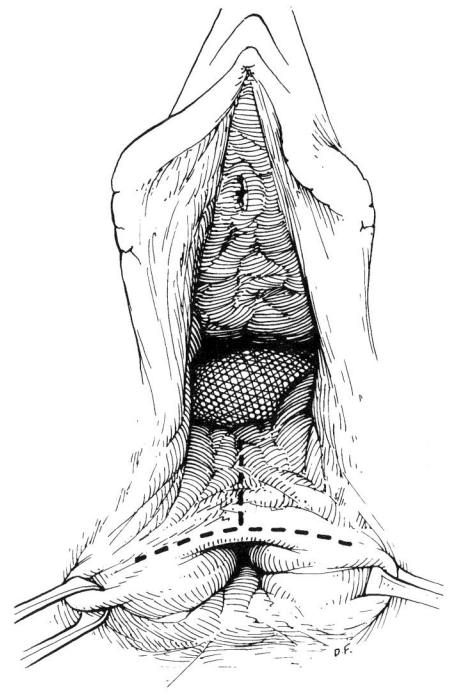

Fig. 20-3 A transverse elliptical perianal incision is made connecting the bisected external sphincter. This is done to avoid dissecting initially on top of the scar tissue present on the posterior aspect of the vagina.

anesthesia. An elliptical incision is then made from the 3 o'clock to the 9 o'clock position around the anterior edge of the anus (Fig. 20-3; Color Plate 15). Then, by sharp dissection with Metzenbaum scissors, the posterior vaginal mucosa is dissected away from the rectum. Because there is really no perineal body or rectovaginal space separating the rectum from the vagina, one must be extremely careful in this area to avoid perforating the rectum. The sharp dissection must be carried as high as possible on the posterior vaginal wall. Placing a finger in the rectum helps identify the rectum in order to avoid causing injury to it.

Then one must begin to dissect laterally, searching for remnants of the perirectal fascia (Fig. 20-4). This is the same technique used to repair a rectocele. It is important to dissect this perirectal fascia freely from any area of the vagina or the rectum to relieve tension. Throughout the repair it is important that all muscles and planes be freely dissected so as to reapproximate them without undue tension. It is also necessary to remove any devascularized area in order to promote faster healing.

After identifying the perirectal fascia, one must search for the transverse perineal muscles, the levator ani, the bulbocavernosus muscles, and the external sphincter. The torn ends of the external sphincter and the transverse perineal muscles are usually identified by the dimpling effect that they have on the tissue. Once identified they must be dissected to allow for proper mobilization. Any small rectal tears or inner vaginal fistula should be repaired at this time.

If a small anal fistula is identified, it must be excised so that the devascularized tissue is removed. Any tear in the rectal mucosa is repaired with a continuous suture of No. 3-0 polyglycolic acid (Dexon) or polyglactin (Vicryl) or, better yet, with a new monofilament, fast-absorbing poliglecapron 25 (Monocryl). The perirectal fascia is then again identified and reapproximated without tension with continuous sutures of No. 3-0 polyglyconate (Maxon) or polydiaxonone (PDS). All bleeders should be carefully ligated with No. 4-0 Dexon or electrocoagulation to prevent hematoma formation. The anal canal itself is reconstructed with interrupted sutures of No. 3-0 Dexon. At this point, the external sphincter is reapproximated by placing interrupted sutures of No. 0 Monocryl or Vicryl (Fig. 20-5). Monocryl is a monofilament, extremely inert, reabsorbable suture. The levator ani is then integrated into the perineal body with a No. 2-0 Monocryl.

A finger is placed in the rectum, and the repair is checked to test for the strength of the sphincter. The finger is removed. The whole area is washed with normal saline. At this point the transverse perineal body is attached in the midline, on top of the external sphincter (Fig. 20-6). The ends of the bulbocavernosus muscles are also identified and attached to the transverse perineum and the perineal body (Fig. 20-7). It is vital that all these structures be attached together, because if they are separated, the repair may not be successful. A perineorrhaphy is done by ap-

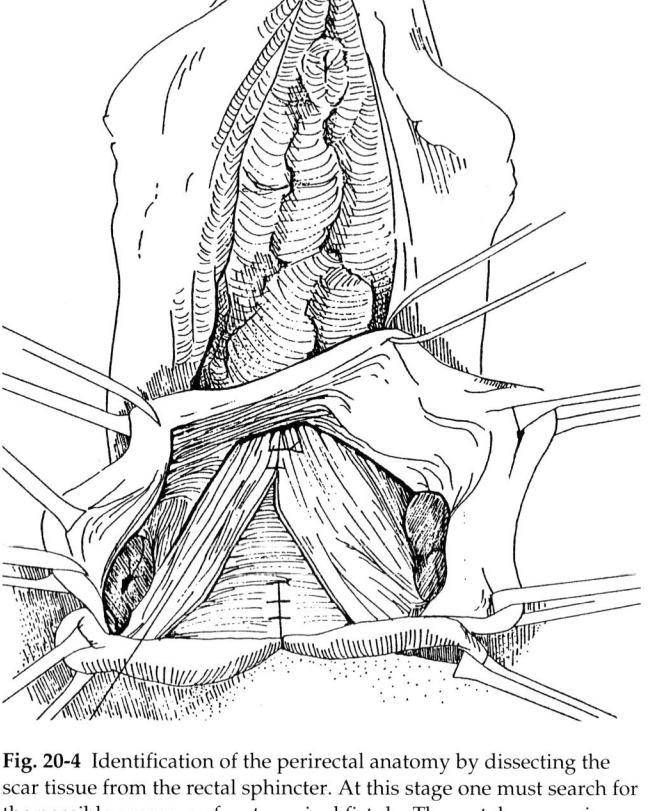

Fig. 20-4 Identification of the perirectal anatomy by dissecting the scar tissue from the rectal sphincter. At this stage one must search for the possible presence of rectovaginal fistula. The rectal mucosa is reapproximated with a continuous suture of 3-0 Vicryl or Dexon.

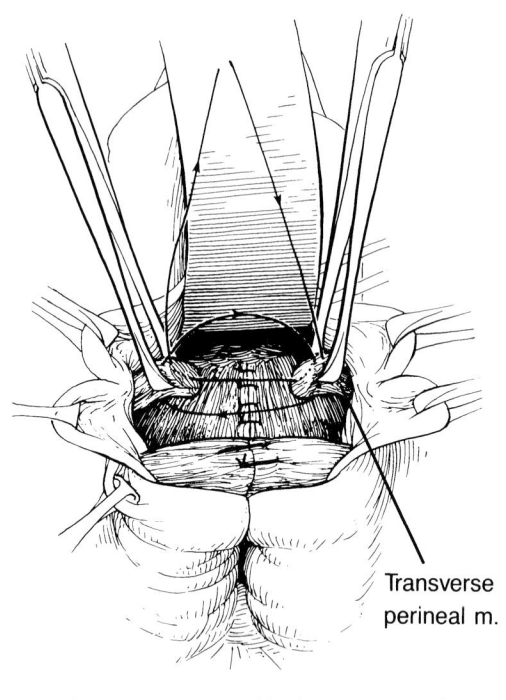

Transverse perineal m.

Fig. 20-6 Attach transverse perineal body: coaptation of transverse perianal muscle with 2-0 PDS or Maxon.

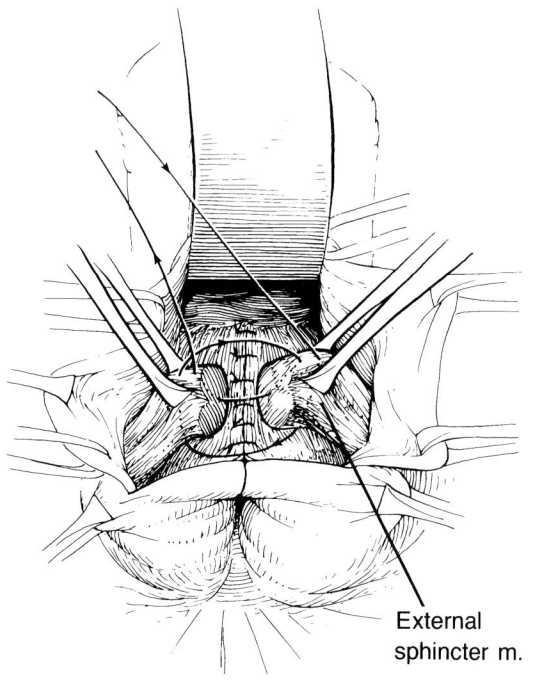

External sphincter m.

Fig. 20-5 Reapproximate external sphincter. The perirectal fascia is closed with continuous sutures of 3-0 Maxon or PDS. The external sphincter is loosely approximated with a figure-of-eight suture of 2-0 PDS or Maxon. The external sphincter must be well dissected to avoid devascularizing the tissue.

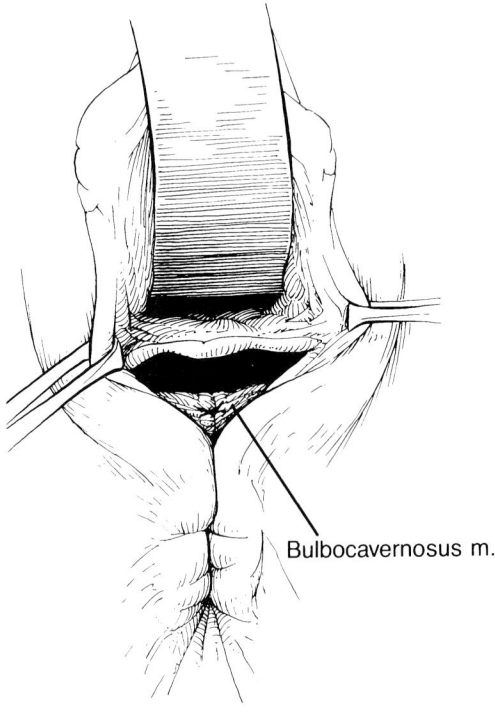

Bulbocavernosus m.

Fig. 20-7 Perineoplasty with formation of a new perineum and attachment of bulbocavernosus muscle to transverse perineal muscle.

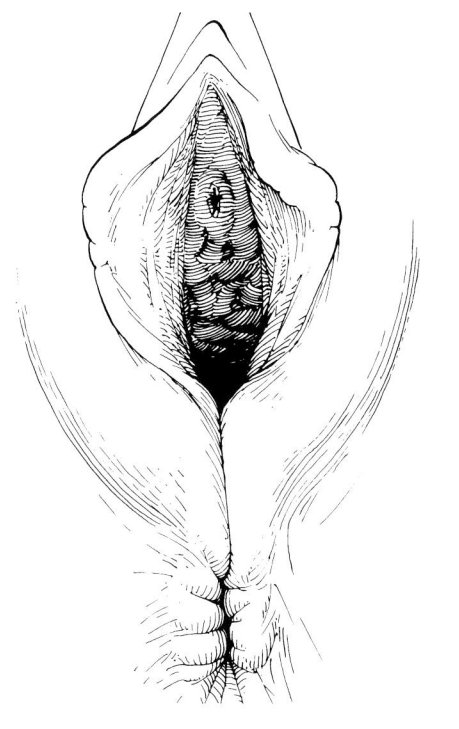

Fig. 20-8 Closure of posterior vaginal mucosa and subcuticular closure of perineal skin.

proximating loosely the perineal body with continuous sutures of No. 2-0 or 3-0 Monocryl or Vicryl.

The vaginal mucosa is then trimmed if necessary. It is then reapproximated with a continuous suture of No. 3-0 Monocryl. The vagina should allow the entrance of two or three fingers (Fig. 20-8). The perianal skin is then closed with a subcuticular closure using No. 5-0 Dexon or Vicryl. At the conclusion of the operation, the anal sphincter should demonstrate good contraction and strength, yet allow enough patency for a digital rectal examination.

Complications

Complications are difficult to handle and may lead to breakdown of the repair. It is easiest to avoid them by following good surgical techniques and preparation. The most common complications are infection, bleeding, hematomas, and breakdowns. Infections tend to occur early and late; therefore, the patient should be seen in the office on a weekly basis. As soon as an infection, induration, increased tenderness, or cellulitis is detected, one must begin treatment with antibiotics and sitz baths. If needed, one must incise and drain any abscess. Early bleeding can be controlled by a pressure ice pack after the surgery. A large hematoma will have to be drained. In my series of 27 patients, the most common complication was delayed infection. There was one failure with the formation of a rectovaginal fistula, but

this was more a failure of the patient to comply with postoperative instructions.

Postoperative measures

Place an ice pack to the perineum to decrease swelling and bleeding. Permit ambulation after 24 hours and administer a stool softener immediately postoperatively. Diphenoxylate with atropine (Lomotil) may be used during the first few days to avoid a bowel movement. Ketorolac tromethamine (Toradol) or Acetominophen (Tylenol No. 3) can be used for pain control. Place the patient on a liquid diet and advance to a low-residue diet on the third postoperative day. Tailor the regimen to avoid diarrhea and constipation. Sitz baths should be started on the second postoperative day.

Summary

Anal incontinence is a socially debilitating problem that may result from many causes. The choice of treatment is usually dictated by etiology. If surgical correction is indicated, the technique described above provides a successful means for the restoration of continence. It is important to remember that there must be an appropriate vascular supply, no evidence of infection, and no tension when approximating tissue. As much scar tissue as possible must be removed. It is also important that all these structures be repaired layer by layer. Complications, then, are minimal, and long-term success can be anticipated. Although the operation is tedious and the preoperative and postoperative care of the patient can be time-consuming, surgical correction of anal incontinence is one of the most rewarding operations.

References

1 West JB. Physiologic basis of medical practice. Baltimore: Williams & Wilkins, 1985.
2 Fry RD, Dockner IJ. Anorectal disorders. CIBA 1985; 37(6).
3 Snell RS. Clinical anatomy. Boston: Little, Brown, 1983.
4 Pritchard JA, MacDonald PC, Gant NF, eds. Williams obstetrics, 17th ed. Norwalk, Conn: Appleton-Century-Crofts, 1985.
5 Russell TR. Anorectum, In: Current surgical diagnosis and treatment. Los Altos, Calif: Lange Medical Publications, 1983.
6 Hauth JC, Gilstrap CC III, Ward SC, et al. Early repair of an external sphincter ani muscle and rectal mucosal dehiscence. Obstet Gynecol 1987;67:806.
7 Sanz LE, Blank KA. Repairing rectovaginal fistulas with the Martius graft. Contemp Obstet Gynecol 1986;68:95.

Suggested readings

Aronson P, Lee R, Berquist T. Anatomy of anal sphincters and related structures in continent women studied with magnetic resonance imaging. Obstet Gynecol 1990;76:846.

Part 3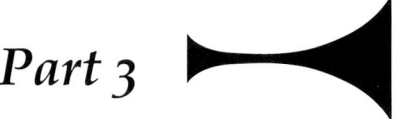

Gynecologic Urologic Surgery

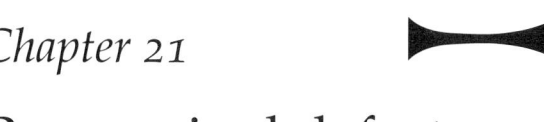

Chapter 21

Paravaginal defect repair for stress urinary incontinence: the A. Cullen Richardson procedure

James P. Youngblood

Nearly all abdominal and vaginal operative procedures currently used for treatment of stress urinary incontinence (SUI) have an eventual failure rate of approximately 15% to 25%. Abdominal procedures include the Marshall-Marchetti-Krantz urethropexy, featuring periurethral fixation to the retropubic periosteum, and the Burch procedure, characterized by paravaginal fascia suspension to Cooper's ligament (1,2). Vaginal procedures are anterior colporrhaphy and Kelly plication. Among combined procedures are those of Pereyra and Stamey (3–5).

Modifications of these various repairs are almost as many as the number of practicing gynecologic surgeons (6). However, all have in common production of a surgical defect to correct an anatomic one. All such techniques, said A. Cullen Richardson, who pioneered a different approach, rely on creation of a "compensatory abnormality" (7).

To my knowledge, this is the first time a description of the paravaginal defect repair for SUI has had affixed the name of A. Cullen Richardson. Even though Dr. Richardson has humbly refrained from using his name in the past, it is time that we honor this man for his basic anatomic research as well as his description of the repair that he so cleverly devised for the treatment of SUI.

Basic anatomy

To grasp Richardson's procedure one must understand the anatomic interrelations of the female bony pelvis (especially the symphysis pubis and coccyx), supporting muscles and fascia, and enclosed organs such as the bladder, urethra, ureters, vagina, cervix, and rectum (Fig. 21-1). Reflecting the bladder medially shows its relation and that of the pubocervical fascia to the lateral pelvic sidewalls and local muscles and vessels (Fig. 21-2). The bladder rests on the pubocervical fascia, which incorporates the entire vagina, whose anterolateral sulci are attached anterolaterally to the pelvic fascia's tendinous arch (white line). The obturator foramen is traversed by the obturator vessels and nerve.

Removing all but the bladder trigone and vagina and transecting the rectum more graphically illustrates the vaginal pubocervical fascia's anterolateral attachment to the white line, which is the tendinous aponeurosis of the obturator internus muscle anteriorly and of the levator ani complex posteriorly (Fig. 21-3). The pubocervical fascia incorporating the anterior vagina acts as a suspending hammock for the bladder and urethra. Childbirth trauma that avulses the vaginal fascia's anterolateral attachment to the white line can allow a collapse of one side of the vagina. If trauma is bilateral, the entire vagina collapses, thereby allowing the proximal urethra and distal bladder (urethrovesical junction) also to collapse.

Removing the bladder and unroofing the vagina, including its anterolateral attachments, causes the vagina to be suspended only by the levator plate and to completely lack anterolateral attachments (Fig. 21-4). Avulsion of the anterolateral vaginal fascia from the arcus tendineus results in a collapse of the urethra and bladder, thereby contributing to SUI (Fig. 21-5).

In Figure 21-6, a right paravaginal defect has caused the attachment of the vagina's anterolateral sulcus to avulse away from the white line. The longitudinal veins overlie the vagina's anterolateral sulcus.

The obturator foramen is positioned about 1.5 to 2 cm above the white line. This is an important landmark, as the white line is often not visible; the "key" stitch (described below) is placed 1.5 to 2 cm below the foramen.

Correcting the defect

In the early 1970s, Richardson, frustrated with his failure rate, reasoned that perhaps proper anatomic restoration could produce continence. His subsequent dissection of both nulliparous and parous fresh cadavers in the Atlanta morgue indicated that SUI was related to a transverse injury at the anterior cervix, or to a central defect, or to a paravaginal defect (Fig. 21-7).

The most common injury, occurring more than 75% to 80% of the time, is the paravaginal defect. It is, in essence,

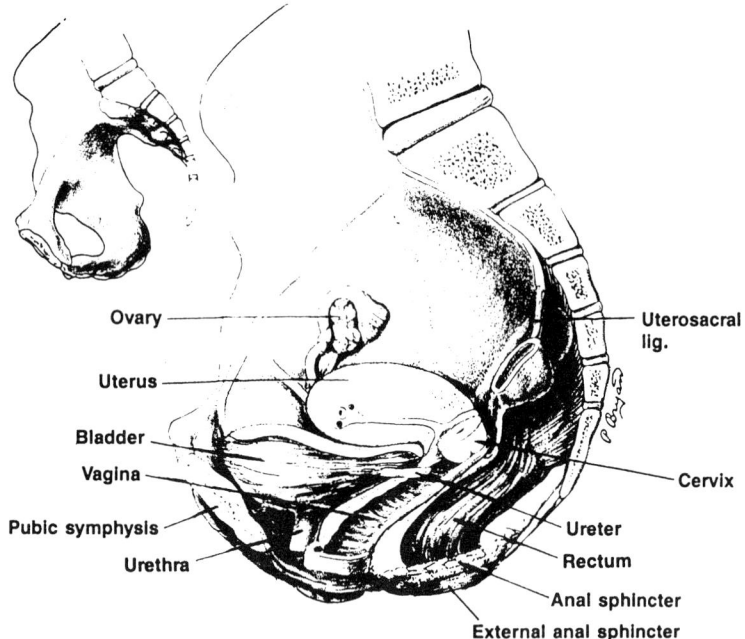

Fig. 21-1 A sagittal view of the female pelvis shows the relationship of the pelvic organs. (Reproduced with permission from Youngblood JP. Paravaginal defect repair for SUI. Contemp Obstet Gynecol 1990; 28–35.)

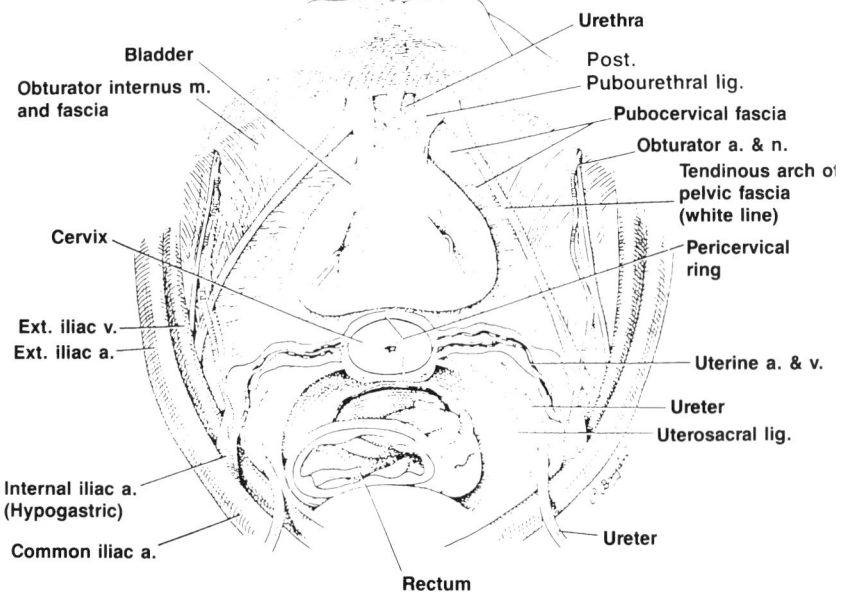

Fig. 21-2 With the bladder reflected medially, note the pubovesical fascia enveloping the vagina and its attachment to the white line. (Reproduced with permission from Youngblood JP. Paravaginal defect repair for SUI. Contemp Obstet Gynecol 1990; 28–35.)

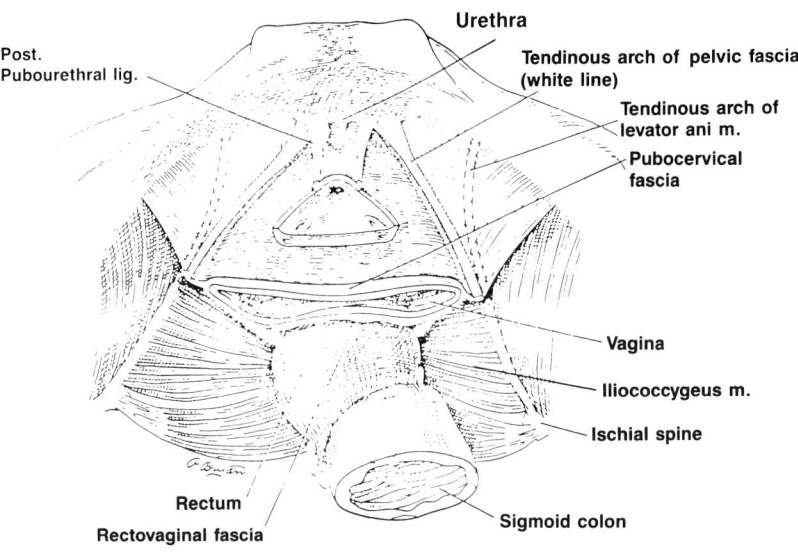

Post.
Pubourethral lig.

Urethra

Tendinous arch of pelvic fascia
(white line)

Tendinous arch of
levator ani m.

Pubocervical
fascia

Vagina

Iliococcygeus m.

Ischial spine

Rectum

Rectovaginal fascia

Sigmoid colon

Fig. 21-3 The pubocervical fascia acts as a suspending hammock for the bladder and urethra. (Reproduced with permission from Youngblood JP. Paravaginal defect repair for SUI. Contemp Obstet Gynecol 1990; 28–35.)

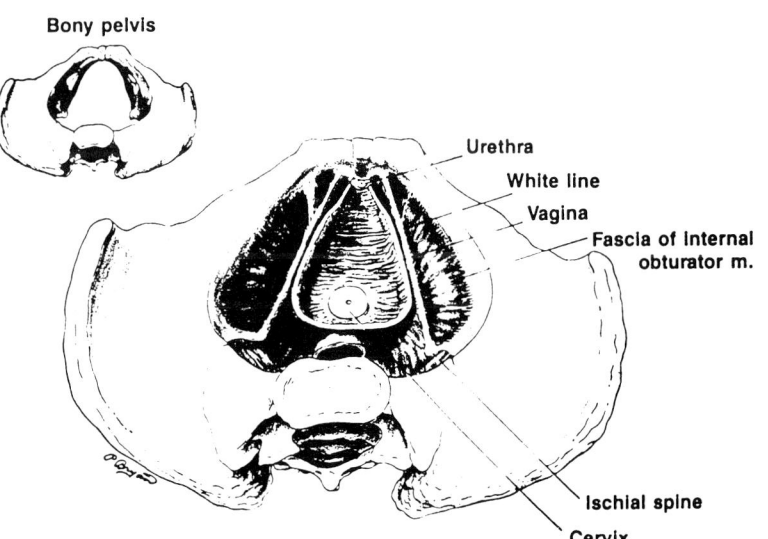

Bony pelvis

Urethra

White line

Vagina

Fascia of internal
obturator m.

Ischial spine

Cervix

Fig. 21-4 With the bladder removed and the vagina's anterior lateral attachments unroofed, the vagina is suspended only by the levator plate. (Reproduced with permission from Youngblood JP. Paravaginal defect repair for SUI. Contemp Obstet Gynecol 1990; 28–35.)

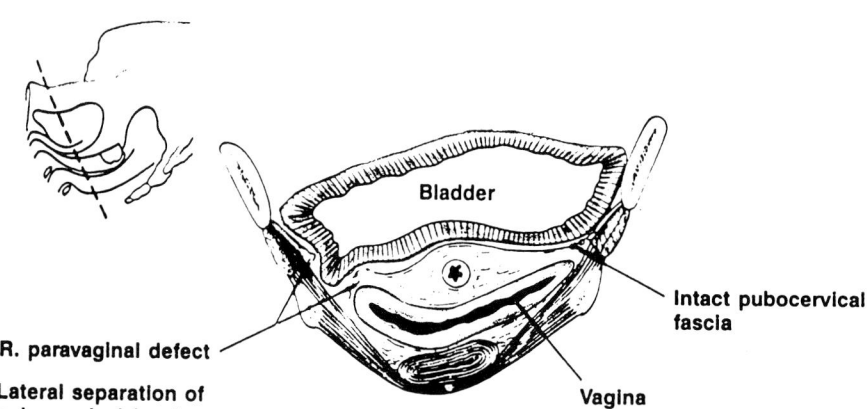

Bladder

Intact pubocervical
fascia

R. paravaginal defect

Lateral separation of
pubocervical fascia

Vagina

Fig. 21-5 Shown is collapse of the urethra and bladder as a result of avulsion of the anterolateral vaginal fascia from the arcus tendineus. This condition contributes to stress urinary incontinence. (Reproduced with permission from Youngblood JP. Paravaginal defect repair for SUI. Contemp Obstet Gynecol 1990;28–35.)

an avulsion of the anterolateral vaginal sulcus from its attachment along the endopelvic fascia's arcus tendineus.
Richardson noted that this defect was almost always on
the right. Between 15% and 20% of the time it was either
on the left or bilateral. Hence, he subsequently developed
the paravaginal defect repair. (Obviously, if one of the
other defects mentioned above is found to be the problem,
specific repair, rather than paravaginal defect repair, is appropriate.)

In 1981, Richardson and coworkers published their experiences with the new procedure (7). They concluded that
it was anatomic, that it almost never resulted in either
short- or long-term urinary retention requiring indwelling
catheterization, and that patients remained continent over
time. (The series, now extending 21 years, has an approximate cure rate of 95%.) Experience at our institution cor-
roborates the group's conclusions.

The procedure

To perform paravaginal defect repair, proceed as follows:
• If the uterus is present, perform total hysterectomy, if indicated, and carry out careful cuff suspension.
• Use uterosacral ligament plication to prevent enterocele formation.
• Next enter the space of Retzius.
• After reflecting the bladder medially and exposing the anterior lateral vaginal wall, place a strategic ("key") stitch opposite the vesical neck in the anterolateral vaginal sulcus after
inserting the left forefinger into the vagina to direct the needle. Place the suture through-and-through the vaginal mucosa, taking care to avoid large longitudinal vessels (Fig. 21-8).
• Pass the needle through the arcus tendineus about 1.5 to
2 cm below the obturator foramen (Fig. 21-9). This action
completes the "key" stitch.

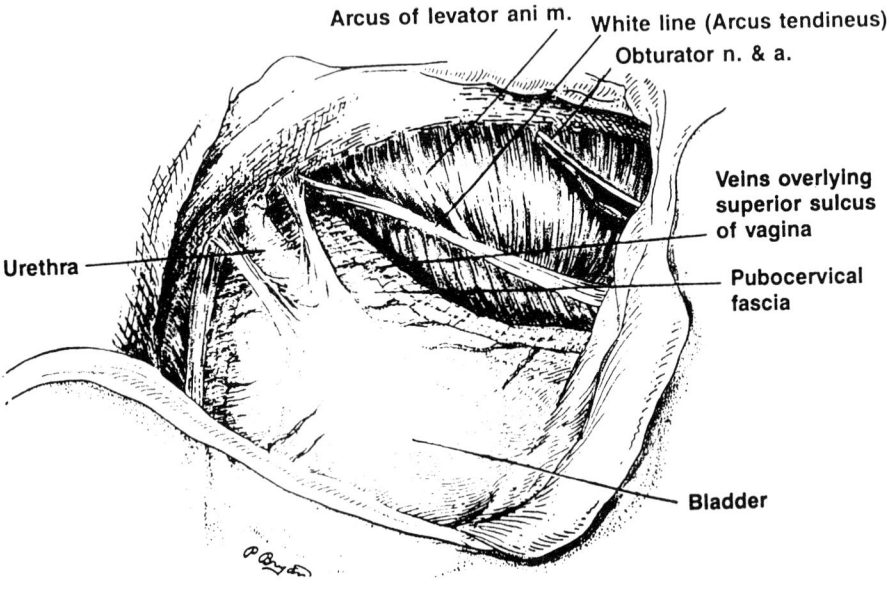

Fig. 21-6 Shown is a right paravaginal defect with the vagina's anterolateral sulcus
avulsed away from the white line. The obturator foramen is depicted 1.5 to 2 cm
above the white line. (Reproduced with
permission from Youngblood JP. Paravaginal defect repair for SUI. Contemp Obstet
Gynecol 1990;28–35.)

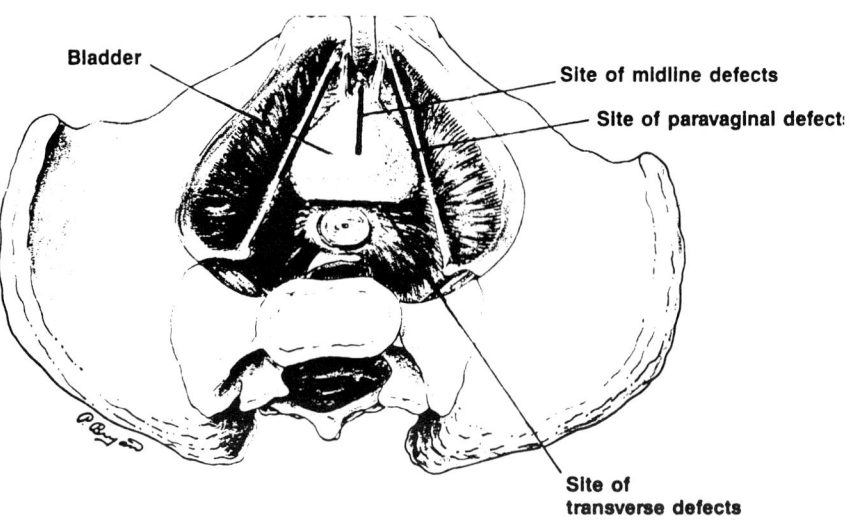

Fig. 21-7 Among injuries that contribute to
stress urinary incontinence, the most important are paravaginal defects. (Reproduced with permission from Youngblood
JP. Paravaginal defect repair for SUI. Contemp Obstet Gynecol 1990;28–35.)

• Similarly, place two to four similar sutures distally and one or two sutures proximally.
• Tie down all of the sutures at one time (Fig. 21-10).
• Use permanent 2-0 polyester braided-plain (Dacron) sutures and small needles.

Not unduly difficult

Although the procedure appears initially to be somewhat more complex than the average urethropexy operation, after observing an experienced operator, we found it was not unduly difficult. Therefore, we heartily endorse it for anatomic surgical treatment of SUI related to a paravaginal defect.

Central and transverse defects are best addressed by anterior colporrhaphy or Kelly plication or both.

If both central and paravaginal defects are present with a very large cystocele, volume reduction may be attained either by abdominal approach (Macer's technique) or by accompanying vaginal anterior colporrhaphy.

Currently under development in many centers by multiple investigators is a vaginal approach to paravaginal defect repair. Shortly there should be many reports regarding this technique. Early indications are that it should be successful. At this time, however, it is not clear whether it will address SUI as well as the abdominal approach. If, indeed, stress incontinence is as well controlled by the vaginal approach to paravaginal defect repair, the woman suffering from cystourethrocele will be well served.

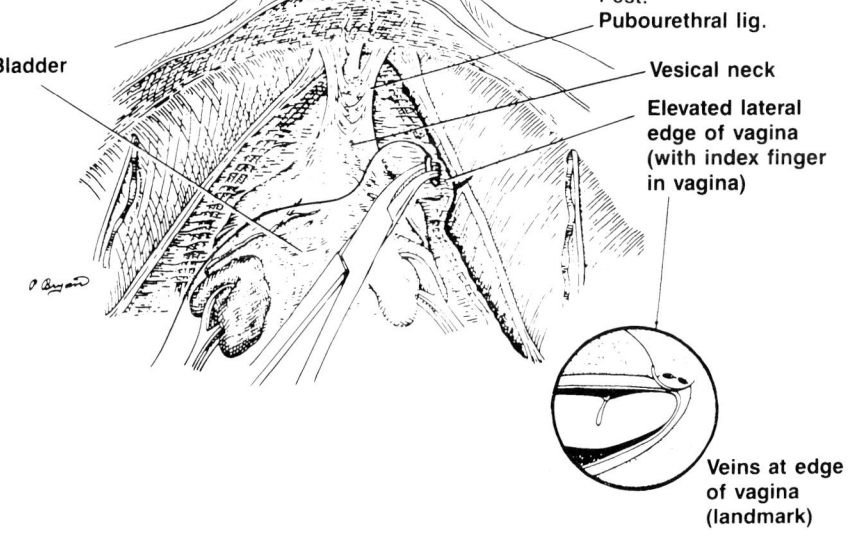

Fig. 21-8 With the left forefinger in the vagina directing the needle (inset), place the "key" stitch. (Reproduced with permission from Youngblood JP. Paravaginal defect repair for SUI. Contemp Obstet Gynecol 1990; 28–35.)

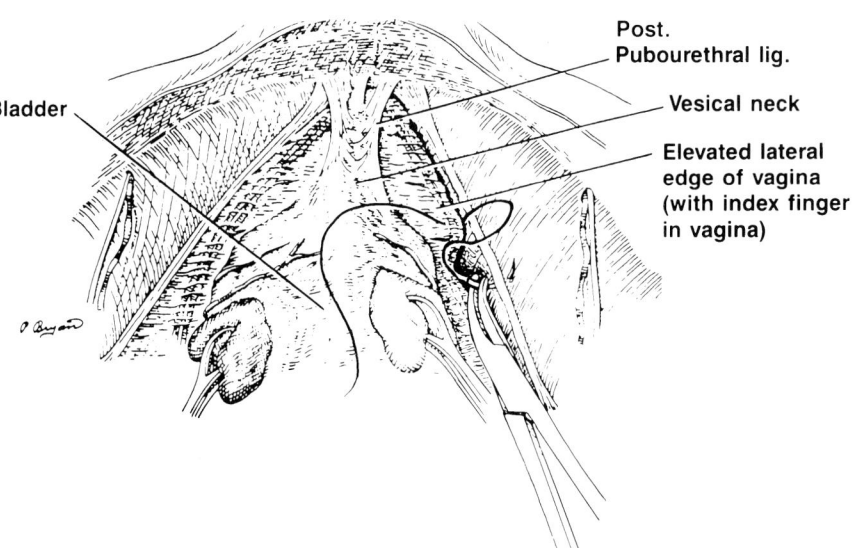

Fig. 21-9 Complete the "key" stitch after passing the needle through the arcus tendineus 1.5 to 2 cm below the obturator foramen. (Reproduced with permission from Youngblood JP. Paravaginal defect repair for SUI. Contemp Obstet Gynecol 1990; 28–35.)

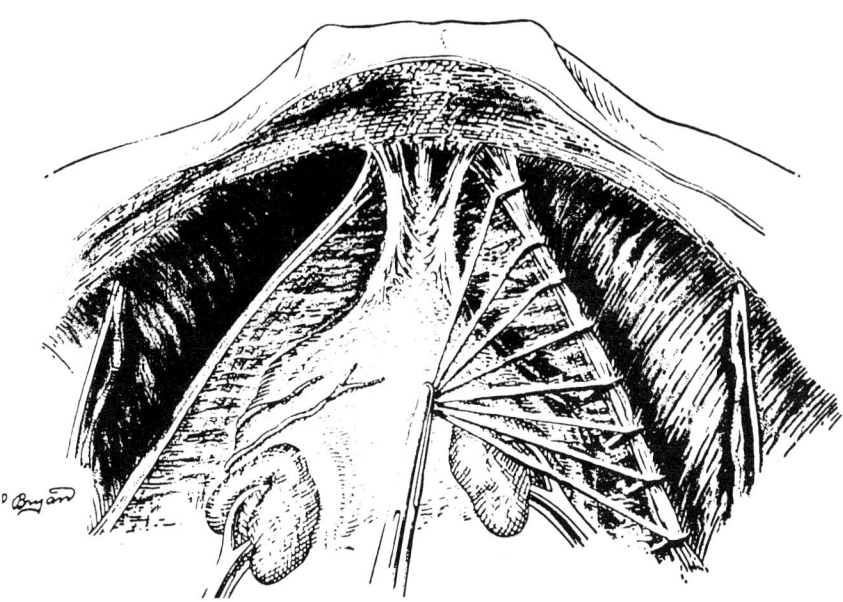

Fig. 21-10 Shown here is complete repair of a right paravaginal defect. (Reproduced with permission from Youngblood JP. Paravaginal defect repair for SUI. Contemp Obstet Gynecol 1990;28–35.)

References

1 Marshall VT, Marchetti AA, Krantz KE. The correction of stress incontinence by simple vesico-urethral suspension. Surg Gynecol Obstet 1949;88:509–518.

2 Burch JC. Urethro-vaginal fixation to Cooper's ligament for correction of stress incontinence, cystocele and prolapse. Am J Obstet Gynecol 1961;81:281–290

3 Schaeffer AJ, Stamey TA. Endoscopic suspension of vesical neck for urinary incontinence. Urology 1984;23:484–494.

4 Asken MH, Abrams PH, Lawrence WT. Stamey endoscopic bladder neck suspension for stress incontinence. Br J Urol 1984;56:629–634.

5 Huland H, Bucher H. Endoscopic bladder neck suspension (Stamey-Pereya) in female urinary stress incontinence. Eur Urol 1984;10: 238–241.

6 Poliak A, Daniller AI, Liebling RW. Sling operation for recurrent stress incontinence using the tendon of the palmaris longus. Obstet Gynecol 1984;63:850–854.

7 Richardson AC, Edmonds PB, Williams NL. Treatment of stress urinary incontinence due to paravaginal fascial defect. Obstet Gynecol 1981;57:357–362.

Chapter 22

Evolution of surgery for stress urinary incontinence

Steven E. Swift and Donald R. Ostergard

Over the years, more than 100 surgical procedures have been devised to cure genuine stress urinary incontinence (SUI), and more than 150 are currently being evaluated and tested. The urethra has been elevated, twisted, kinked, slung, and elongated—both fore and aft. The number of procedures and conflicting opinions on which operation is the most effective, as well as under which circumstances, is bewildering.

The surgical approach to treating genuine SUI began in the late nineteenth century with diversionary procedures and attempts to increase the outflow resistance by twisting and kinking the urethra. In 1907, Giordano introduced a technique utilizing the gracilis muscle to encircle the urethra and act as a sphincter (1). In 1910, Goebell modified this technique by using the pyramidalis muscle and introducing the concept of a suburethral sling (2). This marked the beginning of the modern era in anti-incontinence procedures. Although slings were one of the earlier forms of surgery to correct incontinence, their use was limited to complicated cases of congenital incontinence and never gained acceptance as a primary treatment for uncomplicated SUI.

Howard Kelly, in 1914, was the first to introduce a simple technique for treatment of primary uncomplicated SUI (3). At that time, it was felt that SUI was due to an incompetent urethral sphincter, and this procedure was a simple plication to reinforce the muscle. For many subsequent years, gynecologic dogma held that a vaginal procedure—Kelly plication or the Kennedy modification—was the primary procedure of choice. The disappointing long-term results of this procedure gradually became apparent, particularly when contrasted to the success of retropubic procedures that were subsequently developed.

The introduction of retropubic surgery by Marshall, Marchetti, and Krantz in 1949 was a major breakthrough in the treatment of SUI (4). Since that time, several procedures have been developed and modified around the central concept of elevating the urethrovesical junction (UVJ) and proximal urethra above the pelvic diaphragm. These include the Burch retropubic urethropexy, the paravaginal repair, and a plethora of needle suspension procedures.

As the understanding of the mechanisms of genuine SUI grew, it became apparent that a small group of patients had scarred fixed urethras that did not respond to any of the standard anti-incontinence procedures. In 1947, Foley suggested that a prosthetic sphincter could be devised (5). Early in the development of the artificial urinary sphincter (AUS) there were problems with erosion of the urethral mucosa and mechanical failures. However, the model currently in use has overcome these problems and is a viable option in a small, select group of patients.

The following is a discussion on the development of the different anti-incontinence procedures and their intended benefits. We will also present the current indications for each technique.

Early history of anti-incontinence procedures

In the late nineteenth century, there were two types of procedures described in the literature for curing urinary incontinence—diversionary procedures and techniques to increase the outflow resistance. In his original paper on the plication named for him, Howard Kelly described the procedures in practice at that time (3). The diversion procedures involved either creating a vesicoabdominal fistula then sewing the urethra closed or an elaborate procedure, described by Rose, in which a rectovaginal fistula was surgically developed then the introitus was sewn closed so that the urethra emptied into the vagina, which overflowed through the fistula, allowing the anal sphincter to act as the continence mechanism. These procedures seem barbaric by current standards and fortunately never gained popularity. However, they do show the lengths to which women would go to correct urinary incontinence.

The various techniques to increase the outflow resistance of the urethra were equally as varied and bizarre by current standards. Generally they involved resecting a portion of the UVJ by removing an elliptical piece of vagina with the underlying urethral and bladder mucosa, then reapproximating and closing the defect. In essence, they were constricting the urethral lumen. Other techniques required the urethra to be completely dissected free of the surrounding tissue and then twisted, forming a corkscrew effect. One can only imagine the incidence of vesicovaginal fistulas following such repairs.

Kelly-Kennedy plication

In 1914, Kelly (Fig. 22-1) borrowed on the technique of resecting a portion of the UVJ by plicating the pubourethral fascia beneath the UVJ to constrict the lumen and correct stress incontinence (3). This remained the operation of choice for primary SUI for several decades with subjective cure rates reported at 85% to 90%. In the 1960s, investigators began questioning its effectiveness in curing SUI. Since then, several prospective studies have shown that using long-term objective data, the cure rates run in the 40% to 60% range (6,7). However, there remain proponents of this procedure for correcting mild to moderate SUI, and it still appears in textbooks on gynecologic surgery as an anti-incontinence operation (8).

When Kelly introduced his repair as an anti-incontinence procedure, the thinking was that SUI was due to an incompetent or incomplete urethral sphincter mechanism. Through the trauma of labor and vaginal delivery or as the result of a congenital defect, the sphincter was incomplete or horseshoe-shaped and could not effectively constrict the urethra when contracted. The Kelly plication, as originally described, was the imbrication or plication of the pubocervical fascia underlying the UVJ and bladder base with interrupted sutures of fine silk or linen. This seemed a logical

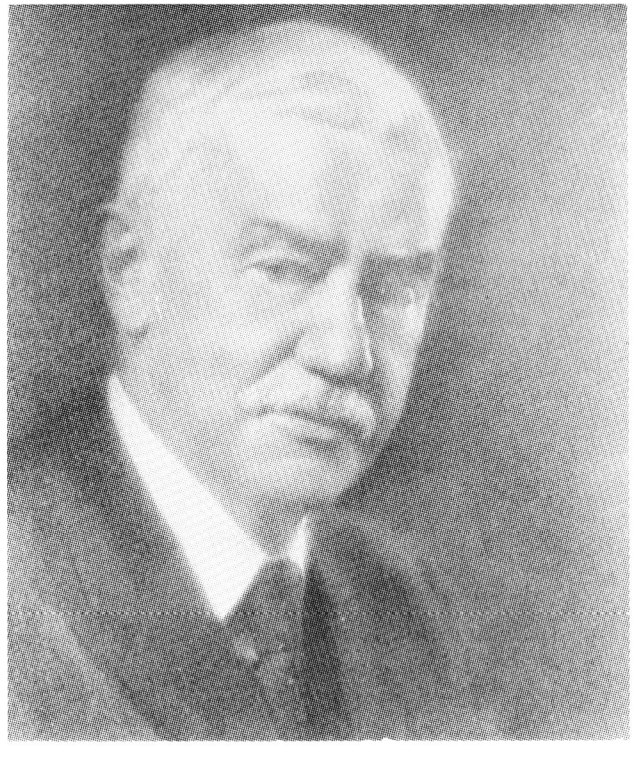

Fig. 22-1 Howard A. Kelly. (Reproduced by permission from Davis AW. Dr. Kelly of Hopkins. Baltimore: Johns Hopkins Press, 1959.)

procedure for strengthening and tightening the sphincter by reapproximating the free ends and restoring its circumferential configuration. He reported that 16 of 20 patients were cured of their incontinence, but he gave no information on how the patients were diagnosed, and follow-up was by patient report with no mention of examinations.

In 1937, Kennedy introduced a modification to Kelly's repair (9). He felt that part of the problem with the urethral sphincter mechanism in SUI was lateral scarring that occurred with childbirth. This caused the urethra to be attached laterally to the inferior border of the descending rami of the pubic bone, and the sphincter was now essentially tented laterally and unable to freely contract. His modification was to extend the lateral dissection and free the periurethral tissue from the inferior pubic rami. He is also credited with introduction of a second layer of imbricating sutures beneath the urethra (now referred to as the Kelly-Kennedy plication). However, earlier in 1922 Young described placing a second layer of imbricating sutures beneath the urethra to reinforce and bolster the sphincter in patients with simple incontinence whose onset was late in life (10). Kennedy also advocated placing three interrupted vertical mattress sutures of silver wire as far lateral as possible in the periurethral tissue to hold this area medially. This was done to prevent the sphincter from reattaching to the pubic rami during the healing process. The silver wire sutures were removed on postoperative day 12. He reported 26 of 28 patients cured with this technique. Again, there was no mention of how patients were diagnosed or how patients were followed and what their criteria for cure were.

In the late 1960s, investigators began questioning the efficacy of the Kelly-Kennedy plication as more objective criteria were used to document cures. Low, in 1967, performed one of the first objective studies of patients with SUI treated with a Kelly-Kennedy plication (11). They evaluated patients objectively before and after the procedure by clinical examinations, cystometry, and radiographic studies. They reported a cure rate of only 46%. This was one of the earliest reports to suggest that this procedure may be inappropriate for correcting SUI.

Our current concept of SUI has changed since Kelly and Kennedy's work. The importance of replacing the proximal urethra to a high retropubic position, so that any rise in intra-abdominal pressure is fully transmitted to the urethra, is now stressed. Also, our knowledge of the anatomy has increased, and the "scar tissue" that Kennedy was taking down probably represented the pubourethral ligaments that are now considered an important part of the support mechanism.

A further modification of the Kelly-Kennedy plication has been described taking the current knowledge of SUI into account (8,12). Here subjective success rates of 80% are reported with this technique in which the UVJ plicating sutures are placed through the pubourethral ligament at its attachment to the periosteum of the inferior border of the pubic symphysis (Fig. 22-2). In reality, this is an attempt to perform a Marshall-Marchetti-Krantz procedure vaginally, thus providing increased support for the UVJ. However, even with this technique, there are no good long-term objective studies that demonstrate its efficacy.

Currently, the anterior repair with the Kelly-Kennedy bladder neck plication should not be used as an anti-incontinence procedure, as the objective success rates are only in the 50% to 60% range, and there are other procedures with objective cure rates in the 85% to 90% range (6,7). The mechanism of action with this repair is probably simply to constrict the urethral lumen and increase outflow resistance. This is similar to the method of action with UVJ bulking agents, and it is interesting that the cure rates are similar (13).

Twenty years ago, gynecologic dogma held that in patients with uncomplicated SUI, one should first perform a vaginal procedure and then, if this failed, go above. However, the current thinking is that the best chance of curing SUI is with the first procedure, so that procedure should be selected carefully.

Retropubic urethropexies

The first major breakthrough in anti-incontinence surgery occurred in 1949 with the introduction of a retropubic urethropexy by Marshall, Marchetti, and Krantz (Fig. 22-3)

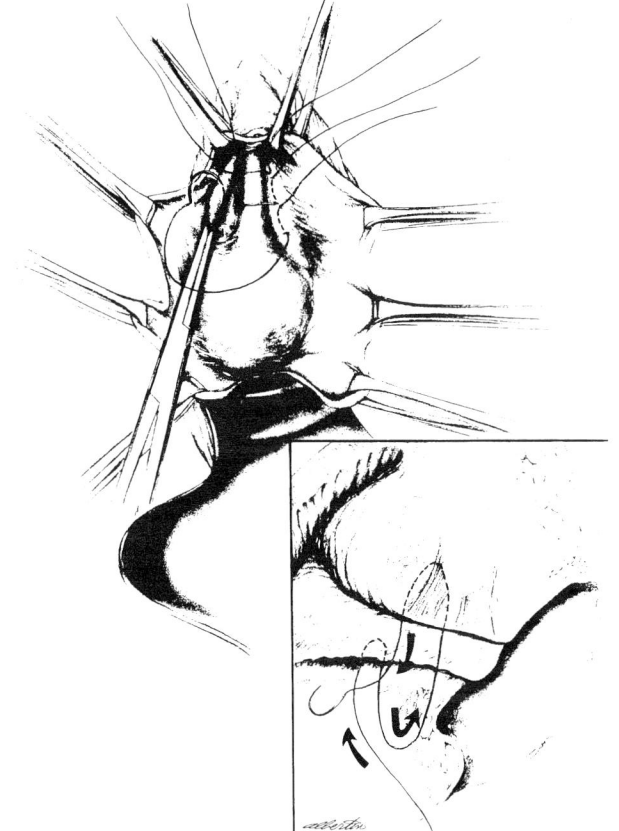

Fig. 22-2 This demonstrates the plication of the proximal urethra and UVJ using a permanent suture. Inset: note that the UVJ suture is placed deep and incorporates the pubourethral fascia where it attaches to the periosteum of the pubic bone. (Reproduced by permission from Thompson JD. TeLinde's operative gynecology, ed 7. Philadelphia: JB Lippincott, 1992.)

(14). Although a similar technique had been described some 20 years earlier by Hepburn, who used it to correct prolapse of the female urethra in children, they were the first to describe its use as an anti-incontinence procedure (15). Their application came out of observations in males. They noted a subset of men who had stress incontinence of urine following transurethral revision of the vesical outlet done to correct obstructive voiding that resulted from resection of the rectum. These individuals had excessive sagging of the perineum after an abdominal-perineal resection of the rectum. This often resulted in obstruction. Many of these patients underwent transurethral resection of their prostates or vesical necks, and a few mysteriously developed incontinence despite apparently normal function of the urethral sphincter. They described the following case, which seemed to integrate all of these observations and led directly to the development of the Marshall-Marchetti-Krantz procedure:

A 54-year-old male had complete urinary retention following abdominoperineal removal of the rectum. Neu-

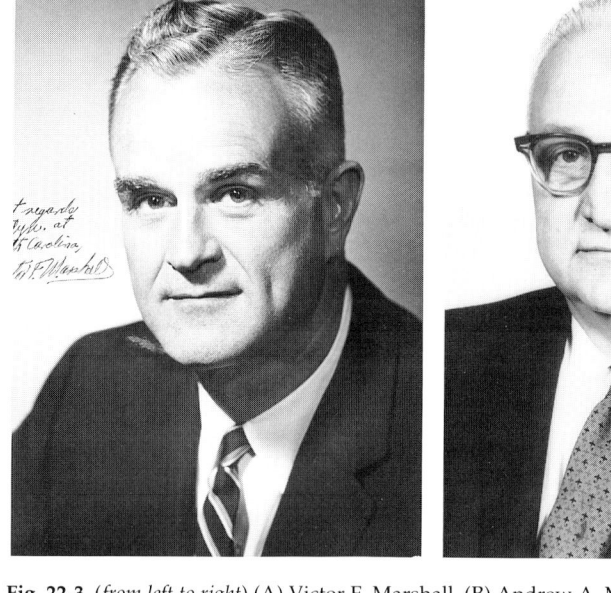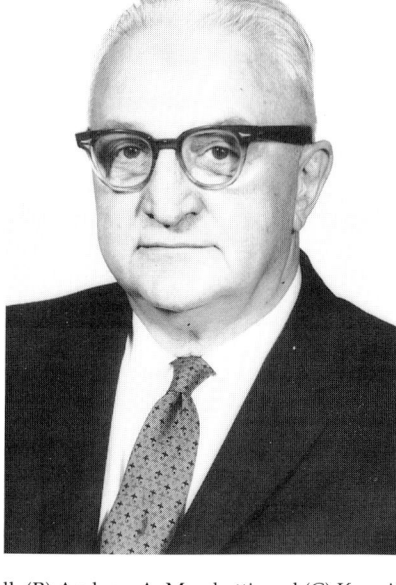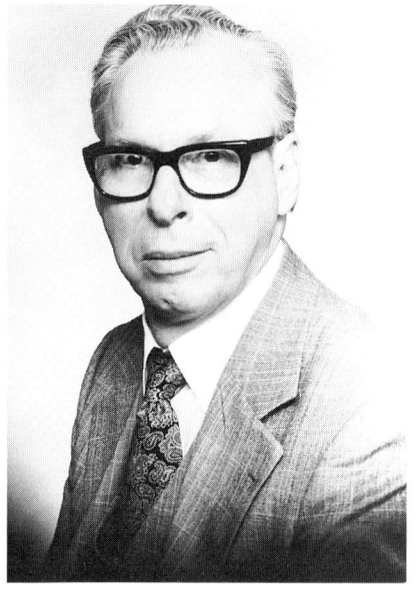

Fig. 22-3 (*from left to right*) (A) Victor F. Marshall, (B) Andrew A. Marchetti, and (C) Kermit E. Krantz.

rologic changes in the urinary apparatus could not be demonstrated. Two transurethral resections resulted in total incontinence, even though the external sphincter had not been damaged. Perineal pressure would provide good control. Simple suprapubic suspension of the vesical outlet corrected his urinary control, which has remained normal for 46 months.

The first Marshall-Marchetti-Krantz urethropexy was performed on a male by a urologist, and in Marshall, Marchetti and Krantz's original report, 4 of the 50 patients were men.

Their procedure required suprapubic dissection into the space of Retzius. Sutures of No. 1 chromic catgut were placed through the pubocervical fascia just lateral to the urethra, and included the wall of the urethra, on either side along its entire length. These were then placed through the periosteum of the pubic rami adjacent to the symphysis pubis, effectively suspending the urethra from the back of the pubic bone (Fig. 22-4). Several sutures were also placed in the dome of the bladder to attach it to the underside of the rectus fascia.

They reported that 82% of patients had an excellent result, meaning that the patients had no complaints of urine loss despite pursuing normal activities. They could not explain why simple elevation of the urethra and vesical neck cured SUI, but they felt that this was a major factor in maintenance of urinary control. However, in keeping with the dogma of that time, they recommended this procedure only when previous surgery (Kelly-Kennedy plication) had failed.

In 1961, Burch improved on the technique of the Marshall-Marchetti-Krantz by utilizing Cooper's ligament (16). While performing the procedure, they had difficulty

with sutures pulling out of the periosteum. They noted that the anterior vaginal wall was easily elevated to the arcus tendineus levator ani (white line), so the periurethral sutures were placed there. They used this technique in seven cases and obtained excellent results. Eventually, they felt this would not provide adequate support, so they went in search of a sturdier structure and settled on Cooper's ligament, which was well known to surgeons as a strong ligament used for repairing inguinal and femoral hernias.

The procedure is similar to the Marshall-Marchetti-Krantz, except that the pubocervical fascial sutures do not incorporate the wall of the urethra and are taken up to Cooper's ligament instead of the pubic symphysis (Fig. 22-4). They also used No. 1 chromic catgut. They reported a 100% cure rate in 45 patients with SUI. It is noteworthy that they used this technique in eight patients who only had a cystocele but no SUI and reported excellent results here as well.

There have been several modifications to the Burch retropubic urethropexy. However, other than using permanent suture, the procedure as it is currently performed remains true to Burch's original description.

The Burch procedure has gained widespread acceptance, and it or one of its modifications is the abdominal procedure of choice for most surgeons doing anti-incontinence surgery. It has two main advantages over the Marshall-Marchetti-Krantz: there is no associated osteitis pubis, and it is more effective in correcting mild to moderate cystoceles. However, cure rates for both procedures are in the 85% to 95% range and are consistent from one institution to another (6,7,17).

The greatest problem with the Burch is that the anterior vaginal wall is tented anteriorly, and this opens the posterior compartment to enterocele formation. The incidence of

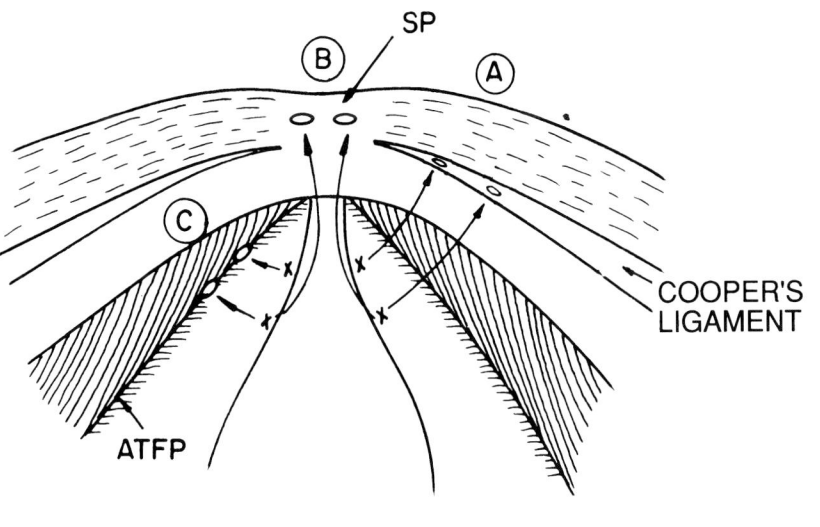

Fig. 22-4 (A) Burch colposuspension with sutures attached to Cooper's ligament. (B) Marshall-Marchetti-Krantz procedure with sutures attached to the periosteum lateral to the symphysis. (C) The paravaginal repair with sutures attached to the arcus tendineus levator ani. SP, symphysis pubis; ATFP, arcus tendinous fascia pelvis. (Reproduced with permission from Richardson DA. Evaluation of different surgical procedures. In: Ostergard DR, Bent AE, eds. Urogynecoloy and urodynamics: theory and practice, ed 3. Baltimore: Williams & Wilkins, 1991.)

this ranges from 7% to 17%, but generally less than half of these patients will require surgical correction (18,19). The paravaginal repair as originally described by Burch and reintroduced by Richardson may be a way to avoid this problem (20). This procedure involves suturing the endopelvic fascia lateral to the urethra and along the bladder base to the arcus tendineus levator ani (white line) (Fig. 22-4). This does not appear to pull the anterior vaginal wall forward as much as the Burch procedure, and the incidence of enterocele formation may be less. There are no long-term data to document cure rates with the paravaginal repair; therefore, it is not known how it compares with other accepted procedures for correcting SUI.

Currently, several investigators are attempting to perform Burch retropubic urethropexies through the laparoscope. If this becomes an accepted procedure, it will most likely reduce postoperative morbidity but will probably not improve the cure rates. Laparoscopic procedures should be considered experimental until appropriate studies are done to document their effectiveness.

The retropubic urethropexies are the gold standard in anti-incontinence surgery. The fact that in almost all objective studies their cure rates are superior to those of other procedures for primary uncomplicated SUI makes them the procedure of choice.

Needle urethropexies

In 1956, Armand Pereyra (Fig. 22-5) became the chief medical officer of the hospital at the California Institution for Women and was presented with the opportunity for close long-term follow-up of his patients. He had several patients who had recurrent SUI following Marshall-Marchetti-Krantz urethropexy. Secondary retropubic dissection and repair revealed fibrous strands between the pubic bone and the pubocervical fascia. He postulated that the traction produced by coughing and Valsalva was in an undesirable vec-

tor to the suture placement with the Marshall-Marchetti-Krantz, and that connecting the sutures to the rectus fascia would transmit forces in a more desirable direction. He also felt that retropubic dissection was unnecessary as he wanted to connect, by suture, two areas of tissue that were both superficial. Thus was born the idea for the needle urethropexies (21).

There is now a plethora of needle procedures bearing names of many individuals. These are all modifications of the Pereyra procedure that center on the idea of suspending the periurethral pubocervical fascia from the rectus fascia (Fig. 22-6). Pereyra modified his procedure many times. The current modified Pereyra procedure evolved from observations throughout his career. Most of the modifications that have been introduced over the years were previously tried and reported on by him. The only major modification introduced by another physician was Stamey's addition of cystoscopy to evaluate placement of the sutures (22).

The original Pereyra procedure involved making a small suprapubic transverse abdominal incision. The special needle and cannula were then passed through the rectus fascia at its insertion into the pubic bone and guided through the space of Retzius, staying close behind the pubic bone and emerging through the vaginal mucosa just lateral to the urethrovesical junction. Stainless steel wire was threaded through the needle. Two passes were made through the mucosa on either side, and the two ends of the wire were brought back up through the rectus fascia, lifted until the anterior vaginal wall was appropriately elevated, and then tied across the midline (23). This is very similar to the current Gittes technique, except that No. 2 hydroxypropylene is used instead of wire and a helical suture technique is used in the vaginal mucosa (Fig. 22-6) (24).

The use of wire has been dropped, and currently all of the needle procedures are done with permanent sutures. The other major modifications involve dissection into the retropubic space from below and the introduction of en-

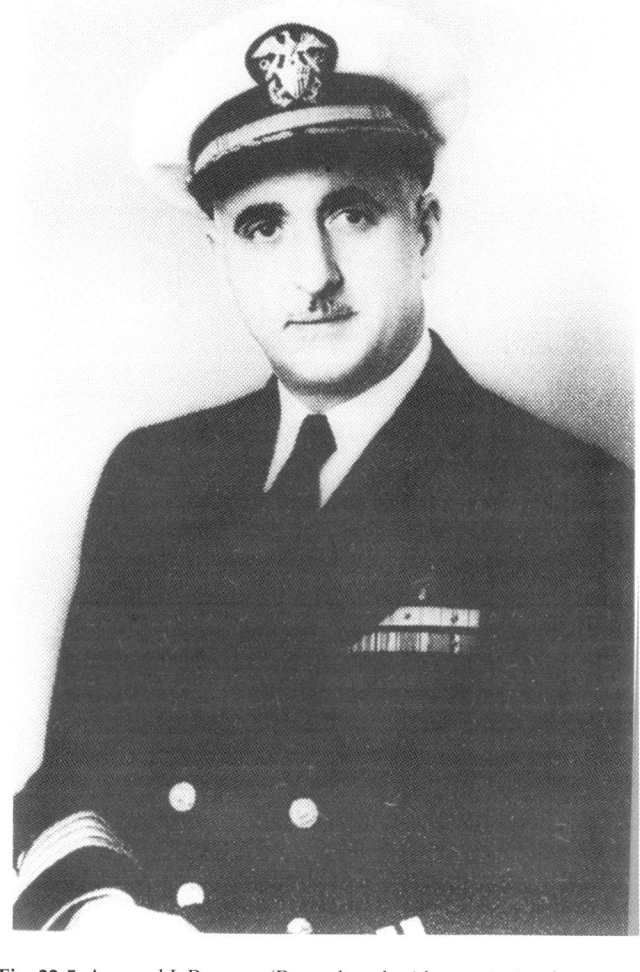

Fig. 22-5 Armand J. Pereyra. (Reproduced with permission from Cornella JL, Pereyra AJ. Historical vignette of Armond J. Pereyra, MD, and the modified Pereyra procedure: the needle suspension for stress incontinence in the female. Int Urogynecol J 1990;1:25–30.)

doscopy. Pereyra serendipitously discovered that transvaginal penetration of the urogenital diaphragm and dissection of the space of Retzius would allow for easier and safer passage of the needles. This occurred accidentally one day during vaginal dissection. He realized it aided in mobilization of the tissues and allowed for delivery of the needle with less risk of perforation of the bladder, so he repeated it on the other side. From then on, he incorporated it into his procedure (21). It may also increase scarification of the bladder neck and surrounding tissue to the posterior aspect of the pubic bone and give more durable long-term results. This is very similar to the Raz technique except that he uses an inverted U incision on the anterior vaginal wall instead of a simple midline incision and incorporates the vaginal wall in the helical sutures (25).

Stamey introduced the use of endoscopy in 1973 to assist with suture placement and with suture tension (22). He has also been credited with introducing Dacron buttresses on the vaginal loop to prevent suture pullthrough. However, Pereyra used these between 1968 and 1971 and abandoned

this practice because of problems with infection (21). Stamey's technique does not call for retropubic dissection. He advocates using the endoscope to ensure placement of the sutures at the urethrovesical junction and to assess the tension required to close the UVJ when tying down the sutures. In his original article, he placed the Dacron buttresses only in patients who had weak pubocervical fascia. However, he stated that in the future "the sleeve of knitted Dacron should be used to buttress the vaginal loop of nylon in every patient" (Fig. 22-6) (22). He did not encounter any problems with infection, although others have reported a 5% rate of infection or foreign body reaction requiring removal (26). The Stamey procedure, as it is currently performed, requires the use of the Dacron buttresses.

Needle urethropexies are a common procedure used to correct SUI. Their popularity stems from their low morbidity, short hospital stay, and short convalescence time. The problem with these procedures is that their results are inconsistent, as noted in the literature. Most of the studies with objective, long-term follow-up report cure rates in the 40% to 85% range, and when they are compared with retropubic urethropexies, they are consistently poorer (27–30). Also, unlike the retropubic urethropexies, their results vary widely between institutions, with subjective cure rates as low as 40% and as high as 96% (22,23). A recent multicenter study of the modified Pereyra procedure documented a one-year objective (urodynamic studies before and after operation) cure rate of 63%, which is similar to that of a Kelly-Kennedy plication (31). At present, the low urodynamically validated success rates would seem to contraindicate their use in patients with uncomplicated SUI. They have been shown to be effective in patients with potential incontinence (SUI that is noted in patients with severe uterovaginal prolapse only when the prolapse is reduced during preoperative evaluation, but otherwise have no complaints of urine loss). Bergman used the modified Pereyra in these patients and, at 6 months, noted an objective cure rate of 100% (32).

Regarding retropubic procedures for correcting SUI, it is curious that, overall, urologists seem to prefer a needle procedure (which was developed by a gynecologist) while gynecologists seem to prefer a retropubic urethropexy (which was developed in part by a urologist stemming from observations in males).

Suburethral sling procedures

In the early part of the twentieth century, there were several reports in the German literature on the use of suburethral sling procedures to correct SUI. In 1910, Goebell described a procedure for detaching the pyramidalis muscle and suturing the free ends beneath the urethra, thus forming a muscular sling (2). This technique had its origins in a previous report by Giordano, who used a gracilis muscle flap to form a circular sphincter around the urethra (1). Initially a

MODIFIED PEREYRA   GITTES   STAMEY

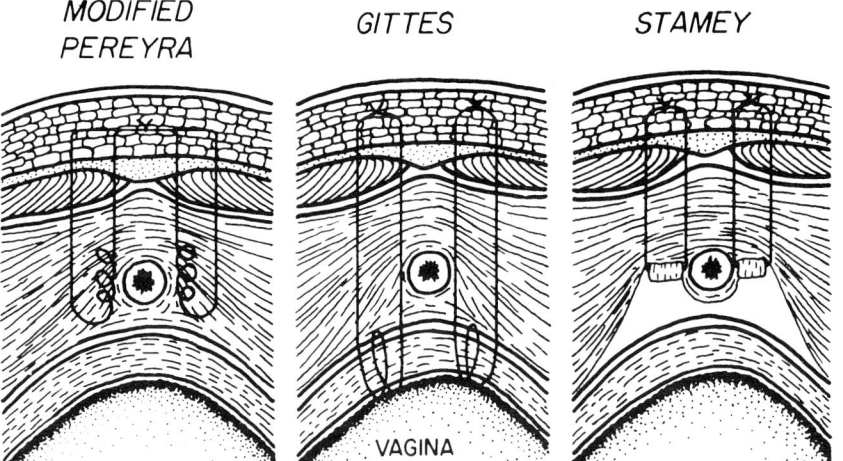

VAGINA

Fig. 22-6 Three variations of the needle urethropexy procedures. (Reproduced with permission from Richardson DA. Evaluation of different surgical procedures. In: Ostergard DR, Bent AE, eds. Urogynecology and urodynamics: theory and practice, ed 3. Baltimore: Williams & Wilkins, 1991.)

muscular sling was used as it was intended to act as a sphincter as well as a sling to support the urethra. Stoekel modified this in 1917 by developing a strip of rectus fascia attached to the pyramidalis muscle and securing this beneath the urethra (33). By the late 1920s and early 1930s, it was recognized that the muscular portion of the sling was unnecessary and only added bulk, making for a difficult dissection and placement of the graft underneath the urethra.

Price, while working in China in 1933, was the first to introduce an autologous fascia lata graft for the sling procedure (34). He described the case of a young Chinese girl with congenital absence of the coccyx, who was incontinent of both stool and urine. She underwent a procedure to correct her fecal incontinence using a fascia lata graft looped around the anus and attached to the gluteal muscles. This was so successful that he devised a procedure using a fascia lata graft looped under the urethra, brought up through the space of Retzius, and attached to the underside of the rectus muscles. They felt attaching the graft to the rectus fascia would provide too much tension and kink the urethra, making it impossible to void. This was the first report of a fascial suburethral sling not employing a muscular component. Aldridge improved on this by utilizing a graft of rectus fascia that was left attached on one end, looped under the urethra, and attached to the rectus fascia on the opposite side (35). All of the active slings are currently brought up to or over the anterior rectus fascia. This technique appeared as effective as the muscular slings, and since then investigators have abandoned the use of transposed muscle.

Other modifications were introduced, but these proved ineffective and, for the most part, have been abandoned. Passing the sling anterior to the pubic symphysis was tried, but not adopted, because it provided the wrong angle of support beneath the urethra (36). There were also concerns regarding infection with the vaginal incision, and in 1948 Millin advocated tunneling under the urethra without any vaginal dissection (37). This technique, which resulted in

increased incidence of bladder and urethral injury, is rarely used today.

Currently, the techniques used for suburethral slings vary greatly but can be divided into two main types. Most of the slings are active, meaning that the graft is passed beneath the urethral vesical junction and then brought up through the space of Retzius and either sutured to the rectus fascia or brought anterior to it and the free ends are sutured to each other (Fig. 22-7). Therefore, whenever the patient contracts her abdominal wall, the sling is pulled up, kinking the proximal urethra and preventing urine loss. The other type of sling can be termed passive. The free ends of the graft are attached to a fixed structure, such as Cooper's ligament, and the sling acts as a shelf under the proximal urethra. When there is an increase in abdominal pressure, the bladder rotates posteriorly and the proximal urethra remains fixed so that it is compressed against the sling, obstructing the flow of urine. Currently, there are too many different techniques for any one to be discussed in detail.

Several materials have been used as a sling, while the search continues for a material that will not be rejected, will provide long-term strength, and can be easily removed or adjusted if the patient becomes obstructed. So far this has proved to be a difficult task, and most of the modifications over the past 40 years have revolved around this issue. While autologous fascia may seem an ideal choice, it can be difficult to obtain a large enough piece of rectus fascia, especially if the patient has had an abdominal procedure. There are also problems with obtaining fascia lata, and it requires a separate procedure for harvesting. There are data suggesting that individuals with genuine SUI and genitourinary prolapse have an inherent defect in their connective tissue, so long-term durability may also be a problem (38,39). We prefer the use of Goretex® (W. L. Gore, Flagstaff, Ariz), as it is easy to work with, durable, and easy to remove; however, it has a high rejection rate. Others have used nylon, Marlex mesh® (Davol Rubber Co., Providence, RI), and Mersilene strips® (Ethicon, Somerville, NJ).

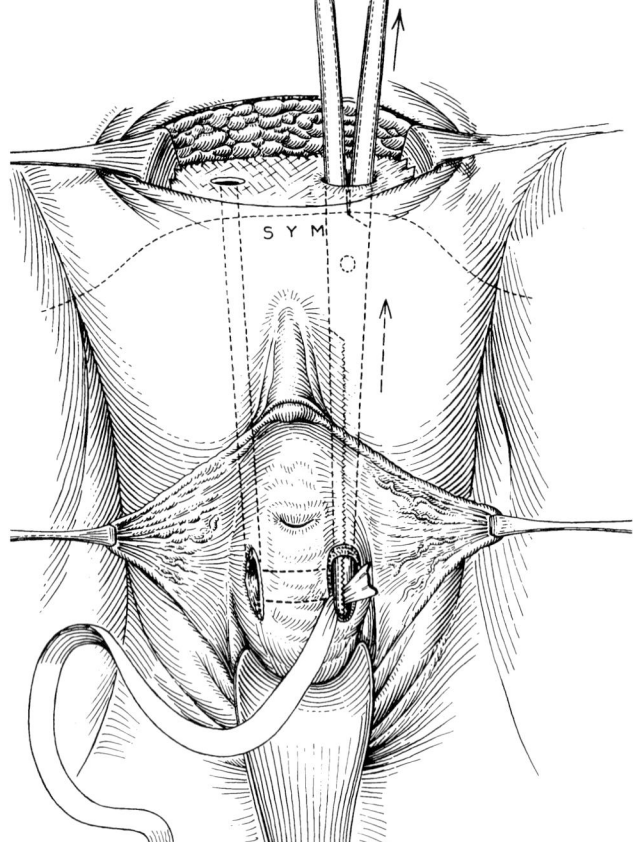

Fig. 22-7 Active suburethral sling with the dashed line showing where the graft will lie once in place. The sling loops underneath the urethrovesical junction, is brought up over the anterior rectus fascia, and is fixed in place. (Reproduced by permission from Ridley JH. Te Linde's operative gynecology, ed 7. Philadelphia: JB Lippincott, 1992.)

Another controversy surrounding suburethral slings is under what circumstances they should be used. In the past, slings were used only as a salvage procedure in patients with recurrent incontinence or as a primary surgery in young girls with a congenital defect responsible for their SUI (8,37,40). Currently, many investigators feel that the sling has a role as a primary procedure in patients with a low pressure or a nonfunctioning urethral sphincter mechanism (41).

In 1981, McGuire evaluated his patients who failed standard anti-incontinence procedures and found that the majority had relatively low urethral closure pressures, suggesting a poorly functioning sphincter mechanism (42). In 1987, Sand found a recurrence rate of 54% in patients who underwent a Burch procedure and had a maximal urethral closure pressure of less than 20 cm of water (43). In this group of patients, a suburethral sling should be considered as a primary procedure.

Over the years, suburethral sling procedures have undergone many modifications in technique, graft material, and indications for their use. However, regardless of the

procedure used, they remain an excellent option for certain individuals with SUI and have objective cure rates between 85% and 95% (41,43,44).

Artificial urinary sphincters

The artificial urinary sphincter (AUS) was first introduced by Foley in 1947 as a means of controlling incontinence in men with a defective external sphincter (45). His device was an inflatable cuff applied externally to the penile urethra. Obviously this could not be used in the female, but the idea of implanting an inflatable cuff had its origins with this device. Through the 1960s, several implantable devices were developed for the penile urethra, but it was not until 1973 that Scott and associates introduced a device for the female urethra (46).

The early device had a silicone cuff that was implanted around the urethra. This was connected to a reservoir balloon by two tubes with one-way valves. The valves were implanted into either labia and were used to inflate or deflate the cuff manually. The patient would squeeze the valve in the labia to deflate the cuff, allowing micturition and reinflation by squeezing the other valve. The maximal cuff pressure was set below tissue perfusion pressure, and while this maintained continence under normal circumstances, it could not always prevent urine loss under conditions of significant physical activity. There were also problems with mechanical failures requiring reoperation, which led to further modifications and developments (47).

The AUS now used (AS-800®, American Medical Systems, Minnetonka, Minn.; Fig. 22-8) is quite different from the original device introduced by Scott. It has overcome several of the problems with mechanical failures with design changes and simplification of the mechanical workings so that there are fewer parts to fail. The mechanism regulating cuff pressure has also been changed to a dynamic system that can increase under periods of stress. The device currently uses a balloon implanted in the space of Retzius to regulate the cuff pressure. Therefore, any increase in abdominal pressure (i.e., cough, sneeze, Valsalva) will be applied to the balloon, which will transmit it to the cuff and increase the pressure applied to the urethra. Also, now there is only one valve implanted into the labium that allows for deflation of the cuff for micturition. Reinflation occurs by a slow leak-back mechanism, so the patient has about 3 minutes to void, or she will need to deflate the cuff again.

The patients in whom an AUS is indicated are those with a defective urethral sphincter and normal urethral support (48). These are individuals that have normal anatomic positioning of the urethra, but a scarred open or drainpipe urethra. In this select group of patients, success rates range from 75% to 95%. The major drawback to the AUS is mechanical failure, with up to 19% of patients requiring reoperation to repair or replace the components (48,49).

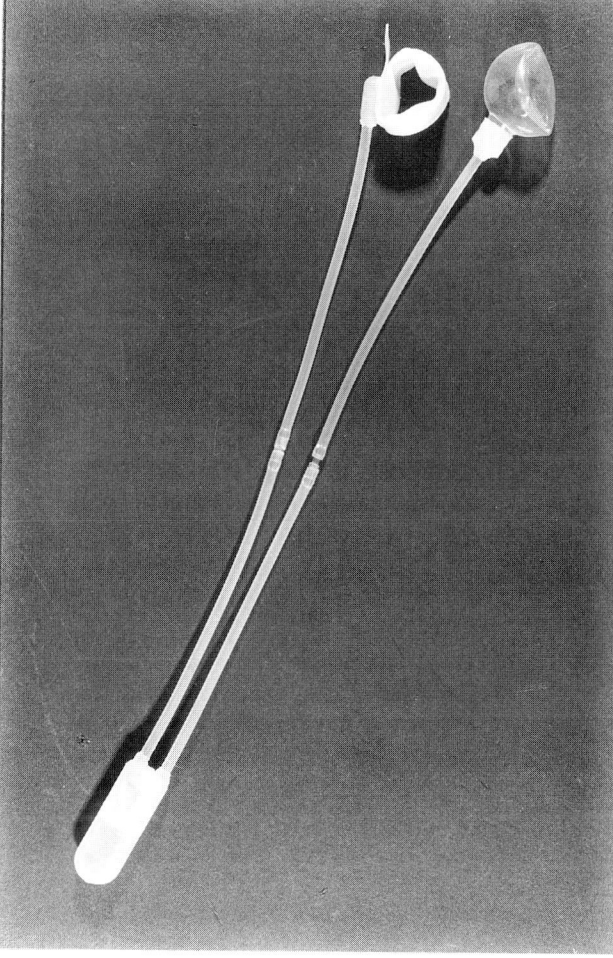

Fig. 22-8 AS-800® artificial urinary sphincter (American Medical Systems, Minnetonka, Minn.).

The AUS is currently an option in treating patients with severe incontinence when there are few alternatives available. It is one of the few methods of treating patients that have a scarred, drainpipe urethra, with the alternatives being urinary diversion or possibly the utilization of UVJ bulking agents. If the UVJ bulking agents become popular and the initial success rates are borne out in further studies, an AUS may be indicated only in patients who have failed injectable therapy.

Urethrovesical bulking agents

Recently, there has been an interest in injecting bulking agents around the urethra at the UVJ to restore continence. The earliest report of periurethral injections in the treatment of SUI was from Murless in 1938 (50). He reported on 20 patients with SUI treated with injections of a 5% solution of sodium morrhuate solution (a sclerosing agent) in the periurethral tissue 1 cm proximal to the external urethral meatus. He noted cure in 60% of his patients at one year, with the only major complication being a sloughing of a patch of vaginal mucosa at the injection site in most of his patients. The first report of using a true bulking agent injected at the UVJ was in 1973 by Berg, who described the use of polytetrafluoroethylene, (Teflon®, E. I. DuPont de Nemours Co., Ft. Lauderdale, Fla.) in three patients (51). He did a pretreatment injection with glycerine (which is absorbed in 36 hours) to determine if patients would obtain continence with a bulking agent to increase urethral resistance. Since then many have described its use in patients who failed standard anti-incontinence surgery, or who have severe incontinence with drainpipe urethras, and have reported long-term subjective cure rates of 20% to 50% (52,53). The problem with Teflon® is that there have been many reports of it migrating to other parts of the body and setting up a granulomatous reaction; therefore, its use has been questioned, and other agents have been sought.

The use of cross-linked collagen was first reported in 1989 (54). However, as for Teflon®, the cure rates were disappointing, with only 24% cured or greatly improved. Other investigators who tried the collagen injections for SUI have shown similar results. Although most of these studies used subjects who had drainpipe urethras or failed previous surgery, there is one report of its use as a primary form of therapy (55). However, the authors did not report on this group separately, so we do not know its effectiveness in this subset of patients. They did report on its success by type of incontinence and noted an objective cure rate of 50% in patients with a normal urethral sphincter mechanism. The problem with collagen is that eventually the body will absorb it, and the patients will require reinjection. Other agents are being evaluated, such as bioglass, whose use was reported in dogs and pigs (56).

The greatest advantage to UVJ bulking agents is the low associated morbidity. The technique for injecting the agents is simple and can be done in the office with little anesthesia. A 0-degree urethroscope is placed such that the UVJ can be seen in its entirety. The material is then injected transvaginally to add bulk to the UVJ. Generally, three or four injections are made around the circumference of the urethra to cause the mucosa to bulge into the canal and just occlude the UVJ opening at rest. Frequently, at least two series of injections are required for patient satisfaction.

The use of injectable bulking agents has not found widespread use, and whether or not it becomes a primary treatment depends on future studies. It will probably have a place as a treatment for type III incontinence, and the trial of an injectable bulking agent may be appropriate before placement of an AUS, which is one of the few alternatives for these patients.

Summary

Currently there are more than 100 procedures used to correct stress urinary incontinence. They have been developed and refined over the past century so that now one can offer acceptable cures to most patients with SUI. However, there are still many failures and patients who are not candidates for any of these procedures. Therefore, new and alternative procedures must be developed and evaluated. One of the most important lessons that can be gleaned from this history is that we must evaluate, in an objective fashion, all of our current techniques so that we can offer the best procedure to the individual patient. This means that multichannel urodynamics or radiographic studies must be done both preoperatively and at least one year postoperatively to document cure rates. Subjective data such as telephone follow-up or mailed questionnaires are not sufficient evidence on which to base a surgical decision. Also, trying to use one procedure to correct all patients with SUI will lead to an unacceptably high failure rate and a loss of trust on the part of the patient.

In patients with uncomplicated SUI and an intact intrinsic sphincter mechanism, we believe the retropubic urethropexy is the best procedure with excellent long-term cure rates. The needle procedures have inconsistent results and poor objective cure rates; therefore, we cannot recommend their use in patients with uncomplicated SUI. However, they have been shown to be effective in patients with potential incontinence. The anterior repair should no longer be considered as an anti-incontinence procedure, as the cure rates at long-term follow-up are poor. The role of the suburethral sling as a primary procedure for patients with poor urethral support and an intrinsically defective sphincter mechanism is becoming better recognized and accepted. The artificial urinary sphincter remains one of a few options for patients with a fixed, scarred urethra, but this is an one area in which the injectable agents may have a significant impact.

Acknowledgments

Special thanks to H. O. Williamson, MD, for his insights and review of this manuscript.

References

1 Hohenfellner R, Petrie E. Sling procedures in surgery. In: Stanton SL, Tanagho E, eds. Surgery of female incontinence, ed 2. Berlin: Springer-Verlag, 1986:105–113.
2 Goebell R. Zur operativen beseitigung der angeborenen. Incontinentia Vesicae Z Gynakol Urol 1910;2:187–192.
3 Kelly HA, Dumm WM. Urinary incontinence in women without manifest injury to the bladder. Surg Gynecol Obstet 1914;18:444–450.
4 Marshall VR, Marchetti AA, Krantz KE. The correction of stress incontinence by simple vesicourethral suspension. Surg Gynecol Obstet 1949;88:509–518.
5 Foley FEB. An artificial sphincter: a new device and operation for control of enuresis and urinary incontinence. J Urol 1947;58:250–259.
6 Van Geelen JM, Theeuwes AGM, Eskes TKAB, Martin CB. The clinical and urodynamic effects of anterior vaginal repair and Burch colposuspension. Am J Obstet Gynecol 1988;159:137–144.
7 Bergman A, Ballard CA, Koonings PP. Comparison of three different surgical procedures for genuine stress incontinence: prospective randomized study. Am J Obstet Gynecol 1989;160:1102–1106.
8 Thompson JD. Selected operations for genuine stress incontinence. In: Thompson JD, Rock JA, eds. TeLinde's operative gynecology, ed 7. Philadelphia: JB Lippincott, 1992:904–940.
9 Kennedy WT. Incontinence of urine in the female, the urethral sphincter mechanism, damage of function, and restoration of control. Am J Obstet Gynecol 1937;34:576–589.
10 Young EL. Urinary incontinence in the female. JAMA 1922;79:1753–1756.
11 Low JA. Management of anatomic urinary incontinence by vaginal repair. Am J Obstet Gynecol 1967;97:308–315.
12 Beck RP, McCormick S. Treatment of urinary stress incontinence with anterior colporrhaphy. Obstet Gynecol 1982;59:269–274.
13 Kieswetter H, Fischer M, Wober L, Flamm J. Endoscopic implantation of collagen (GAX) for the treatment of urinary incontinence. Br J Urol 1992;69:22–25.
14 Marshall VF, Marchetti AA, Krantz KE. The correction of stress incontinence by simple vesicourethral suspension. Surg Gynecol Obstet 1949;88:509–518.
15 Hepburn TN. Prolapse of the urethra in female children. Surg Obstet Gynecol 1927;44:400–401.
16 Burch JC. Urethrovaginal fixation to Cooper's ligament for correction of stress incontinence, cystocele, and prolapse. Am J Obstet Gynecol 1961;81:281–290.
17 Mainprize TC, Drutz HP. The Marshall-Marchetti-Krantz procedure; a critical review. Obstet Gynecol Surv 1988;43:724–729.
18 Burch JC. Cooper's ligament urethrovesical suspension for stress incontinence. Am J Obstet Gynecol 1968;100:764–768.
19 Stanton SL, Williams JE, Ritchie B. The colposuspension operation for urinary incontinence. Br J Obstet Gynaecol 1976;83:890–896.
20 Richardson AC, Edmonds PB, Williams NL. Treatment of stress urinary incontinence due to paravaginal fascial defect. Obstet Gynecol 1981;57:357–362.
21 Cornella JL, Pereyra AJ. Historical vignette of Armond J. Pereyra, MD, and the modified Pereyra procedure: the needle suspension for stress incontinence in the female. Int Urogynecol J 1990;1:25–30.
22 Stamey TA. Endoscopic suspension of the vesical neck for urinary incontinence. Surg Gynecol Obstet 1973;136:547–554.
23 Pereyra AJ. A simplified surgical procedure for the correction of stress incontinence in women. West J Surg Obstet Gynecol 1959;67:223–226.
24 Gittes RF, Loughlin KR. No-incision pubovaginal suspension for stress incontinence. J Urol 1987;138:568–572.
25 Raz S. Modified bladder neck suspension for female stress incontinence. Urology 1981;17:82–85.
26 Richardson DA, Bent AE, Ostergard DR, Cannon D. Delayed reaction to Dacron buttress used in urethropexy. J Reprod Med 1984;29:689–692.
27 Mundy AR. A trial comparing the Stamey bladder neck suspension procedure with colposuspension for the treatment of stress incontinence. Br J Urol 1983;55:687–690.
28 Weil A, Reyes H, Bischoff P, Rottenberg RD, Krauler F. Modification of the urethral rest and stress profile after different types of surgery for stress incontinence. Br J Obstet Gynaecol 1984;91:46–55.
29 Bhatia NN, Bergman A. Modified Burch versus Pereyra retropubic urethropexy for stress incontinence. Obstet Gynecol 1985;66:255–261.
30 Bregman A, Ballard CA, Koonings CA. Comparison of three different surgical procedures for genuine stress incontinence: prospective randomized study. Am J Obstet Gynecol 1989;160:1102–1106.
31 Karram MM, Angel O, Koonings P, Tabor B, Bergman A, Bhatia N. The modified Pereyra procedure; a clinical and urodynamic review. Br J Obstet Gynaecol 1992;99:655–658.

32 Bergman A, Koonings PP, Ballard CA. Predicting postoperative incontinence development in women undergoing operation for genitourinary prolapse. Am J Obstet Gynecol 1988;158:1171–1175.

33 Stoekel W. Uber die verwendung der musculi pyridimale beider operativen behandlung der incontinentiaurinae. Zentrabl Gynakol 1917;41:11–16.

34 Price PB. Plastic operations for incontinence of urine and feces. Arch Surg 1933;26:1043–1053.

35 Aldridge AH. Transplantation of fascia for relief of urinary stress incontinence. Am J Obstet Gynecol 1942;44:398–411.

36 Miller NF. The surgical treatment of urinary incontinence in the female. JAMA 1932;98:628–632.

37 Millin T, Read C. Stress incontinence of urine in the female: Millin's sling operation. Postgrad Med J 1949;24:51–58.

38 Sayer TR, Dixon GL, Hosker GL, Warrell DW. A study of paraurethral connective tissue in women with stress incontinence of urine. Neurourol Urodyn 1990;9:319–320.

39 Norton P, Baker J, Sharp H, Warenski J. Genitourinary prolapse: relationship with joint hypermobility. Neurourol Urodyn 1990;9:321–322.

40 Kennedy C. Stress incontinence of urine: a survey of 34 cases treated by the Millin I sling operation. Br Med J 1960;3:263–267.

41 Horbach NS, Blanco JS, Ostergard DR, Bent AE, Cornella JL. A suburethral sling procedure with polytetrafluoroethylene for the treatment of genuine stress incontinence in patients with a low urethral closure pressure. Obstet Gynecol 1988;71:648–652.

42 McGuire EJ. Urodynamic findings in patients after failure of stress incontinence operations. Prog Clin Biol Res 1981;78:351–360.

43 Sand PK, Bowen LW, Panganiban R, Ostergard DR. The low pressure urethra as a factor in failed retropubic urethropexy. Obstet Gynecol 1987;69:399–402.

44 Stanton SL, Brindley GS, Holmes DM. Silastic sling for urethral sphincter incompetence in women. Br J Obstet Gynaecol 1985;92:747–751.

45 Foley FEB. An artificial sphincter: a new device and operation for control of enuresis and urinary incontinence. J Urol 1947;58:250–259.

46 Scott FB, Bradley WE, Timm GW. Treatment of urinary incontinence by implantable prosthetic sphincter. Urology 1973;1:252–259.

47 Montague DK. Evolution of implanted devices for urinary incontinence. Cleve Clin Q 1984;51:405–409.

48 Duncan HJ, Diane EN, Mundy AR. Role of artificial urinary sphincter in the treatment of stress incontinence in women. Br J Urol 1992;69:141–143.

49 Webster GD, Perez LM, Khoury JM, Timmons SL. Management of type III stress urinary incontinence using artificial urinary sphincter. Urology 1992;39:499–503.

50 Murless BC. The injection treatment for stress incontinence. J Obstet Gynecol 1938;45:67–73.

51 Berg S. Polytef augmentation urethroplasty. Arch Surg 1973;107:379–381.

52 Politano VA, Small MP, Harper JM, Lynne CM. Periurethral Teflon injection for urinary incontinence. J Urol 1974;111:180–183.

53 Beckingham IJ, Wemyss-Holden G, Lawrence WT. Long-term follow-up of women treated with periurethral Teflon injections for stress incontinence. Br J Urol 1992;69:580–583.

54 Shortliffe LMD, Freiha FS, Kessler R, Stamey TA, Constantinou CE. Treatment of urinary incontinence by the periurethral injection of glutaraldehyde cross-linked collagen. J Urol 1989;141:538–541.

55 Herschorn S, Radomski SB, Steele DJ. Early experience with intraurethral collagen injections for urinary incontinence. J Urol 1992;148:1797–1800.

56 Walker RD, Wilson J, Clark AE. Injectable bioglass as a potential substitute for injectable polytetrafluroethylene. J Urol 1992;148:645–647.

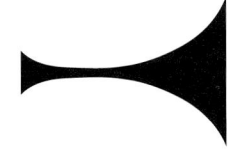

Chapter 23

Procedures for correcting urinary incontinence

Raymond A. Lee

Several surgical procedures are advocated as cures for recurrent stress urinary incontinence (SUI). No single operation is universally effective, yet each has advantages in selected patients. Standard approaches include variations of the suburethral sling procedure (Marshall-Marchetti-Krantz) and anterior vaginal wall suspension (Burch). A newer and less invasive procedure, frequently combining a vaginal phase with a semiblind passage of periurethral needles, apparently results in fewer complications, shorter hospital stays, and improved outcome in the properly selected patient.

Examination immediately after any of these procedures would probably show a remarkable similarity. Common to all patients would be a high retropubic position of the bladder neck, no rotational descent of the anterior vaginal wall, and correction of any funneling that might have been present in the proximal urethra.

Physicians often develop a preference for a specific method as a result of training or experience. However, the pelvic surgeon must be prepared to improvise or alter steps during operation in order to tailor the procedure for an individual patient. Long-term results depend on the accurate and meticulous performance of a sound surgical procedure, adapted to correct specific anatomic defects of each patient.

Retropubic operations

Sling methods

Ridley prefers the Goebell-Fragenheim-Stoeckel type of sling procedure, for which he uses fascia lata obtained from the lateral aspect of the thigh (1). He emphasizes that one of the difficulties of the operation is obtaining proper tension when placing the sling beneath the urethra. He suggests having the sling rather loose (Fig. 23-1).

McGuire's group, in favoring this approach, emphasize that some patients cannot benefit from other retropubic procedures (2,3). Those with fixed, open, nonfunctional urethral continence mechanisms at rest, those with large cystoceles or rectoceles, and those with uterine prolapse or an enterocele would not be suitable candidates for sling procedures. Relative contraindications they mention include the presence of residual urine, a reflux vesical dysfunction, severe detrusor instability, and spontaneous bladder contraction. They state that when a woman has detrusor instability, there is no way of predicting whether it will disappear, persist, or get worse after an operation that is successful in correcting SUI. They estimate that 70% of women who have both these conditions are relieved of both by operation. Another 10% will gradually be cured of their detrusor instability during the first 6 to 8 weeks after surgery.

The problems with the pubovaginal sling include urinary retention, erosion of the urethra or bladder, difficulty with intermittent catheterization during the postoperative period, pain at the site of the sling attachment at the rectus fascia, exacerbation of detrusor instability, and obstructive uropathy.

Parker and coworkers also prefer a urethrovesical suspension using fascia lata for recurrent SUI unresponsive to more conservative attempts at surgical management (4). They believe that fascia lata support of the proximal 1 to 2 cm of the urethra ensures continued elevation of the urethra and, with stress, provides a pulling-up effect. Further, the fascia lata serves as a tight, lasting support over the attenuated and weakened pubocervical fascia.

The material is simple to obtain, is easy to work with, and, when properly placed, does not cut through the urethra. It rarely causes any tissue reaction. The Parker team prefers fascia lata over tissue from the aponeurosis of the abdominal wall, because it is easier to get the required 18 to 20 cm of length, it is thicker, and it does not predispose the patient to a ventral hernia. At the site of the fascial graft on the lateral aspect of the leg, bleeding is rare, pain is minimal, and muscle herniation is not a problem.

Generally, surgeons consider the sling procedure the best choice for patients who have recurrent stress incontinence, especially those who have previously had retropubic procedures. The most frequent complication is the inability to void satisfactorily and to empty the bladder completely. For such problems, the Parker group suggests gentle dilation of the urethra to the caliber of a 28-F sound, prolonged antibiotic coverage, and voiding on a schedule of every 2 to 3 hours (4). They state that it is seldom necessary to cut the sling but add that if it becomes necessary, the fascia lata may be cut transversely high on the lateral vaginal wall. With this relief from tension, scar tissue will form, and most patients will remain continent.

Long-term success, obtained in 90% of patients, is attributed to the exceptional strength and durability of the fascia, which can provide a pulling-up effect for years, even when the patient coughs or sneezes. The outstanding success of this technically demanding operation can be attributed to the vast clinical experience and excellent surgical technique of its advocates.

Suspension

Various modifications of the Burch procedure elevate the bladder neck and urethra by suspending the anterior vaginal wall to Cooper's ligament by means of permanent or absorbable sutures (5). The technique is less complex than the sling procedure and does not require suburethral dissection. Hysterectomy is generally done, with a posterior colpoperineorrhaphy in selected patients. The suspension may be advantageous in the patient who has a short, scarred urethra. In such a patient, only a single pair of the Marshall-Marchetti-Krantz type of suture can be inserted adjacent to the urethra.

As in any operation in which the vagina is displaced anteriorly, a posterior enterocele may occur. The more recent emphasis on obliteration of the cul-de-sac, further enhanced

by securing the sigmoid colon to the anterior peritoneum, will reduce this postoperative complication. Because of the wide or lateral position of the sutures, one is relying on the inherent tone and quality of the elastic tissue within the anterior vaginal wall to support a long, hammock-like suspension of the urethra. Eventually, as these supportive tissues degenerate and lose elasticity, the anterior vaginal wall may relax. With recurrent rotational descent of the bladder neck, the urinary incontinence will return.

Stamey procedure

This method combines a suprapubic with a vaginal incision (6). A needle is passed through the anterior rectus fascia to the anterosuperior border of the symphysis pubis and is guided along the undersurface to the urethrovesical junction. The needle should exit in the vaginal incision immediately in front of the Foley balloon and to the lateral side of the vesical neck. The Foley catheter is then removed at a right angle, and the cystoscope is introduced. The bladder is inspected for any inadvertent perforation by the needle, and the cystoscope is placed at the vesical neck. If the needle is positioned properly, its movement causes a corresponding movement of the bladder neck.

A No. 2 monofilament suture is threaded through the eye of the needle, and the needle is withdrawn, leaving one free end in the vaginal incision. The needle is passed a second time 2 cm lateral to the first passage (Fig. 23-2). The No. 2 nylon suture is passed through a 1-cm tube of 5-mm Dacron before the nylon is threaded into the eye of the needle, and the needle is withdrawn into the suprapubic incision.

Stamey stresses the importance of keeping the second passage of the needle lateral—exactly at the bladder neck—and not down the urethra distal to the first suture. In this way, the internal vesical neck—not the urethra—is suspended into position behind the symphysis pubis. The nylon loop is buttressed to prevent it from tearing through the pubocervical fascia.

The identical procedure is repeated on the contralateral side. Two separate suspending sutures, each with a vaginal Dacron tube buttress, are thus positioned on either side of the internal vesical neck without passage beneath the neck. Three steps must be checked as each suspending loop is individually pulled superiorly: that the closure occurs exactly at the internal vesical neck; that both suspending loops are symmetrically placed; and that minimal tension is used to close the vesical neck, which serves as a guide to how tightly the sutures will have to be tied suprapubically.

At this time, the accuracy of the operation can be assessed through the panendoscope (Fig. 23-3). As the instrument is removed, fluid will gush from the urethra. With gentle elevation of either suspending suture, the flow of fluid should abruptly cease (if the bladder is overfilled, considerable suprapubic elevation may be required). If the leaking does not stop, the sutures should be replaced. The

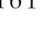

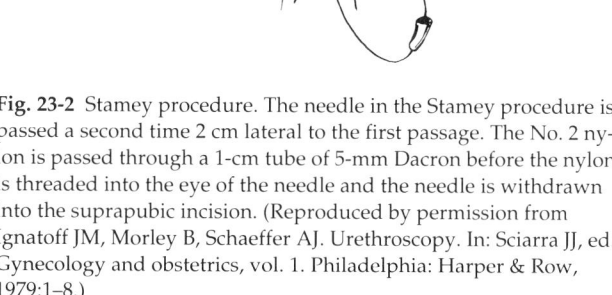

Fig. 23-1 Sling procedure. In this procedure, the fascia lata strap passes beneath the urethra at the bladder neck. The strap is anchored to the anterior abdominal fascia on the patient's right side, drawn into the vagina, and secured with proper tension at the other slitlike incision in the fascia. (Reproduced with permission from Ridley JH. Surgery for stress urinary incontinence. In: Ridley JH, ed. Gynecologic Surgery: errors, safeguards, and salvage. Baltimore: Williams & Wilkins, 1974:114–154.)

Fig. 23-2 Stamey procedure. The needle in the Stamey procedure is passed a second time 2 cm lateral to the first passage. The No. 2 nylon is passed through a 1-cm tube of 5-mm Dacron before the nylon is threaded into the eye of the needle and the needle is withdrawn into the suprapubic incision. (Reproduced by permission from Ignatoff JM, Morley B, Schaeffer AJ. Urethroscopy. In: Sciarra JJ, ed. Gynecology and obstetrics, vol. 1. Philadelphia: Harper & Row, 1979:1–8.)

nylon sutures are then tied with enough tension to elevate the bladder neck effectively.

Complications have been few. Of 300 patients, 10 required removal of a suprapubic suture under local anesthesia because of pain or infection or both. Most of these patients had had silk or braided nylon as the suspending suture. In one patient, the Dacron tube eroded into the vagina, where it was cut free from the nylon suture. Generally, these patients have remained continent even after removal of the suture or supporting material.

Stamey offers the following five factors as advantages of endoscopic rather than retropubic suspension of the vesical neck: endoscopy accurately identifies the internal vesical neck for suture placement; permanent monofilament heavy nylon No. 2 and vaginally placed Dacron buttresses afford stronger support of the pubocervical fascia that must be used to suspend the internal vesical neck; functional closure of the internal vesical neck is confirmed during the operation by observing complete cessation of urinary leakage before permanently tying the suspending sutures; anatomic closure of the internal vesical neck and not the urethra is confirmed by endoscopy before the operation is completed; and postoperative morbidity is less because open-bladder surgery is avoided.

Stamey believes that the operation is particularly well adapted to obese patients as well as those who have had pelvic fractures, retropubic surgery, or radiation incontinence. Perforation of the bladder and urethra by the blind passage of a needle would seem to be more likely when previous retropubic procedures resulted in scarring and the intimate fixation of the anterior surface of the urethra and bladder to the back of the symphysis pubis and rectus fascia. Stamey, however, has not reported this problem.

The only experience that my colleagues and I have had with this procedure involved patients who had recurrence of incontinence several weeks or months after they had

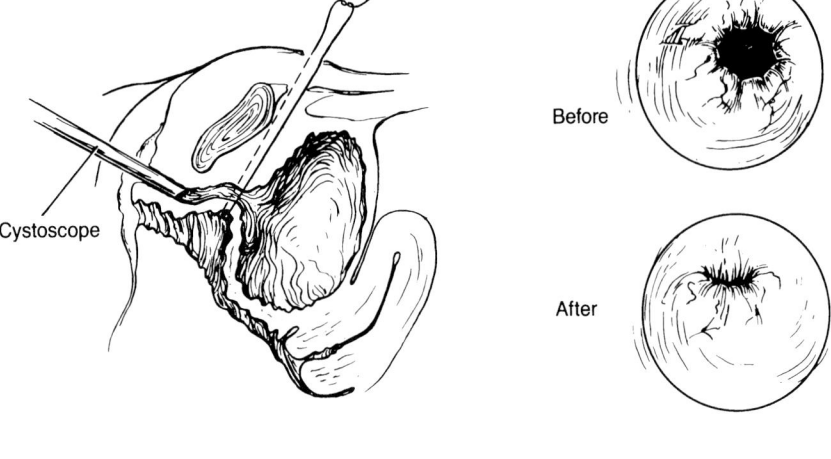

Cystoscope

Before

After

Fig. 23-3 Assessment through panendoscope. The pubovesicocervical fascia on one side of the urethrovesical junction is suspended in a broad loop. The same procedure is repeated on the other side. A cystoscope with wide-angle viewing is introduced into the distal third of the urethra. The vesical neck appears patulous (*before*) but is closed (*after*) exactly at the urethrovesical junction when the assistant pulls vertically on either nylon loop. (Reproduced with permission from Ignatoff JM, Morley B, Schaeffer AJ. Urethroscopy. In: Sciarra JJ, ed. Gynecology and obstetrics, vol. 1. Philadelphia: Harper & Row, 1979:1–8.)

this operation done with absorbable sutures. Other patients have had sinus formation and urinary tract fistulas when the permanent material to buttress the nylon suture became a source of infection. Surgeons who favor procedures of this type have reported favorable results and can state that complications rarely occur when the operation is properly performed.

Mayo approach

My colleagues and I prefer a modification of the Marshall-Marchetti-Krantz procedure accomplished through a lower midline incision with the dome of the bladder open (7,8). If this is the first such procedure for the patient, the space is developed in a few moments. If the patient has had a previous retropubic operation, sharp dissection is needed to free scarring and fixation of the bladder and urethra to the posterior aspect of the rectus muscle and symphysis pubis. Often, only the upper anterior bladder wall and bladder neck have been suspended in the previous operation. The absence of adhesions along the periurethra and bladder neck suggests the patient with recurrent stress incontinence has not had a true urethral and bladder neck suspension.

Opening the dome of the bladder permits direct visualization and palpation of the bladder neck and proximal urethra (Fig. 23-4). Usually, with a No. 22 Foley catheter in place, the surgeon's right index finger can be inserted alongside the catheter, through the bladder neck, and down the proximal urethra for 2 to 3 cm. Further, this maneuver facilitates the accurate placement of the suspending sutures. Before closing the abdominal incision, the experienced surgeon can assess the operative result after the sutures have been tied. A second glove is placed on the surgeon's left hand. The left index and middle fingers are inserted into the vagina to permit the accurate placement of the periurethral permanent sutures. The surgeon's fingers, rather than a sponge stick, retractor, or assistant's fingers, are preferred to help elevate the vaginal wall and identify the urethra.

Figures 23-5, 23-6, and 23-7 show the correct placement of the sutures after the periurethral region has been identi-

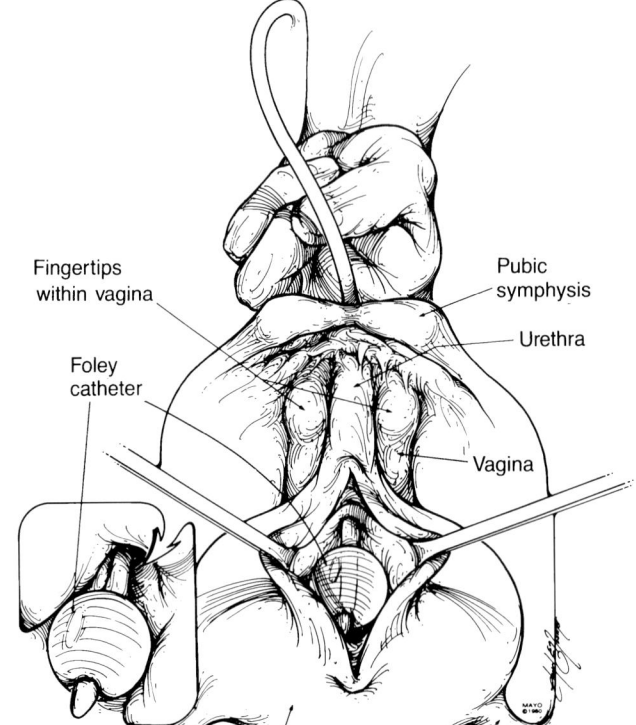

Fingertips within vagina

Foley catheter

Pubic symphysis

Urethra

Vagina

Bladder   Ureter

Fig. 23-4 Mayo approach. When using the Mayo approach, the dome of the bladder is opened longitudinally approximately 2 to 3 cm from the vesical neck to permit direct visualization and palpation of the tone and quality of the bladder neck. Inset: Funneling of the bladder neck with patulous noncontractile proximal urethra. (Courtesy of the Mayo Foundation.)

fied. This not only aids in determining the thickness, quality, and mobility of the anterior vaginal wall and the appropriate position for its suspension to the pubic symphysis, but also permits the accurate location of the urethra, which can then be avoided as the sutures are placed.

Once the periurethral region is identified, one to three nonabsorbable sutures are inserted lateral to the side of the

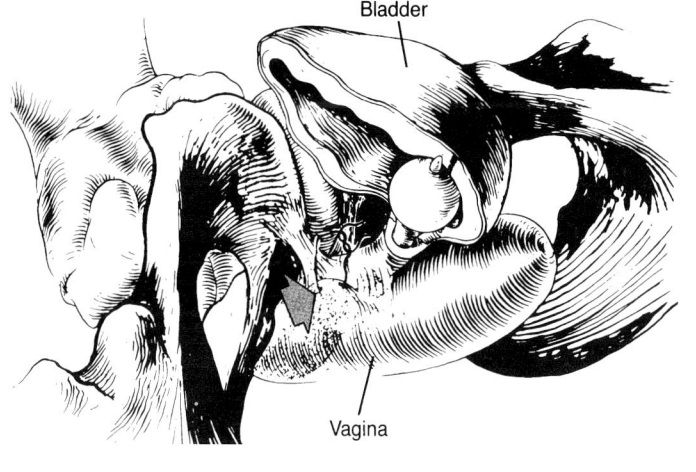

Bladder

Vagina

Fig. 23-5 Placement of first suture. The first suture on the left side of the urethra is being placed (*arrowhead*). The midline finger of the surgeon's left hand identifies the urethra and aids in determining the depth of penetration into the the vagina wall. (Reproduced by permission from Lee RA. Correcting recurrent stress incontinence. Contemp Obstet Gynecol 1978;12:33.)

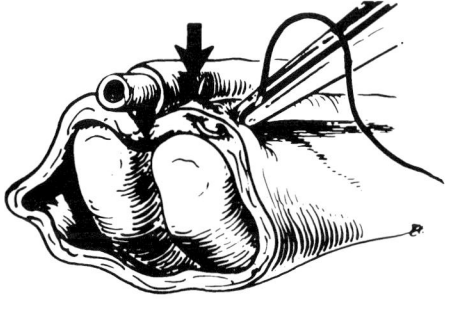

Fig. 23-6 Suturing vaginal wall. Almost the entire thickness of the patient's vaginal wall is included in the suturing, with the needle brought closely (3 to 5 mm) to the urethra (*arrow*). (Reproduced by permission from Lee RA. Correcting recurrent stress incontinence. Contemp Obstet Gynecol 1978;12:33.)

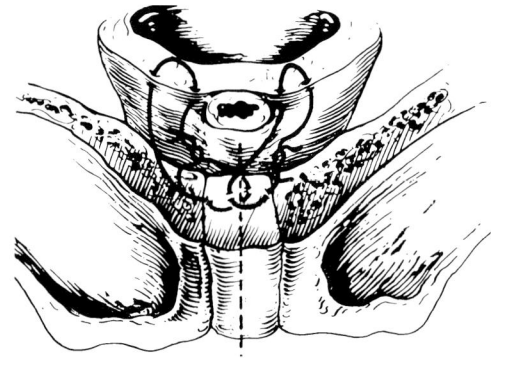

Fig. 23-7 Companion sutures. This shows a companion set of sutures, including essentially full thickness of anterior vaginal wall a few millimeters lateral to the urethra and fixed into the cartilage of the symphysis pubis, not the periosteum. (Courtesy of the Mayo Foundation.)

urethra; these are placed so that almost the entire thickness of the anterior vaginal wall is included with each suture. The number of sutures is governed by the length of the available urethra. Sutures are placed securely and deeply in the fibrocartilage of the symphysis, not the periosteum, with a sturdy No. 6 Mayo needle. A lighter needle cannot penetrate the cartilage of the symphysis without risk of breakage.

If periurethral sutures are placed too far lateral to the urethra, they will not provide the desired support, and some incontinence may persist. Conversely, if sutures are inserted too close to the urethra, mechanical urethral and bladder neck obstruction may occur, causing long-term urinary retention. In more than 90% of the patients, two sets of sutures generally have proved sufficient. Rarely, because of unusual vaginal shortening after radical hysterectomy, radiation therapy, or partial vaginectomy, there is room for only a single set of sutures. Occasionally, because of unusual mobility of the anterior vaginal wall, three sets of sutures will be beneficial.

After all suspending sutures have been placed, they are tagged with an instrument and placed laterally. The surgeon then changes gloves and ties the suspending Marshall sutures in the order of their placement (Fig. 23-8). Once all the sutures have been tied, the surgeon inspects and palpates the proximal urethra and bladder neck through the cystostomy with the urethral catheter in place. If the surgeon is satisfied, the urethral catheter is removed and the bladder neck may be assessed further. The repaired neck should appear to be tight, like the anus of a newborn, and it will feel remarkably similar when palpated with the index finger. If needed, a curved forceps may be passed through the bladder neck and proximal urethra and gently opened to assess the tension therein. When satisfied with the repair, the surgeon places a No. 16 Foley catheter in the cystostomy and closes it with two layers of running No. 2-0 chromic suture. A suction catheter is rarely indicated in the primary procedure, but, in general, patients who have had previous retropubic dissection will require a Hemovac suction catheter.

Complications and results

Postoperative problems with our procedure have been few. My colleagues and I have not had a complication that could be attributed to the cystostomy. There have been no fistulas or retropubic collection or abscess, nor has the operation needed to be repeated because of urinary retention.

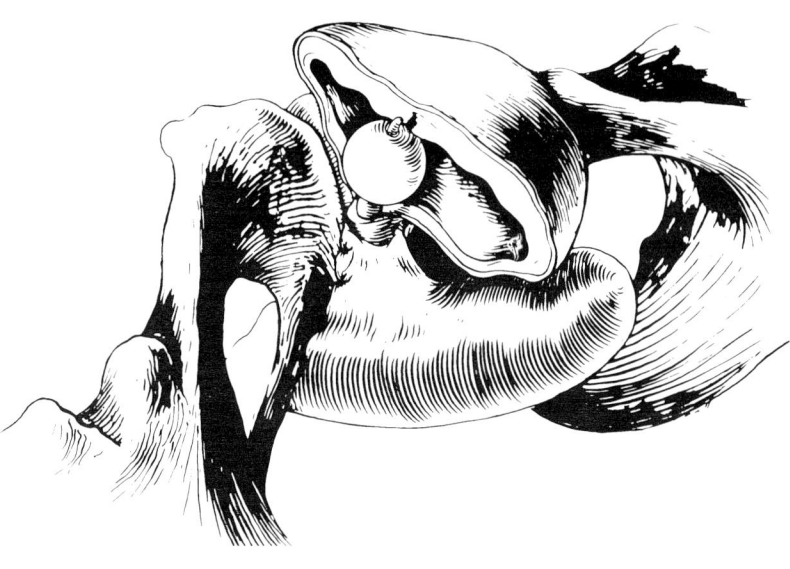

Fig. 23-8 Tying Marshall sutures results in a high retropubic position of the vesical neck, with a tight (hammock) effect on the entire urethra. (Reproduced by permission from Lee RA. Correcting recurrent stress incontinence. Contemp Obstet Gynecol 1978;12:33.)

Some bacteriuria and urinary tract infections have occurred. Also, in 2% of our patients, osteitis pubis, a condition of unknown cause, has developed. The severity of its symptoms and the obvious clinical findings would make this condition difficult to overlook. The inflammation seems to occur with equal frequency after the use of permanent or absorbable sutures and is not associated with chronic infection.

Despite these few problems, overall success has been good. Of more than 600 patients undergoing the operation, after a mean follow-up of 8 years, 89% have had their disabling stress incontinence corrected.

Making a choice

No single operative procedure is universally effective, yet each has its advantages in selected patients. With the various sling techniques or bladder neck suspensions, excessive pressure or tension is placed on a relatively short segment of the urethra, which may produce persistent mechanical obstruction. This pressure can be unrelenting, and the urinary retention that results may be difficult to correct.

The Stamey procedure and its various modifications emphasize accurate placement of paraurethral-bladder neck sutures, which is commendable. However, the "hanging" of these tissues by permanent sutures to the rectus fascia seems poorly conceived. In time, support may be lost and urinary incontinence may recur.

To avoid these problems, my colleagues and I prefer the Marshall-Marchetti-Krantz variation I have described. It offers the advantage of broad suburethral support with effective plication of the urethra and high retropubic position of the vesical neck. Open cystostomy ensures the accurate placement of the proximal sutures and permits assessment and correction of the funneled, patulent bladder neck. The technique is relatively simple when compared with other approaches.

Summary

In the final analysis, long-term correction of stress urinary incontinence in the properly selected patient depends on choosing a sound surgical procedure and performing it with meticulous technique. Success requires attention to correcting the anatomic defect coupled with good surgical judgment during and after the operation.

References

1 Ridley JH. Surgery for stress urinary incontinence. In: Ridley JH, ed. Gynecologic surgery: errors, safeguards, and salvage. Baltimore: Williams & Wilkins, 1974:114–154.

2 McGuire EJ, Lytton B. Pubovaginal sling procedure for stress incontinence. J Urol 1978;119:82.

3 McGuire EJ, Lytton B, Kohorn EI, et al. The value of urodynamic testing in stress urinary incontinence. J Urol 1980;124:256.

4 Parker RT, Addison WA, Wilson CJ. Fascia lata urethrovesical suspension for recurrent stress urinary incontinence. Am J Obstet Gynecol 1979;135:843.

5 Burch JC. Urethrovaginal fixation to Cooper's ligament in the treatment of cystocele and stress incontinence. Prog Gynecol 1963;4:591.

6 Stamey TA. Endoscopic suspension of the vesical neck for urinary incontinence in females: report on 203 consecutive patients. Ann Surg 1980;192:465.

7 Lee RA, Symmonds RE, Goldstein RA. Surgical complications and results of modified Marshall-Marchetti-Krantz procedure for urinary incontinence. Obstet Gynecol 1979;53:447.

8 Blute ML, Symmonds RE, Lee RA. Repeat Marshall-Marchetti-Krantz procedures for genuine stress urinary incontinence. Obstet Gynecol (in press).

9 Ignatoff JM, Morley B, Schaeffer AJ. Urethroscopy. In: Sciarra JJ, ed. Gynecology and obstetrics, vol. 1. Philadelphia: Harper & Row, 1979:1–8.

10 Lee RA. The modified Marshall-Marchetti-Krantz operation as a primary procedure in urinary stress incontinence. In: Buchsbaum HJ, Schmidt JD, eds. Gynecologic and obstetric urology, ed 2. Philadelphia: WB Saunders, 1982:250–258.

11 Lee RA. Correcting recurrent stress incontinence. Contemp Obstet Gynecol 1978;12:33.

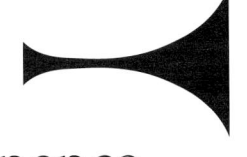

Chapter 24

Treating incontinence transvaginally

David H. Nichols and Stephen F. Ponchak

Factors in stress urinary incontinence

Causes

An involuntary loss of urine may occur along with increases in intra-abdominal pressure caused by laughing, coughing, sneezing, or position changes. The involuntary escape of urine is produced when intravesical pressure temporarily exceeds intraurethral pressure and no detrusor contraction takes place. The loss of urine ceases as soon as the cause of increased pressure ceases.

When support from the urogenital diaphragm is weak, the vesicourethral junction may be outside the range of response to increases in the intra-abdominal pressure. Intra-abdominal pressure changes may be transmitted to the bladder but not to the urethra. When intravesical pressure temporarily exceeds intraurethral pressure, urine is again involuntarily lost. When the increased intra-abdominal pressure is withdrawn, as it is at the end of a cough, laugh, or sneeze, intraurethral pressure once again exceeds intravesical pressure and the involuntary loss of urine ceases.

Urethral funneling is another factor. When it is present, the physiologic vesicourethral junction lies at the bottom of the funnel, often effectively displacing it outside the true pelvis.

Types of cystocele

The supporting structures of the bladder, urethra, and vagina are complex. The urethra is both suspended by the urogenital diaphragm and supported by the vagina. A cystocele may result if the anterior vaginal wall is damaged. Before operating, determine which specific supporting tissues have been altered and how the damage has affected the patient's urinary function.

Descent of the vagina and urethra anterior to the vesicourethral junction is called an anterior cystocele, and descent posterior to the interureteric ridge is called a posterior cystocele (1).

Anterior cystocele is generally associated with rotational descent of the bladder neck. In this case, stress urinary incontinence (SUI) occurs when intraurethral pressure cannot exceed intravesical pressure. This defect may or may not be combined with posterior cystocele.

Posterior cystocele may be due to distention, displacement, or a combination of the two problems. In the distention type, the defect is produced by primary intrinsic damage to the vaginal wall from within. In displacement cystocele, the damage is concentrated in the lateral connective tissue and muscular supports outside the vagina. A combination of the two defects usually follows childbirth and progresses as the patient ages.

To correct a distention cystocele, excise the weakened portion of the anterior vaginal wall and plicate the subepithelial tissue. Displacement cystocele must be treated by restoring vaginal depth and providing support to the vaginal vault.

If lateral or paravaginal supports have been damaged or avulsed, they may also be restored by transvaginal reattachment to the arcus tendineus of the pelvic diaphragm.

Before embarking on a treatment plan, establish an appropriate diagnosis in every case of incontinence. Reconstructive surgery has three specific goals: to relieve symptoms, restore normal anatomy, and achieve normal function.

Establishing cause

Suspect a fistula if the patient constantly loses urine through the vagina whether or not transabdominal pressure increases. There may be detrusor dysfunction if she urinates while walking, when exposed to the sound or feel of water, or when lying down or asleep. Leakage may result from spontaneous detrusor hyperirritability. Occasionally, however, cystitis, anxiety, chemicals such as caffeine, or systemic medication may be the trigger.

Urinary incontinence often has more than one cause. In our practice, about one third of these patients have a demonstrable pure primary SUI. Another third have distinct detrusor dysfunction with uninhibited bladder contraction. The rest have a mixture of the two factors. In a few cases the disability has a definite neurologic origin, occasionally it is congenital (e.g., spina bifida), or it may be acquired coincident with straining or obstetric damage, or related to disc herniation and sometimes to bladder denervation after pelvic surgery.

A careful history and physical examination, including examination of the patient when she is standing, should pinpoint the most likely cause or causes of the incontinence. For some women, an anticholinergic may relieve the detru-

sor dysfunction so that the stress component no longer warrants surgery. If there is doubt about the cause of the incontinence, or the patient has recurrent SUI, sophisticated urodynamic testing is recommended, especially the urethrocystometrogram, obtained in both the standing and lithotomy position as the bladder fills.

A bladder drill of reeducation is helpful (voiding at 2-hour intervals during the waking hours, but not in between), along with a program of Kegel's isometric perineal resistive exercises, or if the patient is interested, a course of electrical pulsating stimulation to the pelvic musculature.

Correction attempts

When detrusor dysfunction is strongly suspected, elimination of any contributing detrusor stimulants, such as caffeine, may be helpful. A trial of total dietary caffeine restriction should include coffee, tea, cola drinks, and chocolate, as both caffeine and theobromine in some persons appear to irritate the detrusor muscle.

The patient can also be placed on a clinical trial of an anticholinergic drug. The effects of these measures on function may be assessed by the patient's responses to questioning on a subsequent office visit.

Once one determines that the patient's disability is primarily from detrusor dysfunction and SUI, it is important that the initial treatment be directed toward relief of the detrusor dysfunction. For many patients, a course of bladder reeducation exercises is useful, and the bladder drill exercise is easily instituted.

It is important that the patient develop and exercise cerebral dominance of detrusor contraction over spinal reflex contraction. This may be accomplished by asking the patient to void "by the clock." During waking hours, the pa-

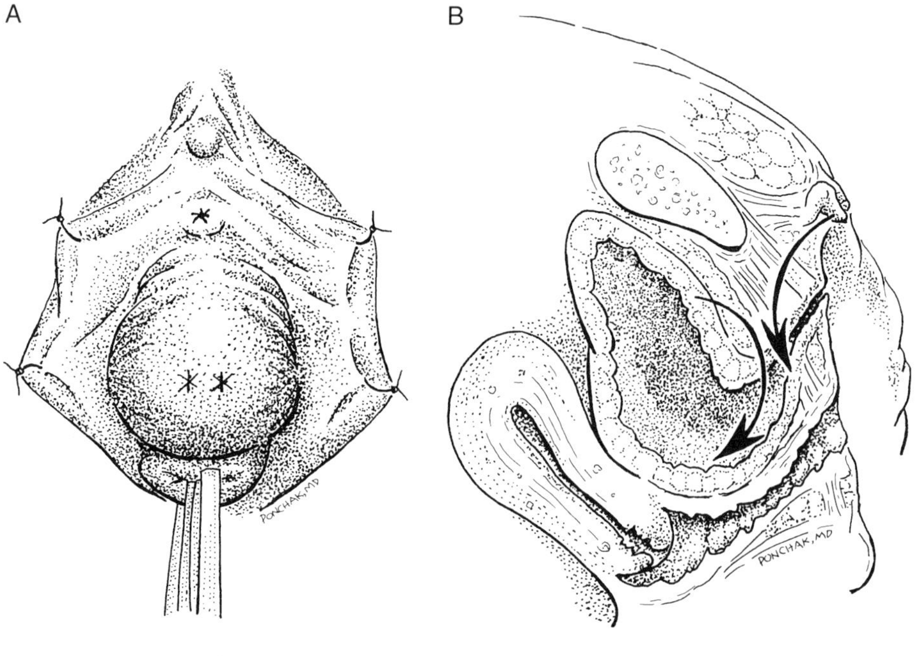

A

B

Fig. 24-1 (A) Clamp placement. The asterisks mark the site for placing Allis clamps before opening the anterior vaginal wall of a patient with a large cystocele. (B) Rotational descent of the vesicourethral junction and demonstrable funneling of the resting urethra are evident. The hypermobile vesicourethral junction is caudal to the pubis, and there is some posterior cystocele.

tient urinates every hour on the hour whether or not the stimulus to void is present. She must deliberately refrain from voiding at other times.

When the patient is consistently dry, the interval between voiding should be lengthened until a duration of 2 1/2 to 3 hours without voiding has been reached. Administering a supplemental anticholinergic drug may help to increase urethral tone, and in the postmenopausal patient, the administration of vaginal estrogen for a long period of time may be helpful.

Surgical correction

If the patient's SUI is disabling and fails to respond to drugs or exercise, consider surgery to restore normal anatomy and physiology. Appropriate plication of the urethra will correct funneling. Replacement within the pelvis may be necessary when the vesicourethral junction is dislocated. Marked pelvic relaxation mandates repair of all the demonstrated sites of damage. In most instances, the transvaginal route is effective for handling these indications.

Transvaginal approach

Begin repair of a cystocele by placing a No. 16 silicone-coated transurethral Foley catheter in the bladder. Inflate the bulb. Make an incision directly into the vesicovaginal space through the full thickness of the vaginal wall as shown in Figures 24-1 and 24-2.

Carry the dissection to the lateral limits of the vesicovaginal space. Next, open the remainder of the anterior vaginal wall in the suburethral area to within 1 cm of the external urethral meatus. Lay the vaginal walls back by sharp dissection (Fig. 24-3).

Locate the vesicourethral junction by exerting gentle traction on the Foley catheter. Note the relation of the lower margin of its inflated bulb to the posterior surface of the pubic symphysis. In the continent, this junction is where the lower third of the pubis meets the upper two-thirds. In SUI patients, however, it is often caudal to the inferior margin of the pubis.

Grasp the tissue of the urogenital diaphragm lateral to the urethra in the tips of Kocher hemostats. Place one clamp at each side of the urethra, incorporating the paraurethral supporting tissues of the urogenital diaphragm, the so-called pubourethral ligaments, as shown in Figures 24-4, 24-5, and 24-6.

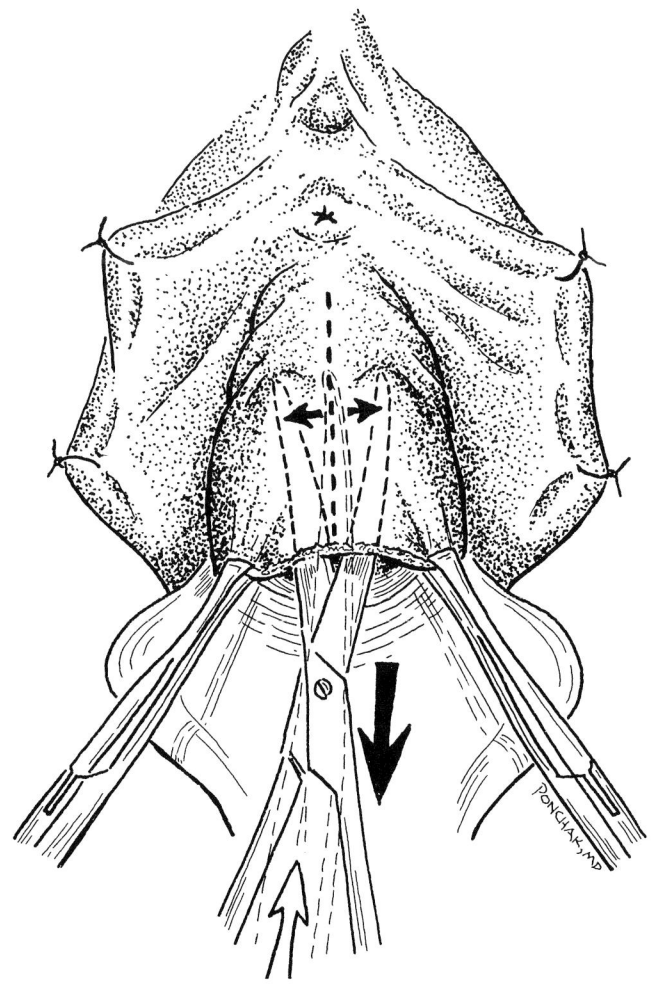

Fig. 24-2 Perform Incision. The incision in the anterior vaginal wall is carried cranially to within 1 cm of the external urethral meatus. Mayo scissors undermine the full thickness (*open arrow*). Scissors are opened (*small closed arrows*) and withdrawn (*large closed arrow*). Incise vagina (*dashed line*).

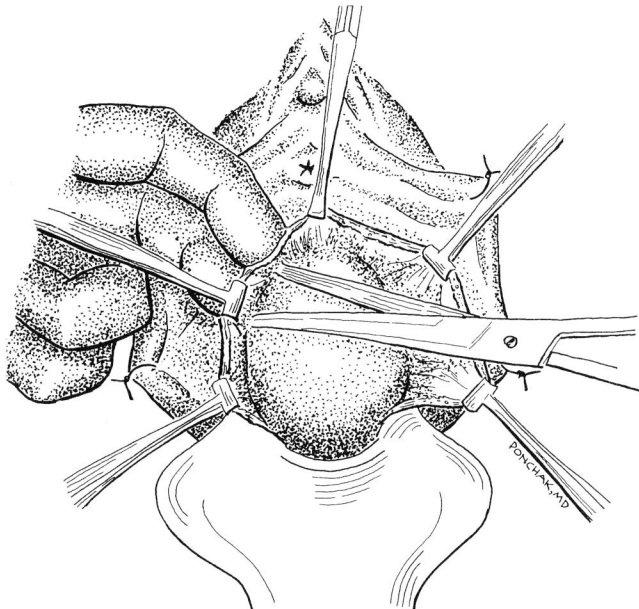

Fig. 24-3 Separate vagina from bladder. Sharp dissection is required to separate the vagina from the bladder. Incise first on one side and then on the other.

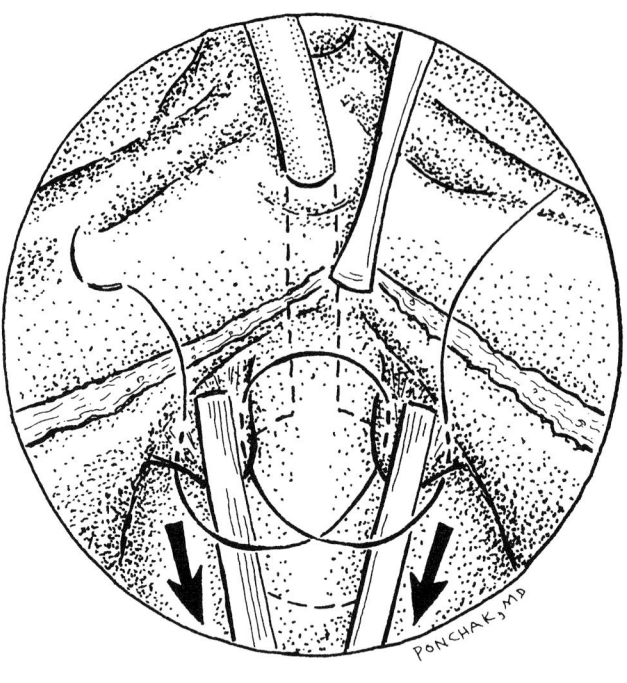

Fig. 24-4 Pull tissues. The dotted line indicates the position of the inflated bulb on a transurethral Foley catheter. The tissues lateral to the bulb are grasped in a Kocher hemostat and gently pulled in the direction of the arrow.

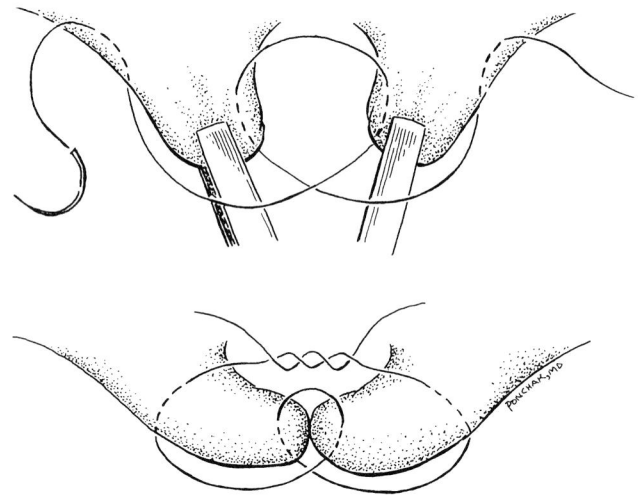

Fig. 24-5 Place sutures at the top. The drawing at the top shows placement of a far-near–near-far suture; the bottom, how the tissues are brought together when the suture is tied.

If there is urethral funneling, place suburethral Kelly-type plication stitches of polyglycolic acid (PGA) suture (Dexon, Vicryl).

To determine whether the hemostats are properly placed—in the tissues continuous with the pubourethral ligament portion of the urogenital diaphragm—tug them in the same direction as the ligaments are attached to the posterior surface of the pubis. Pulling should move the patient

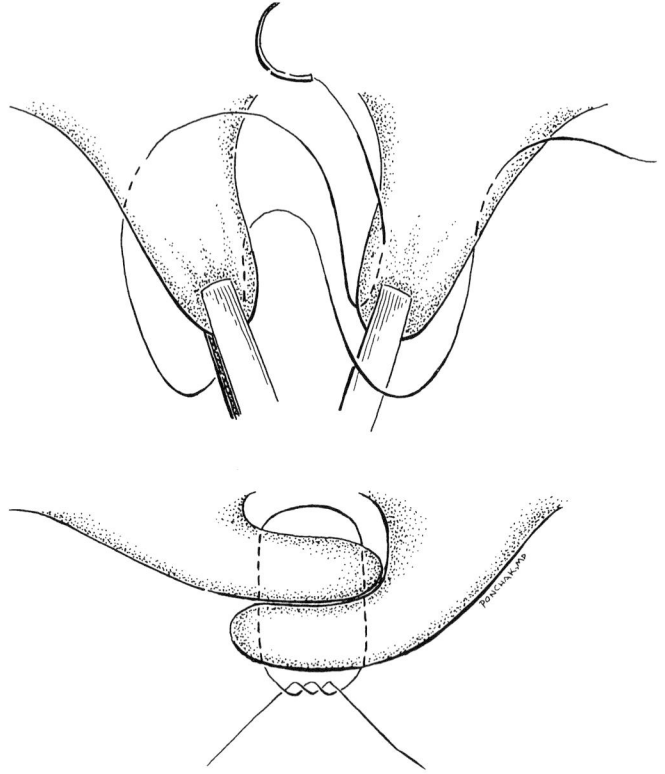

Fig. 24-6 Markedly elongated tissues may require alternative placement. When the sutures are tied, one of the tissue condensations overlaps the other, as shown in bottom drawing.

a little. If the positioning is satisfactory, replace these hemostats by transfixion ligatures. Use sutures of No. 00 polydi-axanone (PDS, Maxon). The elevation of the vesicourethral junction should return to normal as one ties these sutures. If it does not, place and tie another stitch lateral to the first to bring the vesicourethral junction to its proper level. Then reestablish fusion with the undersurface of the vagina by taking a bite on the undersurface of the vaginal wall on each side of the urethra (Fig. 24-7).

Now, approximate the connective tissue capsule of the bladder from side to side with interrupted mattress sutures of No. 00 PGA (Figs. 24-8, 24-9, and 24-10). If the width is excessive, place a second, more superficial layer of mattress sutures. Bring the "bladder pillars" together with a series of interrupted No. 00 PGA sutures. Trim the excess full thickness of the *unsplit* anterior vaginal wall appropriately on each side. Approximate it, from one side to the other for the full length of the vagina, by a subcuticular suture tied without tension (Fig. 24-11). Before this step, some may want to divide the vaginal wall into its fibromuscular and epithelial components and repair each layer separately. In the postmenopausal patient, however, this approach may interfere with the nutrition and blood supply of these layers.

When a large cystocele is associated with an abnormal thinning of the vaginal wall, usually among postmenopausal patients, a patch of full-thickness vaginal wall cut from one of

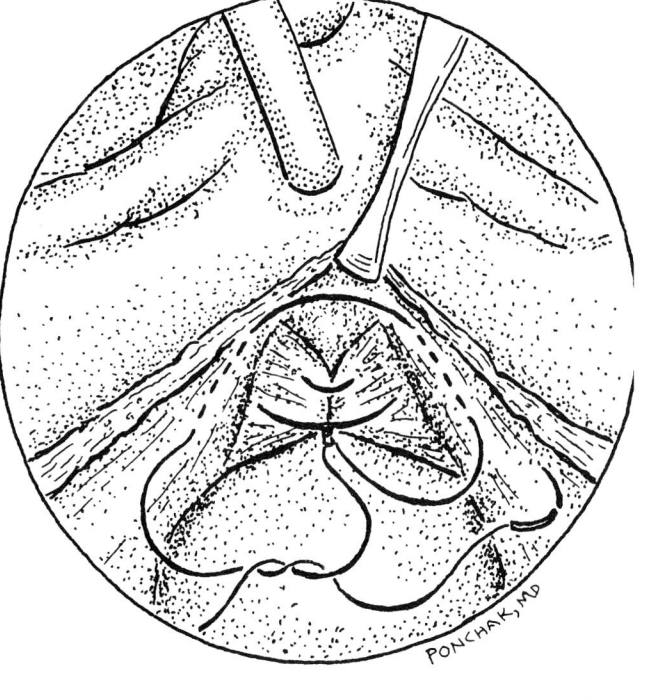

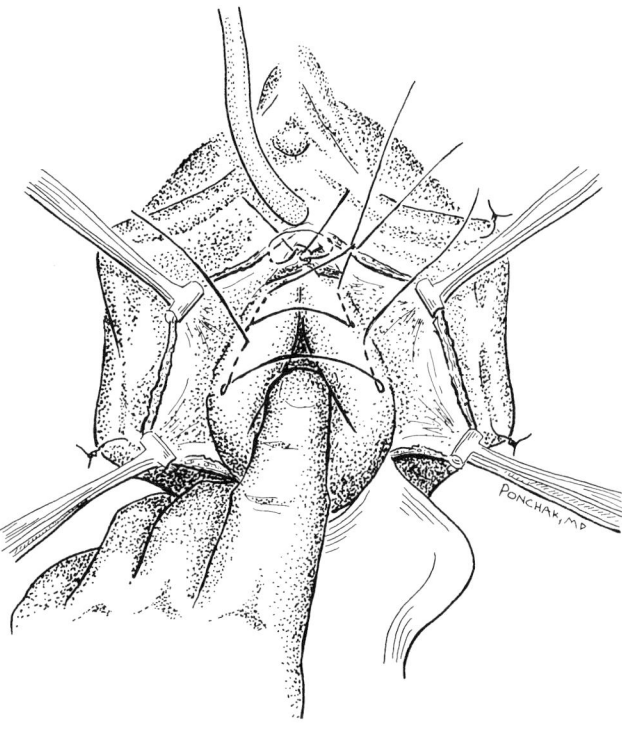

Fig. 24-7 Fusion is reestablished. The pubourethral plication stitch has been tied, and a second bite taken from the undersurface of the anterior vaginal wall on each side. When this suture has been tied, fusion between vagina and urogenital diaphragm will be reestablished in this area.

Fig. 24-9 Further reduction. Interrupted mattress stitches placed in the connective tissue capsule of the bladder further reduce the size of the cystocele.

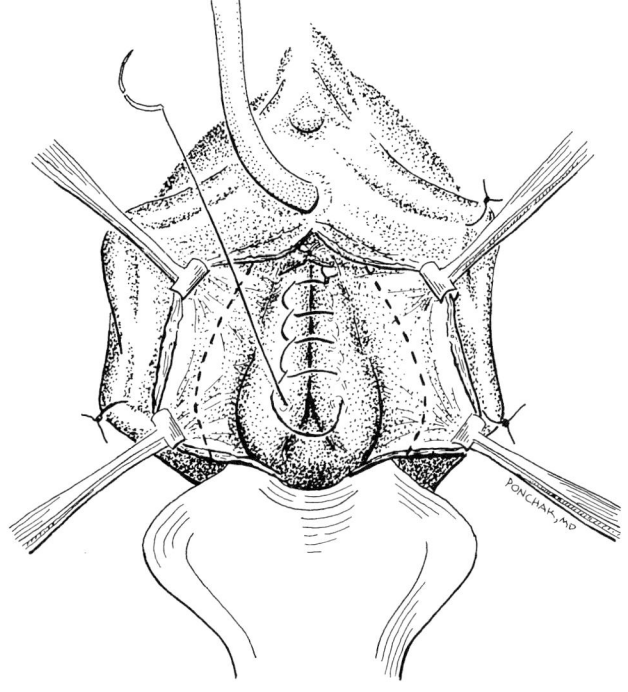

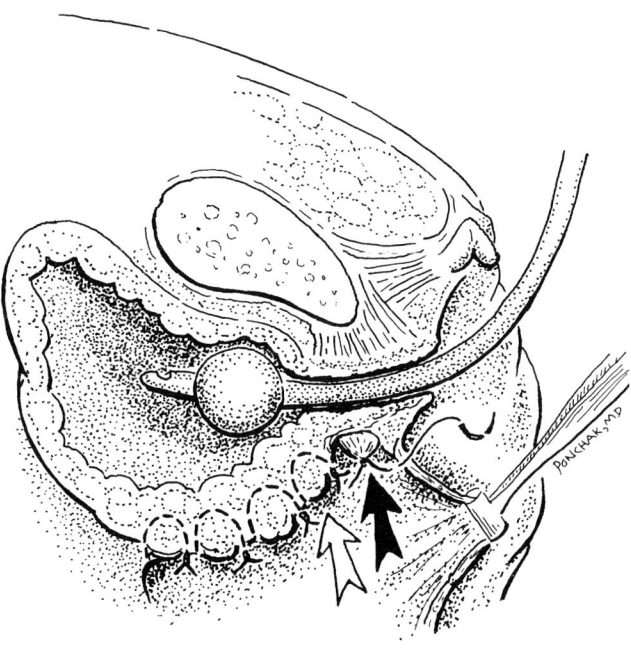

Fig. 24-8 Reducing the size of the cystocele. The fibromuscular capsule of the bladder is made smaller by a layer of running locked mattress stitches. The excess vaginal wall to be trimmed is shown by the dashed line.

Fig. 24-10 End result. Sagittal view shows the effect of plication of the pubourethral ligaments and urogenital diaphragm (*closed arrow*) beneath the vesicourethral junction. Tied, the Kelly stitch corrects the funneling (*open arrow*).

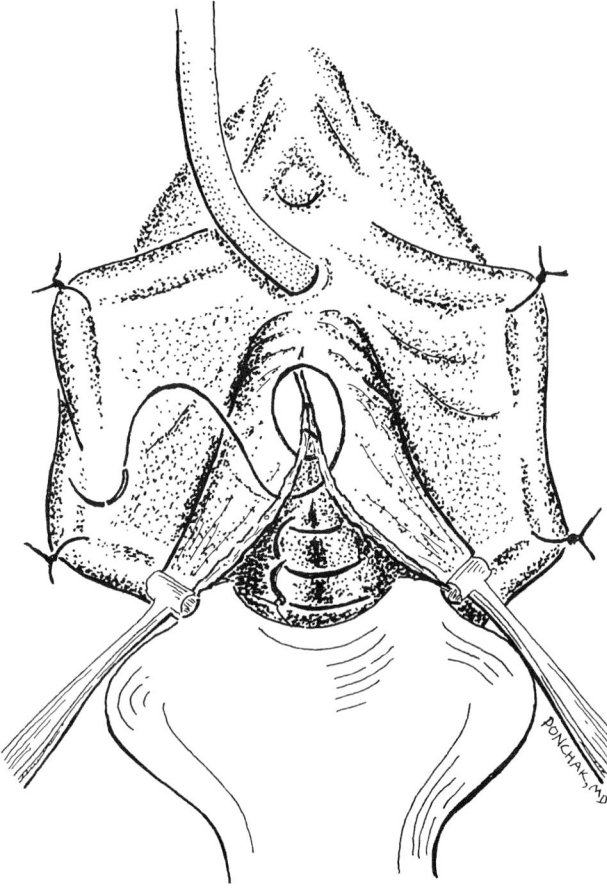

Fig. 24-11 Approximate the vaginal wall. Excess anterior vaginal wall has been trimmed and the full thickness of anterior vaginal wall is being approximated one side to the other with a running subcuticular suture.

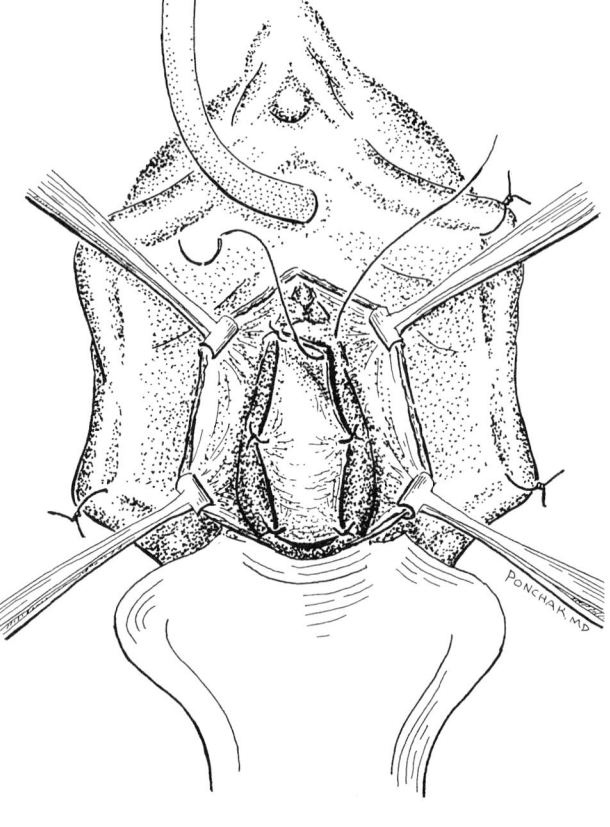

Fig. 24-12 Implantation of vaginal patch. A patch of resected anterior vaginal wall has been tacked to the surface of the fibromuscular layer of the vagina with a series of interrupted stitches as shown.

the resected flaps may be tacked to the surface of the bladder muscularis by a series of interrupted stitches (as shown in Figure 24-12), as suggested by Zacharin (2). The trimmed cut edges of the remaining anterior vaginal wall are closed over this patch without tension. This patch is most likely converted to collagen within a few months, and no epithelial inclusion cysts have been reported (3; Fig. 24-13).

Detachment or stretching of one or both vaginal sulci from their attachment to the arcus tendineus can be identified both preoperatively and intraoperatively and are known as paravaginal defects. When present, the defect should be remedied by reattachment of the lateral sulci to the fascia of the obturator internus at the site of the arcus tendineus (4; Figs. 24-14 through 24-17) to aid in restoration of the support of the vagina by both bladder and urethra. When this is coincident with demonstrable midline weakness, the latter should be repaired simultaneously (5).

The urethra and bladder, and the anterior vaginal wall beneath them, rest on the posterior vaginal wall. Therefore, repair any wall defect by posterior vaginal colporrhaphy or perineorrhaphy.

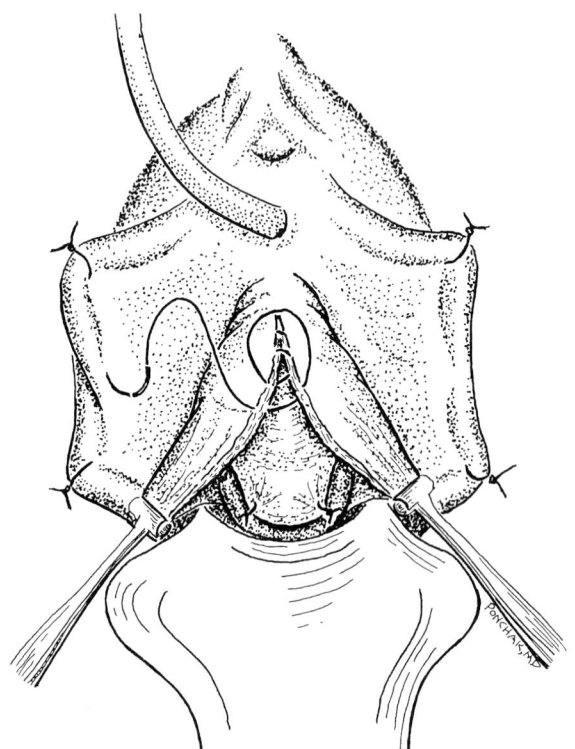

Fig. 24-13 Closure of vaginal incision. The cut edges of the anterior vaginal wall are closed over the patch, but without tension.

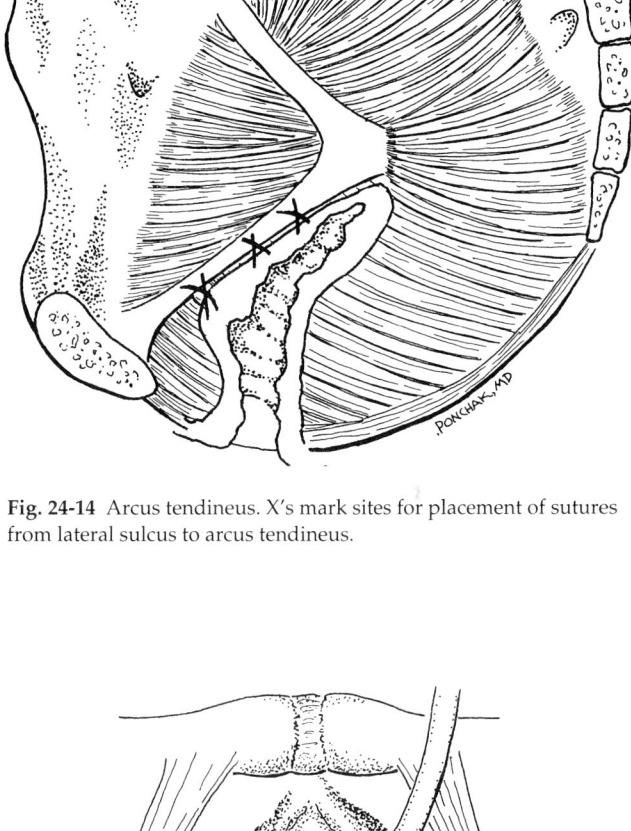

Fig. 24-14 Arcus tendineus. X's mark sites for placement of sutures from lateral sulcus to arcus tendineus.

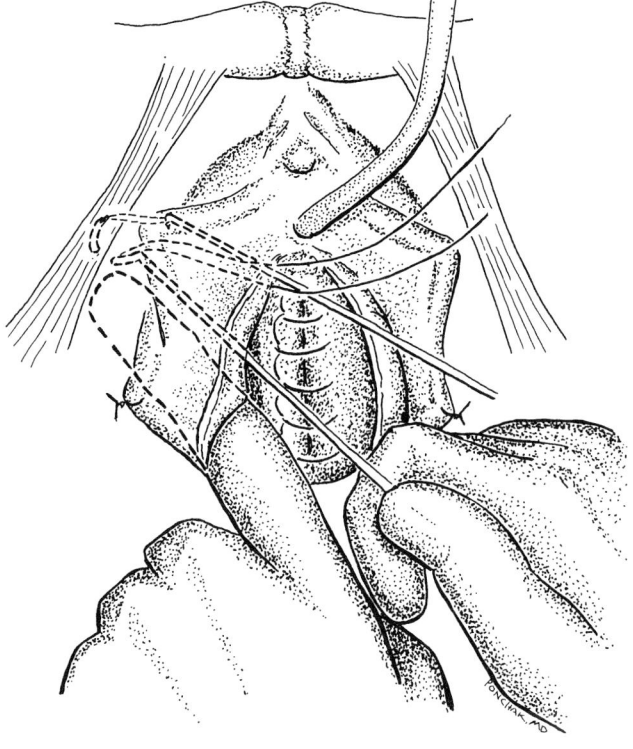

Fig. 24-16 Stitching the obturator fascia. Using the Deschamps ligature carrier, sutures are placed in the arcus tendineus and obturator fascia at the sites shown in Fig. 24-14.

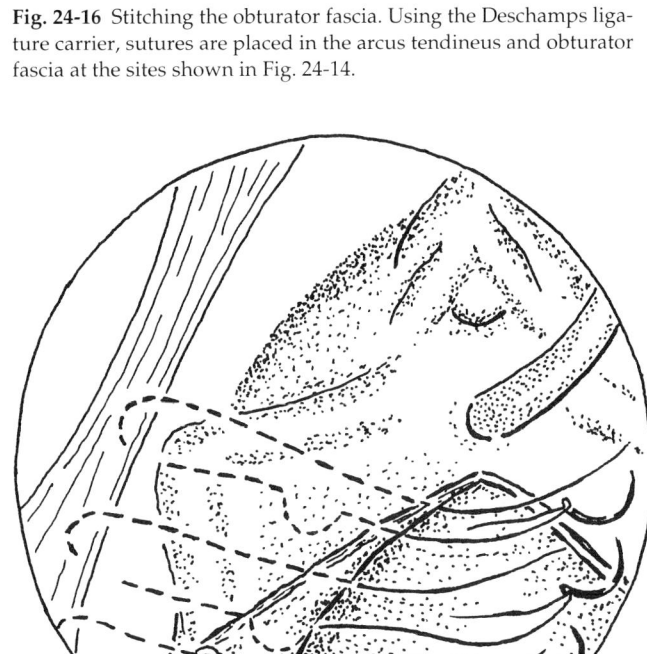

Fig. 24-15 Opening the space of Retzius for correction of paravaginal defect. The vaginal wall has been opened in the midline and dissected laterally beyond the limits of the vesicovaginal space opening directly into the space of Retzius. The surface of the obturator fascia is cleared by blunt dissection from both bladder and urethra.

Fig. 24-17 Stitching the sulci. Interrupted stitches are placed in the obturator fascia at the site of the arcus tendineus, and these are sewn beneath the anterior vaginal wall at the site of the sulci, as shown. When these paravaginal fixation knots have been tied, the sutures are cut, burying the knots beneath the vaginal epithelium. Correction of any midline vaginal defect is accomplished and the excess anterior wall is trimmed and closed without tension.

Summary

We have satisfactorily used this method, with modifications, since 1968. In some cases it is not possible to use the pubourethral ligament portion of the urogenital diaphragm to elevate the vesicourethral junction. Two alternatives are the Franz-Ingleman-Sundberg pubococcygeus muscle transplant and the Martius bulbocavernosus fat pad transplant (3,6).

By using the newer, long-acting synthetic sutures, such as polydiaxanone, we have successfully achieved long-term restoration of continence in more than 90% of patients who needed primary repair.

References

1 Ball TL. Anterior and posterior cystocele: cystocele revisited; of some antifascialists and fascialists as I knew them. Clin Obstet Gynecol 1964;9:1062.

2 Zacharin RF. Free full-thickness vaginal epithelium graft in correction of recurrent genital prolapse. Aust N Z J Obstet Gynaecol 1992;32:140–148.

3 Nichols DH. Gynecologic and obstetric surgery. St. Louis: Mosby-Yearbook, 1993:334–362.

4 White GR. Cystocele—a radical cure by suturing lateral sulci of vagina to the white line of the pelvic fascia. JAMA 1909;53:1707–1709.

5 Baden WF, Walker T. Surgical repair of vaginal defects. Philadelphia: JB Lippincott, 1992.

6 Nichols DH, Randall CL. Vaginal surgery, ed 3. Baltimore: Williams & Wilkins, 1989.

Chapter 25

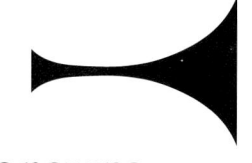

The modified Pereyra procedure for stress urinary incontinence

William A. Growdon and

Thomas B. Lebherz

The fact that there are more than 50 variations of surgical technique for correction of anatomic stress urinary incontinence (1) suggests that, for one reason or another, surgeons have been dissatisfied with the techniques that have been developed through the years and have tried to improve them. Of the factors considered in evaluating any surgical technique—versatility, reliability, safety, and ease of performance—one or another has always seemed to require improvement.

Surgeons who prefer the vaginal approach for most gynecologic surgery have relied in past years on the anterior colporrhaphy, the Kennedy-Kelly plication; however, they have been confronted with failure rates of 40% to 50% (2,3). Abdominal retropubic procedures such as the Marshall-Marchetti-Krantz procedure and the modified Burch procedure improved results, but did not fit well with vaginal surgery, requiring another large incision and, basically, another procedure separate from the vaginal approach.

The prototype "retropubic needle" suspension procedure was a new vaginal approach introduced in 1959 by Dr. Armand J. Pereyra (4). The procedure has since been reevaluated, and changes in instrumentation and technique have culminated in the modified Pereyra procedure, developed in association with Dr. Pereyra at the University of California, Los Angeles Medical Center (5). The procedure specifies a vaginal approach to the space of Retzius described by Studdiford (6). This surgical dissection paravesically at the urethrovesical junction (UVJ) allows for identification of the posterior pubourethral ligament at the proximal urethra so that this substantial support of the UVJ may be used for suspension to the anterior rectus sheath. Several authors have pointed out this structure's importance (7–9), especially in the surgical restoration of continence. The modified Pereyra procedure is our procedure of choice for the surgical correction of anatomic stress urinary incontinence. In addition to its high success rate, the procedure combines continued utilization of the vaginal approach with ease of surgical technique and is reliable, safe, and versatile.

Patient selection

All patients who complain of urinary incontinence must be thoroughly evaluated to ensure that the problem is due to anatomic factors and is not secondary to uninhibited bladder contractions, neurogenic bladder, or another anatomic problem such as diverticuli (10).

A thorough preoperative evaluation is mandatory. A medical history is obtained with the use of the Hodgkinson questionnaire (11), and pelvic examination, including both observation of pelvic relaxation during Valsalva efforts and the Q-tip test, is performed in the initial screening. More thorough urologic evaluation using volumetric stress testing, cystometrics, and cystourethroscopy with standing and supine evaluation will help to identify other factors that may cause incontinence. Lateral strain voiding cystourethrography helps to objectively demonstrate bladder neck competence and abnormal vesical neck anatomic relations. Patients in whom anatomic findings demonstrate rotation descent of the UVJ, with or without significant cystocele, are excellent candidates for the modified Pereyra procedure. If detrusor instability is elucidated in the initial evaluation, it should be treated before surgical correction is attempted. Likewise, postmenopausal patients with estrogen insufficiency should be given estrogen therapy, and an adequate objective response should precede surgery.

Advanced age and obesity, which often contraindicate or at least complicate abdominal retropubic procedures, are not contraindications to the use of the modified Pereyra procedure. Due to the limited surgical dissection required for the modified Pereyra procedure, patients who would otherwise have been denied retropubic abdominal procedures have been successfully treated by use of the modified Pereyra procedure.

Versatility of the procedure

We have used the modified Pereyra procedure in both primary and recurrent stress urinary incontinence. The procedure may be used in conjunction with vaginal hysterectomy, anterior-posterior colporrhaphy, and such specialized procedures as the Le Fort procedure or sacrospinous colpopexy. In most cases, when a vaginal approach is being used and when stress urinary incontinence is a problem manifested by rotational descent of the UVJ, this anatomic change is easily corrected with the use of the modified Pereyra procedure.

Although general or regional anesthesia is preferred for other major surgery such as vaginal hysterectomy, local anesthesia can be used for the modified Pereyra procedure (12). Table 25-1 indicates the various local nerve blocks required to achieve patient comfort. Preanesthetic doses of narcotic and amnestic agents are given as usual prior to injection of local anesthesia, and additional small doses of these agents administered by the anesthesiologist help to make the patient more comfortable during the procedure. Appropriate dosing should enable the patient to retain the ability to respond to verbal commands.

Table 25-1 Anesthetic technique

Nerve	Anesthetic (with epinephrine*)
Pudendal nerve	10 cc (l,r) 0.5%
Posterior femoral cutaneous nerve	5 cc (l,r) 0.5%
Ilioinguinal branch of genitofemoral nerve	5 cc (l,r) 0.5%
Suprapubic/perifascial	10 cc 1%
Vaginal epithelium at UVJ	10 cc 1%

*Epinephrine = 1:200,000

Surgical technique

The patient should be positioned as for vaginal hysterectomy in the modified dorsolithotomy position, avoiding overflexion of the hips. Vaginal hysterectomy is carried out if indicated. When cystocele is present, anterior repair is begun as usual, with midline incision of the anterior vaginal epithelium to a point that is 1 cm above the UVJ. The UVJ may be easily identified by inserting an indwelling Foley catheter and palpating the vesical neck while placing gentle traction on the catheter.

After the vaginal epithelium has been reflected, attention is directed toward blunt and sharp dissection of the tissues of the inferior urogenital diaphragm from the pubic rami bilaterally, dissecting laterally at a 45-degree angle from the UVJ; this procedure can usually be accomplished without difficulty by blunt dissection. Continued digital exploration of the retropubic space in this plane will bring the fingertip to a point of resistance approximately 2 to 3 cm lateral to the midline. Ventral digital pressure against the undersurface of the pubic ramus generally enables the digit to break through the tissues of the urogenital diaphragm and into the retropubic space. Sharp dissection may be necessary.

The pubic tubercle is easily palpated and can be used as a landmark after entry into the retropubic space. The finger normally can course over the UVJ unimpeded if previous retropubic procedures have not been performed. When previous surgery has been performed, minimal blunt or sharp dissection is usually all that is necessary to release the adhesions. Once the bladder neck is encircled with the index finger and pulled medially and caudad toward the operator, the sharp bands of tissue representing the lateral expansion of the posterior pillar of the pubourethral ligament and tissues of the urogenital diaphragm may be palpated and drawn into view. An Allis Adar forceps may be placed on the edge for identification and suturing. Once identified, 0 polypropylene suture is used to incorporate these structures in a continuous helical suture of three to five loops. Premeditated sharp traction on the completed suture should cause the patient to move on the table—convincing evidence of strong support. A partial-thickness vaginal suture incorporated in the helical suture at an appropriate distance from the edge of the vaginal incision may be used for additional support if thin tissues are apparent. The same procedure is carried out on the contralateral side.

A small incision, approximately 3 to 4 cm in transverse length, is made in the suprapubic space at the superior margin of the symphysis pubis and carried through the subcutaneous tissue to the anterior rectus sheath. The anterior rectus sheath is identified and rendered free of adipose tissue by blunt dissection. At this point, one digit placed alongside the vesical neck and into the retropubic space through the previously created lateral defect abuts the anterior rectus sheath from below through the retropubic space of Ret-

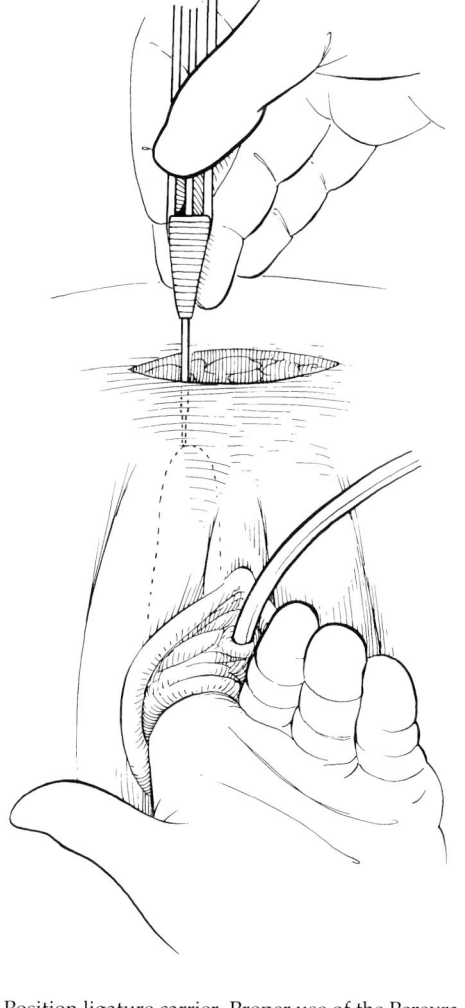

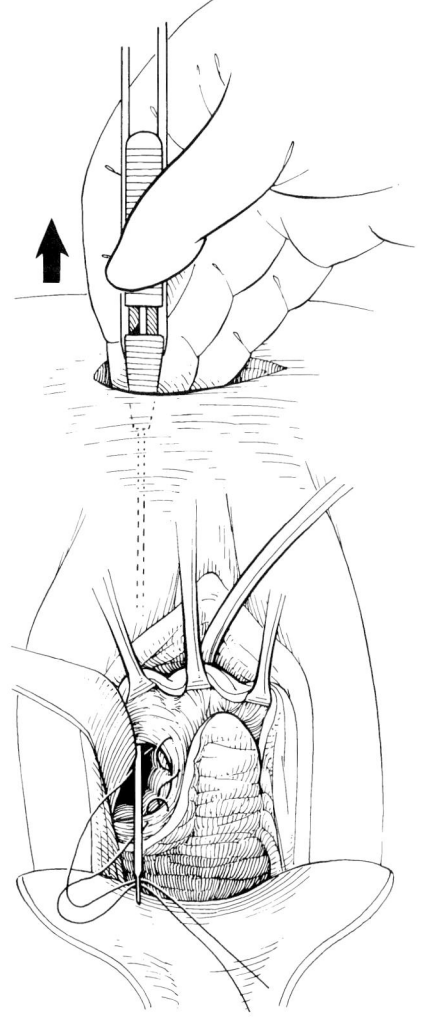

Fig. 25-1 Position ligature carrier. Proper use of the Pereyra ligature carrier is of great importance to avoid bladder neck injury. The operator's finger is in the retropubic space extending to the underside of the anterior rectus sheath through the space of Retzius. Once the Pereyra ligature carrier needle point has pierced the fascia, it should not leave the fingertip of the surgeon but should be guided upon extension sheathed by this finger until direct visualization of the end of the instrument is noted vaginally.

Fig. 25-2 Place suture and withdraw carrier. Two suture ends from an ipsilateral helical suture are threaded through the eye of the ligature carrier. The instrument is then withdrawn abdominally, thus transporting the suture. Before suture fixation, the cystocele and vaginal epithelium are repaired.

zius, while the Pereyra ligature carrier '75 (Cook Ob/Gyn, Spencer Ill.) simultaneously pierces the anterior rectus sheath onto the finger approximately 2 cm lateral to the midline (Fig. 25-1). The needle is extended vaginally, while sheathed with the vaginal finger, into direct vision. After the two ends of the helical suture on that side are threaded through the ligature carrier, the carrier is simply drawn back through its course (Fig. 25-2), and the suture ends are transposed through the abdominal incision. The same maneuver is performed on the contralateral side. It is important to lift the sutures and directly view the elevation of the vesical neck and UVJ. Once hemostasis is adequate and *before fixing the sutures abdominally*, the cystocele is repaired, the vaginal epithelium is trimmed, and the vaginal incision is closed. These procedures are cumbersome if not accom-

plished before suture fixation from above, because the surgical field is prematurely pulled away from the operator. After these repairs have been made, pancystoscopy is performed to demonstrate ureteral function, with 5 cc of indigo carmine administered intravenously.

Sutures may be abdominally fixed in two ways. The suture ends on each side may be tied together across the midline with eight knots; we prefer to place a hemostatic metal clip on the free ends of the suture above the last knot to prevent unraveling. Alternatively, and especially in patients in whom there is concern about the integrity of the abdominal fascia, the two ipsilateral sutures may be separated one from another on each side by the use of an aneurysm needle. The needle is driven from a point approximately 2 cm above on the anterior rectus sheath, moving one of the su-

Table 25-2 Steps to the modified Pereyra procedure

1. Vaginal incision with Foley in place

2. Release of UVJ from vaginal epithelium

3. Dissection at 45-degree angle from UVJ with release of UVJ from pubic rami

4. Enter space of Retzius

5. Identification of pubourethral ligament (PUL)

6. Helical suture (0 polypropylene) of PUL to edge of tissues of the urogenital diaphragm

7. Suprapubic transverse incision

8. Passage of ligature carrier

9. Transposition of sutures

10. Cystoscopy

11. Closure of vaginal incision

12. Fixation of sutures abdominally

13. Closure of abdominal incision

14. Vaginal pack

ture pairs to that level. Each side is thus separately suspended. After the abdominal wound is irrigated, it is simply closed with a subcuticular closure.

The optimal angle of elevation should be determined through a combination of modalities. The first method requires *palpation* of the UVJ and its relationship to the inferior aspect of the pubic ramus such that the UVJ is elevated above this level. Second, it is important to *visually observe* the urethrovesical angle and the vaginal retropubic orientation while palpating. Once the optimal angle is achieved, palpation of the urethra and vesical neck should allow for some lateral mobility of the tissues. Third, internal meatal closure of the urethra can be observed during the procedure through *urethroscopy* while the sutures are elevated. Last, if a regional or local anesthetic has been administered, the patient will be able to *make Valsalva efforts* to demonstrate incontinence with a full bladder; continence can then be achieved by exerting upward tension on the sutures to the appropriate level.

If surgery is contemplated for anatomic stress urinary incontinence in the absence of need for other repairs such as cystocele or hysterectomy, the Pereyra procedure can be easily performed using a curvilinear incision, or inverted U, described by Raz (13). This incision allows for easy access to the retropubic space with minimal surgical dissection of the vaginal epithelium. When indicated, the Pereyra procedure can be easily incorporated into the Le Fort procedure after the anterior vaginal epithelium has been dissected off the prolapsed vagina, since the most proximal transverse incision to the urethra is near the vesical neck. After all incisions have been closed vaginally, elevation and fixation of the vesical neck should complete the procedure.

Avoidance of pitfalls

Absence of ligament

Dissection too close to the vesical neck may avulse the fascial attachments to the proximal urethra such that no medial attachments to the proximal urethra will be available to suture; this may be recognized on digital palpation by the lack of a sharp fascial band coursing into the anterior proximal urethra. In such cases, the space may be closed, and the appropriate space dissected slightly laterally may allow for identification of more substantial fascial elements. Alternatively, the helical suture may be placed solely in the detached tissues of the urogenital diaphragm on that side. Clinical experience has shown that this technique works well for patients in whom the pubourethral ligaments are not well delineated.

Avoiding injury to the bladder neck

If suture placement through the bladder neck is to be avoided, the most important aspect of the procedure is the placement of the vaginal finger into the retropubic space to guide the Pereyra ligature carrier down into the operator's field. A suprapubic catheter should not be placed before passing the Pereyra ligature carrier, for this may pin the bladder neck against the anterior rectus sheath, thus positioning it in the area of greatest potential injury. Alternatively, if the vaginal finger elevates the bladder neck, rather than coursing lateral to the bladder neck and into the retropubic space, the bladder neck may be pushed against the Pereyra needle tip. Therefore, it is important that the operator feel the retropubic anatomy to locate the pubic tubercle and ensure that no soft tissues, such as the bladder neck, are insinuated between the fingertip and the undersurface of the anterior rectus sheath. However, if cystoscopy shows that a suture has entered the bladder, the suture need only be removed and replaced in the appropriate position. Recognition of injury at the time of surgery is important because release of the suture after surgery may impair long-term results.

Abdominal Pereyra sutures too far lateral or medial

If the Pereyra needle is driven through the anterior rectus sheath too far lateral to the midline, the genitofemoral branch of the ilioinguinal nerve may be entrapped, causing pain in the suprapubic area. It is also possible that such lateral placement will cause opening, rather than closure, of the internal urethral meatus when tension is placed on the vesical neck. Therefore, it is important that these sutures be elevated parallel to the sagittal plane with as little medial or lateral tension as possible on the internal urethral meatus.

Premature elevation and fixation of the Pereyra sutures

If the UVJ is elevated and fixed into the retropubic space before closure of vaginal incisions, closure becomes almost impossible; 2- to 3-cm elevation of the UVJ draws the incisions severely into the retropubic space and out of view. Thus, these incisions must be closed before the sutures are fixed.

Use of nonabsorbable sutures

The use of nonabsorbable suture material for the fixation sutures is associated with a higher rate of failure (5). Polypropylene suture has been very effective for this procedure, with no foreign-body reaction in our series. The two disadvantages to this type of suture are the tendency for knots to unravel, a problem that can be overcome by *placing a metal hemostatic clip above the last knot,* and the tendency for the "pigtail" of knots in the suprapubic area to be palpable in thin patients. The latter complaint can be avoided by using a separate suture to pin the length of knots to the anterior rectus sheath cephalad in the anterior rectus fascia. Thus, the pointed edges of the end of the tied suture will be situated as deep as possible in the subcutaneous tissues.

Perioperative and postoperative management

Because we favor intermittent self-catheterization as a postoperative alternative to suprapubic or urethral drainage, we begin before the surgery to instruct patients in intermittent self-catheterization techniques. Simple hand-mirror techniques or palpation while in the shower can help the patient to identify digitally and visually the urethral meatus. Once patients are confident in the identification of the external meatus, they usually learn intermittent self-catheterization easily.

Perioperatively, we administer prophylactic antibiotics and, in postmenopausal patients, subcutaneous heparin. A medicated vaginal pack is placed immediately after surgery and an indwelling Foley catheter is allowed to drain overnight. The pack is removed on the first postoperative day. Intermittent self-catheterization is used if the patient has an increasing volume of residual urine, or finds that she is unable to void spontaneously after the transurethral catheter is discontinued on the first or second postoperative day.

In selected patients, intraoperative suprapubic catheterization is performed as the last procedure in the operating room. Less than 10% of patients will require these techniques of postoperative urinary drainage for a prolonged period of time.

Evaluations of success with the modified Pereyra procedure suggest that the majority of patients are satisfied with the result of the procedure. Lower cure rates are sometimes reported in series using nonabsorbable sutures, the "old" Pereyra procedure, and when definition of cure is based on effective urodynamic studies as an endpoint (i.e., the patient thinks she is cured, but urodynamic testing disproves the patient's satisfaction). Highly successful personal series may reflect some bias, but also may reflect consistent selection criteria and operative performance. Satisfaction in our experience suggests that the modified Pereyra procedure will not fall by the wayside due to a lack of efficacy.

Finally, we urge all who use the old Pereyra needle and the procedure originally described by Dr. Pereyra to abandon them. Reports of high failure rates and injuries to the bladder neck suggest that they should not be used.

Summary

The modified Pereyra procedure is a simple and useful technique evolved over many years of evaluation (Table 25-2). While the original Pereyra technique and needle are associated with the disadvantages of blind periurethral manipulation and unacceptable long-term failure rates, the modified Pereyra procedure is an open technique that is anatomically precise yet easy to perform. Success rates have been highly acceptable in both primary and recurrent stress urinary incontinence (5,12–16).

The modified Pereyra procedure has been our procedure of choice for both primary and recurrent stress urinary incontinence since 1976. More than 600 surgical procedures have been performed, and our continued evaluation of the procedure reveals it to be safe, reliable, and well suited to use in a teaching institution. We achieve long-term cure rates of approximately 90%. The procedure itself, including cystoscopy, can be performed in approximately 45 minutes, and general, regional, or local anesthesia can be used. Approximately 20 minutes are added to standard anterior colporrhaphy to complete the procedure when it is performed along with vaginal hysterectomy and anterior-posterior colporrhaphy. Because of the limited scope of surgical dissection, patients tolerate the procedure well and recover rapidly; the technique is therefore especially useful in patients of advanced age or those with debilitating medical illness.

With his report in 1959 of a simplified surgery for stress urinary incontinence, Dr. Armand J. Pereyra was the first to successfully stimulate interest in these kinds of techniques. The impact of his procedure on both the gynecologic and urologic specialties is already apparent.

References

1 Graber EA. Stress incontinence in women: a review, 1977. Obstet Gynecol Survey 1977;32:565.

2 Cullen KR, Welch JS. Stress incontinence. Surg Gynecol Obstet 1961;113:85.

3 Green TH. The problem of urinary stress incontinence in the female. Obstet Gynecol Survey 1968;23:603.

4 Pereyra AJ. A simplified procedure for the correction of stress incontinence in women. West J Surg Obstet Gynecol 1959;67:223.

5 Pereyra AJ, Lebherz TB, Growdon WA, et al. Pubourethral supports in perspective: modified Pereyra procedure for urinary incontinence. Obstet Gynecol 1982;59:643.

6 Studdiford WE. The problem of stress incontinence and its surgical relief. Surg Gynecol Obstet 1946;83:742.

7 Zacharin RF. The suspensary mechanism of the female urethra. J Anat 1963;97:423.

8 Zacharin RF. Abdominoperineal urethral suspension: a ten-year experience in management of recurrent stress incontinence of urine. Obstet Gynecol 1977;50:1.

9 Milley PS, Nichols DH. The relationship between pubourethral ligaments and urogenital diaphragm in the human female. (Anat) Rec 1971;170:281.

10 Shingleton HM, Kerr-Wilson R, Davis RO. Office assessment of urinary incontinence. Contemp Obstet Gyencol 1984;24:71.

11 Hodgkinson CP. Stress urinary incontinence. Am J Obstet Gynecol 1970;108(suppl):1149.

12 Growdon WA, Lebherz TB. The modified Pereyra procedure: use of local anesthesia. Obstet Gynecol 1986;68:272.

13 Raz S. Modified bladder neck suspension for female stress incontinence. Urology 1981;17:82.

14 Quigley GJ, King SK. Transvaginal retropubic urethropexy—the "revised Pereyra procedure": a report of 50 cases. Am J Obstet Gynecol 1981;139:268.

15 Roberts JA, Angel JR, Thomas R, et al. Modified Pereyra procedure for stress incontinence. J Urol 1981;125:787.

16 Bhatia NN, Bergman A. Modified Burch versus Pereyra retropubic urethropexy for stress urinary incontinence. Obstet Gynecol 1985;66:255.

Suggested readings

Bergman A, Ballard CA, Koonings PP. Comparison of three different surgical procedures for genuine stress incontinence: prospective randomized study. Am J Obstet Gynecol 1988;160:1102.

Bergman A, Koonings PP, Ballard CA. Primary stress urinary incontinence and pelvic relaxation: prospective randomized comparison of three different operations. Am J Obstet Gynecol 1989;161:97.

Karram MM, Angel O, Koonings P. The modified Pereyra procedure: a clinical and urodynamic review. Br J Obstet Gynaecol 1992;99:655.

Park GS, Miller EJ. Surgical treatment of stress urinary incontinence: a comparison of the Kelly plication, Marshall-Marchetti-Krantz and Pereyra procedures. Obstet Gynecol 1985;71:575.

Riggs J. Retropubic cystourethropexy: a review of two operative procedures with long-term followup. Obstet Gynecol 1986;68:98.

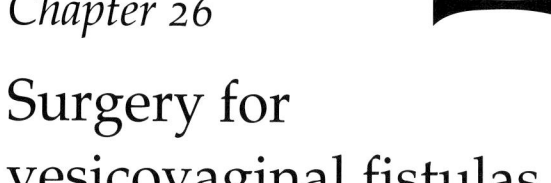

Chapter 26

Surgery for vesicovaginal fistulas

Hans Georg Bender and Lutwin Beck

Managing genitourinary fistulas taxes more than our surgical skills. As important for success as effective surgical performance is choosing the proper strategy and procedure. A precise diagnostic workup, careful preparation for surgery, and optimal timing are also vital. Establishing the patient's trust during early management helps prevent the conflicts that, all too often, lead to legal action.

According to a 1980 survey of postoperative complications in gynecologic surgery from 85 gynecology departments in Germany, intraoperative lesions of the urinary bladder after total abdominal hysterectomy occurred at a rate of 0.6%. The frequency was about 1% after vaginal hysterectomy, whether or not vaginal repair had been done for pelvic relaxation (1). The figure was higher—1.5%—in patients who had undergone radical hysterectomy. One (1%) of 16 bladder lesions in abdominal hysterectomy resulted in a vesicovaginal fistula. Two (1.5%) of 16 bladder lesions in 1300 vaginal hysterectomies resulted in vesicovaginal fistulas, as did 5 (1.5%) of 334 radical hysterectomies (2).

Statistics indicate that few gynecologic surgeons have the necessary experience and expertise to treat fistulas. It is therefore appropriate to consider transferring those patients who develop them to gynecologic centers.

Preventing lesions

Because most ureter and bladder injuries occur after routine hysterectomies, place particular emphasis on preventing lesions when planning such procedures. Key in gynecologic surgery are visualization of the ureters and a clear delineation of the bladder wall, which must be dissected free of the anterior aspect of the uterus and vagina. This point is particularly well observed by Symmonds and Lee in their explanation of total abdominal hysterectomy technique (3). Following these principles for every routine abdominal hysterectomy will provide excellent preparation for more difficult situations.

Managing urinary bladder lesions

As soon as one has evidence that the urinary bladder has been injured, locate and close the lesion. Using suture material with prolonged absorption time, create a two-layer closure without tension. It is sometimes a good idea to cover the suture row in abdominal procedures with a peritoneal flap mobilized from the anterolateral paravesical serosa. This step may be especially helpful when lesions occur in the lower part of the dorsal bladder wall. In vaginal hysterectomies, pulling down the anterior peritoneum serves the same purpose.

The sutures used for repair of lesions in the bladder dome usually heal without any problem. Inserting a suprapubic catheter lowers the tension on the bladder sutures and speeds healing.

Surgical repair of fistulas

The timing, strategy, and final results of surgical repair differ substantially for simple and complicated postoperative lesions of the urinary bladder. Closing recurrent and radiogenic fistulas is often difficult. Performing a complete preoperative workup should include cystoscopy, intravenous pyelogram, laboratory and bacteriologic analysis of urine specimens, and, in cancer patients, biopsies from the fistula wall.

When to intervene is a delicate question. If the fistula has not spontaneously healed after the bladder has been drained by catheter for 4 to 6 weeks, surgery is usually indicated. There is general agreement that vesicovaginal lesions should be closed immediately, within the first 48 hours, or later, after 1 to 4 months. The reason for the long delay if closure cannot be performed promptly is that conditions deteriorate once an inflammatory reaction sets in. This complicates dissection of the fistula's borders and, ultimately, wound healing.

Waiting until conditions improve is difficult for the patient, who naturally wants to become dry as soon as possible. Nevertheless, before closure can be accomplished, the fistula margin must be cleared of inflammation and necrosis so that the sutures can be applied into solid tissue without disrupting the fragile wound borders. During this waiting period, administer antibiotics as long as a Foley catheter is in place. Systemic estriol may be useful, especially if atrophy is obvious.

We generally do not apply systemic cortisone. Whether to use the vaginal or abdominal approach depends on the location and the size of the fistula, the width of the vagina, and the surgeon's experience. Gynecologists tend to prefer the vaginal procedure; urologists, the abdominal. Table 26-1 summarizes success rates of several techniques.

Vaginal procedures

A wide operating field is mandatory for the vaginal approach. If such a field does not already exist, create one with a lateral episiotomy or a Schuchardt incision. In Germany, surgeons tend to favor the techniques proposed by Füth and Mayo and the proximal colpocleisis as suggested by Latzko (4).

The Füth and Mayo method

This approach works best in small and medium-sized fistulas—those with a maximum diameter of 1 to 2 cm—that are not located in the highest aspect of the anterior vaginal wall (Fig. 26-1). The fistula is optimally exposed by speculum and traction sutures, which guarantee countertraction for dissection in the vesicovaginal septum after the fistula itself has been circumcised. This creates a 0.5- to 1-cm broad cuff of vaginal epithelium around the fistula opening.

From the outer aspect of the cuff, begin by performing sharp dissection in all directions. Stay closer to the vaginal

Table 26-1 Success rates for various closure techniques

Technique	No. of patients with successful closure (%)
Vaginal route	
Döderlein	29 (96%)
Sims-Simon	157 (94%)
Latzko	38 (92%)
Füth-Mayo	34 (76%)
Moir	40 (70%)
Abdominal route	
Omental flap	27 (100%)
Peritoneal flap	54 (91%)
Rotation flap of urinary bladder	56 (87%)
Suprapubic	54 (75%)

Reproduced by permission from Friedberg V, Altwein JE, Petri E. Vaginaler oder abdominaler Verschluss von Blasen-Scheiden-Fisteln? In: Petri E, ed. Gynäkologische urologie. Stuttgart: Georg Thieme, 1983:73–85.

epithelium than to the bladder wall. It is essential to transect all scar tissue that interferes with closure.

After appropriate mobilization, invaginate the fistula and the newly created cuff of vaginal epithelium into the urinary bladder. Close the bladder wall with atraumatic absorbable No. 3-0 sutures. Carry the stitches through the fascia and bladder musculature, but do not include bladder epithelium.

The suture, which usually extends transversely, may be longitudinal instead. Using the same material, cover the suture with a second layer of the same stitches. Place all stitches in both rows to avoid the intramural part of the ureter. Finally, one may close the vaginal epithelium—an optional procedure. Insert a suprapubic or indwelling Foley catheter for 7 to 10 days; administer antibiotics until the catheter has been removed.

We used this technique in 24 patients. Of these, 21 healed after the first closure. In three others, a second attempt with a bulbocavernosus flap was necessary.

The Sims and Simon technique

This approach differs from the Füth-Mayo procedure in that all scar tissue, including the fistula itself, is excised. The surgeon sutures the bladder wall, excluding the bladder epithelium, in one or two layers, to close the hole (Fig. 26-2) (5).

The Latzko technique

In this procedure, a partial colpocleisis, the surgeon approximates the upper part of the anterior and posterior vaginal walls (Fig. 26-3). It is used for fistulas high in the vaginal vault, which occur most commonly after hysterectomy. Mobilization, as described for the Füth-Mayo proce-

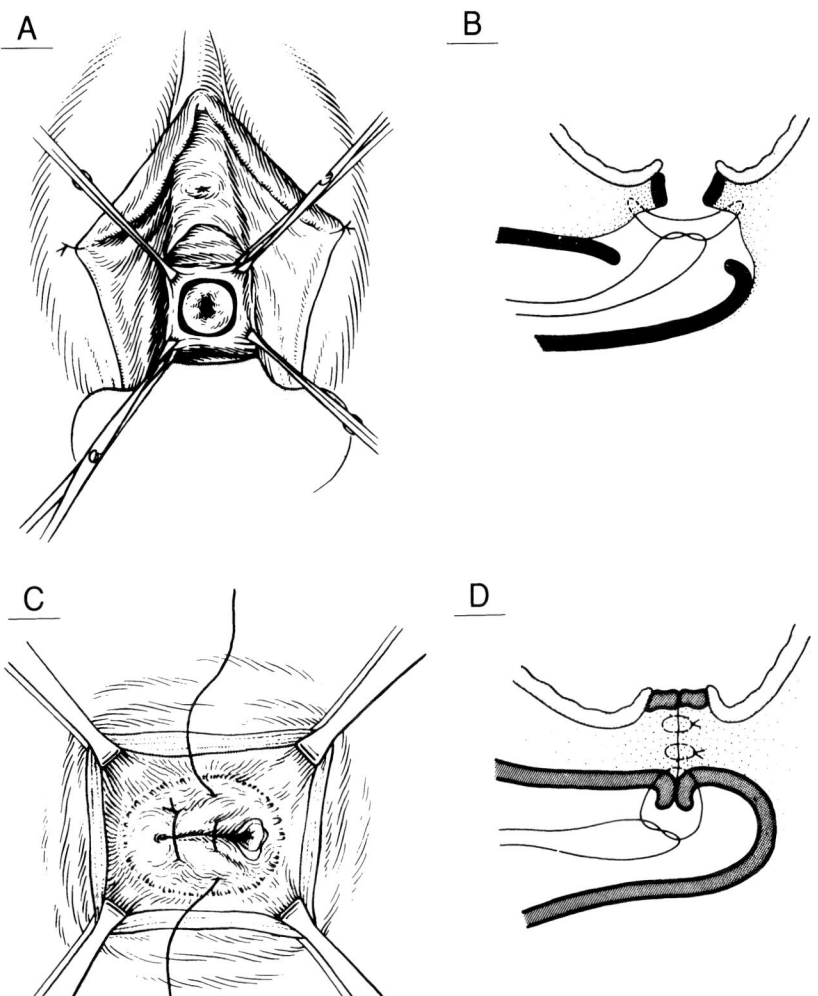

Fig. 26-1 In the Füth-Mayo technique, the fistula is circumcised (A); initial sutures are placed (B), invaginating the cuff around the fistula and opening into the bladder; the first two sutures of the first row are applied (C); three-layer closure (D). (Reproduced by permission from Friedberg V, Altwein JE, Petri E. Vaginaler oder abdominaler Verschluss von Blasen-Scheiden-Fisteln? In: Petri E, ed. Gynäkologische urologie. Stuttgart: Georg Thieme, 1983:73–85.)

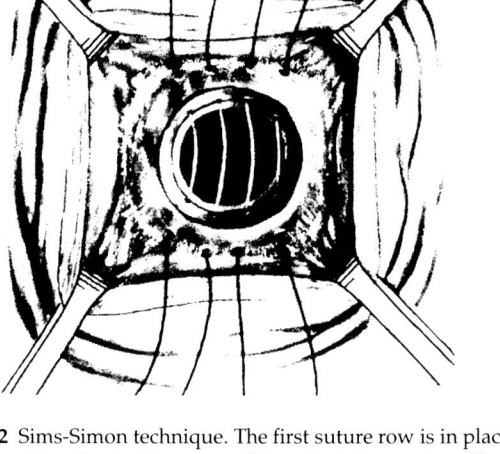

Figure 26-2 Sims-Simon technique. The first suture row is in place in a fistula closed by this highly successful method. (Reproduced by permission from Käser O, Iklé FA, Hirsch HA. Atlas der gynäkologischen Operationen. Stuttgart: Georg Thieme, 1983.)

dure, is impossible. The minor shortening of the vagina that occurs with the Latzko technique rarely interferes with function. Good exposure with specula and traction sutures is essential.

Begin by circumcising the opening of the fistula, creating a radius of vaginal epithelium of about 1.5 cm anteriorly and 2 cm posteriorly. Subdivide the cuff with incisions in four parts of epithelium. These sections are usually removed from the outer aspect toward the fistula, which is also stripped of epithelium. Apply atraumatic absorbable No. 3-0 sutures. A second row is occasionally used for safety. Close the vaginal epithelial wound with sutures.

We used the Latzko procedure for 32 patients. In 29, one attempt was sufficient to close the fistula.

An alternative route

One should use abdominal procedures for the following:
• large fistulas (diameter greater than 2 cm);
• fistulas that require ureteral reimplantation;
• complex or multiple fistulas (ureteral-vesicovaginal);

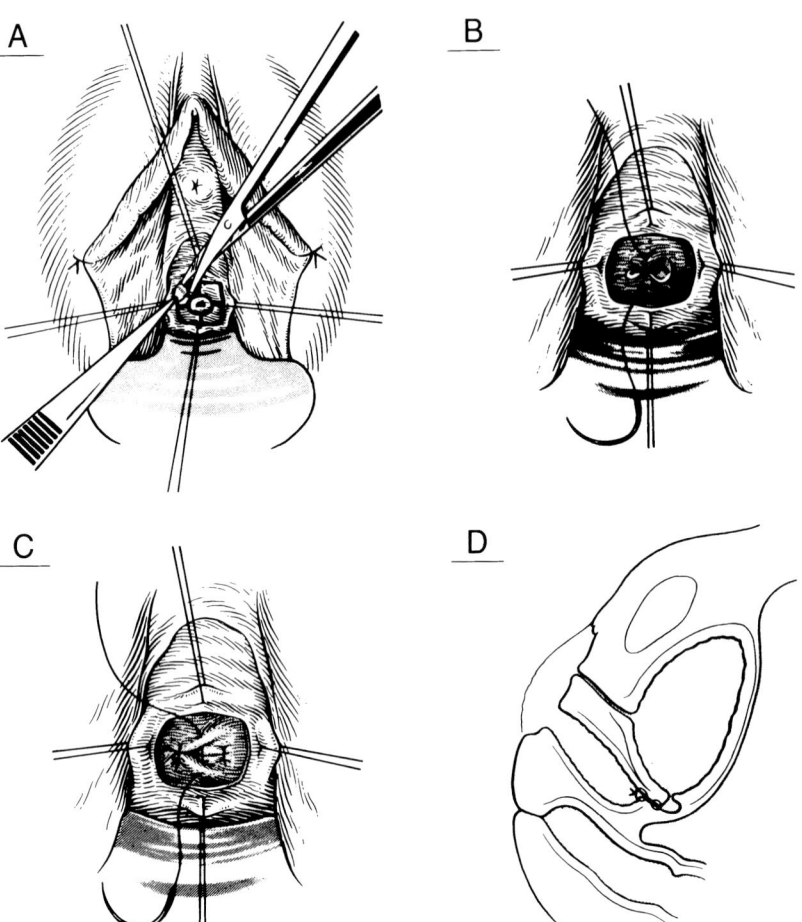

Fig. 26-3 The Latzko technique is essentially a high vaginal occlusion. Shown are crosswise incision and deepithelialization (A); first suture row (B); and second suture row (C), which covers the first. Last is a schematic of the technique (D). (Reproduced by permission from Friedberg V, Altwein JE, Petri E. Vaginaler oder abdominaler Verschluss von Blasen-Scheiden-Fisteln? In: Petri E, ed. Gynäkologische urologie. Stuttgart: Georg Thieme, 1983:73–85.)

- vesicouterine fistulas;
- selected cases of recurrent fistulas, and
- conditions characterized by poor vascularization, such as radiation and diabetes.

Figure 26-4 illustrates the principles of an abdominal fistula closure. Make an abdominal incision wide enough to permit sufficient movement. Delineate the urinary bladder and separate it from the vagina. Place a pad in the vagina to identify the appropriate layer. Incise the posterior bladder wall 4 to 5 cm into the area of the fistula. Excise the fistula itself as well as all surrounding scar tissue, so that one can close well-vascularized tissue without creating scars or tension.

Close the isolated edges of the vaginal wall around the fistula opening with everting interrupted sutures of No. 2-0 polyglactin (Vicryl) or chromic catgut. Before suturing the bladder incision, one may wish to interpose a 4- to 6-cm pedicled peritoneal flap, raised from the paravesical area, between the suture rows in the vagina and the urinary bladder. Attach the peritoneal flap to the vagina with one side or the other. If the course of one or both ureters runs into the fistula, perform an implantation through a subepithelial tunnel to prevent reflux. Finally, close the bladder wall with interrupted sutures, using everting atraumatic No. 3-0 polyglactin or chromic catgut.

To help ensure closure, one may wish to stitch a second row with a running No. 2-0 polyglactin suture. The peritoneal flap separates the suture rows in the bladder and vagina and prevents a recurrence of the fistula. The flap will soon occlude the two wounds completely. We successfully applied a peritoneal flap in 15 patients, either after closing a fistula, or as added protection for the suture closing a lesion in the urinary bladder.

For transabdominal closure use the pedicled omentum (Fig. 26-5; 2). The omental flap can improve vascularization, especially in high-risk patients who have had radiation, necrotic damage, or severe inflammation. The procedure leads to closure even if sharp dissection of the communicating organs is impossible. However, the pedicled omentum technique has a higher complication rate than the peritoneal flap technique. It also takes longer and bears a higher risk of bleeding and bowel obstruction. This method was successful in the three patients in whom we attempted it.

Muscle flaps

In patients who have had radiation therapy, the main problem is to reestablish normal vascularization in the area surrounding the fistula. If this cannot be done by using adjacent

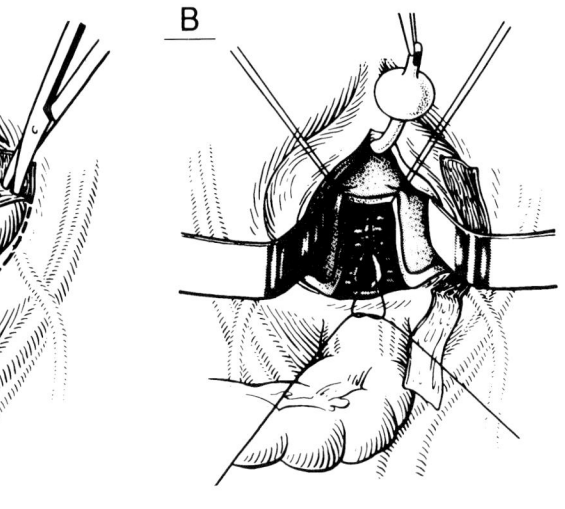

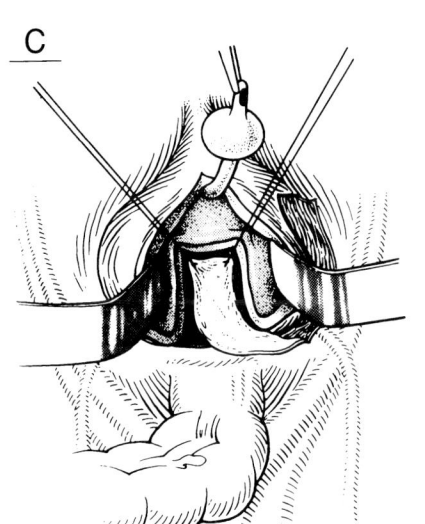

Fig. 26-4 Abdominal peritoneal flap technique. Major steps in this method: Incision lines are made (A) for opening the bladder (medial) and mobilizing the peritoneal flap. Next, the urinary bladder is opened; here, the suture row in the vagina is visible (B). The peritoneal flap is interposed (C) before the bladder is closed. (Reproduced by permission from Friedberg V, Altwein JE, Petri E. Vaginaler oder abdominaler Verschluss von Blasen-Scheiden-Fisteln? In: Petri E, ed. Gynäkologische urologie. Stuttgart: Georg Thieme, 1983:73–85.)

structures, attach healthy tissue to the fistula closure; this will prevent breakdown of the wound. Vascularization can be achieved not only with peritoneal or omental flaps but also with flaps made with any of several different muscles.

Martius first proposed the bulbocavernosus flap, which is easily mobilized (Fig. 26-6). The major limitation is the shortness of the pedicle. The flap can therefore be used only for fistulas in the lower part of the anterior vaginal wall. One variation is to create a pedicled muscular strip from the rectus abdominis muscle (6). Frequently, however, the abdominal wall will have been included in the radiation field. As a result, the muscle may be damaged or difficult to mobilize (see Chapter 16).

Another useful transplant for large vesicovaginal fistulas is the gracilis muscle. It can be mobilized after one has extended a skin incision down from the pubic tubercle to the inner aspect of the thigh. In this way, the muscular insertion can be transected above the medial aspect of the knee. Preserve the vascular pedicle that curves laterally into

the muscle at the distal end of the proximal third. The muscle is then pulled with its distal end through the obturator foramen and fixed under the fistula closure. The vagina is closed over the gracilis transplant.

One disadvantage of this method is that the resulting subtotal occlusion of the vagina will interfere with sexual function. In many such patients, however, sexual relations have already been affected by urine leakage and other problems related to damage from radiation.

Bladder problems

The ultimate aim of all these surgical efforts is not merely to close the bladder lesion but also to reestablish urinary continence. One of the most difficult preoperative tasks—particularly important after radiation—is to evaluate bladder capacity and urinary continence. One problem is that fibrosis of the bladder wall may result. Another is the diffi-

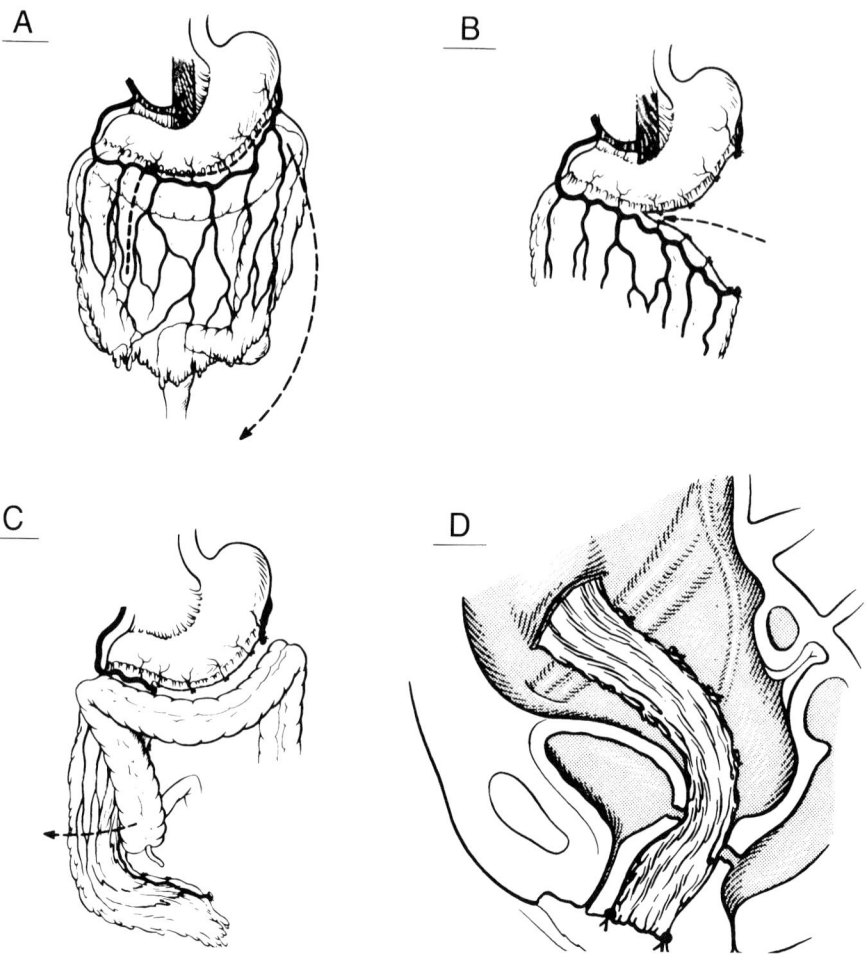

Fig. 26-5 Omental pedicle technique. Shown is the stepwise mobilization of left part of omentum and retrocolic pull-through into the true pelvis (A, B, C) and fixation of the omental pedicle (D). (Reproduced by permission from Friedberg V, Altwein JE, Petri E. Vaginaler oder abdominaler Verschluss von Blasen-Scheiden-Fisteln? In: Petri E, ed. Gynäkologische urologie. Stuttgart: Georg Thieme, 1983:73–85.)

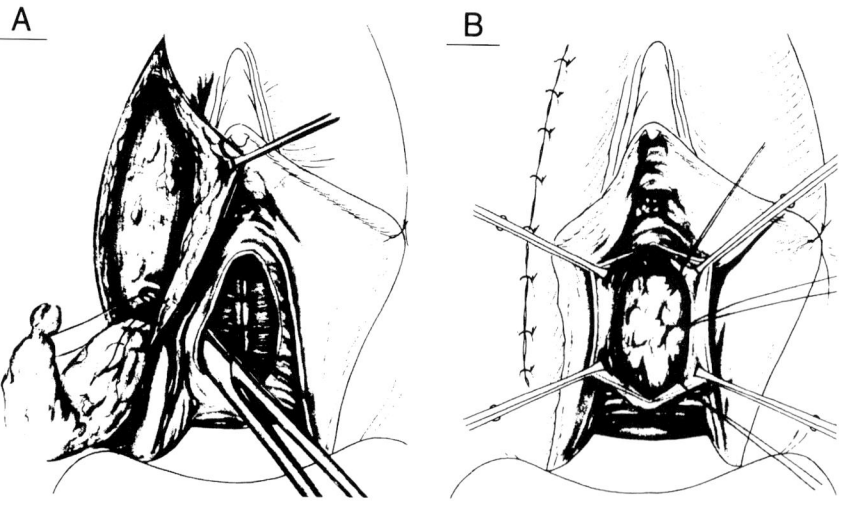

Fig. 26-6 Martius bulbocavernosus flap is mobilized (A), then affixed (B). It covers the paravesical fascia. (Reproduced by permission from Käser O, Iklé FA, Hirsch HA. Atlas der gynäkologischen Operationen. Stuttgart: Georg Thieme, 1983.)

culty of maintaining continuous drainage without inducing bladder distention. Bladder leakage complicates urodynamic examinations in these patients. Pulling a condom over the catheter tip may facilitate matters.

A broad lesion in the bladder neck and the urethral junction may indicate that urinary continence is unlikely or impossible. In some patients, stress incontinence after fistula closure can be corrected with a retropubic suspension (7). Large defects with gross scarring and loss of the whole urethra may defy all attempts at repair. In these circumstances urinary diversion will be required. The permanent abdominal stoma of an ileal conduit, however, is not acceptable in developing countries, so ureterocolic anastomosis is unavoidable. A Kock pouch with umbilicus stoma and emptying by catheter is acceptable and may help control reservoir function.

References

1 Stark G. Problematik der Qualitätssicherung in der Gynäkologie. Grafelfing, 1980:18.

2 Kiricuta J, Goldstein AHB. The repair of extensive vesicovaginal fistulas with pedicled omentum: a review of 27 cases. J Urol 1972;108:724.

3 Symmonds RE, Lee RA. Abdominal hysterectomy—simple. In: Nyhaus LM, Baker RJ, eds. Mastery of surgery. Boston: Little, Brown, 1985.

4 Friedberg V, Altwein JE, Petri E. Vaginaler oder abdominaler Verschluss von Blasen-Scheiden-Fisteln? In: Petri E, ed. Gynäkologische urologie. Stuttgart: Georg Thieme, 1983:73–85.

5 Käser O, Iklé FA, Hirsch HA. Atlas der gynäkologischen Operationen. Stuttgart: Georg Thieme, 1983.

6 Ingelman-Sundberg A. Surgical treatment of urinary fistulae. Zentralbl Gynakol 1978;100:1281.

7 Lawson J. Vaginal fistulas. Int J Gynecol Obstet 1993;40:13–17.

8 Lawson J. The management of genito-urinary fistulae. Clin Obstet Gynecol 1978;5:221.

9 Symmonds RE. Incontinence: vesical and urethral fistulas. Clin Obstet Gynecol 1984;27:499.

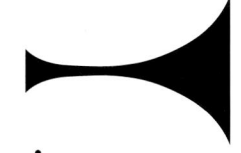

Chapter 27

The Latzko technique for repairing vesicovaginal fistulas

John F. Bresette and James A. Patterson

The sources of vesicovaginal fistulas are multiple. Before cesarean section became prevalent, obstetric trauma was the leading cause of fistulas. Now it is second, with gynecologic surgery at the head of the list. Fistulas that occur following urologic procedures, pelvic trauma, pelvic malignant disease, and pelvic irradiation are rare and seldom seen by the general gynecologist.

Making the diagnosis

The usual history of painless and continuous vaginal leakage of urine after hysterectomy is strongly suggestive. Table 27-1 lists the standard diagnostic procedures. On occasion, severe stress incontinence or bladder instability can mimic a fistula. The tampon test often will confirm the diagnosis of urine loss from stress incontinence in the patient who has anatomic descent of the bladder neck. In this test, one inspects a tampon after filling the bladder with methylene blue solution and having the patient cough and exercise. If there is stress incontinence, the intravaginal portion of the tampon will be clean, while the portion near the introitus will be stained blue. If the vaginal portion of the tampon is blue, probably there is a vesicovaginal fistula. Cystometric studies will rule out unstable bladder.

Fistulas usually are easily identified. Filling the bladder with sterile milk or methylene blue solution makes it possible to see the site or sites of vaginal leakage (Fig. 27-1). Minute fistulas can be discovered by filling the bladder with carbon dioxide and the vagina with water, and identifying the vaginal opening and the source of the rising bubbles. An intravenous pyelogram is essential to exclude concomitant ureteral injury or ureterovaginal fistula, and the ectopic ureter that starts to leak because of pelvic changes consequent to a previous hysterectomy.

When bladder testing is negative, carefully inspect the vagina after intravenous methylene blue administration. Very small fistulas may be evident only on colposcopy,

Table 27-1 Diagnostic procedures

To make the diagnosis:

Cystography. R/O reflux.

Cystoscopy. With patient in knee-chest position, determine site and number of fistulas and condition of tissues.

Dye or milk test. Fill bladder with methylene blue solution or milk; inspect vagina for sites of leakage.

Flat tire test. Fill vagina with water and bladder with carbon dioxide; watch for rising bubbles.

Tampon test. Fill bladder with methylene blue solution; inspect tampon. If there is a fistula, the intravaginal portion will stain blue.

To exclude ureterovaginal fistula:

Intravenous pyelogram; retrograde pyelogram; tampon test with intravenous methylene blue

R/O, rule out.

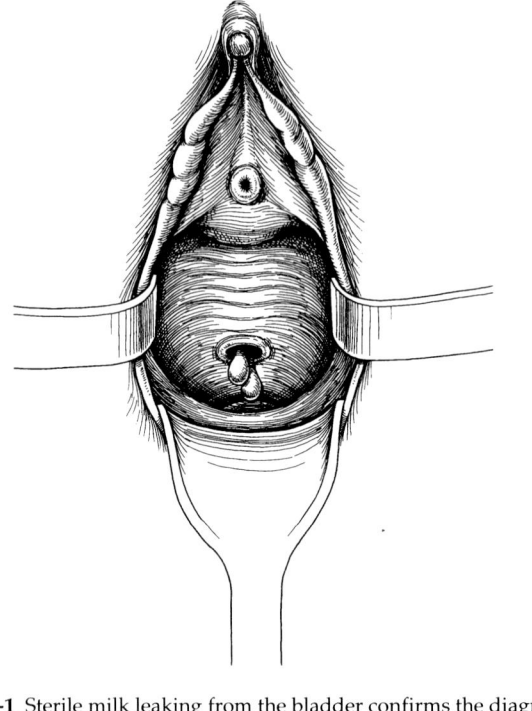

Fig. 27-1 Sterile milk leaking from the bladder confirms the diagnosis of vesicovaginal fistula and marks the site.

even after the injection. Retrograde pyelography is occasionally necessary; a cystogram may help document the fistula and exclude a ureterovaginal fistula in a refluxing ureter. In irradiated patients, the cystogram may reveal a small, contracted bladder. A more extensive repair will then be necessary, including enterocystoplasty with an intestinal patch. Cystoscopy is essential to determine the site and number of fistulas, and to assess the health of the tissue around the fistula opening.

Timing repair

Most experts recommend delaying surgery 4 to 6 months after discovery, to allow maturation of the fistula tract (Table 27-2). However, delay is a hardship for the patient, who usually is continually wet and often infected. In such

Table 27-2 Survey of repair results

Studies	No. of cases	Average delay	Recommended timing	Success rate
Bresette JF	15	1 month	Immediate	15/15 (100%)
O'Connor VJ Jr (4)	42	3 months	3 months	37/42 (88%)
Persky L, Herman G, Guerrier K (2)	7	1–10 weeks	On referral	7/7 (100%)
Tancer ML (3)	43	8–16 weeks	8–16 weeks	40/43 (93%)
Wein AJ, Malloy TR, Carpinello VL, et al. (5)	34	10–12 weeks	10 weeks	30/34 (88%)

cases, the clinician will find it difficult to fit appropriate drainage devices, and the patient will become more and more frustrated. A lawsuit is often the result.

Collins and Prent reported 16 cases of operations within 4 weeks for discovering the fistula (1). Several more recent articles in the literature indicate renewed enthusiasm for early repairs (2,3). We believe repair is advisable as soon as the bladder and vaginal site are nonfriable and free of edema, as determined by endoscopy and actual testing of the vaginal tissue by teasing with the Allis clamp.

Repair technique

We prefer to approach all uncomplicated vesicovaginal fistulas by the vaginal route. Our choice of procedure is the Latzko technique, which avoids excision of the tract and allows early repair.

Preoperative preparation consists of catheter drainage equivalent, specific antibiotic therapy, and estrogen vaginal cream (Table 27-3). We reassess the bladder and vagina for resolution of edema and inflammation and, if the tissue appears healthy, proceed to operate.

Regional anesthesia is satisfactory for vaginal repair. With the patient in the lithotomy position, place traction sutures through the labia to maintain an open vagina. Use a paravaginal displacement incision (Schuchardt's) if the vagina is small or contracted. Of paramount importance is complete denudation of the vagina mucosa around the fistula. To facilitate the dissection and limit bleeding, inject dilute epinephrine for 3 cm in all directions around the fistula (Fig. 27-2A). Do not excise the fistulous tract, but strip its surrounding vaginal mucosa by sharp dissection to prepare a vaginal–bladder bed to invert over the fistula (Fig. 27-2B). A small Foley catheter inserted into the fistula tract allows one to pull the operative field upward for ease of dissection.

Remove the catheter and invert the fistula using 3-0 polyglycolic sutures (Figs. 27-2C and 27-2D). Suture the denuded surfaces of the anterior and posterior vaginal walls from above downward, being extremely careful not to enter the bladder or the fistula tract. Extend the suture lines beyond each lateral end of the tract. Invert two vaginal–bladder fascial layers. Finish the closure by approximating the remaining vaginal mucosa (Figs. 27-2E and 27-2F).

Table 27-3 Preoperative steps

Institute urethral catheter drainage, 10 days to 2 weeks before the procedure.

Give appropriate antibiotics for documented infection.

Apply estrogen vaginal cream.

Reassess by vaginal examination and cystoscopy.

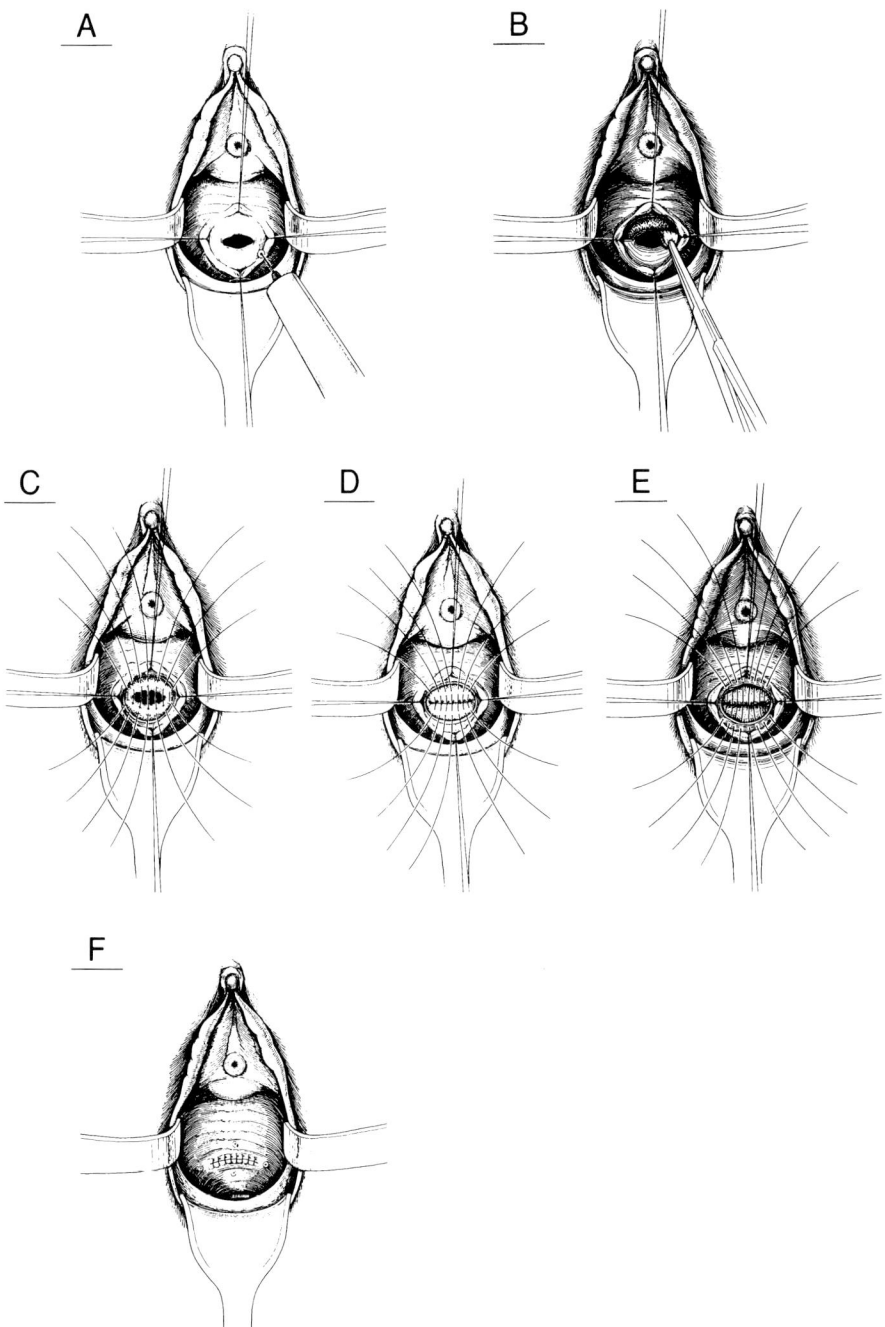

Fig. 27-2 Essentials of repair technique. Begin repair by placing traction sutures around the fistula site, after injecting normal saline (A). Next, dissect the surrounding vaginal mucosa (B). Invert the submucosa and close with interrupted sutures (C), and then repeat the inversion step (D). Finally, close the vaginal mucosa (E, F) to complete the procedure. (Reproduced by permission from Ostergard DR. Gynecologic urology and urodynamics: theory and practice. Baltimore: Williams & Wilkins, 1980.)

In irradiated patients, obtain a Martius bulbocavernosus patch from under the labia majora and transpose it over the first two inverted layers, then cover it with vaginal mucosa. After placing the first row of sutures, fill the bladder with sterile milk and reinforce any leaking area. It is important that a Foley catheter drain the bladder continuously throughout the procedure; otherwise, the bladder will distend and thin out, making it difficult to invert the fistula tract. At the conclusion of the procedure, insert a suprapubic tube and leave it in place for 7 days. Obtain cultures before removing the catheter and prescribe appropriate antibiotics. Caution the patient against having intercourse or douching for 2 months.

When the problem is complex

Contraindications to early fistula repair are listed in Table 27-4. For complicated fistulas, a longer delay may be indicated before operating. A variety of procedures have been used for these cases. We favor a transabdominal approach with complete mobilization of the vagina and bladder, excision of the fistula tract, and interposition of a flap of viable omentum between the vaginal and bladder closures. Patients with contracted bladders or with very large fistulas may require bladder patching or augmentation with sigmoid colon, cecum, or ileum. For patients who have had several repair failures, especially after high-dose radiotherapy, a staged reconstruction is advisable. The first stage consists of supravesicle diversion, using a sigmoid or ileal conduit with transabdominal fistula repair. If the fistula heals, then the urinary tract is reconstructed, and the conduit is implanted into the bladder dome.

Table 27-4 Reasons to avoid transvaginal repair

Excessive vaginal scarring

Fistulas associated with high-dose radiation (relative)

Inaccessible location

Involvement of other organs (ureter, bowel, uterus)

Multiple previous repairs (relative)

Small contracted bladder

Suspicion of recurrent cancer

Very large fistula (relative)

References

1 Collins CG, Prent D. Results of early repair of vesicovaginal fistula with preliminary cortisone treatment. Am J Obstet Gynecol 1960;80:1005.
2 Persky L, Herman G, Guerrier K. Nondelay in vesicovaginal fistula repair. Urology 1979;13:273.
3 Tancer ML. The post-total hysterectomy (vault) vesicovaginal fistula. J Urol 1980;123:839.
4 O'Connor VJ Jr. Review and experience with vesicovaginal fistula repair. J Urol 1980;123:367.
5 Wein AJ, Malloy TR, Carpinello VL, et al. Repair of vesicovaginal fistula by a suprapubic transvesical approach. Surg Gynecol Obstet 1980;150:57.

Chapter 28

Correcting urethral diverticula

Jack R. Robertson

Successful gynecologic surgery for urethral diverticula depends primarily on accurate diagnosis and secondarily on endoscopy during operation. Incidence between 1.85% and 4.7% has been reported in the literature (1,2). Urethral diverticula may be one of the most overlooked diagnoses in urology. This condition is found in direct proportion to the avidity which it is sought (3). Blind resection of diverticula through the anterior vaginal wall accounts for the 17% complication rate and unsatisfactory cure rate associated with the procedure of enucleation, supposedly long since mastered (4).

Urethroscopy

Diverticula vary in size from a few millimeters to 8 cm in diameter, and their ostia from 1 mm to more than 1 cm in diameter. Most ostia are located in the urethra's middle third, on the posterior wall between the 5 o'clock and the 7 o'clock positions.

The diagnosis is made by voiding cystography, urethrography with a Davis or Tratner catheter, ultrasound, or urethroscopy. I prefer urethroscopy because of its simplicity and accuracy.

For urethroscopy, insufflate the bladder with 150 ml of carbon dioxide. With two fingers in the vagina, occlude the vesical neck by compressing it against the symphysis pubis. This will trap gas in the urethra (Fig. 28-1).

Then massage the anterior vaginal wall, as in prostatic massage. Pus or urine will exude from the ostium. Occasionally, stones are present. Rarely, malignancy is seen.

Determine the peak closure pressure site by slowly withdrawing the endoscope through the urethra (Fig. 28-2). If the ostium is proximal to this site, it will be visible.

In such cases, to avoid making the patient incontinent, dissect the diverticulum, using conventional enucleation, and close the urethra in layers.

If the ostium is distal to the peak pressure site, gas will be heard escaping from the meatus. For these cases, marsupialize the diverticulum, using the Spence procedure.

Dissection techniques

In 1935, Furniss incised the diverticulum transvaginally, packed the sac with gauze, and in a second stage excised the resultant urethrovaginal fistula and the granulated sac (5). In 1938, both Young (6) and Hunner (7) passed a sound through the urethra to stabilize it and excised the diverticulum transvaginally. Hunner was also first to create a vaginal flap to cover the incision line and avoid superimposed suture lines.

Other early transvaginal excision techniques are those of Hyams and Hyams, who first packed the diverticulum transurethrally with gauze (8), and of Cook and Pool, who passed a ureteral catheter into the diverticulum transurethrally, so that it coiled up to aid excision (9). In 1952,

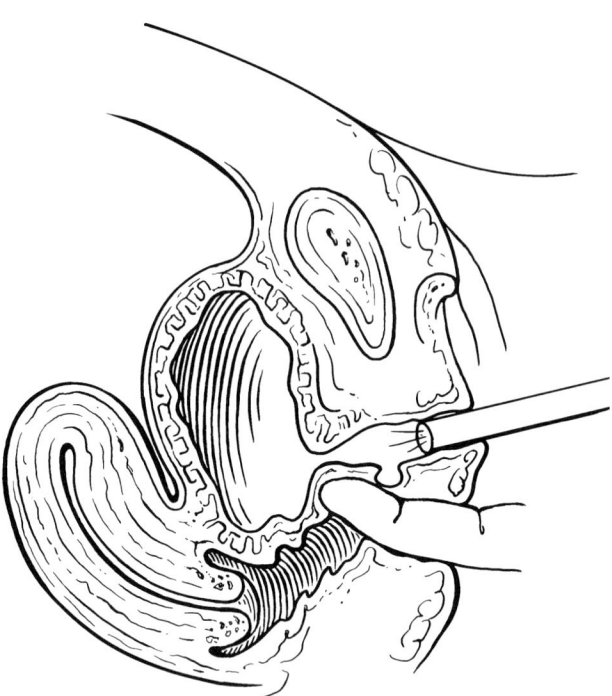

Fig. 28-1 Urethroscopic diagnosis. Occlude the vesical neck by placing fingers in the vagina to distend urethral diverticula.

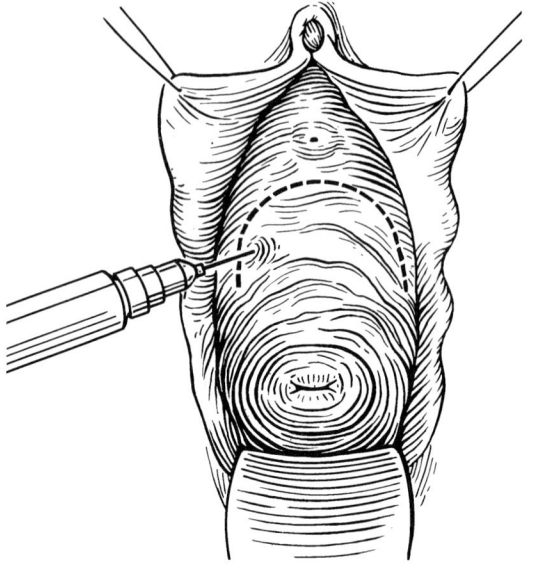

Fig. 28-3 Infiltrate the vaginal mucosa with normal saline for hemostasis and make a half-moon incision.

Moore exposed the diverticulum transvaginally, incised it, and inserted into the sac a Foley catheter with the tip removed (10). Inflating the balloon and purse-string suturing the opening allowed traction during resection.

In 1955, Edwards and Beebe incised the urethral and vaginal wall to include the diverticulum and repaired the incision with a urethroplasty (11). Ellik, in 1957, incised the sac transvaginally near the bladder neck, packed it with oxidized cellulose, and oversewed the incision (12). The surrounding tissues healed by fibrosis.

More recently, Hirschhorn injected liquid dimethicone into the diverticulum before excising it (13), and O'Connor and Kropp filled it with a firm fibrin clot formed from human fibrinogen (14).

In contrast with these various excision methods, Spence and Duckett, using a technique analogous to marsupialization of a Bartholin's cyst, marsupialized the diverticulum and the distal urethra to the external meatus. They lockstitched the edges to the vaginal mucosa, creating a generous meatotomy (15). Lichtman and Robertson were the first to report using this technique in the literature (4). They confirmed the low complication of Spence and Duckett.

A long-term follow-up study of the Spence procedure, with a mean of 5 years, reported that 53 patients considered the operation successful (16). Four patients had complications, three had minimal incontinence, and one had recurrent urinary tract infection. The researchers concluded that the Spence marsupialization procedure has a high success

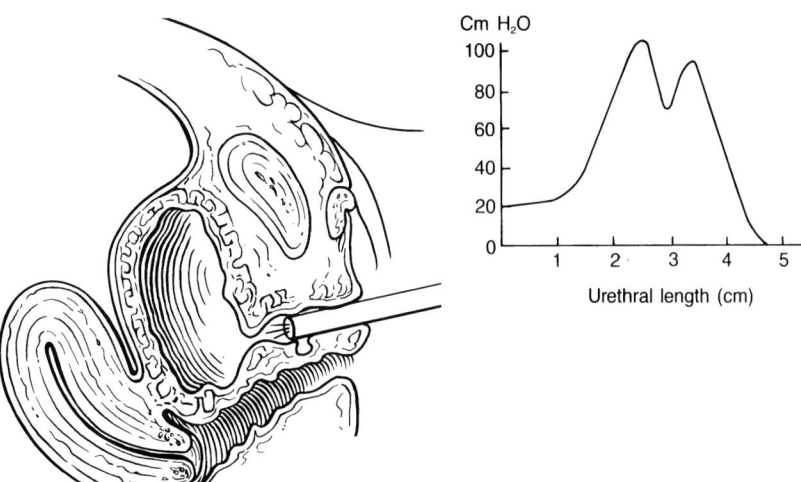

Fig. 28-2 Slowly retract the endoscope with the gas flowing. If the dip in pressure is distal to the peak pressure, marsupialize the diverticulum.

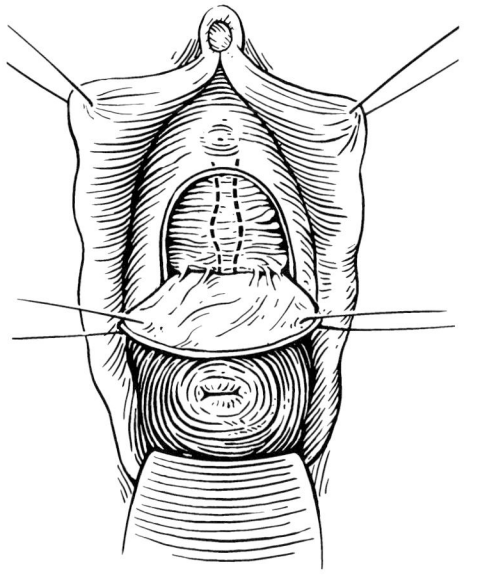

Fig. 28-4 Reflect the vaginal flap inferiorly to expose the diverticular sac.

rate and low morbidity, making it applicable for the treatment of most cases of urethral diverticula in women.

Standard vaginal enucleation

The fusion of the urethra to the anterior vaginal wall, associated infection, and the tendency of the diverticulum to surround the urethra make the dissection difficult. Cleavage planes do not exist, and a tedious, time-consuming operation is required.

In a large series of 108 patients, incontinence was observed in 2 patients immediately after surgery (17). However, incontinence was noted in 14 patients, for an overall incontinence rate of 15%. Also, there was a 9% recurrence rate of the diverticulum.

For conventional removal, as currently practiced, first inject normal saline submucosally to identify tissue planes and promote hemostasis. Then make a half-moon incision in the anterior vaginal wall 1 to 2 cm below the urethral meatus (Fig. 28-3). Develop the vaginal flap over the diver-

ticulum and reflect it inferiorly (Fig. 28-4). Follow with a transverse incision in the periurethral fascia and reflect the tissue superiorly and inferiorly down to the diverticulum.

Insert the urethroscope through the urethra to determine the size of the ostium, the condition of intraurethral tissues, and the presence or absence of other diverticula. Next, open the diverticulum and thoroughly inspect its interior with the endoscope.

If there is any periddiverticulitis, do a partial ablation rather than separate the friable mucosa of the diverticulum from the vaginal mucosa and fascia. Otherwise, if the ostium is small and not fixed, use sharp dissection to separate the sac from the vagina and urethral floor. Take care not to remove mucosa from the urethral floor.

Close the urethral defect with interrupted sutures of No. 3-0 chromic catgut, inverting the edges, and bury this row with another row of mattress sutures by approximating the periurethral fascia. Trim the vaginal flap and close it with interrupted catgut sutures. Following the procedure, fill the bladder with 300 ml of saline and insert a suprapubic catheter. Suprapubic drainage avoids both injuring the suture line with an indwelling urethral catheter and complications resulting from intermittent catheterization.

Partial ablation

Indications for this procedure, devised by Tancer and associated, are periddiverticulitis and a lesion in the proximal urethra (18). First, dissect the vaginal mucosa free, leaving the diverticulum intact (Fig. 28-5A). Enter the sac longitudinally, identify the urethral opening, and excise that portion of the sac that is easily accessible (Fig. 28-5B). Try not to enucleate the sac at its neck, and close the opening side to side with No. 3-0 chromic catgut (Fig. 28-5C). Then place a second layer of sutures, imbricating the previous urethral defect. Close the remainder of the diverticular wall in double-breasted fashion and close postoperative suprapubic bladder drainage exactly as for conventional enucleation.

The average hospital stay is 6 days. Tancer and associates reported no urinary incontinence, fistula formation, or recurrence (18).

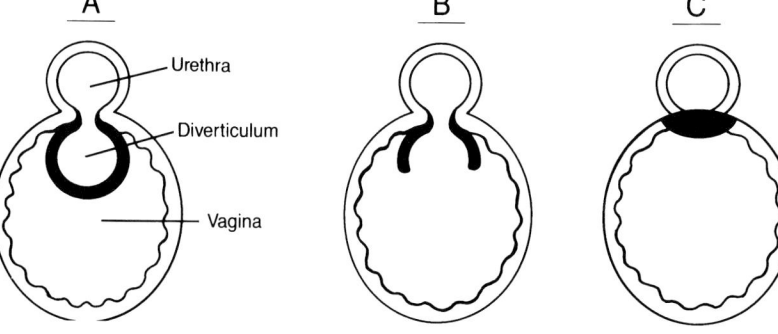

Fig. 28-5 If the ostium is small and the periurethral tissue is not inflamed, do a standard enucleation (A), but if periddiverticular and urethral inflammation is present, do a partial ablation (B). Close the urethral opening without compromising the urethral floor (C).

Marsupialization

Locate the urethral diverticulum with the endoscope and place a Kelly clamp on the anterior vaginal wall opposite the diverticular orifice (Fig. 28-6). Placing one blade of a sharp pair of scissors in the urethra and the other blade in the vagina, cut through and divide the floor of the urethra (Fig. 28-7). Grasp the divided structures with an Allis clamp and, to secure hemostasis, place a running-locking stitch of No. 3-0 chromic suture from the apex of the incision to the external meatus (Fig. 28-8). The procedure takes from 20 to

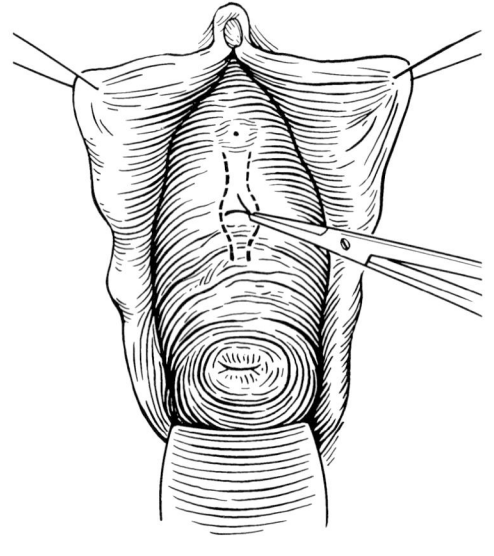

Fig. 28-6 Locate the diverticular ostium with the endoscope and place a Kelly clamp on the vaginal side.

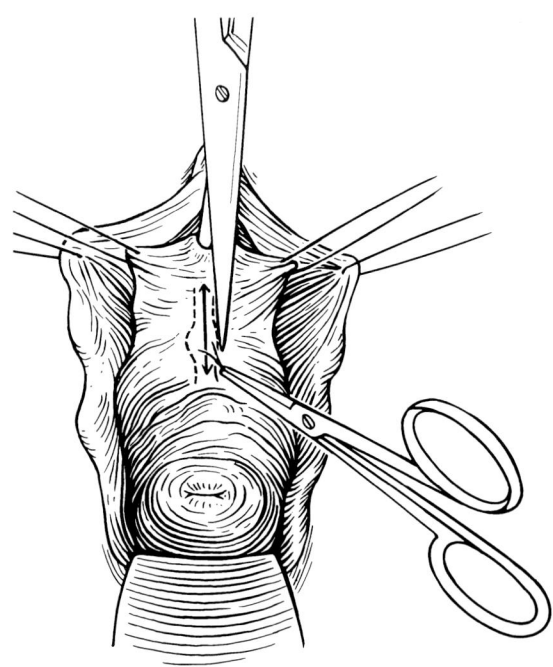

Fig. 28-7 Use a sharp pair of scissors to divide the urethral floor to the ostium.

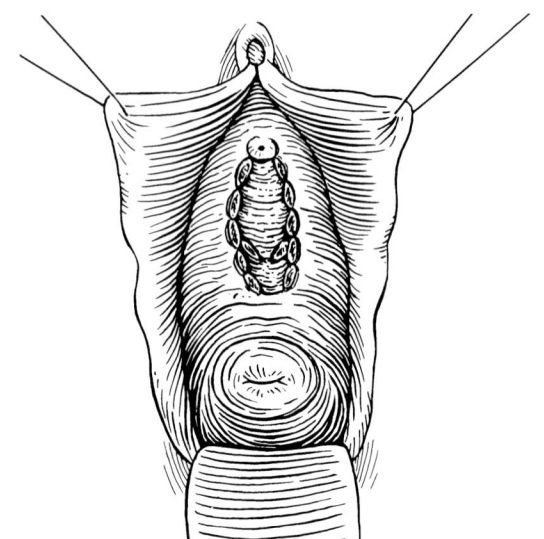

Fig. 28-8 Using a running-locking stitch of No. 3-0 chromic suture from the incision's apex to the external meatus, create a generous meatotomy.

30 minutes. Do not place a vaginal pack or insert a catheter. The patient can be discharged within 24 hours.

Strictures may result from removing too much of the urethral mucosal floor. Another common problem is urethral fistula, which occurs in about 5% of patients.

Greater use of endoscopy in the future should reduce complications. Meanwhile, treatment of stricture is by gradual urethral dilation postoperatively. Fistulas may be prevented by antibiotic infection control. A fistula located distal to the continence zone is an indication for a corrective Spence procedure.

Summary

My observation of more than 100 cases of urethral diverticula is that the most common surgical procedure used was marsupialization, for which the complication rate was only 4%. Most complications involved minimal postoperative bleeding that responded to a vaginal pack. Only one patient required suturing for hemostasis, and there were no urethral fistulas.

Patients did not spray during voiding, have dyspareunia, or get recurrent urinary tract infections. Two patients were incontinent postoperatively but regained continence after using estrogen vaginal cream.

References

1 Davis BL, Robinson DG. Diverticula of the female urethra: assay of 120 cases. J Urol 1970;104:850.
2 Adams WE. Urethrography. Bull Tulane Med Fac 1964;23:107.
3 Hanno PH, Wein AJ. Female urethral diverticula. Am Urol Assoc Update Series 1968;5:Lesson 3.

4 Lichtman AS, Robertson JR. Suburethral diverticula treated by marsupialization. Obstet Gynecol 1976;47:203.

5 Furniss HD. Suburethral abscesses and diverticula in female urethra. J Urol 1935;33:498.

6 Young HH. Treatment of urethral diverticulum. South Med J 1938;31:1043.

7 Hunner GL. Calculus formation in a urethral diverticulum in women. Report of three cases. Urol Cutan Rev 1938;42:336.

8 Hyams JA, Hyams MN. New operative procedures for treatment of diverticulum of female urethra. Urol Cutan Rev 1939;43:573.

9 Cook EN, Pool TL. Urethral diverticulum in the female. J Urol 1949;62:495.

10 Moore TD. Diverticulum of female urethra: an improved technique of surgical excision. J Urol 1952;68:611.

11 Edwards EA, Beebe EA. Diverticula of the female urethra. Obstet Gynecol 1955;5:729.

12 Ellik M. Diverticulum of the female urethra: a new method of ablation. J Urol 1957;77:234.

13 Hirschhorn RC. A new surgical technique for removal of urethral diverticula in the female patient. Urology 1964;92:206.

14 O'Connor VJ Jr, Kropp KA. Surgery of the female urethra. In: Glenn JF, Boyce WH, eds. Urologic surgery. New York: Harper & Row, 1969.

15 Spence HM, Duckett JW. Diverticulum of the female urethra: clinical aspects and presentation of a simple operative technique for cure. J Urol 1970;104:432.

16 Roehrborn CG. Long term follow-up study of the marsupialization technique for urethral diverticula in women. Surg Gynecol Obstet 1988;167:191.

17 Lee RA. Diverticulum of the urethra. Clin Obstet Gynecol 1984;27:490.

18 Tancer ML, Mooppan MMU, Pierre-Louis C, et al. Suburethral diverticulum: treatment by partial ablation. Obstet Gynecol 1983;62:511.

Part 4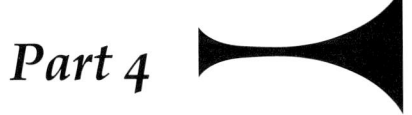

Infertility Surgery

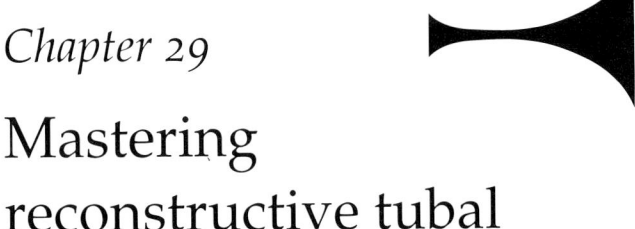

Chapter 29

Mastering reconstructive tubal microsurgery

Victor Gomel and Timothy C. Rowe

The use of microsurgery to repair or reconstruct the fallopian tube has been a major part of infertility therapy over the past two decades. Since the first use of magnification for salpingostomy more than a quarter century ago, the techniques of microsurgery have been developed and refined for use in other reconstructive procedures.

The development of in vitro fertilization and embryo transfer (IVF-ET) offered another treatment option for the management of tuboperitoneal disease causing infertility. Despite 15 years of continuing development, pregnancy rates after IVF-ET continue to average 15% to 20% per treatment cycle (1,2).

The lifetime pregnancy rates after most microsurgical procedures are higher than this. In addition, microsurgical management allows control of conception to be returned to the couple, in contrast to the dependence on technology in IVF-ET. Clearly, microsurgery will continue to be a major form of management for infertile couples for the foreseeable future.

The choice between IVF and microsurgery will be influenced by both nontechnical and purely technical considerations (3). The nontechnical considerations include the respective costs of surgery and IVF, the age of the woman, and the couple's perceptions of the various procedures. The costs of treatment may be considerable, and the extent of health insurance coverage may vary significantly. The age of the woman is important, given that fertility begins to decline at about age 31. The perceptions that the couple have regarding gamete manipulation will be a product of their own values, ethical views, and other influences. Some women will wish to avoid surgery if at all possible.

The technical considerations in choosing between IVF and microsurgery will depend, at first, on whether or not microsurgical treatment is even possible. For example, only IVF is possible when both tubes have been removed, are damaged severely, or are involved in tuberculous salpingitis. If both IVF and microsurgery are possible, the choice between them should be based on the probability of pregnancy expressed in a standardized fashion. The results of microsurgical treatment usually are expressed as crude pregnancy rates (percentage of patients pregnant after one, two, or three years) or as a cumulative probability of pregnancy at a fixed point (usually two years after surgery) following life table analysis. The results of IVF-ET are usually expressed as the pregnancy or live-birth rate after embryo transfer in a single treatment cycle. The difference between the two treatments in the measurement of outcome must be understood (3).

Determine the cause of infertility

Even when tubal or peritoneal defects are suspected, always investigate all possible causes. Start with a semen analysis and ovulation testing. When necessary, evaluate sperm-mucus interaction and other hormonal and im-munologic factors.

To assess tubal patency, first perform hysterosalpin-gography (HSG) to check the uterine cavity and intratubal architecture. We use an aqueous contrast medium (Hy-paque-M60%, Winthrop). Water-soluble medium is better tolerated by the patient. It disperses easily and coats ep-ithelial surfaces. Thus it provides excellent radiologic de-tail of intratubal architecture and disease.

When tubal occlusion is terminal, the presence of longitudinal rugal markings is a good prognostic sign. Con-versely, intratubal adhesions usually indicate an unfavor-able prognosis. By using HSG, one can also assess length, internal patency, and architecture of proximal segments in women who either have midtubal obstruction or seek re-versal of sterilization (4).

If there is evidence of proximal tubal occlusion, HSG permits assessment of the intramural tubal segment. How-ever, a tube may be patent even if dye does not pass at HSG, the apparent obstruction being due to cornual spasm, the presence of a mucus plug, synechiae in the cornu obstruct-ing entry of dye, or simply poor technique. The use of tubal cannulation (using radiologic, hysteroscopic, or ultrasound guidance) will usually allow determination of whether or not the obstruction is real. Some cases of true proximal tubal obstruction may also be overcome by cannulation, al-though this has yet to be proved. In fact, the value of tubal cannulation in the treatment of tubal factor infertility has yet to be proved in a randomized study, but because it is a relatively innocuous procedure, it is reasonable to attempt cannulation in women when HSG suggests proximal occlusion (5).

Laparoscopy should complement HSG. We recommend laparoscopy be done second. It is important to know the status of the fallopian tubes and their patency at the time of laparoscopy; this information is most valuable should laparoscopic surgery appear feasible. Because initial HSG may be therapeutic, delay laparoscopy for a few months when HSG shows patent oviducts. By using laparoscopy, one can assess the nature and extent of pelvic and peri-adnexal adhesions. Moreover, laparoscopic surgery fre-quently makes laparotomy unnecessary, and it has become our primary approach in peritubal and distal tubal disease (4,6–8).

If HSG reveals uterine synechiae, submucous fibroids, or polyps, perform hysteroscopy at the same time as lap-aroscopy. If HSG has shown cornual occlusion and cannu-lation is not performed using imaging (x-ray or ultrasound), then hysteroscopy and tubal cannulation can be performed at the same time.

Be mindful of basic principles

Microsurgery's success depends on gentle tissue handling, meticulous hemostasis, careful dissection with delicate in-struments and fine sutures, and accurate approximation of tissues (9). Equally important is keeping foreign material out of the peritoneal cavity.

Peritoneal trauma, whether mechanical, thermal, chem-ical, or bacterial, induces an inflammatory reaction that can lead to adhesions. The exudate resulting from inflam-mation contains fibrinogen, which is converted into fibrin. Adhesions form when fibroblasts proliferate over the fib-rin matrix.

Handle tissues gently, elevating, retracting, or grasping them with rounded polytetrafluoroethylene (Teflon) rods or the gloved fingers. To prevent desiccation, always keep exposed peritoneal surfaces moistened with an irrigating solution. Adding heparin to the solution (5000 U/L lactated Ringer's solution) minimizes both clot formation during surgery and collection of fibrin in the peritoneal cavity.

Reperitonealize denuded serosal surfaces *without tension* and using always fine inert suture material. To reestablish function properly be sure to excise diseased tissues totally and approximate tissue planes accurately.

Magnification enhances one's ability to prevent tissue trauma and recognize pathologic changes and serosal disturbances. It also allows precise hemostasis with pin-point electrocoagulation, to minimize destruction of adja-cent tissue (10).

Instruments needed

The basic microsurgery kit requires a microneedle driver, plain and toothed platform microforceps, and microscis-sors. The needle driver and forceps should have rounded rather than pointed tips, and the needle driver should have a concave-convex jaw configuration to provide a firm grip on the needle. Use iris scissors for tubal transection and Teflon-coated rods with rounded tips to retract tissues and elevate adhesions. An irrigator with a sliding sleeve (Gomel Irrigator, Martin, Germany) allows fingertip control of irri-gation to prevent desiccation of tissue and permit identifi-cation of individual bleeders (10).

We recommend using an insulated microelectrode with a 100-μm-diameter shaft and conical tip to divide adhesions and coagulate bleeders. One may also coagulate with a bipo-lar microforceps that resembles a jeweller's instrument.

Some clinicians routinely use a carbon dioxide laser for dividing adhesions and tubal transection. However, no cur-rent data suggest that this laser is functionally superior to using electromicrosurgery (11–13).

We prefer to use an electrosurgical unit (Valleylab, Boul-der, Col.) that works with a microelectrode such as the one described above. This unit delivers a steady current at the low levels that are required for use with a microelectrode. The handle's rocker switch permits fingertip control for cut-ting and coagulation.

The suturing combination that we find best is No. 8-0 ab-sorbable polyglactin 910 (Vicryl) on a tapercut needle 130 μm in diameter and 4 or 5 mm long (Ethicon, Somerville, NJ). Using a fine needle is important to avoid the trauma associated with an inappropriately large needle, which would negate the benefits of using fine sutures (9,10,14).

Magnification methods

An operating microscope allows high magnification, clear vision with coaxial illumination, and a constant visual field. To leave adequate working distance between lens and pelvic organs, use an objective with a focal length of 275 or 300 mm. Hand or foot controls alter magnification, focus, and direction of the microscope. It is important to reserve magnifying loupes for dividing adhesions at their distal extremities on the pelvic sidewall and cul-de-sac, excising endometriotic lesions located deep in the pelvis, and making subsequent repairs.

Setting up

Before inducing anesthesia, be sure all necessary instruments are available and in working order. Check the microscope and adjust it for surgery. Make sure that any ancillary equipment, such as the television camera and monitor—if used—and the electrosurgical unit, are working properly. After anesthetizing the patient, insert a Foley catheter into the bladder.

For intraoperative chromopertubation, also place a pediatric Foley catheter into the uterine cavity. Connect one end of a sterile extension tube to this catheter and the other end to a syringe filled with dilute dye solution. This maneuver makes it possible to bring the syringe into the sterile field. Place a pack in the vagina to elevate and antevert the uterus. Finally, to minimize introduction of starch and foreign bodies into the peritoneal cavity, all personnel scrubbed for the case should first wash their gloves thoroughly (9,10).

Operative preliminaries

Subcutaneous tissues are infiltrated with 0.25% bupivacaine (Marcaine) before the initial incision is made. We have for some years favored a suprapubic incision that is short (minilaparotomy) and transverse or midline (if there already is a scar). The fascia is incised vertically in the midline after stripping the subcutaneous fat from it. The recti muscles are separated in the midline, and the peritoneum is incised vertically (5). Good hemostasis of the abdominal incision is important to prevent blood dripping into the peritoneal cavity.

Before entering the cavity, rinse gloves again. Once it is entered and the abdominal organs are examined, insert a wound protector and apply a Dennis-Brown retractor. Displace the bowel into the upper peritoneal cavity, and keep it in place with a Kerlex pad soaked in irrigation solution. Keep manipulation of bowel to a minimum.

The table should be placed in a 10- to 15-degree Trendelenburg position and tilted toward the surgeon. Elevate the uterus and adnexa by packing the pouch of Douglas loosely with soaked fluffy gauze (Kerlex) pads.

Next, bring the microscope over the operative field. We do not drape the microscope but have it cleaned before surgery and place sterile neoprene caps on the controls. In thousands of such procedures performed by several surgeons in Vancouver since 1968, no postoperative morbidity has been associated with this practice.

Salpingo-ovariolysis

Our primary approach to periadnexal disease when tubes are patent is laparoscopic salpingo-ovariolysis (6,8,15). However, if adhesions are present in a patient requiring a reconstructive tubal procedure, than lysis of these adhesions will be undertaken at laparotomy, if laparoscopic salpingo-ovariolysis has not already been performed during the preliminary laparoscopy.

Periadnexal adhesions commonly encapsulate parts or all of the tube and ovary and extend to the lateral pelvic wall, the posterior aspect of the broad ligaments, and uterus. Begin salpingo-ovariolysis by exposing the adhesions at their distal margins with Teflon rods. Then divide them electrosurgically over a Teflon rod using a microelectrode, one layer at a time, without damaging adjacent pelvic peritoneum. Attaching an elongating adaptor to the electrosurgical unit's handle facilitates division deep in the pelvis (9,10,14,15).

Divide with the unit set in the blend mode, which adds coagulating current to the cutting current to accomplish hemostasis. When necessary for additional hemostasis, use pure coagulating current on individual bleeders. Magnification with loupes and proper illumination enhance accuracy.

After freeing adhesions from their distal attachments, elevate the adnexa by packing the pouch of Douglas loosely with Kerlex pads soaked in irrigating solution. Then bring the microscope over the operating field. Excise the adhesions by dividing them— as already described—at the level of the tubal serosa or ovarian surface, taking care not to damage these tissues (9,10,14,15).

Salpingostomy

Our primary approach to surgical treatment of distal tubal obstruction is by laparoscopy. The results of laparoscopic treatment approximate those achieved by means of a microsurgical approach. This indicates that the outcome of surgical treatment depends largely on the extent of tubal damage rather than on the surgical method used (3,5,10).

It is now uncommon to perform a primary microsurgical salpingostomy (16), but it may be indicated in selected cases and as a unilateral procedure combined with another operation on the contralateral tube.

When a tube's fimbrial end is totally occluded, forming a hydrosalpinx or sactosalpinx, salpingostomy or salpingoneostomy creates a new ostium. Depending on anatomic location, the procedure may be terminal or ampullary. Terminal salpingostomy is preferable, because it conserves the entire tube and maintains the tubo-ovarian relationship.

Adhesions within the distal tube may make it necessary to excise this portion of the oviduct and perform ampullary salpingostomy. Reversal of previous fimbriectomy (Kroener sterilization) may also require ampullary salpingostomy. We do not perform isthmic salpingostomy, as the chance of successful outcome is extremely low (3,5,10).

Before beginning terminal salpingostomy, examine the tube, ovary, and tubo-ovarian ligament. It is essential that the tube—especially the fimbrial end—be free. If it is ad-

hering to the ovary or another structure, free it, using sharp or blunt dissection or electrosurgery.

Once normal anatomic relations are restored, distend the tube by transcervical chromopertubation and examine its occluded terminal end through the microscope. Usually one will see relatively avascular lines extending radially from a central point (Fig. 29-1A).

Enter at this point, using the microelectrode and blended current, and continue the incision toward the ovary over an avascular line to create a new fimbria ovarica and maintain the tubo-ovarian relation (Fig. 29-1B). Make additional incisions along the tube's circumference over avascular areas by everting the mucosa and working from within the tube (Fig. 29-1C). This technique avoids cutting through the tube's vascular mucosal folds, which will be shaped as fimbriae, and minimizes bleeding.

Seal bleeding points individually with the microelectrode, using coagulating current. Once a satisfactory stoma

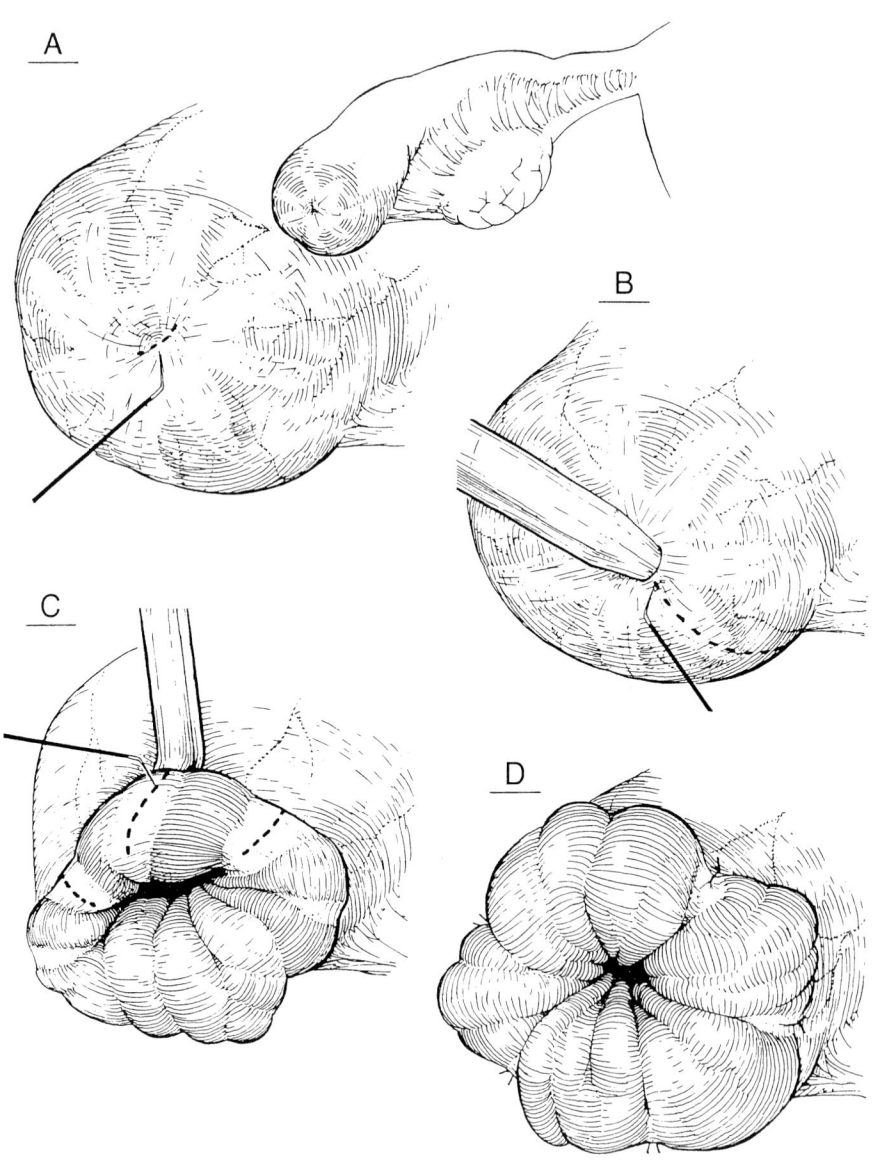

Fig. 29-1 Salpingostomy. (A) Locate the central dimple at the end of the occluded tube. (B) Enter this point with the microelectrode, and extend the incision toward the ovary over an avascular line. (C) Working from inside the tube, make additional incisions along the avascular areas of its circumference to create a stoma. (D) Evert and suture mucosal edges to secure the stoma.

is fashioned, evert the mucosal edges slightly, without tension, and secure them with interrupted No. 8-0 Vicryl sutures placed at the angles of the everted flaps (9,10,14,15,17,18) (Fig 29-1D).

Special circumstances making it necessary to modify this technique have been described elsewhere (10,17).

Terminal salpingostomy for hydrosalpinx offers an intrauterine pregnancy rate of approximately 30% (9,10, 14,15,17–20). Ampullary salpingostomy (other than for reversal of Kroener sterilization) is less likely to be followed by pregnancy. Other factors that affect the outcome include the presence or absence of vertical mucosal folds, thickness of the tubal wall, and the extent and nature of the pelvic adhesions. In view of the relatively modest success rate associated with salpingostomy and the option of in vitro fertilization, reconstructive surgery should now be used for those who appear to have a favorable prognosis (3).

Tubocornual anastomosis

Pathologic cornual occlusion (proximal tubal occlusion) caused by such conditions as infection, salpingitis isthmica nodosa, or endometriosis has been treated in the past by tubouterine implantation, but this operation is now considered obsolete. Instead, a microsurgical approach allows anastomosis after removing the affected tubal segment (9,10,14,15,21–23). However, before surgery is undertaken, it is reasonable to undertake tubal cannulation first. This will allow identification of women who have true cornual occlusion (3,5).

Before beginning tubocornual anastomosis, inject the uterine cornua superficially along a circle 1 cm proximal to the uterotubal junction with a dilute vasopressin solution (100 ml of normal saline with 10 U of vasopressin). This will minimize bleeding. Then incise the tube at the uterotubal junction, taking care not to divide the arteriovenous arcade at its mesosalpingeal margin. Assess patency of the tube's intramural portion by transcervical chromopertubation, and examine the cut surface under maximal magnification for abnormal changes.

Excise the intramural tube 1 or 2 mm at a time until patent normal oviduct is reached. Using the microelectrode, first dissect the portion of intramural tube to be excised from the surrounding uterine musculature (Fig. 29-2A). Then grasp it with a strong-toothed microforceps and transect it with the curved Gomel Cornual Blade (Spingler-Tritt, Jestetten, Germany) (Fig. 29-2B). This approach prevents the creation of a large defect in the cornu. Depending on the length of intramural tube that has been excised, the anastomosis site may be positioned juxtamural, intramural, or juxtauterine (Figs. 29-2C and D).

Normal tube will be free of fibrosis, exhibit normal muscular architecture, and possess intact mucosal folds showing a pristine vascular pattern (Fig. 29-2E). Excise the occluded and affected isthmic segment by making serial incisions with straight iris scissors, starting at the uterotubal

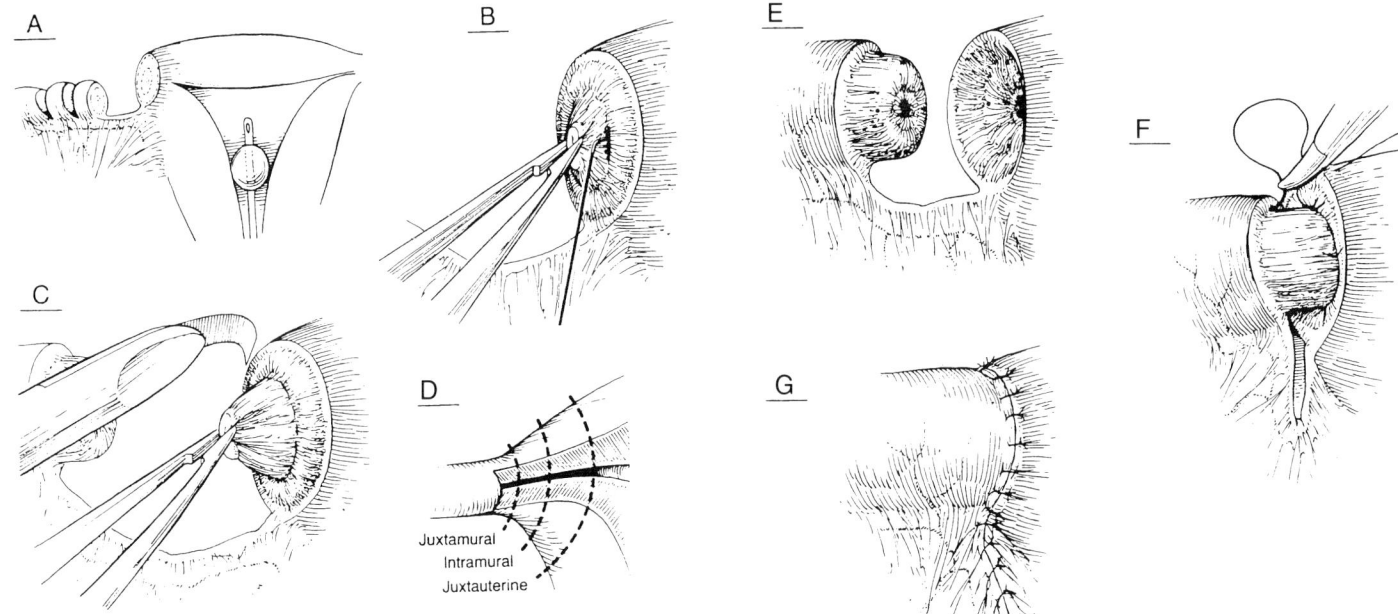

Fig. 29-2 Tubocornual anastomosis. To reach the patent normal intramural oviduct, dissect the portion to be excised from the surrounding uterine musculature (A), grasp the tube with a toothed forceps (B), and transect with a curved Gomel Cornual Blade (C). A tubocornual anastomosis may be juxtamural, intramural, or juxta- uterine, depending on how much intramural tube is removed (D). Patent oviduct is free of fibrosis and exhibits normal muscular architecture and intact mucosal folds (E). After excising the diseased portion, complete the anastomosis with suture knots tied on the outside (F, G).

junction and continuing until normal isthmus is reached. Remain close to the tube to spare tubal vessels. Confirm the distal segment's normalcy under high magnification and verify patency by injecting irrigation solution through the tube's fimbriated end (descending hydropertubation).

Avoid devitalizing the anastomosis site by overzealous electrocauterization. Achieve hemostasis by coagulating only significant bleeders, which are located under the serosa. Now effect end-to-end anastomosis between the apparently healthy intramural and isthmic segments. Approximate the muscularis and epithelium with interrupted No. 8-0 polyglactin 910 (Vicryl) sutures placed at cardinal points with knots external (Figs. 29-2F and G).

Except when doing juxtamural anastomosis, place all sutures before tying them. Otherwise, tying the first suture will make it difficult or impossible to place others.

Place the first suture at the 6 o'clock position. Identify it with a Weck clip. Then place the others using a single strand of material. This approach facilitates placement and prevents the individual sutures from getting tangled.

Hold the isthmus close to the intramural segment and tie the 6 o'clock suture. Divide the loop between the succeeding muscularis sutures and tie each in turn. To tie without undue tension, it may be necessary first to approximate the isthmic mesosalpinx to the uterus with a single No. 7-0 suture.

After apposing the epithelium and muscularis, approximate the cornual seromuscularis to the tubal serosa with No. 8-0 polyglactin sutures. Similarly, join the mesosalpinx to the uterus.

One can also do tubocornual anastomosis for sterilization reversal. In such cases, the anastomosis is usually juxtamural, as the tube's intramural segment commonly is intact (24).

Tubotubal anastomosis

Occlusions associated with disease processes are rare at sites other than the cornu and the fimbriated end. Therefore, the most frequent reason for performing tubotubal anastomosis is to reverse a previous tubal sterilization (9,10,14,15,24).

First resect the occluded segment or, if reversing sterilization, the occluded ends (Figs. 29-3A and B). Transect the tube with iris scissors, and excise the occluded stump from the mesosalpinx electrosurgically. While excising, remain close to the tube to avoid broaching the mesosalpingeal vessels. Confirm patency of the proximal and distal segments by transcervical chromopertubation and descending hydropertubation, respectively, and examine the cut surfaces under high magnification to ascertain normalcy (Fig. 29-3C).

Perform end-to-end anastomosis of the tubal segments in two layers, as for tubocornual anastomosis, again using No. 8-0 suture material (Figs. 29-3D through G). Place the first musculoepithelial suture at the 6 o'clock position, at the tube's mesosalpingeal edge, and tie it. These sutures, incorporating the muscularis and submucosa, should be placed such that their knots remain peripheral.

Depending on the tubal segment's luminal caliber, place three or more additional sutures to complete approximation of the muscularis and epithelium. Using the same techniques and material, appose the serosa and mesosalpinx to complete the anastomosis.

If there is a significant difference between the caliber of the lumen in the two segments of tube, it is best to fashion an opening into the lumen of ampulla that matches the lumen of the isthmus. To accomplish this, excise the serosa over the occluded ampullary end to expose the muscularis. Incise the muscularis and epithelium at the tip of the occluded end using microscissors and fashion a small opening (9,10,15,24).

Postoperative management

Before closing the abdomen, we leave 150 ml of lactated Ringer's solution containing 1000 mg of hydrocortisone sodium succinate (Solu-Cortef) in the pelvis. We do not use prostheses or stents during the procedure. At the close of the procedure subcutaneous tissues are again infiltrated with local anesthetic, and a local nerve block is established. Because of these measures and very minimal bowel manipulation during the procedure, the patients require little postoperative analgesia (5).

Postoperative morbidity is rare. One can usually discharge patients from the hospital on the first postoperative day. Depending on the procedure, we perform HSG 3 to 6 months postoperatively to assess the surgical outcome.

For most patients, we do not recommend early second-look laparoscopy. Exceptions are late-reproductive-age women who have undergone salpingostomy or had extensive pelvic adhesions. If a postsalpingostomy patient fails to become pregnant in 12 to 18 months, second-look laparoscopy can be considered to reassess the pelvis (25).

Conservative management of ectopic pregnancy

Earlier identification of ectopic pregnancy by quantitative β-subunit human chorionic gonadotropin (β-hCG) and serum progesterone assays and ultrasound (especially using vaginal transducers) has made laparoscopy less important in diagnosis. However, one can still use laparoscopy to confirm diagnosis and to remove the gestation surgically.

A conservative surgical approach is appropriate for patients who want to become pregnant again (10,25,26). Although more common when the gestational sac is intact, it is also appropriate for treating ruptured ectopic pregnancy, provided sufficient tube can be salvaged. Always follow conservative management by serial determinations of plasma β-hCG to ensure complete removal of the trophoblast.

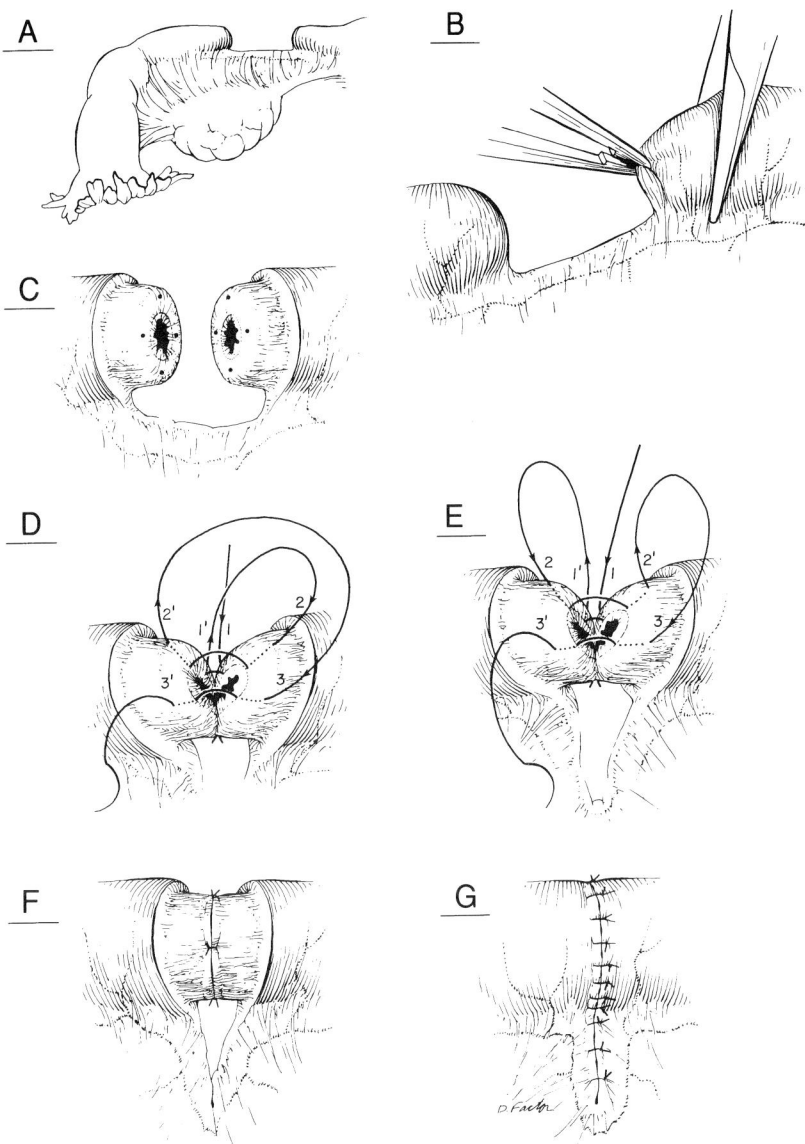

Fig. 29-3 Tubotubal anastomosis. Resect the occluded segment or ends (A, B), and confirm patency of proximal and distal segments (C). In the suture placement technique using a single strand of suture, the loop between two sutures is divided and each suture is tied individually (D, E). Perform end-to-end anastomosis in two layers (F, G).

Laparoscopic procedures

Do not attempt laparoscopic conservative management of tubal pregnancy without proper training. We recommend a multiple-puncture technique. This separates the visual and operative axes, allows greater precision, and reduces the incidence of complications. Once diagnosis is confirmed by laparoscopy, one will need to assess thoroughly the gestational site and the condition of the tube, ipsilateral ovary, and contralateral adnexa (9,10,25,26).

Segmental ablation

One can laparoscopically destroy an unruptured isthmic or proximal ampullary pregnancy of 1.5-cm diameter or less. Grip the segment containing the tubal pregnancy with a bipolar grasping forceps and thoroughly destroy it by electrodesiccation. Subsequent reconstruction by tubotubal anastomosis is possible.

Linear salpingotomy

Laparoscopic salpingotomy may be used to treat an unruptured ampullary or isthmic gestation or one with an early rupture. Introduce a grasping forceps through a second puncture placed suprapubically in the midline. Using a 22-gauge spinal needle inserted transabdominally, inject 2 to 3 ml of a dilute vasopressin solution (10 U in 100 cc of normal saline) under the serosa of the adjacent mesosalpinx. Then make a third puncture in the right iliac fossa, at McBurney's point, and through it introduce the hooked scissors.

Immobilize the tube with the forceps. Using the scissors, make a longitudinal incision on the affected tubal segment's antimesosalpingeal edge (the incision can also be made electrosurgically using a needle electrode). Replace the scissors by a second grasping forceps, and carefully use it to compress the tube gently and extrude the products of conception. Then gently tease out the conceptus.

Next, replace the second grasping forceps with a suction irrigation cannula. Irrigate the opening into the tube and the incision's edges with warm, heparinized lactated Ringer's solution. Seal any bleeders using bipolar or unipolar desiccation. Capillary oozing usually ceases spontaneously. Remove products of conception from the peritoneal cavity and perform pelvic lavage (27).

Segmental excision

Immobilize the tube with a bipolar grasping forceps inserted suprapubically and introduce a pair of scissors through a cannula inserted at McBurney's point. Desiccate the oviduct immediately proximal and distal to the gestational site using bipolar current and divide it with the scissors. Grasp and elevate the edge of the cut tubal segment, electrodesiccate and divide the adjacent exposed mesosalpinx, and remove the excised segment from the peritoneal cavity (9,10,25–27). Segmental excision is the approach of choice with pregnancies of isthmic location. In the event of persistent bleeding after salpingotomy, it is possible to resort to segmental excision, if tubal conservation is desired.

Laparotomy

Treatment by laparotomy is necessary only if the patient has severe hemoperitoneum and is hemodynamically unstable, or if the necessary laparoscopic equipment or skills are not available.

Magnification is not mandatory, although low-power loupes are useful to ensure precision in treating the patient who wishes to retain fertility. Observe tenets of microsurgical technique, excise all gestational tissue, establish hemostasis, conserve as much healthy oviduct as possible, suction all blood, and perform pelvic lavage. A minilaparotomy incision (as described previously) is usually adequate (10,25).

Elevate the tube containing the pregnancy on a Kerlex pad soaked in lactated Ringer's solution. We use linear salpingotomy for ampullary gestation and use segmental excision for isthmic and ruptured tubal pregnancies when tissues appear devitalized.

Although some have used tubal abortion—milking the pregnancy through the tube's fimbriated end—for gestations in the distal ampulla, this approach carries an unacceptable rate of postoperative bleeding from retained trophoblastic tissue. Therefore, linear salpingostomy is also preferable for these pregnancies, even if the incision extends to the fimbrial extremity (28).

Segmental excision

For this segmental excision, ligate the tube immediately proximal and distal to the gestational site with No. 3-0 or 4-0 Vicryl sutures (Fig. 29-4). Excise the affected tubal segment after ligating its mesosalpinx.

Linear salpingotomy

Using a needle electrode and blended cutting and coagulating current, make a longitudinal incision on the involved tubal segment's antimesosalpingeal edge (Fig. 29-5). Hold the tube between finger and thumb; the prod-

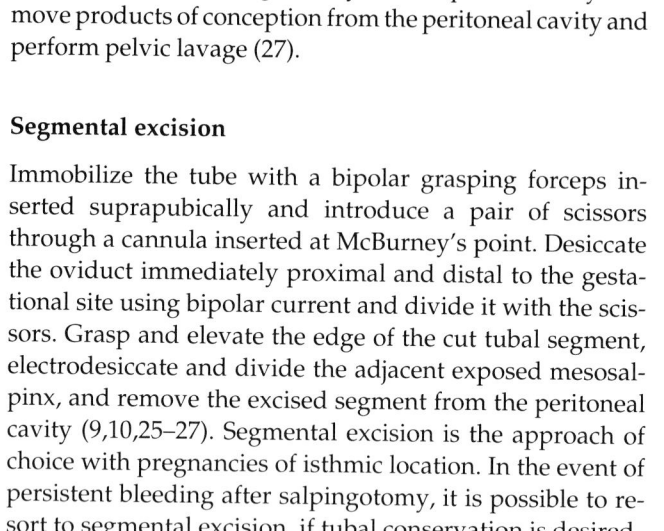

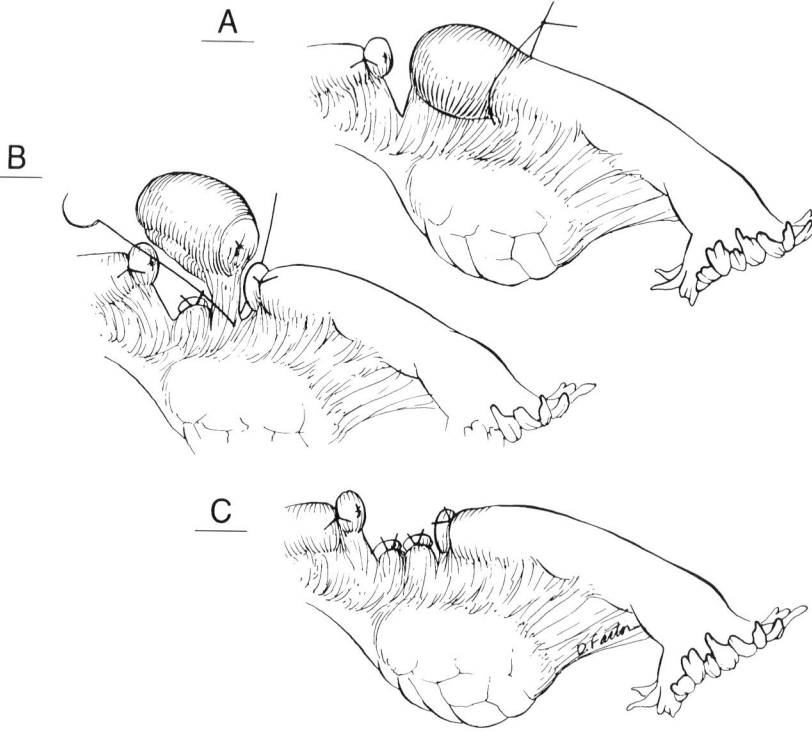

Fig. 29-4 To perform segmental excision, ligate and transect the tube proximal and distal to the gestation (A, B). The affected segment is removed after ligating and dividing the adjacent mesosalpinx (C).

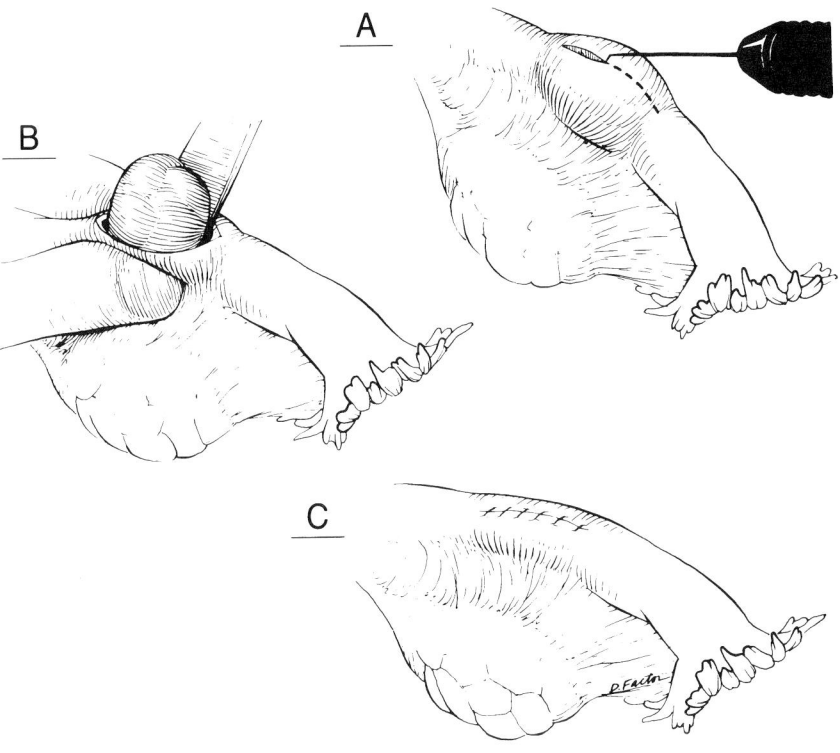

Fig. 29-5 For linear salpingotomy, make a longitudinal incision on the antimesenteric surface (A). After removing products of conception (B), close the incision with No. 6-0 polyglactin 910 (Vicryl) suture (C).

ucts of conception extrude through the incision by gentle pressure. Shell out products either with the back of a scalpel handle or by guiding the tissue through the incision with a pair of forceps. Irrigate the implantation site to ensure complete removal.

Mild venous oozing from the tubal incision's margins usually stops spontaneously. If necessary, electrodesiccate individual bleeders. Treat persistent bleeding from the implantation site after compression, by injecting a dilute solution of vasopressin subserosally on the tube's mesosalpingeal margin. No. 6-0 Vicryl sutures may be used to close the salpingostomy incision. Linear salpingotomy for a gestation near the fimbrial extremity is similar to that described above (Fig. 29-6).

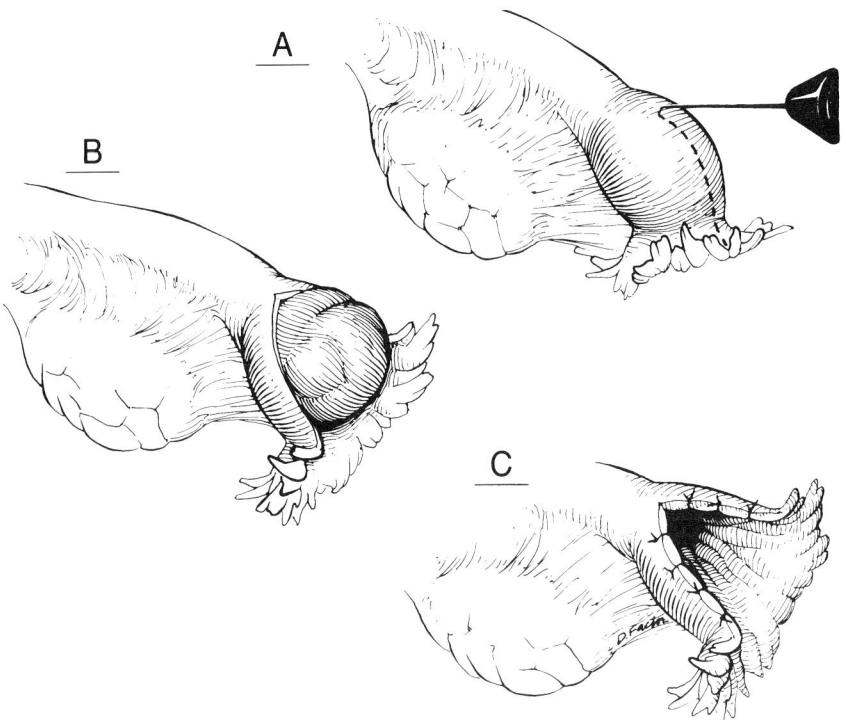

Fig. 29-6 Use linear salpingotomy also to remove a gestation in the distal ampulla, even if the incision extends to the fimbrial extremity.

References

1 FIVNAT 1989 et bilan general 1986–1989. Contrib Fertil Sexual 1990;18:588–600.

2 Medical Research International Society for Assisted Reproductive Technology. The American Fertility Society. In vitro fertilization–embryo transfer (IVF-ET) in the United States: 1989 results from the IVF-ET registry. Fertil Steril 1991;55:14–23.

3 Gomel V, Taylor PJ. In vitro fertilization versus reconstructive tubal surgery. JARGE 1992;4:306.

4 Rowe TC, Gomel V, McComb P. Investigations of tuboperitoneal causes of female infertility. In: Insler V, Lunenfeld B, eds. Infertility: male and female. Edinburgh: Churchill Livingstone, 1993: 253–282.

5 Gomel V, Taylor P. Reconstructive tubal surgery in the female. In: Insler V, Lunenfeld B, eds. Infertility: male and female. Edinburgh: Churchill Livingstone, 1993:481–503.

6 Gomel V. Laparoscopic tubal surgery in infertility. Obstet Gynecol 1975;46:47.

7 Gomel V. Laparoscopy. Can Med Assoc J 1974;111:167.

8 Gomel V. Salpingo-ovariolysis by laparoscopy in infertility. Fertil Steril 1983;40:607.

9 Gomel V. Recent advances in surgical correction of tubal disease producing infertility. Curr Probl Obstet Gynecol 1978;1:1.

10 Gomel V. Microsurgery in female infertility. Boston: Little, Brown, 1983.

11 Daniell J. The role of lasers in infertility surgery. Fertil Steril 1984;42:815.

12 Filmar S, Gomel V, McComb P. Effectiveness of CO_2 laser and electromicrosurgery in adhesiolysis: a comparison. Fertil Steril 1986; 45:407.

13 Fayez J, McComb J, Harper M. Comparison of tubal surgery with the CO_2 laser and the unipolar microelectrode. Fertil Steril 1983; 40:476.

14 Gomel V. An odyssey through the oviduct. Fertil Steril 1983;39:144.

15 Gomel V. Reconstructive surgery of the oviduct. J Reprod Med 1977;18:181.

16 Gomel V. Salpingostomy by laparoscopy. J Reprod Med 1977; 18:265.

17 Gomel V. Salpingostomy by microsurgery. Fertil Steril 1978;29:380.

18 Gomel V, Swolin K. Salpingostomy: microsurgical technique and results. Clin Obstet Gynecol 1980;23:1243.

19 Boer-Meisel ME, teVelde ER, Habbema JD. Predicting the pregnancy outcome in patients treated for hydrosalpinx: a prospective study. Fertil Steril 1986;45:23.

20 DeCherney AH, Mezer HC, Naftolin F. Analysis of failure of microsurgical anastomosis after midsegment, noncoagulation tubal ligation. Fertil Steril 1983;39:618.

21 Gomel V. Tubal reconstruction by microsurgery. Proceedings of the 8th World Congress on Fertility and Sterility, Buenos Aires, Argentina, 1974.

22 Gomel V. Tubal anastomosis by microsurgery. Fertil Steril 1977; 28:59.

23 McComb P, Gomel V. Cornual occlusion and its microsurgical reconstruction. Clin Obstet Gynecol 1980;23:1229.

24 Gomel V. Microsurgical reversal of female sterilization: a reappraisal. Fertil Steril 1980;33:587.

25 Gomel V, et al. Laparoscopy and hysteroscopy in gynecologic practice. Chicago: Year Book Medical Publishers, 1986.

26 Gomel V. Operative laparoscopy: time for acceptance. Fertil Steril 1989;52:1.

27 Zouves C, Urman B, Gomel V. Laparoscopic surgical treatment of tubal pregnancy. J Reprod Med 1992;37:205–209.

28 Bruhat MA, Manhes H, Mage G, et al. Treatment of ectopic pregnancy by means of laparoscopy. Fertil Steril 1980;33:41.

Chapter 30

Managing ectopic pregnancy in young patients

Albert Altchek

Managing ectopic pregnancy in young patients requires the following considerations:

1 The ectopic pregnancy incidence continues to increase because of early sexual activity with exposure to pregnancy and sexually transmitted disease and salpingitis.

2 The diagnosis is more difficult in the adolescent.

3 Ectopic pregnancy is the second leading cause of maternal mortality and the leading cause early in pregnancy.

4 The teenage group, especially among underprivileged blacks, has the highest mortality rate.

5 Early diagnosis permits conservative surgery (salpingostomy rather than salpingectomy) or even nonsurgical options in an effort to preserve fertility as well as reduce mortality.

6 Early diagnosis and vigorous therapy of salpingitis reduce later chances of ectopic pregnancy.

7 The adolescent may not be reliable in follow-up after surgery or for nonoperative management.

Recent advances have emphasized early diagnosis by transvaginal ultrasound, laparoscopy for therapy as well as diagnosis, and nonsurgical options.

Approaches to further improvement include adolescent behavioral modification to reduce the incidence of salpingitis and pregnancy by postponing sexual activity, use of effective contraception, early medical care, and increased awareness of ectopic pregnancy by the patient and the physician.

Public health aspects

The Centers for Disease Control has been collecting national data on ectopic pregnancy since 1970. Unfortunately, the data have not been precise because of underestimations of the total number and of 10% of fatal cases, because of improving technologic recognition, and because of variable sampling estimates that do not include federally funded hospitals. To further confuse the incidence, three different denominators have been used: ectopic pregnancies per live births, per women ages 15 to 44, and per all pregnancies.

In 1970 there were 17,800 ectopic pregnancies in the United States. In 1989 there were 88,400, representing a relative stabilization from 88,000 in 1987, but still an increase of almost fivefold overall (1; Table 30-1).

The highest incidences are in women 30 years of age or older, and they are almost 40% higher for blacks and other minority groups and in the South (2).

Despite the increased incidence of ectopic pregnancy, the risk of death in the United States dropped 90%, from 35.5 per 10,000 cases in 1970 to 3.8 in 1989 (1).

There were even greater decreases, however, in maternal mortality from the other traditional causes of hypertensive disease, hemorrhage, and infection. Therefore, the relative significance of ectopic pregnancy has increased from 7.8% in 1980 to 12% in 1987 (3), making it the second leading cause of maternal mortality and the leading cause of early pregnancy mortality (1).

Table 30-1 Number and rates of ectopic pregnancy in the United States, by year: 1970–1989

Year	No. estimated*	Per 1000 reported pregnancies	Per 1000 live births	Per 10,000 women ages 15–44
1970	17,800	4.5	4.8	4.2
1971	19,300	4.8	5.4	4.4
1972	24,500	6.3	7.5	5.5
1973	25,600	6.8	8.2	5.6
1974	26,400	6.7	8.4	5.7
1975	30,500	7.6	9.8	6.5
1976	34,600	8.3	11.0	7.2
1977	40,700	9.2	12.3	8.3
1978	42,400	9.4	12.8	8.5
1979	49,900	10.4	14.3	9.9
1980	52,200	10.5	14.5	9.9
1981	68,000	13.6	18.7	12.7
1982	61,800	12.3	17.0	11.5
1983	69,600	14.0	19.2	12.6
1984	75,400	14.9	20.6	13.6
1985	78,400	15.2	20.9	14.0
1986	73,700	14.3	19.7	12.8
1987	88,000	16.8	23.1	15.3
1988	80,700	15.1	20.7	14.4
1989	88,400	16.1	22.0	15.5
Total	1,047,900	11.3	14.8	10.3

*Estimated from the National Hospital Discharge Survey conducted by the Centers for Disease Control, National Center for Health Statistics; rounded to the nearest 100.
Reproduced by permission from Centers for Disease Control. Ectopic pregnancy—United States, 1988–1989. MMWR 1992;41(32):591–594.

care, socioeconomic factors, and possibly cultural attitudes. In addition, misdiagnosis occurs because ectopic pregnancy is often not considered in the young patient.

Ectopic pregnancies usually occur in the fallopian tube ampulla (78%), in the isthmus (12%), and in the fimbria (5%). About 2% are cornual or interstitial, and the remaining 3% are abdominal, cervical, or ovarian. The rare latter four (total 5%) have the greatest mortality (5).

Interstitial and rudimentary uterine horn ectopic pregnancies, although rare, cause 20% of the ectopic gestation fatalities. There is a relatively late onset of symtoms because of the presence of a uterine muscle wall unlike the usual tubal ectopic site. Rupture tends to occur in midtrimester with massive intra-abdominal bleeding. Diagnosis can be made by ultrasonography in the first trimester before rupture because of an unusual pregnancy location, a thin sur-

Table 30-2 Deaths per 10,000 ectopic pregnancies

	1970–1976	1977–1983	Decrease (%)
Age			
15–19	30.7	9.5	69
20–24	19.4	8.2	57
25–29	18.8	6.4	66
30–34	20.2	7.1	64
35–44	17.5	8.6	54
All races	19.9	7.4	63
White	11.9	4.3	64
Black and other	39.9	16.1	60

Adapted from Atrash HK, Friede A, Hogue CJR. Ectopic pregnancy and mortality in the United States, 1970–1983. Obstet Gynecol 1987;70:817–822.

Table 30-3 Risk of death per 10,000 ectopic pregnancies

	1970–1976			1977–1983		
	White	Black and other	Relative risk	White	Black and other	Relative risk
Total	11.98	39.9	3.4	4.3	16.1	3.8
Age						
15–19	15.9	58.9	3.7	4.0	31.7	8.0
20–24	10.9	40.8	3.7	5.1	16.0	3.2
25–29	14.2	31.4	2.2	4.4	12.4	3.2
30–34	11.1	40.9	3.7	3.7	16.6	4.5
35–44	6.5	43.5	6.7	3.5	18.4	5.3

Adapted from Atrash HK, Friede A, Hogue CJR. Ectopic pregnancy and mortality in the United States, 1970–1983. Obstet Gynecol 1987;70:817–822.

Most ectopic pregnancy deaths are due to hemorrhage, 59% without surgery and 28% with surgery. Surprisingly, 59% occurred in a hospital, while 27% were at home, and 8% in transit (4).

There is a lack of awareness that the risk of death from ectopic pregnancy in the United States is highest in the group 15 to 19 years of age (see Table 30-2).

The risk of death for "black and other" races is markedly increased, even more than by age alone (Table 30-2).

According to Atrash et al., "during 1977 to 1983 the most notable disparity was that teenage women of black and other races had a risk eight times that of white teenagers" (4) (Table 30-3). The risk of death for the former in 1988 was more than three times the risk for whites and in 1989 almost five times the risk (1).

Part of the reason is probably because these two groups have less prenatal care, especially in the first trimester of pregnancy. This is related to inadequate access to medical

rounding uterine wall with an incomplete myometrial layer, and an empty uterus (6).

Ultrasound can also detect the rare but dangerous cervical pregnancy, which sometimes requires hysterectomy to stop bleeding. There are extremely rare cases of ectopic pregnancy following hysterectomy with ovaries present.

Ectopic pregnancy causes a significant economic burden. In 1990 is was estimated as a total cost of $1.1 billion, with direct costs of 77% including an average individual hospital cost of $6079. Public payment covered the largest portion of direct costs incurred by teenage patients (7).

Some claim that at least 80% of ectopic cases could be treated by laparoscopy. This is a theoretical exaggeration based on many assumptions. If valid, in 1987 there would have been a theoretical savings of about $139 million (8). Laparoscopy is available for less than 30% of ectopic pregnancies.

Risk factors

The chance of ectopic pregnancy increases after salpingitis, reconstructive tubal surgery, previous ectopic pregnancy, perhaps in utero exposure to diethylstilbestrol, when pregnancy occurs despite an intrauterine device or sterilization, and with ovulation-inducing agents.

Women with pelvic inflammatory disease who delayed seeking care were three times more likely to experience subsequent infertility and ectopic pregnancy, especially with chlamydia. Prompt treatment can prevent these sequelae (9).

Although ectopic fallopian tube cultures may be negative for chlamydia, there may be a chronic salpingitis and serum antibodies induced by plasma cell chlamydia (10).

After an episode of acute inflammatory disease confirmed by laparoscopy, there was a 9.1% ectopic pregnancy rate compared with a 1.4% rate in control subjects (11).

It is thought that salpingitis isthmica nodosa, which is usually acquired, is associated with ectopic pregnancy and infertility.

All previous pelvic operations increase the risk of ectopic pregnancy, from a twofold increase for appendectomy to a ninefold increase for previous ectopic pregnancy (12).

The risk of an ectopic pregnancy is less after in vitro fertilization and embryo transfer than after microsurgical tubal reconstruction. In one report the chance of ectopic pregnancy was 12% after tubal reconstruction, but was 28% considering all pregnancies. This risk persisted for at least 5 years after surgery. The risk for those undergoing in vitro fertilization was only 3% (others reporting 2% to 9%), suggesting that it is preferable when there is a high risk of ectopic pregnancy (13).

Midfundal uterine transfer for in vitro fertilization yielded 14.2% intrauterine pregnancies per cycle with a 0.4% ectopic rate. Deep fundal transfer yielded 12.4% in-

trauterine and 1.5% ectopic pregnancies. Thus midfundal transfer may reduce the chance of ectopic pregnancy, perhaps by being farther from the tubes (14).

Ovulation induction increases the chance of ectopic pregnancy (15). Assisted reproduction technology might also increase the chance of rare forms of ectopic and heterotopic pregnancy (16,17).

Increased chances of ectopic pregnancy also occur with pregnancy after progestin-only oral contraceptives, previous infertility, and cigarette smoking (18).

There might be an association with douching, season (19), and exposure to antineoplastic drugs (20).

Compared with the noncontraceptors, intrauterine device (IUD) users had fewer ectopic pregnancies (21).

The use of an IUD for 3 or more years doubles the risk of ectopic pregnancy for many years after the IUD is removed, even with copper IUDs (22).

Progestin-only IUDs have a ratio of ectopic to total accidental pregnancies of 171 to 1000, while copper IUDs have a ratio of 39 to 1000. Although IUDs protect against ectopic pregnancy, with copper and nonmedicated IUDs the age-specific ectopic pregnancy ratios are six times those of noncontraceptors (23).

Diagnosis

The classic symptoms of unruptured ectopic pregnancy are amenorrhea, and sometimes unilateral lower abdominal discomfort and slight vaginal bleeding. The signs are sometimes a unilateral tender adnexal mass and a normal or slightly enlarged soft uterus with a blue-tinted cervix. With leaking or rupture there may be severe unilateral or bilateral lower abdominal or generalized abdominal pain, shoulder pain, vertigo, fainting, and shock. Examination may show a tender tense abdomen, pain on motion of the cervix, a very tender adnexal mass and cul-de-sac fullness.

The symptoms and signs are variable. Early ectopic pregnancy may not have any symptoms or palpable adnexal mass. Conversely, with normal intrauterine pregnancy there may be a unilateral palpable tender cystic corpus luteum (which may bleed), physiologic staining from placental invasion of the uterus, or threatened miscarriage bleeding. There may also be an incomplete uterine abortion or missed abortion. Salpingitis or an ovarian cyst may result in a tender unilateral adnexal mass.

Based on clinical examination, the frequent problems of differential diagnosis of ectopic pregnancy include threatened abortion, salpingitis (especially unilateral, which may be associated with an IUD), intraperitoneally bleeding corpus luteum cyst, appendicitis, and torsion of an ovarian cyst.

The less common problems of differential diagnosis include endometriosis, dysfunctional uterine bleeding, urinary tract infection, gastroenteritis, and congenital anomalies with retrograde menstruation.

Ectopic pregnancy has occurred despite amenorrhea after transcervical resection of the endometrium.

There is a newly described syndrome of tubal sterilization followed by endometrial ablation (postablation–tubal sterilization syndrome) resulting in a proximal hematosalpinx, which may simulate ectopic pregnancy. Cornual area endometrium regenerates, resulting in retrograde menstruation, pain, and vaginal spotting (24).

It is more difficult to diagnose ectopic pregnancy in the adolescent than in the adult woman. Health providers are lax in their suspicion because older differential diagnosis teaching (before the increase in adolescent sexual activity) did not include ectopic pregnancy.

Adolescents often have irregular and skipped menses because of anovulatory dysfunctional uterine bleeding. Not infrequently nonspecific abdominal pain occurs. Salpingitis causes pain. With ovulation, dysmenorrhea develops. Adolescents may consciously or unconsciously deny sexual activity because of parental disapproval. Adolescents tend to be poor contraceptors and may feel that infrequent sex is not sufficient to cause pregnancy.

Until 20 years ago ectopic pregnancies were usually diagnosed after rupture. The diagnostic approaches included observation, culdocentesis, dilatation and curettage of the uterus, and exploratory laparotomy.

In recent years ectopic pregnancies are being diagnosed before rupture or with only leakage because of precise serum human chorionic gonadotropin (hCG) testing of suspects, pelvic ultrasound, and laparoscopy. Early diagnosis avoids life-threatening rupture and gives the opportunity for conservative surgery to preserve fertility and the option of nonsurgical management. Rather than wait for signs and symptoms, surveillance is increased for high-risk asymptomatic cases.

Ideally, ectopic pregnancy (or pregnancy complication) should be considered in any adolescent (or any female of appropriate age) with abdominal pain, abnormal bleeding, or missed menstrual period.

The most reliable test for the possibility of ectopic pregnancy is a positive serum β-subunit hCG. It occurs in at least 95% of all ectopic pregnancies and is rarely negative (25). Older urine pregnancy tests were positive in only 50% of cases. New urine tests with a sensitivity of 50 to 250 mIU/ml are positive in more than 80% of cases.

If one suspects unruptured early ectopic pregnancy, carefully examine the patient and do a quantitative serum radioimmunoassay β-hCG test. In most cases, ectopic hCG levels will be above the normal nonpregnant limit but below 6500 mIU/ml. At the same time, it might be wise to obtain a complete blood count (to have a baseline hemoglobin-hematocrit) and an erthrocyte sedimentation rate (ESR). The ESR is slightly elevated in pregnancy but markedly elevated (over 50 mm/hour) in cases of acute salpingitis, which may present a problem for differential diagnosis.

The level of serum hCG doubles about every 2 to 3 days through the first 6 weeks of pregnancy (8 weeks from the last menstrual period [LMP]) and then levels off. Between weeks 4 and 5 (around 6.5 weeks from the LMP), mean hCG is about 10,000 mIU/ml. Failure to achieve the appropriate level by a certain time after the LMP on a single hCG reading suggests a pregnancy is ectopic. Failure of hCG to almost double in 48 hours is even more suggestive. Of course, late ovulation or intrauterine fetal death could result in a lower than expected hCG level, and the latter would also cause failure to rise rapidly.

With normal intrauterine pregnancy, pelvic (lower abdominal) sonography will reveal a gestational sac when the quantitative hCG level is 6000 to 6500 mIU/ml (about 6 weeks from the LMP). Sonography before that time is unreliable in intrauterine pregnancy. After that time it is about 85% reliable, with a false-positive rate of 10% and a false-negative rate of 5%. Suggestive sonographic findings of ectopic pregnancy are absence of a uterine gestational sac or presence of an adnexal mass or cul-de-sac fluid. Newer real-time sonography is better than older static sonography. The recently developed transvaginal sonography is better than pelvic (lower abdominal) sonography.

Culdocentesis is being used less because it is awkward in the nulliparous adolescent and because of a high false-negative rate (14.8%) (26). Nevertheless, it can be a method of rapid confirmation of hematoperitoneum (90% positive). There may be a false-positive rate of 15% due to a bleeding corpus luteum cyst, retrograde menstruation, or miscarriage. An 18- or 20-gauge spinal needle is used. A positive test is free-flowing, nonclotting blood. If there is clinical evidence of a ruptured ectopic pregnancy and impending shock, proceed to an immediate laparotomy rather than delay for a culdocentesis.

If the pelvic sonogram shows a uterine sac but the hCG level is less than 6000 mIU/ml, it suggests a missed abortion or "blighted ovum" or perhaps late ovulation. If there is evidence of a missed intrauterine abortion by hCG or ultrasound, or if the patient wants a pregnancy interruption, then a dilatation and curettage may be done. Trophoblastic tissue will diagnose a previous intrauterine pregnancy. Heterotopic pregnancy (intrauterine and extrauterine) is rare. Although it is assumed that with ectopic pregnancy the endometrium is always decidual, in fact it is decidual in only about 60%. About 30% have a secretory or proliferative endometrium, and 9% have an Arias-Stella reaction. Occasionally, uterine curettage after spontaneous complete abortion may not show even microscopic evidence of chorionic villi.

Diagnostic laparoscopy is considered for one or more of the following:

1 Serum hCG over 6500 mIU/ml without a uterine sac on pelvic ultrasound.

2 Lack of appropriate rise in hCG.

3 No trophoblastic tissue on curettage with a persistent positive hCG.

4 Positive pelvic sonography.

5 Clinical signs of intraperitoneal bleeding, positive culdocentesis. If there is impending shock, do an immediate laparotomy.

6 Clinical picture of ectopic pregnancy with an adnexal mass.

Despite the high accuracy of laparoscopy, ectopic tubal pregnancies can be missed if they are very early and are not leaking, if there is also salpingitis, and if there are difficulties in visualization because of adhesions. There may be up to 3% false-negative and false-positive rates. The unruptured ectopic pregnancy appears as an oval, smooth enlargement of the tube with a dusky blue cyanotic discoloration. An early 0.5 cm ectopic pregnancy may mimic a normal tube variation and is easily missed. A clue to the ectopic condition is bleeding from the fimbria, either spontaneously or by stroking the tube at laparoscopy.

Recently there have been attempts at early diagnosis using serum tests, particularly progesterone. Serum progesterone is decreased in ectopic pregnancy at 16 days after conception, even before there is a reduction of serum hCG, compared with intrauterine pregnancy (normal and with blighted ovum). This suggests that another unknown factor of uterine pregnancy, besides hCG, maintains luteal function (27).

At 4 weeks the progesterone threshold for viable and nonviable ectopic pregnancy versus intrauterine pregnancy was 5 ng/ml: at 5 weeks, 10 ng/ml; and at 6 weeks, 20 ng/ml. The differences were most distinct at 4 weeks, when ectopic pregnancies cannot be visualized by ultrasound (28).

A mean single serum progesterone level for normal pregnancy was 32.8 ± 4.25 ng/ml; for ectopic pregnancy, 7.8 ± 0.79; and for spontaneous abortion, 8.1 ± 0.91. A cutoff of 24 ng/ml would exclude ectopic pregnancy in 99% of cases (29).

Another study found that a single serum progesterone level could differentiate between ectopic and normal pregnancy in more than 80% of patients. No normal pregnancy was found to have a progesterone level less than 8 ng/ml, and no ectopic pregnancy had a progesterone level over 15 ng/ml. Others have reported a "gray zone" from 10 to 25 ng/ml. A combination of progesterone, hCG, estradiol (high in normal pregnancy), and α-fetoprotein (higher in ectopic pregnancy) predicted ectopic pregnancy with 98.5% specificity and 94.5% accuracy while clinical diagnosis was less than 75% accurate (30).

Not all agree on whether there is a minimum progesterone threshold (31). A London commentary downplays progesterone because with ovarian hyperstimulation progesterone is always high; a low progesterone level cannot distinguish between a miscarriage and an ectopic pregnancy; a single progesterone report cannot reliably predict

the presence or absence of ectopic pregnancies, and progesterone determination requires at least 2 to 4 hours. A rapid qualitative hCG test with a sensitivity of 25 to 50 IU/L (First International Reference Preparation [IRP]) was recommended. With a positive test and a suspicion of pregnancy, expert transvaginal ultrasound should be done. This may give the diagnosis in 90% of cases before rupture. The ectopic fetal heart activity can be detected in 21% at 6 to 7 weeks' gestation. If further biochemical testing is necessary, then a quantitative serum hCG test, and not a progesterone test, should be done. With normal intrauterine pregnancy transvaginal ultrasound should show a gestational sac a few days after a missed period, when the quantitative hCG is at a level of 500 to 1000 IU/L (First IRP). A second quantitative hCG test done after 48 hours should show a doubling in normal pregnancy. Falling levels suggest miscarriage whereas plateauing levels suggest ectopic pregnancy (32).

Transvaginal (endovaginal) ultrasound (TU) has been a marked improvement over transabdominal pelvic ultrasound. A higher frequency transducer is used with better resolution but reduction in penetration. The latter is accommodated by the reduced distance to the fallopian tube. Pregnancy can be identified earlier. In normal pregnancy TU can identify a sac with an hCG level of over 1000 IU/ml, within 2 or 3 weeks after a missed menses. In addition, there is no need for a full bladder (as with the pelvic procedure), and it avoids imaging through the abdominal wall. The disadvantages of the transvaginal approach are change of orientation and an 8 cm limit from the probe tip.

With TU a confident diagnosis of ectopic pregnancy can be made at the initial scan in 74% of cases in contrast to 58% with the first pelvic scan (33). Some believe that a "halo sign," a thin sonolucent area surrounding an "adnexal ring," is suggestive of a living ectopic pregnancy (34).

Experience is required in TU, and errors may occur with other pathology, with bowel segment, and with poor demarcation from the ovary (35).

A recent improvement in TU has been the addition of color flow and Doppler waveform analysis. The normal ovary and tissues generally have a low-amplitude, high-impedance systolic flow because of the arteriolar muscle wall. Trophoblastic tissue has high velocity and low-impedance flow because there are no muscular vascular walls. This is analogous to ovarian malignancies. The corpus luteum is similar to trophoblastic flow but usually with a lower peak amplitude. Thus a high-velocity flow may be found in the ectopic pregnancy, in the ovarium corpus luteum and in the echogenic outer ring of the normal intrauterine pregnancy sac. The pseudo-uterine sac of ectopic pregnancy has no color flow (36).

Adding color flow and pulsed Doppler to endovaginal sonography improved the sensitivity from 71% to 87% for ectopic pregnancy, from 24% to 59% for failed intrauterine pregnancy, and from 90% to 99% for viable intrauterine pregnancy. It increased the percentage of diagnostic initial sonographic examinations from 62% to 82%. The specificities ranged from 99% to 100% (37).

To the present, Doppler waveform analysis required the visualization of the ectopic mass, then its peritrophoblastic circulation was examined. Therefore, it did not permit earlier diagnosis. Increased blood flow in uterine arteries with ectopic pregnancy suggests trophoblastic activity but does not indicate the side. A report from Innsbruck described a new approach using endovaginal triplex color Doppler ultrasonography for qualitative blood flow analysis of both

tubal arteries (tubal branch of the ascending arch of the uterine artery). There was an increase in blood flow on the ectopic side with a mean difference of 20.45%, while control subjects had a mean between-side difference of 2.95% (early normal pregnancy, early uterine pregnancy failure, and nonpregnant). Using an 8% cutoff in difference, the sensitivity was 85%, the specificity was 96%, and the positive predictive value was 93%. The percentage difference between the sides was independent of gestational age or hCG level. This new technique is positive even before clinical signs or ultrasound visualization of the ectopic mass are present. If confirmed, it would be the earliest method of making the diagnosis. The usual case took 15 minutes with results immediately available (38).

A recent review described an algorithm for spontaneously occurring pregnancy (Fig. 30-1). (More testing may be required for pregnancy after pharmacologic induction of ovulation.) Initially a single serum progesterone test and quantitative β-hCG test are done as a screening method.

There is only a small change in progesterone level the first 8 to 10 weeks of pregnancy. If the level equals or is greater than 25 ng/ml, it excludes ectopic pregnancy with a 97.5% sensitivity. If the serum progesterone level equals or is less than 5 ng/ml, it indicates a nonviable pregnancy in any location with 100% sensitivity. This permits a dilatation and curettage to be done. If villi are identified, it indicates the completion of a spontaneous intrauterine abortion. If there are no villi but the β-hCG returns to normal, it suggests a completed abortion. (Although the algorithm does not indicate it, it may also be a spontaneous demise of an ectopic pregnancy.) A stable or rising β-hCG level suggests an ectopic pregnancy. With TU detection of

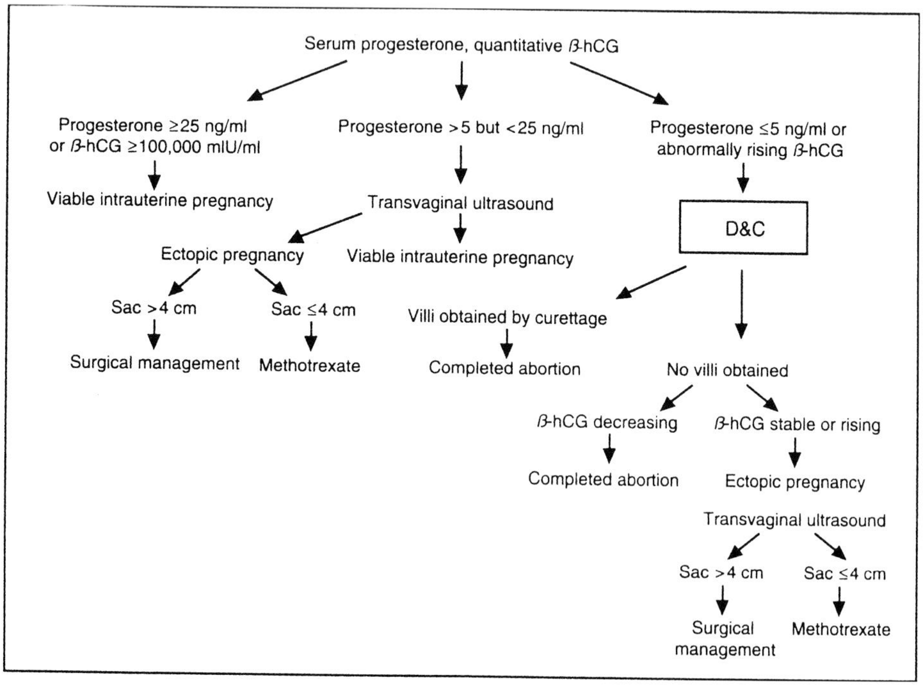

Table 30-4 Single-dose protocol for intramuscular treatment of unruptured ectopic pregnancy

Day*	Therapy
0	hCG, curettage,† complete blood cell count with differential and platelet count, asparate aminotransferase, serum creatinine, blood type, and Rh
1	hCG, intramuscular methotrexate (50 mg/m²)
4	hCG
7	hCG‡

Adapted from Stovall TG, Ling FW. Single-dose methotrexate: an expanded clinical trial. Am J Obstet Gynecol 1993;168:1759–1765.
*In those patients not requiring curettage before treatment initiation day 0 and day 1 were combined.
†Endometrial curettage was performed only in those patients with an hCG titer < 2000 mIU/ml at treatment initiation.
‡If the hCG titer on day 7 decreased to less than 15% from day 4, a second intramuscular methotrexate dose (50 mg/m²) was given on day 7.

Fig. 30-1 Algorithm for the diagnosis of unruptured ectopic pregnancy without laparoscopy. Progesterone measurements increase the sensitivity of the algorithm by inexpensively screening large numbers of patients during the first trimester of pregnancy. The definitive diagnosis is made by transvaginal ultrasound or uterine curettage and does not depend on the serum progesterone concentrations obtained during screening. To convert values for progesterone to nanomoles per liter, multiply by 3.18. D&C, dilation and curettage. (Reprinted by permission from Carson SA, Buster JE. Ectopic pregnancy. N Engl J Med 1993;329:1174–1181.)

an ectopic pregnancy sac larger than 4 cm, surgical management is advised. With a sac up to 4 cm, Carson and Buster recommend intramuscular methotrexate therapy (Table 30-4). If the serum progesterone is between 6 and 24 ng/ml, vaginal ultrasound is advised to determine pregnancy viability (39).

Not all agree with this algorithm. Many would advise routine immediate TU, repeated in one week if necessary. This might identify an intrauterine pregnancy and its viability and later identify an ectopic pregnancy. It might avoid the dilatation and curettage of the uterus but would incur the expense of the ultrasound. Another difference of opinion relates to the reliability of a single serum progesterone as a screening test. In addition, most gynecologists do not favor intramuscular (IM) methotrexate as the primary therapy.

They find that one third of their cases are eligible for methotrexate (39). If laparoscopy is needed for diagnosis, then laparoscopic salpingostomy or salpingectomy is done.

A new protocol at the Mount Sinai School of Medicine in New York City recommends that any suspected unstable ectopic pregnancy be considered a surgical emergency. A stable ectopic suspect with an hCG level over 2000 mIU (Second IRP) undergoes a vaginal ultrasound, which should show an intrauterine sac if there is a normal pregnancy. An abdominal ultrasound requires a level of 6000 mIU. If there is an absence of an intrauterine sac with an appropriate hCG level, the diagnosis is considered ectopic pregnancy, and the patient is admitted for surgical or pharmacologic therapy. Of course, such findings may be present immediately after completed (or incomplete) abortion. Stable ectopic suspects are hospitalized if there is an IUD, fever, pain, or mass palpable on pelvic examination, a debilitating illness, or if the patient is unreliable. Stable suspects with hCG levels too low for ultrasound are followed as outpatients with examination and hCG determination every 2 days. Normal pregnancy should have a 66% rise in hCG, and failure to rise warrants treatment. A falling hCG suggests ectopic pregnancy or impending intrauterine abortion. Falling hCG may be associated with rupture until the level is below 10 mIU. A falling and then level hCG suggests ectopic pregnancy or a trophoblastic neoplasm. Slowly falling hCG levels are treated if there was a previous ectopic pregnancy, if there are symptoms, if there is an adnexal mass, or if there is no gestational tissue on endometrial sampling. After treatment by laparoscopic or laparotomy salpingostomy or methotrexate treatment, serial hCG tests are done every 2 days until the level is below 10 mIU.

Unfortunately, rarely an ectopic pregnancy may rupture even when the hCG level is less than 10 mIU/ml (40).

Management

The rare types of ectopic pregnancy—intramural (cornual), abdominal, ovarian, and cervical—have the highest mortality. They are often diagnosed late. Assisted reproductive technology and ovulation induction increase the incidence of ectopic and heterotopic (intrauterine and ectopic) pregnancy.

Since 1988, there has been a significant change in management approach. Previously, although laparoscopy was the method of choice for diagnosis, the standard treatment was laparotomy with salpingostomy (leaving the tubal incision open), salpingotomy (closing the tubal incision), or salpingectomy. At present, laparoscopic salpingostomy is considered the ideal or gold standard in general, and especially regarding surgical therapy.

With improved earlier diagnosis, nonsurgical options may be considered: observation, since a significant percentage of conceptuses will spontaneously die; methotrexate to end the ectopic pregnancy by systemic injection or by injection into the ectopic region by laparoscopy or TU needle; or injection of other substances into the pregnancy, such as concentrated potassium chloride, hyperosmolar glucose, or prostaglandin. Of course, cases of ruptured and hemodynamically unstable ectopic pregnancy should be treated with immediate laparotomy.

Laparotomy for treatment is done rather than laparoscopy if the surgeon is not comfortable with laparoscopy technique, or if the operating room is not equipped for laparoscopy. For the young patient especially, conservative surgery or salpingostomy is preferred to the past traditional salpingectomy. Salpingostomy does not increase the chance of later repeat ectopic pregnancy and increases the chance of subsequent successful pregnancy compared with salpingectomy. Although in previous years the reproductive endocrinology tubal plastic surgeon was preferred for conservative laparotomy, recent residency training programs have included it in general gynecology.

Conservative surgery for unruptured tubal ectopic pregnancy entails the following:
- removal of all pregnancy tissue
- preservation of normal tube
- meticulous hemostasis
- gentle handling of tissues (avoiding trauma, avoiding sponging to reduce later adhesion formation, keeping tissues moist with irrigation and wet pads, and washing out any clots)
- elevation of tubes for adequate exposure by wet pads or a board in the cul-de-sac
- use of fine absorbable suture material such as 5-0 to 8-0 polyglactin (Vicryl) or polyglycolic acid (Dexon) on the tube, with an atraumatic needle (3-0 for mesentery vessels)
- use of microsurgical instruments and instrument ties
- solid-state electrosurgery, unipolar needle (if possible, microneedle electrode cutting and coagulation, and bipolar coagulation)
- knowledge of tubal anatomy and precise suturing of layers.

Meticulous hemostasis is essential because the involved tube is fragile, friable, and bleeds readily, and because clots predispose to adhesions. To achieve hemostasis, apply one or more of the following measures:

• Gently compress the mesosalpinx vessels with wet gloved fingers (Fig. 30-2A).

• Inject the mesenteric border of the tubal wall or the tube itself with diluted vasopressin (Pitressin) (10 U in 20 ml of saline), using a fine 25-gauge needle (Fig. 30-2B). Hemostatic response may occur with 0.5 ml.

• Irrigate the tube with lactated Ringer's solution using a pencil-like irrigator, Dakin syringe, or intravenous tube with an 18-gauge plastic cannula, to visualize the precise bleeding point and keep the tissues moist (Fig. 30-3A).

• Use unipolar electrocoagulation with a microelectrode needle to control bleeding points (Fig. 30-3B), and bipolar microforceps electrocoagulation for larger bleeders (Fig. 30-3C).

• If necessary, use hemostatic sutures of 6-0, 7-0, or 8-0 absorbable polyglactin in the tubal wall and 3-0 sutures for mesentery vessels.

Handle microsurgical instruments by rotating the needle holder between the thumb and index finger and using a rigid surface to support the ulnar edge of the hand and wrist. In addition, attempt to preserve a comfortable sitting posture. This contrasts with the standard instrument-handling technique, in which the arm, forearm, and wrist move in an arc to pass the needle, while the fingers are held relatively rigidly on the needle holder.

A few microsurgical instruments required include a needle holder delicate enough for a 6-0 suture, forceps, tying forceps, and scissors.

Accessory instruments include glass or polytetrafluoroethylene (Teflon) rod retractors and tubal cannulae. Portable optical hoods or loupes, with either an individual prescription or a nonprescription lens, are also desirable.

The nonprescription Zeiss loupe with headlight attachment and headband works excellently.

One should also use a solid-state electrosurgical unit, ideally with a low-power mode attenuator ("micromode") to keep power under 100 W and voltage no more than 600 V. Such a unit will include a unipolar microelectrode needle for coagulation and cutting and a fine bipolar forceps coagulator.

Besides using lactated Ringer's solution to keep tissues moist and reveal bleeding vessels, one may use it to moisten pads and leave it intraperitoneally (150–200 ml) to reduce adhesion formation. Previously used was 6% dextran 70 in 5% dextrose, or 0.9% sodium chloride (dextran 6% is usually used as a plasma volume expander). Very rarely, and especially when given intravenously, dextran can cause anaphylactoid and allergic reactions, significant plasma or intraperitoneal volume expansion, and transient prolongation of bleeding time. Anaphylactoid reaction has discouraged the use of dextran.

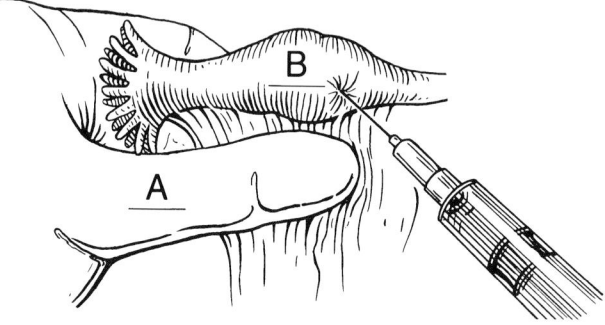

Fig. 30-2 For hemostasis (A) compress mesosalpinx with moistened gloved fingers and inject the tubal wall with diluted vasopressin (B).

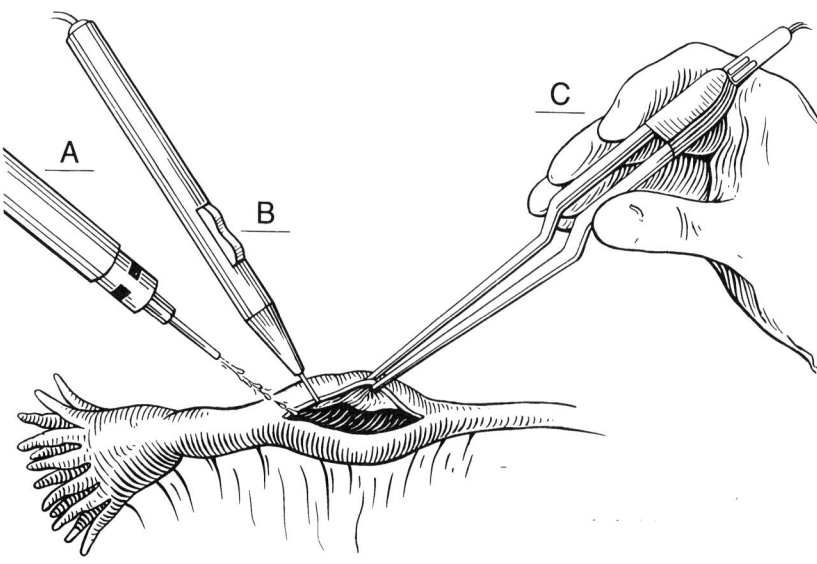

Fig. 30-3 Further methods for effecting hemostasis include irrigation with lactated Ringer's solution or dextran (A), unipolar coagulation for spot bleeding (B), or bipolar coagulation for larger bleeding areas (C).

Tubal anatomy complex

The fallopian tube is 10 to 12 cm long, with an intramural (interstitial) portion in the uterine wall and an extrauterine portion, which is divided unevenly into a shorter (one-third) proximal isthmus and a longer (two-thirds) distal ampulla (Fig. 30-4). The most distal 1 to 2 cm of the tube, the infundibulum, contains the fimbriated ostium.

The ampulla has a large lumen, 1 to 2 cm wide, a thin wall, and an endosalpinx with complex, extensive infoldings. The isthmus, narrower but with a thick muscle wall, has a very contracted lumen, between 0.1 mm and 1.0 mm in diameter, and a few simple longitudinal infoldings of the endosalpinx. The interstitial portion, only about 0.4 mm in diameter, often takes an irregular path through the uterine wall.

How to operate

Ampulla

Most ectopic pregnancies are in the ampulla. Unless the patient is going into shock, either do a Pfannenstiel incision or detach the recti muscles near the symphysis as part of the transverse incision (Fig. 30-5). After opening the abdomen, gently explore the ectopic site, adjacent ovary, opposite tube and ovary, and the corpus luteum. Usually, one can use a four-way, self-retaining retractor.

Gently wall off the intestines with wet laparotomy pads, and place additional wet pads, fluffy gauze (Kerlex), or a plastic Teflon board in the cul-de-sac of Douglas to elevate the tube. One may also use wet pads to wall off the lateral pelvic wall and opposite adnexa (Fig. 30-6).

Make an incision about 2 cm long on the tube's antimesenteric surface over the pregnancy site with a unipolar needle (or microneedle), electrocautery instrument, or laser beam (Fig. 30-7A). Usually, the pregnancy tissue will pop out spontaneously. Gently remove the remainder or scoop it out with the handle of a scalpel or other blunt instrument (Fig. 30-7B).

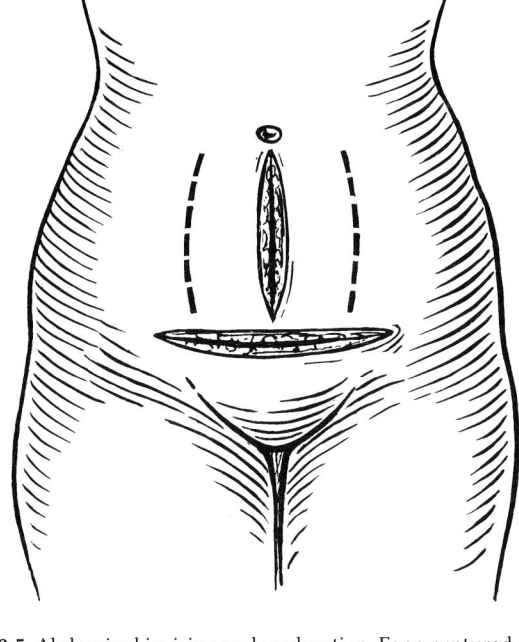

Fig. 30-5 Abdominal incision and exploration. For a ruptured emergency ectopic pregnancy, make a lower abdominal midline or paramedian incision. For an unruptured or leaking nonacute ectopic pregnancy, use a lower abdominal transverse (Pfannenstiel) incision.

Because ectopic pregnancy tissue often infiltrates the tubal wall in and between the muscularis and serosa, making the wall hemorrhagic and friable, some advise debridement to avoid postoperative late bleeding. However, others claim that possible ultimate benefits of debridement fail to justify the immediate bleeding and trauma.

I consider this a judgment matter. Unquestionably, trophoblastic tissue is usually left in the tube, especially since what is considered edema is often infiltration. But postoperative late bleeding is unusual, and trophoblastic neoplastic change (hydatidiform mole) is rare. (See section below on persistent ectopic pregnancy with laparoscopy salpingostomy).

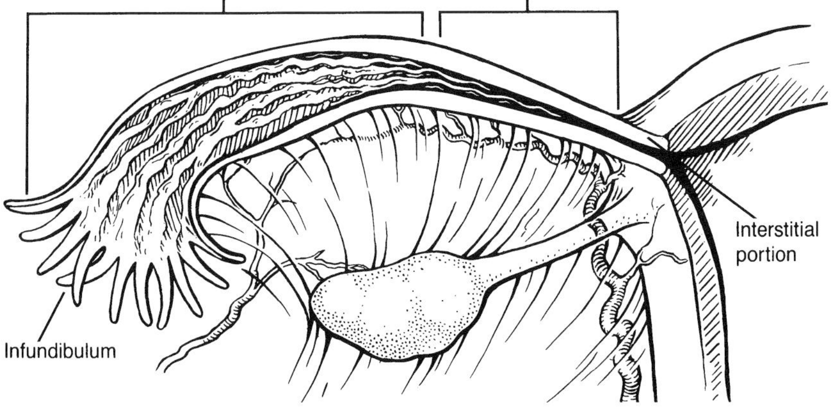

Ampulla   Isthmus

Interstitial portion

Infundibulum

Fig. 30-4 Tubal anatomy. Most ectopic pregnancies occur in the ampulla. There is anastomosis of vessels from the ovarian (infundibulopelvic), to the medial proximal portion of the tube, near the uterus, and then to the uterine.

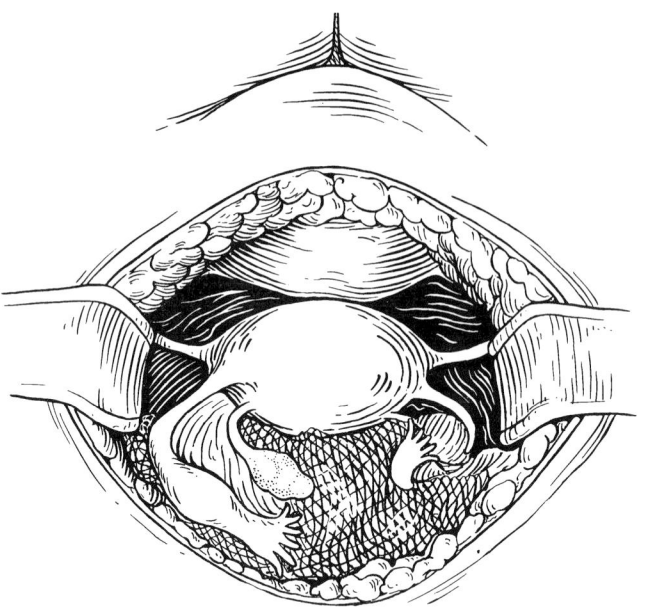

Fig. 30-6 Use moistened loose gauze in the cul-de-sac to support adnexae.

Previously, many recommended primary closure of the tube (salpingotomy), theoretically to reduce chances of adhesions, with one or two layers of interrupted 5-0 to 8-0 polyglactin or polyglycolic acid suture (Fig. 30-7C). Avoid the lumen if possible. After closure, some pass dye through the tubes to test patency. One way of doing this is to clamp the cervix from anterior to posterior with a Siegler-Hellman or Buxton uterine clamp to occlude it, then inject dye (dilute methylene blue or indigo carmine) into the uterine fundus. Another is preoperatively to place a Foley catheter or a cannula through the cervix.

At present most recommend leaving the incision open (salpingostomy) and allowing the tube to close by itself, which occurs within 4 months. If necessary for hemostasis (which is unusual), a running locked suture of 7-0 polyglactin may be placed around the cut edges (Fig. 30-7D). Most do not pass dye. For either salpingotomy or salpingostomy, some recommend leaving about 150 ml of lactated Ringer's solution in the cul-de-sac peritoneum to reduce adhesion formation. Optical magnification, although desirable, is not necessary.

Infundibulum

Here one must decide whether or not to incise the tube. At diagnostic laparoscopy, if the ectopic tissue emerges from the fimbriated end spontaneously or with only slight compression of the distal tube, remove it laparoscopically and observe the tube. If, however, vigorous "milking out" is required, the high risk of late bleeding makes it preferable to perform an incision into the tube. Make a distal antimesenteric linear incision with unipolar electric needle cautery, gently remove the pregnancy tissue, and effect hemostasis (Fig. 30-8). In the past, the incision was left open, or sutured closed in one or two layers. At present it is left open.

Isthmus

If the ectopic pregnancy is in the isthmus, segmental resection is customary, although salpingostomy may be attempted. To avoid fistulas, use a 2-0 nylon or other nonabsorbable suture to ligate the tube proximal and distal to the pregnancy; cut the tube at each site (Fig. 30-9). Ligate the mesosalpinx vessels separately with 3-0 absorbable suture before cutting them.

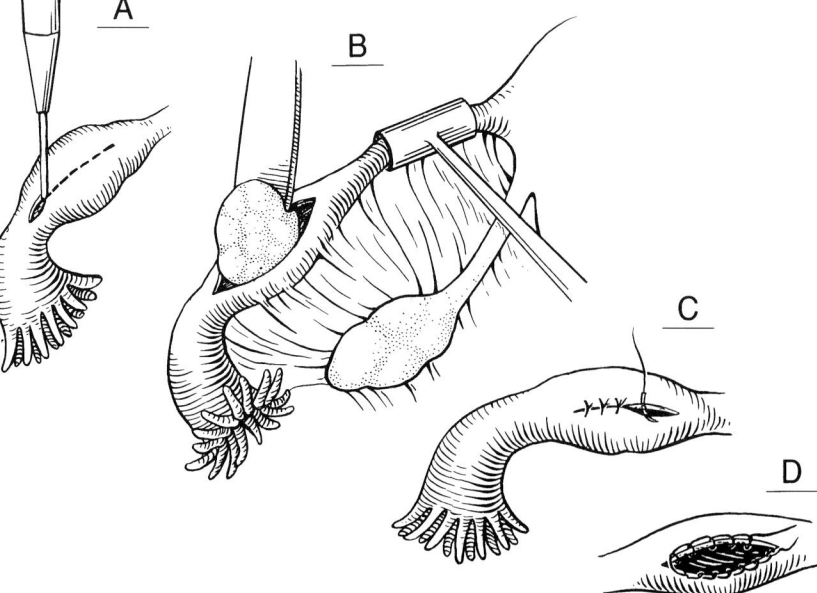

Fig. 30-7 Ampullary site. (A) Make a linear antimesenteric border incision with a needle electrocautery electrode. (B) Scoop out pregnancy tissue; if desired, use a stabilization clamp proximally. (C) Suture the incision site with a 5-0 to 8-0 polyglactin or polyglycolic acid suture in one or two layers, avoiding the lumen. (D) If one chooses salpingostomy, for the unusual necessity of hemostasis a running suture can be placed on the cut edges for hemostasis. At present, salpingostomy without any suturing is preferred, maintaining hemostasis by other means. Salpingotomy is rarely done today. Some (foreign) authors use "salpingotomy" when they mean "salpingostomy."

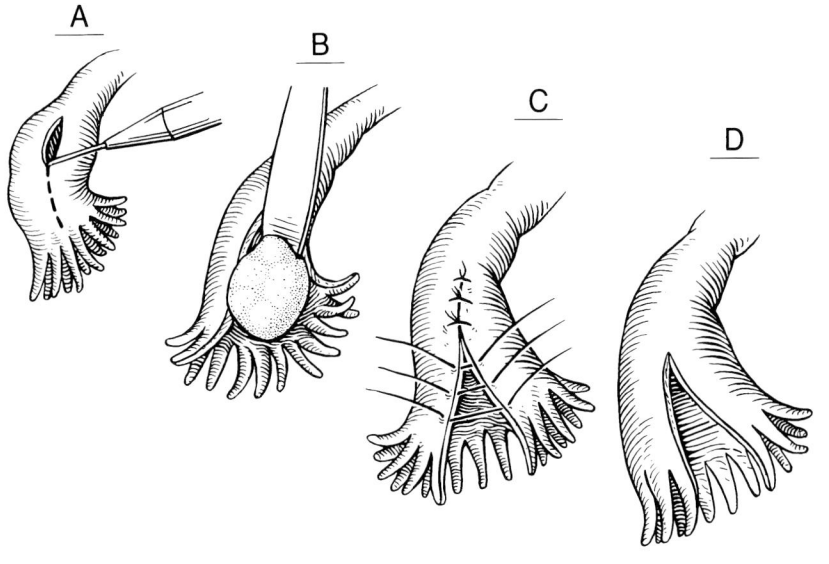

Fig. 30-8 Ectopic pregnancy near infudibulum. Rather than vigorous "milking out," which may cause trauma and postoperative bleeding, make an antimesenteric incision with the needle electrode (A) and scoop out the pregnancy tissue (B). Either close the incision (C) or leave it open (D) in one or two layers.

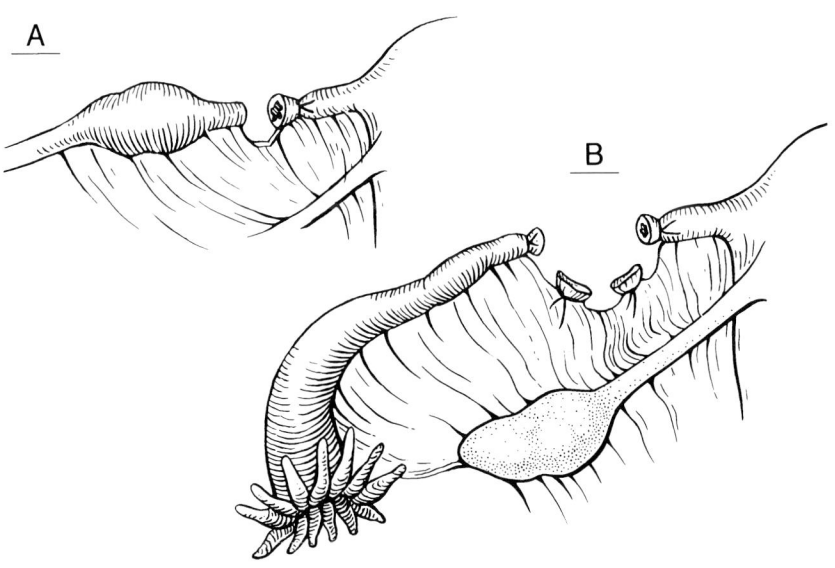

Fig. 30-9 Resection for ectopic pregnancy in the isthmus. (A) Place a nonabsorbable ligature at the proximal cut tube. (B) After resecting the ectopic pregnancy, ligate each end of the tube and the cut vessels of the mesosalpinx.

If the patient subsequently attempts to become pregnant and fails, one can do a tuboplasty anastomosis after one year. An alternative is to have the patient use contraception to avoid a repeat ectopic pregnancy in the resected tube, then after several months do a tubal anastomosis.

Some have successfully done one-stage segmental resections with end-to-end anastomosis of isthmic unruptured ectopic pregnancies, using chromotubation to ensure patency of the proximal and distal portions of the salvaged tube. For this procedure, resect the ectopic area and hold the tube ends together with 6-0 polyglactin suture through the mesentery, and short stabilization or Babcock clamps. Anastomose the ends with three 8-0 polyglactin or polyglycolic acid sutures at 8, 12 and 4 o'clock positions through the serosa (Fig. 30-10).

Resection with simultaneous anastomosis requires a stable patient, an experienced surgeon, and fine instruments. Optical magnification by loupes or microscope is desirable. This is the exceptional instance when it is preferable for an expert tubal plastic surgeon to do the procedure. However, not all authorities advise immediate anastomosis for the isthmus, and none do for the ampulla because of its thin, friable wall and greater potential for bleeding.

If the ectopic pregnancy is in the isthmus just outside the myometrium, remove the involved section of tube either flush with the myometrium or with only a very shallow cornual myometrial resection to obviate the possibility of subsequent uterine pregnancy rupture. If the distal tube is salvageable, there is the possibility of later cornual-tubal anastomosis or reimplantation of the tube into the uterus.

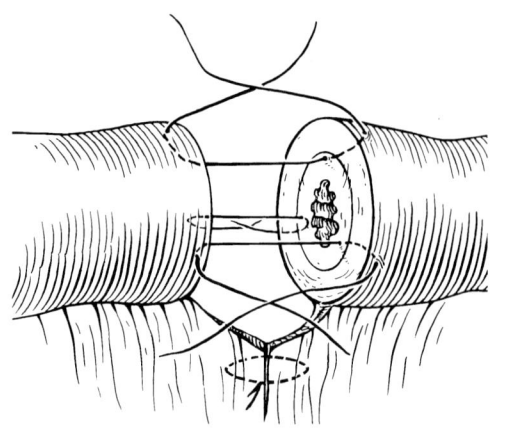

Fig. 30-10 Anastomosis of the resected isthmus. Bring the mesentery together by a suture, and hold each limb of the tube with a stabilization clamp. Use three sutures in the anastomosis, avoiding the lumen. This procedure requires optical magnification and previous experience.

Meticulous hemostasis is necessary. Sutures used to ligate the proximal end of the preserved tube until subsequent reimplantation may be absorbable or nonabsorbable (to prevent recanalization). Some advise contraception between the two stages of the procedure to avoid a repeat ectopic pregnancy in the isolated remaining tube.

Laparotomy for patient in shock

If the patient is in shock or impending shock, have her taken to the operating room at once and do a laparotomy directly while she is being transfused. Usually, general anesthesia with endotracheal intubation is preferred, for speed and better control, to epidural or spinal anesthesia. Enter the abdomen through a lower abdominal midline incision. On incising the peritoneum, one will find everything obscured with blood. Immediately put your hand into the pelvis, grasp the uterine fundus firmly, and pull up. This will enable one to find the site of the ectopic pregnancy and reduce bleeding. Avoid the temptation to reach in and pull up the ectopic site, which will tear tissue and exacerbate bleeding (Fig. 30-11).

Salpingectomy

The traditional operation for ectopic pregnancy, salpingectomy, is done if the patient is in shock, bleeding uncontrollably, has had the entire tube destroyed by a ruptured ectopic pregnancy, or is of mature age and has requested it, usually to effect sterilization. Place a series of overlapping curved Kelly clamps or small hemostats sequentially, beginning distally, across the mesosalpinx, and progressively cut segments of the mesosalpinx up to where the tube enters the uterus. Then replace the hemostatic clamps with a series of 3-0 absorbable polyglactin or polyglycolic acid suture ligatures (Fig. 30-12). In addition, place a figure-of-eight suture in the lateral uterine wall below the tube to occlude the branch from the uterine artery. Make the final cut of the proximal tube, either flush with the uterine wall or excising only a slight amount of the myometrial cornual angle, and close the uterus. Use the round ligament and its adjacent broad ligament to cover the uterine incision if desired.

Previously, cornual angle resection was done to prevent subsequent interstitial ectopic pregnancy. At present it is usually avoided, because interstitial ectopic pregnancy is rare, and because such resection weakens the uterine wall, which may rupture with subsequent uterine pregnancy.

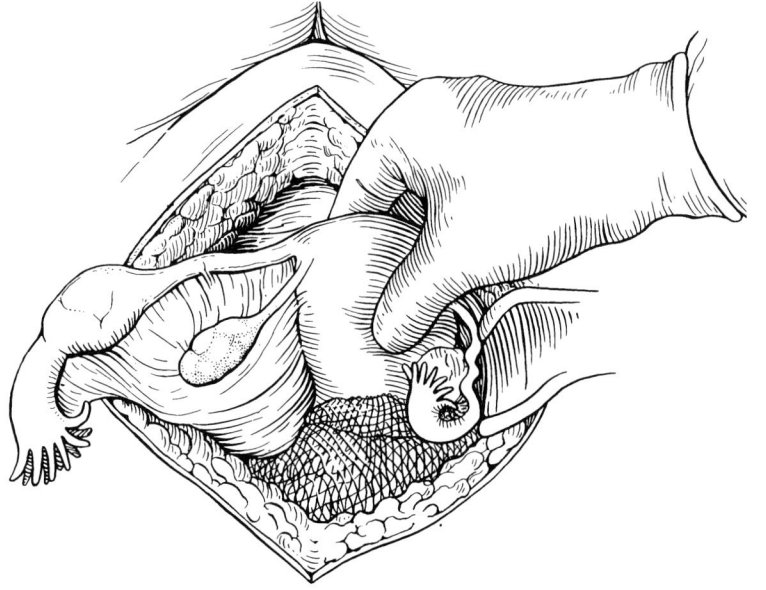

Fig. 30-11 Laparatomy for patient in shock. Hold the uterus to expose the pelvic structures. To avoid fragmentation and severe hemorrhage, refrain from pulling on the site of the tubal ectopic pregnancy. Place loose moist gauze packing or a shelf in the cul-de-sac to support the tube.

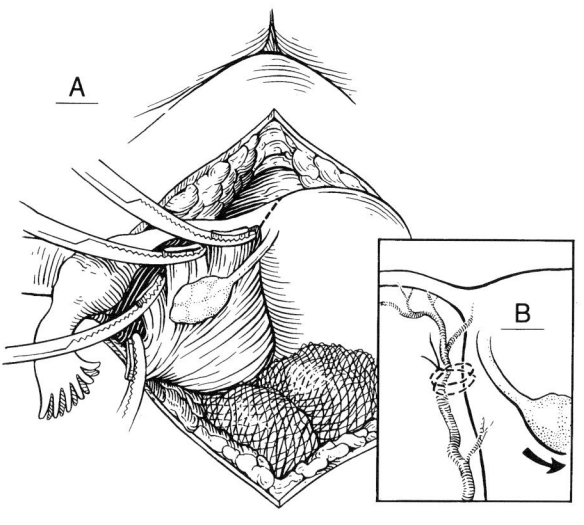

Fig. 30-12 Salpingectomy. (A) Place successive curved clamps on the mesosalpinx and tie off the mesosalpinx vessels following resection of the tube. (B) Tie the branch from the uterine artery below the cornual angle. Do not resect the cornual angle but cover it with the round ligament if desired.

Interstitial pregnancy

An interstitial pregnancy is difficult to diagnose early, especially as the normal pregnant uterus enlarges asymmetrically. There may be staining and localized tenderness. Transvaginal ultrasound can be used to make the diagnosis. Although diagnosis before rupture makes it easier to resect and preserve the uterus and distal tube, discovery may occur after a spontaneous rupture, with severe intra-abdominal bleeding and shock at 12 to 16 weeks from the LMP. In this case, immediate laparotomy is necessary for rupture. Although hysterectomy has been done, for the young patient a conservative procedure is preferred. On entering the peritoneal cavity, hold the uterus up forcefully for inspection and to reduce bleeding. Place a deep figure-of-eight heavy 0 or 2-0 suture in the side of the uterus below the rupture to occlude the branch from the uterine artery. Then excise the intramural cornual angle ectopic site and close the uterus with deep figure-of-eight absorbable 0 or 2-0 sutures on a heavy needle (Fig. 30-13). Clamp across both the proximal part of the tube distal to the interstitial pregnancy and the underlying mesentary to occlude the ovarian branch from the infundibulopelvic vessels. Then carefully ligate the vessels, leaving the distal tube in place (Fig. 30-14). Warn the patient of possible uterine rupture in future uterine pregnancy and probable need for later cesarean section.

For the unruptured case a nonsurgical alternative option for interstitial ectopic pregnancy to avoid weakening the uterine wall is considered. There may be direct injection of the ectopic site at laparoscopy, or when diagnosed by TU by an ultrasound-guided needle using methotrexate or potassium chloride. Systemic IM injection of methotrexate may be used. Another option is observation if the ectopic conceptus has spontaneously died. Nonsurgical options require careful observation.

Ovary and abdomen

About 97% of ectopic pregnancies are tubal. Ovarian sites account for only about 1%. We distinguish between an aborted tubal pregnancy lying on an ovary, and a true ovarian pregnancy, usually in the corpus luteum. Try to preserve part of the ovary by wedge resection and by suturing with 3-0 or finer absorbable material.

For abdominal pregnancy, which is even rarer, remove the fetus and membranes. If the placenta is growing into intestine, cut the cord close and leave the placenta in place to avoid hemorrhage and bowel damage.

If the placenta is small and growing into the uterine serosal surface and bleeding is controlled, one may remove it carefully. However, this involves danger of severe hemorrhage, always the chief problem in abdominal pregnancy. There is always risk of immediate and late maternal morbidity and mortality.

An occasional variant is to leave the placenta in place and suture the membranes to the abdominal wall. However, a placenta so left may (especially if necrotic) later separate, become infected, or cause intestinal obstruction.

Very rarely, one may encounter a term abdominal pregnancy with the fetus relatively high in a transverse or oblique lie and the cervix uneffaced. Sonography is helpful for detection. Occasionally, a live baby is delivered at laparotomy.

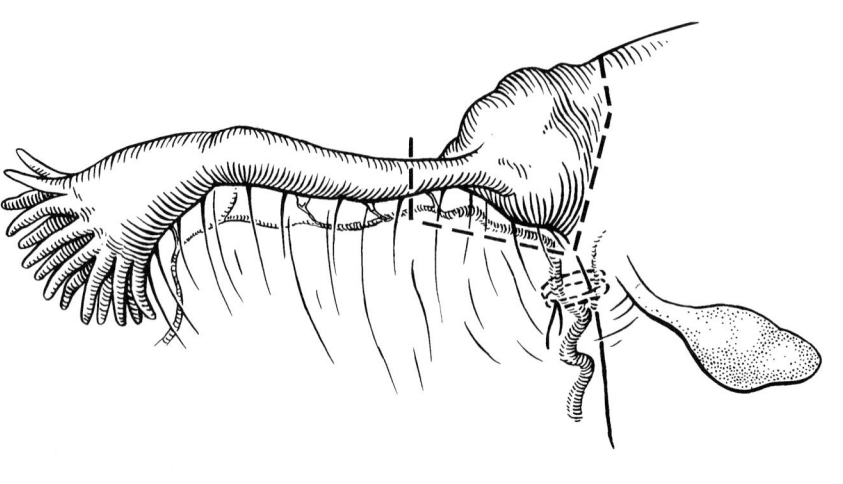

Fig. 30-13 Interstitial ectopic pregnancy. Do a cornual resection, close the uterus with deep figure-of-eight sutures, and ligate the branch of the uterine artery below the cornual angle.

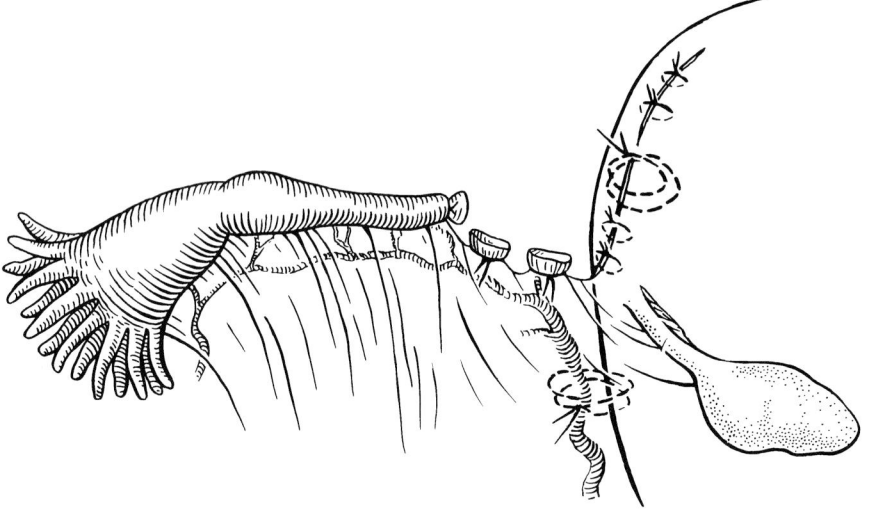

Fig. 30-14 Ligate the branches from the ovarian vessels in the mesosalpinx, close the superficial tissue of the cornual angle, and preserve the distal tube.

Rudimentary uterine horn and broad ligament

A pregnancy may also occur in a rudimentary uterine horn. Follow carefully any patient with a double uterus and cervix or a unicornuate uterus with a pregnancy on one side. When there is intraperitoneal bleeding, pain, and tenderness, do a laparotomy and remove the rudimentary horn.

In addition, ectopic pregnancy may develop in the leaves of the broad ligament, either directly or secondary to tubal rupture. Surgery should be individualized and should reflect concern about hemorrhage and the susceptibility of the ureter to surgical injury. Corrective procedures range from simple removal to unilateral salpingo-oophorectomy, or hysterectomy.

Cervical site and other rarities

The rarest ectopic pregnancy occurs in the cervix, which becomes soft and enlarged and bleeds readily, while fundal size remains normal. Curettage—to terminate a pregnancy or presumed incomplete abortion, or for diagnostic purposes—provokes violent bleeding and shock. Do gentle finger explo-

ration and attempt angle and circumferential suturing; consider Foley catheter balloon tamponade, angiographic uterine artery embolization, or packing. One may leave part of the placenta in place.

If hemorrhage cannot be stopped, one will usually have to do immediate laparotomy with bilateral hypogastric artery ligation, total abdominal hysterectomy, or both, together with transfusion. If one performs a hysterectomy, the dilated cervix will expose the ureters to surgical injury.

To avoid hazardous surgery in the stable patient, one may consider the option of nonsurgical treatment by systemic intramuscular methotrexate.

Early TU diagnosis before symptoms may permit dilatation and curettage of the cervix under abdominal ultrasound guidance without excessive bleeding (40).

Heterotopic pregnancies are rare, with only about 500 cases reported. They have significantly increased since 1988, because of in vitro fertilization. Trophoblastic neoplastic change of ectopic pregnancy, also unusual, had been verified in only 21 cases, as of 1988.

Possible additional measures

Once ectopic pregnancy surgery is completed, consider administration of Rh immunoglobulin to the unsensitized Rh-negative woman; prophylactic antibiotics; repeat quantitative serum β-hCG—it returns to normal in from one to 30 days, with a median of 5 to 8 days; and contraceptive advice.

Prophylactic ipsilateral ovariectomy, although once recommended, is no longer done because it does not reduce the chance of future ectopic pregnancy and because retaining both ovaries enhances the possibility of future in vitro fertilization. Rarely, severe rupture in an old tubo-ovarian inflammatory mass will make it necessary to remove both the ovary and the tube.

Operative laparoscopy

There has been a gradual increase in the use of laparoscopy for treatment as well as diagnosis. It was facilitated by the improvement in laparoscopy instrumentation and the general increased use of laparoscopy for treatment (for example, general surgeons doing laparoscopic cholecystectomies). Laparoscopy compared with laparotomy entails a shorter hospital stay (ambulatory or one day versus 4 or 5 days), results in a lower hospital bill, permits faster recovery and return to work, and gives a better cosmetic result.

The subsequent patency and pregnancy rates of laparoscopic salpingostomy and salpingectomy are comparable to those of the laparotomy procedures.

Of 976 patients who underwent laparoscopic salpingostomies reviewed in the literature from 1980 to 1992, 94% did not require additional therapy, 86% had patent tubes, 66% became pregnant, and 23% of those pregnant had a repeat ectopic pregnancy (39).

It should be pointed out that salpingostomy refers to incision of the fallopian tube and leaving it open. Salpingotomy means incision and then suturing the tubal incision closed. Unfortunately, some reports (usually from non-English-speaking countries) use the word "salpingotomy" when "salpingostomy" is the actual surgery.

In 1992 laparoscopic treatment of ectopic pregnancy was recommended (42).

The present operation of choice for unruptured ampullary ectopic pregnancy (the most common type) is laparoscopic linear salpingostomy without suturing (39,43). There is a satisfactorily rapid learning curve in resident training (44).

One of the factors in laparoscopy that is often not emphasized is the use of the videocamera and screen. This allows the assistant to function spontaneously without constant redirection, permits an audience to view the procedure, permits recording by inexpensive videotape, and magnifies the operative site. It may distort color and decrease the sharpness of image. Laparoscopy requires reeducation of hand-eye coordination and new hand-maneuver skills.

Despite early diagnosis giving the option of nonsurgical management of unruptured ectopic tubal ampullary pregnancy, most gynecologists and most patients prefer laparoscopic surgery as a more immediate, reliable, and less anxiety-producing approach. Surgery is preferred in the patient who cannot be followed closely, for example, because of travel, or for the patient who is not reliable. There is general agreement that if laparoscopy is done for diagnosis, it should also be used for treatment. Nonsurgical therapy is avoided for ectopic pregnancies larger than 4 cm, cardiac activity in the ectopic fetus, and acute intra-abdominal bleeding (39).

Even proponents of methotrexate therapy indicate that only about one third of women with ectopic pregnancies are eligible for this medical treatment (39).

Contraindications to operative laparoscopy usually include the following:

1 Hemodynamically unstable patient, shock.
2 a. Ectopic pregnancy over 4 cm (some limit it up to 6 cm) (43).
   b. Interstitial (and abdominal) ectopic pregnancy.
   c. Hemoperitoneum over 500 ml (some go up to 2000 ml; (43).
   d. hCG over 20,000 IU/L.
3 Extensive pelvic adhesions, marked obesity, technical difficulties.
4 Inadequate surgical experience or operator preference.
5 Lack of equipment.

Laparoscopic salpingostomy parallels the laparotomy procedure.

Bruhat and Pouly (43) use two suprapubic trocars: on the ectopic side (5 mm) a grip forceps is inserted, and on the opposite side (8 mm) a Triton (Microfrance) 7-mm-diameter specially designed instrument is used. It contains an 0.8-mm pressure lavage channel, an insulated retractable monopolar electrode needle, and a 5-mm aspiration channel. The tube is held just proximal to the ectopic site. A 19-gauge spinal needle is pushed through the abdominal wall, and diluted vasopressin is injected into the mesosalpinx at the proximal end of the tube and along the infundibulopelvic ligament. A linear antimesenteric incision is made through to the tubal lumen with a light needle electrofulguration touch. Trophoblastic tissue is removed by lavage, suction, and, if necessary, a scoop or forceps.

Suturing the tubal incision closed (salpingotomy) is not done because it makes no difference in healing and is technically difficult.

Unilateral twin ectopic pregnancy can be managed by laparoscopic salpingostomy (45).

A very small ectopic pregnancy may be obscured by diluted vasopressin injection. In cases of apparent complete tubal abortion, the presence of a hematosalpinx may indicate residual proximal trophoblast. Clinically significant residual trophoblast occurs in about 16% of cases of only tubal "milking" rather than tubal incision, or with very large ectopic pregnancies. Postoperative serum quantitative β-hCG titers are determined until the level is normal. Treatment failure may be detected early if there is no significant decrease of hCG levels (ideally to less than 12%) by the second or third postoperative day. Bruhat and Pouly noted that failures occurred with a hematosalpinx ectopic mass larger than 4 cm, usually greater than 6 cm; with a large hemoperitoneum over 2000 ml; with a high hCG (over 20,000 IU/L); and with transfimbrial "milking" (43).

After conservative surgery, serum β-hCG levels may persist for 12 days because of gradual urinary clearance. The level is observed until it returns to a normal nonpregnant level. If it persists for more than 12 days and then plateaus, or if there are symptoms, then further therapy is needed (46).

One report indicated that after laser laparoscopy an average time of 3 to 4 weeks was necessary for the hCG level to fall to nondetectable levels (47).

Persistent ectopic pregnancy occurred in 15.5% of those undergoing laparoscopy salpingostomy versus in 1.8% of those undergoing laparotomy salpingostomy for intact ampullary ectopic pregnancy (46). Predictive laparoscopy factors were smaller ectopic size and fewer days of amenorrhea. Associated but not predictive factors were histologic absence of products of conception and less frequent hemoperitoneum (more than 50 ml of blood). Incidental factors in that series of laparoscopies were greater use of dilute vasopressin and of laser (rather than electrocautery). All of the persistent ectopic pregnancies were treated successfully by various options (salpingostomy, salpingectomy, methotrexate). Seifer and colleagues concluded that methotrexate as second-line therapy for persistent ectopic pregnancy "allows laparoscopy to remain the preferred surgical approach for the treatment of intact ampullary ectopic pregnancy" (48,49).

It is thought that persistent hCG after salpingostomy is due to a combination of incomplete evacuation of the tubal lumen trophoblast and trophoblast infiltration of the tubal wall. Low-dose oral methotrexate was successful in 15 of 16 cases, with a mean decline of serum hCG to nonpregnant levels in 24 days. Methotrexate (15 mg) was given on days 1, 3, and 5, and citrovorum factor (30 mg) was given on days 2, 4, and 6 (49).

There is no standard definition of *persistent ectopic pregnancy*. One definition is "continued growth of trophoblastic tissue requiring additional treatment after salpingostomy" (46). The need for treatment depends on the physician's anxiety regarding levels of postoperative persistent serum hCG. Some define persistent ectopic pregnancy as increasing β-hCG titers after conservative surgery. With this definition, 19 women were given ambulatory treatment with a single intramuscular injection of methotrexate in a dose of 50 mg/m² (mean dose 80 mg, range 50 to 100 mg). Although β-hCG lev-

els increased the first 3 days afterward, they subsequently declined gradually to a level below 10 IU/L within 18 to 53 days (mean 29 days). Two cases required hospital observation, and one of these had self-limiting hemoperitoneum requiring two transfusions. Therefore close surveillance is required for the rare delayed hemorrhage (50). Repeat surgery is required for active intra-abdominal bleeding.

In the young patient laparoscopic salpingostomy (conservative surgery) is preferred to laparoscopic salpingectomy (radical surgery). The latter may be required for uncontrollable bleeding, hemodynamic instability, second ectopic pregnancy in the same tube, ruptured ectopic pregnancy with irreparably damaged tube, or sterilization. For salpingectomy three suprapubic trocars are recommended: a grip forceps (on the side of the ectopic), a scissors, and a bipolar coagulator (or thermocoagulator). Retrograde successive coagulation and cutting are used (43).

It is possible to perform extracorporeal laparoscopic salpingectomy with only diagnostic equipment through a small suprapubic incision if there is a mobile tube (51).

For isthmus ectopic pregnancies, the tubal segment is usually resected, although occasionally salpingostomy is successful.

Ectopic pregnancy treated at the Mayo Clinic by laparotomy from 1976 to 1985 showed a 68% subsequent fertility with term pregnancy whether treated by salpingostomy or by salpingectomy if there was no previous history of infertility. With a history of infertility, the subsequent fertility was only 25% for salpingostomy and 11% for salpingectomy. The risk of recurrent ectopic pregnancy also was associated with previous infertility: salpingostomy without infertility had a 14% rate, while with infertility there was a 31% rate. The corresponding rates for salpingectomy were 5% and 22%. Thus a previous history of infertility was the most significant factor for fertility potential after surgery for ectopic pregnancy (52).

A Cleveland Clinic study found no difference in future pregnancy rates between laparoscopy and laparotomy surgery for ectopic pregnancy. Those with a normal fertility history had a fourfold higher pregnancy rate than those with a history of infertility (53).

A report from France showed that following laparoscopic salpingostomy the intrauterine pregnancy rate was 67% and the recurrent ectopic rate was 12%. Future fertility and risk of recurrent ectopic pregnancy depended on previous infertility history, ipsilateral adhesions, and the contralateral tubal status (54).

Laparoscopic salpingostomy yielded a 60% subsequent intrauterine pregnancy rate, and salpingectomy gave a similar 54% rate. These are similar to laparotomy rates. When divided according to history of previous tubal damage, the rates for the two laparoscopy procedures were similar for subsequent intrauterine pregnancy: 79% without tubal damage and 42% with tubal damage (55).

Thus there is general agreement that with regard to future fertility the preexisting condition of the tubes is more important than the type of surgery.

Although gamete intrafallopian transfer (GIFT) is associated with an increased risk of ectopic pregnancy, when done in women with a previous ectopic pregnancy with tubes in reasonable condition, the incidence of repeat ectopic pregnancy was no higher than that of infertile women who had a GIFT procedure (6.9%). GIFT has a higher pregnancy rate than in vitro fertilization (56).

If the tube is unsuitable for GIFT, then in vitro fertilization is recommended. Patients have to be monitored for ectopic and heterotopic pregnancy.

Nonsurgical management

According to Stovall, "without doubt, conservative surgical management of ectopic pregnancy remains the mainstay of treatment worldwide" (46).

Nevertheless, if ectopic pregnancy can be diagnosed early before it is too large, before an acute complication, and without laparoscopy, then aside from the traditional surgical treatment (laparoscopy or laparotomy), there are new options of medical management or expectant management.

An empiric, relative pretherapeutic predictive score was developed using six criteria, each measured on a scale of one to three: gestational age, hCG level, progesterone level, abdominal pain, hemoperitoneum value, and hematosalpinx (size of ectopic embryo). A score of 12 or less gave nonsurgical management a success rate of 82%, while a higher score had a 50% rate. The choice between different nonsurgical approaches did not influence the success rate. Despite embryo cardiac activity, nonsurgical treatment is possible with a low score (57).

Medical therapy for ectopic pregnancy usually involves the use of methotrexate in systemic fashion (by intramuscular or intravenous injection or orally) or in local fashion with direct injection into the ectopic site (by TU guidance, laparoscopic-guided injection, or retrograde tubal lumen injection). Only rarely have other medications been used (potassium chloride, hyperosmolar glucose, prostaglandins, and RU-486).

According to Stovall and Ling, "when compared with other treatment protocols available at this time, single-dose intramuscular methotrexate appears to be the best alternative to laparoscopic surgery" (58).

Carson and Buster (39) advise limiting methotrexate to hemodynamically stable cases, with unruptured ectopic pregnancies without acute intra-abdominal bleeding of 4 cm or smaller by ultrasound, without ectopic cardiac activity, and in whom laparoscopy is not needed for diagnosis.

Stovall and Ling (58) have a 3.5-cm size limit. They excluded those that did not desire future fertility, had a twofold elevation of hepatic serum aspartate aminotransferase, had a white blood cell count under $2000/cm^3$, had a platelet count under 100,000, or had a serum creatinine level over 1.5 mg/dl.

Cardiac activity in the ectopic embryo was not considered a contraindication in their series; however, it still "continues to represent a relative contraindication" (58). Their diagnostic algorithm was similar to that of Carson and Buster (39; Fig. 30-1) and was made without laparoscopy using serial hCG titers, serum progesterone, TU, and uterine curettage. Subsequent experience showed that competent TU can identify a viable intrauterine pregnancy with the usual hCG level of 750 to 1000 mIU/ml (and certainly by 2000 mIU/ml to be cautious), thereby reducing the need for curettage.

The single-dose IM methotrexate study of Stovall and Ling (58) is the newest, largest, and best available. Of 270 cases of ectopic pregnancy, 121 or 44.8% were treated with methotrexate. The following were excluded: 24.1% with tubal rupture, 3.6% who did not desire future fertility, 21.5% with a larger than 3.5 cm ectopic embryo in greatest dimension, and 3.3% who elected laparoscopic surgery. They used the protocol in Table 30-5 (58).

Following diagnostic workup, on day 1 (treatment initiation) a repeat hCG was done and one injection of methotrexate (50 mg/m², IM) without citrovorum factor rescue was given on an ambulatory basis. The hCG tests were repeated on days 4 and 7. If there was more than a 15% decline in hCG titers between days 4 and 7, weekly titers were determined until less than 12 mIU/ml. If the decline

Table 30-5 Summary of the methotrexate regimens used

Regimen	Monitor
Multiple-dose (46) Methotrexate, 1 mg/kg of body weight IM every other day (days 1, 3, and so on)	Serum β-hCG levels weekly until undetectable; blood count, platelet count, liver-enzyme levels
Leucovorin, 0.1 mg/kg IM every other day (days 2, 4, and so on)	
Continue treatment until β-hCG levels drop ≥ 15% in 48 hours or 4 doses of methotrexate have been given	
One-dose (58) Methotrexate, 50 mg/m² of body-surface area IM No leucovorin	Serum β-hCG level days 4 and 7, then weekly until undetectable; initial blood count, platelet count, liver-enzyme levels

Adapted from Carson SA, Buster JE. Ectopic pregnancy. N Engl J Med 1993;329:1174–1181.

was less than 15% between days 4 and 7, then a second similar dose of methotrexate was given.

In 59.2% lower abdominal pain was exacerbated after treatment initiation. Four patients were hospitalized overnight for observation and spontaneously improved. The hematocrit and ultrasound were stable.

There was only one original diagnostic pelvic examination, which was never repeated to avoid iatrogenic rupture. Transient pain may occur in 3 to 7 days, lasting 4 to 12 hours, and may be due to tubal abortion. According to Carson and Buster, "perhaps the most difficult aspect of methotrexate therapy is learning to distinguish the transient abdominal pain of successful therapy from that of a rupturing ectopic pregnancy" (39).

Interestingly, in 85.8% the hCG titers increased between days 1 and 4, but only 3.3% had a rising titer between days 4 and 7 requiring a second dose of methotrexate. Of the 121 treated cases, 113 were successfully treated with a mean time to resolution of 35.5 ± 11.8 (8 to 76) days. Seven (5.8%) required surgical management. Of those who desired subsequent pregnancy, 79.6% were successful, and of these, 87.2% were intrauterine and 12.8% were repeat ectopic pregnancies. The failure rate and subsequent reproductive outcome were similar to those with conservative laparoscopic surgery (58). There were only minimal or no side effects of methotrexate.

Thus single-dose methotrexate is as effective as the previously reported multidose regimen. With single-dose methotrexate there is less used, no need for citrovorum recovery, less follow-up and cost, and virtually no side effects (58).

There was no way to predict those who would fail methotrexate therapy since "all treatment failures had falling hCG titers" (57). Routine TU follow-up was not done because hematomas may develop and there can be an increase in ectopic pregnancy size and cul-de-sac fluid (58). Unfortunately, the authors did not study posttreatment pain with ultrasound.

There was a case report of an asymptomatic 10-cm septated hematosalpinx forming after a single IM injection of methotrexate (50 mg/m^2, IM) despite a negative serum hCG and color Doppler analysis. Thus, an apparently closed tube on posttreatment hysterosalpingogram may in fact be an hematosalpinx (59).

In another report following methotrexate treatment, in 10 of 18 cases the mass enlarged during therapy, but this did not predict treatment failure. In seven cases the mass persisted after the hCG became negative (60).

Previously Stovall used multiple-dose methotrexate IM as primary treatment, with 1 mg/kg daily followed by citrovorum factor (0.1 mg/kg/day IM) on alternate days until the hCG titer began to drop (46; Table 30-5).

A review of 306 patients with ectopic pregnancies treated with systemic methotrexate compares favorably with laparoscopic salpingostomy: 94% were treated successfully, 71% became pregnant, and of these 11% had repeat ectopic pregnancies (39).

Single-dose IM methotrexate can be used for persistent ectopic pregnancy as well as for primary treatment.

Oral methotrexate is effective for persistent ectopic pregnancy after salpingostomy, but it is uncertain as primary treatment (46).

Laparoscopy-guided single injection of 25 mg of methotrexate directly into the tubal pregnancy was reported in 77 cases in Israel. This represented 38.5% of 200 ectopic pregnancies with laparoscopically proved unruptured tubal pregnancy. The selection basis was 3 cm or smaller mass and no active bleeding. The authors did not specify whether the injection was by an independent needle or a needle through the laparoscope. There was a failure in 16 of the 77 patients, who required subsequent surgery. The later fertility was comparable to that with IM methotrexate, and with laparoscopy and laparotomy salpingostomy (61).

Among 10 women with laparoscopy-guided methotrexate injection (50 mg in 2 ml) of the ectopic site, 7 had further rising or plateau hCG titers for the following 2 to 7 days (62).

In general, in the United States methotrexate is not used when laparoscopy is done because salpingostomy is recommended at the time. If for some reason salpingostomy could not be done, then methotrexate injection would be considered.

A report from France described 100 cases treated by primary transvaginal injection of methotrexate into the ectopic site under ultrasound control. This represented 42% of all ectopic cases. The dose was 1 mg/kg. There were 83 cures; however, of these, 28 required another dose of IM methotrexate. Among the 17 failures, 4 required emergency salpingectomy for hemoperitoneum, and 13 had laparoscopy surgery because of inadequate regression of hCG. Three patients developed stomatitis after two or more injections of methotrexate. The success rate was highest (92.8%) when the initial hCG level was less than 5000 mIU/mL and when the empiric pretherapeutic score was less than 12.

Of 11 cases involving ectopic cardiac activity, 7 were successfully treated. In the weeks following treatment, there was a transient rise in hCG titer (peak at 4 to 6 days), and some had the onset of unexplained lower abdominal pain. The subsequent fertility was comparable to that with IM methotrexate (63).

My viewpoint is that because the success rate was only 83%, 27.7% required a second dose of IM methotrexate, and transvaginal injection requires special skill (and must have a minimal risk), it is much simpler to use the one dose of IM methotrexate.

A multicenter report from Europe described transcervical tubal cannulation and intraluminal methotrexate injection (up to 50 mg) under fluoroscopic or ultrasound control in 31 cases. There was resolution in 27 cases (87%), with surgery required in 4 cases. Subsequent fertility was satisfactory (64). Another study of 40 cases was successful in

70%; despite declining hCG levels, tubal rupture occurred in 2 cases (65).

Despite this novel approach, IM methotrexate is still a simpler treatment.

Cornual (interstitial) and heterotopic ectopic pregnancy

Cornual (interstitial) uterine ectopic pregnancies may continue development for 12 to 16 weeks before rupture because of a thicker wall than in the usual tubal ectopic pregnancy. When rupture occurs, however, hemorrhage may be severe because larger vessels are torn. The standard treatment is laparotomy with a cornual resection.

In view of the significant weakenings of the uterus by surgical resection with resultant danger of rupture in subsequent pregnancy and the need for later cesarean section, nonsurgical management seems to be a new and very reasonable alternative for the unruptured cornual pregnancy in the young patient. It is true that there is no long-term follow-up, particularly for the residual lesion; still, it seems that the nonsurgical approach would result in less weakening of the uterus. Nevertheless, subsequent cesarean section should still be considered. Of course, nonsurgical management requires continued close monitoring.

Early diagnosis is possible by TU that shows an empty uterine cavity and a separate sac enclosed by a thin layer of myometrium.

Four cases of cornual pregnancy managed nonsurgically and successfully and followed with TU for 47 to 64 weeks were reported from the Ultrasound Division of Columbia Presbyterian Medical Center in New York (66).

In two cases of cornual pregnancy (8 and 10 weeks of gestational age) with inadequate development and low hCG, expectant management was used. Serial TU with color Dopper flow showed the lesion diameters (outer edges of hyperechoic [trophoblastic] ring) to be 1.9 and 2.7 cm. It took 70 and 105 days, respectively, for the hCG levels to return to normal. Nevertheless, the lesions were still present at 1.6 cm 47 weeks after LMP, and at 1.3 cm 64 weeks after LMP. Both cases had resumption of menses, after 3 and 10 weeks, respectively.

In one case with a 2-cm lesion at 7 weeks' gestational age with a developing (live) cornual ectopic pregnancy, 25 mg of methotrexate was injected directly in 1-ml solution with a 21-gauge needle with constant ultrasound guidance. It took 35 days for the hCG level to become normal, however. At 47 weeks after LMP, the lesion was still 1.7 cm. Normal menses returned after 5 weeks.

In one patient with a heterotopic intrauterine and cornual pregnancy, 0.5 ml of potassium chloride (2 mEq/ml) was injected into a 3.5-cm lesion at 9 weeks' gestational age. The hCG level returned to normal in 42 days, but a 1.7-cm lesion was still present 64 weeks after LMP. Normal menses

resumed after 2 weeks. (This was confusing and may have been in error because the intrauterine pregnancy apparently carried.)

The authors recommended, as an alternative to cornual resection, constant TU-guided puncture (salpingocentris) of the early (6 to 8 menstrual weeks) developing cornual ectopic pregnancy with methotrexate, which gives the fastest reduction of hCG. For nonliving cornual ectopic embryos, observation with serial hCG levels and TU was recommended (66).

It was interesting that there were brief initial increases in hCG levels with a tendency to increases in lesion size. It was unexpected that the lesions persisted throughout the time of observation despite resumption of normal menses (66).

Interstitial ectopic pregnancy was successfully treated in one case by methotrexate instillation through the tubal ostium by hysteroscopy (67).

Six cases of interstitial (cornual) ectopic pregnancies were treated by systemic methotrexate (15 mg IM daily for 5 days) or with local injection of 1 mg/kg. Four were successful and two required surgery. In the successful cases the patients had patent tubes at follow-up (68).

Two cases of interstitial pregnancy, one of which was heterotopic, were confirmed 31 and 34 days after in vitro fertilization. Transvaginal-ultrasound-guided injection of methotrexate (and potassium chloride for the heterotopic pregnancy) was uneventful. The woman with an intrauterine pregnancy delivered a 3350-g healthy child at 39 weeks (69).

A report from France described six cases of heterotopic pregnancy with nonsurgical treatment (70). Heterotopic pregnancy is a simultaneous intrauterine and ectopic pregnancy. It has been increasing with assisted reproductive technology associated with multiple ovulation induction, multiple embryos, infertility, and salpingitis. In addition, previously unrecognized cases with spontaneous resolution of the ectopic pregnancy are being discovered with early TU surveillance. These factors explain the difference in incidence from 1 in 30,000 deliveries to 1 in 3000 deliveries. This explains how one hospital had 25 (4.8%) heterotopic pregnancies in 525 ectopic pregnancies in about 7 years. Of the 25 heterotopic cases, six patients with ectopic masses under 3 cm were selected for nonsurgical management: three with selective embryo reduction and three with expectant observation. Of the six, four were cornual heterotopic pregnancies. Three cornual pregnancies had TU-guided needle aspiration and injection of potassium chloride (2 mEq/2 ml) with live embryos. The hCG levels ranged from 15,000 to 25,205 mIU/ml. The cornual ectopic embryos "degenerated" in 6 weeks (range 4 to 7 weeks). Two patients had later spontaneous abortions, and one had a term normal spontaneous delivery. One cornual ectopic patient with an hCG level of 25,000 mIU/ml was managed expectantly (small sac, asymptomatic, no cardiac activity in the embryo) and also had a normal delivery.

Although their policy was laparoscope surgery for the tubal heterotopic pregnancy, two patients were managed expectantly. One was successful, with a term normal delivery. The other had a salpingectomy for pain despite the absence of hemoperitoneum.

There was another case report of successful potassium chloride embryo reduction in an interstitial heterotopic pregnancy with a later normal delivery (71).

Cervix pregnancy

A 5-week cervical pregnancy was successfully treated with four doses of oral methotrexate (1 mg/kg), one every other day, alternating with leucovorin rescue (0.1 mg/kg). A transvaginal sonogram on day 40 still showed a gestational sac despite a negative hCG level. The latter dropped precipitously starting on day 7. Color Doppler analysis showed decreased blood flow. Subsequent suction curettage was uneventful. There have been seven previous cases of methotrexate treatment, in three of which methotrexate was the only therapy. In two cases the cervix was later instrumented. In two cases with gestational size over 12 weeks, laparotomy was required: one with a hysterectomy and one with hypogastric artery ligation. Methotrexate was recommended as the initial treatment of choice for first-trimester cervical pregnancy (72).

Another case was treated with actinomycin D (73).

Ovarian ectopic pregnancy

Ovarian pregnancy is difficult to diagnose and may simulate or be present in a corpus luteum hemorrhagic cyst. A 4-cm ectopic mass was resected at laparotomy (74). A 1.5-cm ovarian ectopic mass was resected with ovarian preservation by laparoscopic unipolar coagulation scissors (75). Ovarian ectopic pregnancy has also been successfully treated with methotrexate (76).

Other medications, local injections

Randomized laparoscopic injection of hyperosmolar glucose solution (10–20 ml of 50% glucose) into an unruptured tubal pregnancy gave results comparable to those with salpingostomy. When hCG levels were less than 5000 mIU/ml and there was no cardiac activity, 13 of 14 cases were successful. In their cases of persistent ectopic pregnancy, it was difficult to find the small amount of residual trophoblastic tissue with relaparoscopy. They recommended systemic methotrexate rather than relaparoscopy repeat salpingostomy (77).

Randomized methotrexate and prostaglandin sulprostone were equally effective by transvaginal injection and systemic administration and gave best results with an hCG less than 5000 mIU/ml (78).

Laparoscopically guided injection of 5 mg of prostaglandin $F_{2\alpha}$ diluted in 9 ml of sodium chloride was in-

jected into tubal ectopic pregnancies in 18 cases with success in 12 cases. With an exclusion of those with hCG levels over 2500 mU/ml, the success rate was 84.6%. "Salpingotomy" (probably salpingostomy) was done in six cases because of rising hCG levels (79).

Direct injection of prostaglandin $F_{2\alpha}$ causes tubular muscle contraction and vasoconstriction. It was successful in only 50 of 71 cases in a dose of 7.5 to 10 mg, and it may have side effects after intratubal injection (39).

Expectant management or careful observation relies on the fact that a significant percentage of ectopic embryos will spontaneously die and resorb. Cases for consideration require a rapidly falling hCG level and hemodynamic stability. Some limit the hCG level to less than or equal to 250 mIU/ml, and to a size of less than or equal to 2 cm, less than or equal to 3 cm, or less than 4 cm.

There is no reliable marker to indicate which ectopic pregnancies will spontaneously resolve. All cases require close observation until the hCG level becomes normal (80). Even then rupture may occur with a low or negative hCG. Carson says, "until a marker exists that identifies which ectopic pregnancies are destined to resolve, observation is probably better replaced by methotrexate treatment" (81).

Spontaneous resolution occurred in 13 patients representing 24% of all ectopic pregnancies. The hCG was less than 1000 IU/L, the size ranged from 1 to 3.5 cm, three had a gestational sac, the hCG became undetectable in 3 to 45 days (mean 15.8 days), and there was complete resolution on ultrasound in 10 to 63 days (mean 30 days). Spontaneous resolution is not uncommon and tends to occur in early and less vascular ectopic pregnancies. Four had transient increase in size and vascularity (81).

Expectant management was used in 83 ectopic pregnancies, representing 26% of all. Spontaneous resolution occurred in 57 cases (69%). Laparoscopy was done in 26 cases because of symptoms or a rise in hCG level after observation for one to 18 days. There was one tubal rupture requiring salpingectomy. The selection criteria were a decreasing hCG level, diameter less than 4 cm, and no rupture or acute bleeding or TU. Repeated sonography and hCG tests are necessary (82).

Both expectant management (12 of 16 successful) and local transvaginal injection of methotrexate or sulprostone (23 of 33 successful) in successful cases resulted in future fertility potential similar to that with surgery (83).

Summary

Extraordinary changes have occurred in the diagnosis and management of ectopic pregnancy. Because of early and increasing sexual activity and sexually transmitted diseases, the number of young patients with ectopic pregnancies continues to increase. There have been dramatic increases in the rare but more dangerous extratubal ectopic pregnancies (cornual [interstitial], cervical, abdominal, and ovarian) and also in the very rare heterotopic (simultaneous intrauterine and ectopic) pregnancies. These unusual varieties are associated with assisted reproductive technology with induced multiple ovulations and embryos and in vitro fertilization combined with previous salpingitis, salpingoplasty, and ectopic pregnancy.

There has been an increase in early diagnosis because of greater physician awareness (consideration of ectopic pregnancy in differential diagnosis in the adolescent) and patient awareness, with early surveillance (especially in high-risk cases) and liberal use of serum quantitative β-hCG. Whereas previously most ectopic pregnancies were diagnosed after an acute rupture, currently most are found before rupture.

Although transvaginal ultrasound was not used previously, it has now replaced transabdominal pelvic ultrasound as standard care. The latter required an hCG titer of 6000 mIU/ml before a normal intrauterine sac could be verified. In addition, it had the discomfort and wasted time associated with the need for a full bladder. The TU can reveal the normal intrauterine sac with an hCG level of 750 to 1000 mIU/ml and, to be even more cautious, certainly with twice the level at 2000 mIU/ml. It has the advantage of the speed and lack of discomfort of the empty bladder. The absence of an intrauterine sac with the appropriate hCG level suggests an ectopic pregnancy outside the uterine cavity. Furthermore, TU gives better definition of the ectopic sac than does pelvic ultrasound. From a research viewpoint, color flow and Doppler waveform analysis can make the TU even more reliable, especially in considering and in monitoring expectant management.

With early diagnosis before rupture there will be a continuing decrease in the mortality rate and a greater use of conservative surgery of salpingostomy rather than "radical" salpingectomy and consideration of the option of nonsurgical management.

Less than 10 years ago laparotomy salpingostomy was the preferred treatment. Now the treatment of choice is laparoscopy salpingostomy. This change is related to early diagnosis, improved laparoscopy technology, and improved physician training. If laparoscopy is done for diagnosis, then laparoscopic salpingostomy should be done at the same time. Laparotomy is still used in cases of hemodynamic instability, technical difficulty with laparoscopy, large ectopic cornual (interstitial) resection, abdominal pregnancy, or to help control bleeding from cervical pregnancy.

If for some reason at laparoscopy an operative procedure cannot be done and the patient is stable, consideration may be given to injection of methotrexate or potassium chloride into the ectopic site (tubal, interstitial, or abdominal).

It is now recognized that there is a greater incidence of "persistent ectopic pregnancy" (usually meaning persistent hCG level) after laparoscopy salpingostomy than after laparotomy salpingostomy. Nevertheless, with systemic methotrexate treatment available, the laparoscopy procedure is still the method of choice. It does mean that closer follow-up is required after laparoscopy and, with it, a judgment call. Subsequent fertility is comparable with laparoscopic and laparotomy salpingostomy.

Early diagnosis of the small unruptured ectopic pregnancy permits consideration of the option of nonsurgical approaches not previously available. These include systemic or local injection of methotrexate and local injection of potassium chloride or hyperosmotic dextrose. Of all of these medical (nonsurgical) management options, the one-dose intramuscular methotrexate method is preferred. It is simple and safe and is comparable to salpingostomy for later fertility. The disadvantage is the frequent transient increase in hCG level and pain and perhaps ectopic enlargement a few days later. One cannot predict the unsuccessful case that might rupture because it could occur despite falling hCG levels. Careful clinical judgment is required for differentiating the frequent benign transient pain (lasting up to 12 hours, with no fall in hematocrit, no increase in culde-sac fluid, and no hemodynamic change) from acute rupture, which requires surgery. Hospitalization may be necessary for a day of observation.

Another type of nonsurgical management is the new option of expectant management for presumed spontaneous embryo demise. Although not unusual, it is difficult to predict, and therefore most tend to "overtreat," often with IM methotrexate.

The previous standard treatment of cornual (interstitial) ectopic pregnancy was laparotomy with surgical excision. This left a residual weakness that might rupture in a subsequent pregnancy and would require a cesarean section. The purpose was to avoid the life-threatening classic midtrimester rupture which might require a hysterectomy. If cornual pregnancy is diagnosed early by surveillance TU, then nonsurgical medical management is the new and ideal approach. This is a completely new concept. Rather than rely on expectant management (based on small size, lack of cardiac activity, low hCG level), most would recommend the one-dose IM methotrexate therapy with close observation. This is easier than TU-guided methotrexate needle injection.

The rare cervix ectopic pregnancy may cause severe bleeding and may require a hysterectomy. Early diagnosis permits the options of curettage and related surgery, expectant management if the embryo has died, or methotrexate with possible later curettage. Direct local injection of methotrexate might provoke bleeding, and therefore the one-dose IM regimen might be safer. The medical management of cervix ectopic pregnancy is a new concept.

Single-dose IM methotrexate is a reasonable option for early abdominal or ovarian ectopic pregnancies.

For heterotopic pregnancy methotrexate is avoided both in IM and direct injection forms. For early, small, unruptured heterotopic tubal pregnancy, laparoscopic salpingostomy is the treatment of choice. This is also true for ovarian (cystectomy) and abdominal heterotopic pregnancies. For early heterotopic cornual (interstitial) pregnancy, although expectant management is an option if the embryo seems dead, most would not wish to take the risk and would advise injection of potassium chloride, probably by a transvaginal route guided by ultrasound. Late diagnosis with rupture results in severe hemorrhage and loss of the intrauterine pregnancy. Early diagnosis with prophylactic embryo reduction gives a reasonable chance of continuing the intrauterine pregnancy and allowing a vaginal term delivery. Again this is a completely new approach.

References

1 Centers for Disease Control. Ectopic pregnancy—United States, 1988–1989. MMWR 1992;41(32):591–594.

2 Centers for Disease Control. Ectopic pregnancy—United States, 1987. MMWR 1990;39(24):401–404.

3 Cartwright PS. Incidence, epidemiology, risk factors, and etiology. In: Stovall TG, Ling FW, eds. Extrauterine pregnancy, clinical diagnosis and management. New York: McGraw-Hill, 1993:27–63.

4 Atrash HK, Friede A, Hogue C. Ectopic pregnancy mortality in the United States, 1970–1983. Obstet Gynecol 1987;70(6):817–822.

5 ACOG. Ectopic pregnancy. Am Coll Obstet Gynecol Technical Bulletin 1990;150:1–7.

6 Achiron R, Tadmor O, Kamar R, Aboulafia Y, Diamant Y. Prerupture ultrasound diagnosis of interstitial and rudimentary uterine horn pregnancy in the second trimester. J Reprod Med 1992;37(1):89–92.

7 Washington AE, Katz P. Ectopic pregnancy in the United States: economic consequences and payment source trends. Obstet Gynecol 1993;81:287–292.

8 Maruri F, Azziz R. Laparoscopic surgery for ectopic pregnancies: technology assessment and public health implications. Fertil Steril 1993;59(3):487–498.

9 Hillis SD, Joesoef R, Marchbanks PA, Wasserheit JN, Cates W Jr, Westrom L. Delayed care of pelvic inflammatory disease as a risk factor for impaired fertility. Am J Obstet Gynecol 1993:168(5):1503–1509.

10 Maccato M, Estrada R, Hammill H, Faro S. Prevalence of active Chlamydia trachomatis infection at the time of exploratory laparotomy for ectopic pregnancy. Obstet Gynecol 1992;79(2):211–213.

11 Westrom L, Joesoef R, Reynolds G, Hagdu A, Thompson SE. Pelvic inflammatory disease and fertility. A cohort study of 1,844 women with laparoscopically verified disease and 657 control women with normal laparoscopic results. Sex Transm Dis 1992;19(4):185–192.

12 Michalas S, Minaretzis D, Tsionou C, Maos G, Kioses E, Aravantinos D. Pelvic surgery, reproductive factors and risk of ectopic pregnancy: a case controlled study. Int J Gynaecol Obstet 1992;38(2):101–105.

13 Tomazevic T, Ribic-Pucelj M. Ectopic pregnancy following the treatment of tubal infertility. J Reprod Med 1992;37(7):611–614.

14 Nazari A, Askari HA, Check JH, O'Shaugnessy A. Embryo transfer technique as a cause of ectopic pregnancy in in vitro fertilization. Fertil Steril 1993;60(5):919–921.

15 Fernandez H, Coste J, Job-Spira N. Controlled ovarian hyperstimulation as a risk factor for ectopic pregnancy. Obstet Gynecol 1991;78(4):656–659.

16 Marcus SF, Brinsden PR. Primary ovarian pregnancy after in vitro fertilization and embryo transfer: report of seven cases. Fertil Steril 1993;60(1):167–169.

17 Svare J, Norup P, Grove-Thomsen S, et al. Heterotopic pregnancies after in vitro fertilization and embryo transfer—a Danish survey. Hum Reprod 1993;8(1):116–118.

18 Phillips RS, Tuomala RE, Feldblum PJ, Schachter J, Rosenberg MJ, Aronson MD. The effect of cigarette smoking, Chlamydia trachomatis infection, and vaginal douching on ectopic pregnancy. Obstet Gynecol 1992;79(1):85–90.

19 Goldenberg M, Bider D, Seidman DS, Lipitz S, Mashiach S, Oelsner G. Seasonal patterns in tubal pregnancy. Gynecol Obstet Invest 1993;35(3):149–151.

20 Saurel-Cubizolles MJ, Job-Spira N, Estryn-Behar M. Ectopic pregnancy and occupational exposure to antineoplastic drugs. Lancet 1993;341(8854):1169–1171.

21 Rossing MA, Daling JR, Voigt LF, Stergachis AS, Weiss NS. Current use of an intrauterine device and risk of tubal pregnancy. Epidemiology 1993;4(3):252–258.

22 Rossing MA, Daling JR, Weiss NS, et al. Past use of an intrauterine device and risk of tubal pregnancy. Epidemiology 1993;4(3):245–251.

23 Sivin I. Dose- and age-dependent ectopic pregnancy risks with intrauterine contraception. Obstet Gynecol 1991;78(2):291–297.

24 Townsend DE, McCausland V, McCausland A, Fields G, Kaufman K. Post-ablation–tubal sterilization syndrome. Obstet Gynecol 1993;82(3):422–424.

25 Maccato ML, Estrada R, Faro S. Ectopic pregnancy with undetectable serum and urine β-hCG levels and detection of β-hCG in the ectopic trophoblast by immunocytochemical evaluation. Obstet Gynecol 1993;81:878–880.

26 Glezerman M, Press F, Carpman M. Culdocentesis is an obsolete diagnostic tool in suspected ectopic pregnancy. Arch Gynecol Obstet 1992;252(1):5–9.

27 Lower AM, Yovich JL, Hancock C, Grudzinskas JG. Is luteal function maintained by factors other than chorionic gonadotrophin in early pregnancy? Hum Reprod 1993;8(4):645–648.

28 Stern JJ, Voss F, Coulam CB. Early diagnosis of ectopic pregnancy using receiver-operator characteristic curves of serum progesterone concentrations. Hum Reprod 1993;8(5):775–779.

29 Williams RS, Gaines IL, Fossum GT. Progesterone in diagnosis of ectopic pregnancy. J Fla Med Assoc 1992;79(4):237–239.

30 Grosskinsky CM, Hage ML, Tyrey L, Christakos AC, Hughes CL. hCG, progesterone, alpha-fetoprotein, and estradiol in the identification of ectopic pregnancy. Obstet Gynecol 1993;81(5):705–709.

31 Choe JK, Check JH, Nowroozi K, Benveniste R, Barnea ER. Serum progesterone and 17-hydroxyprogesterone in the diagnosis of ectopic pregnancies and the value of progesterone replacement in intrauterine pregnancies when serum progesterone levels are low. Gynecol Obstet Invest 1992;34(3):133–138.

32 Grudzinskas JG, Stabile I. Ectopic pregnancy: are biochemical tests at all helpful? Br J Obstet Gynaecol 1993;100:510–511.

33 Russell SA, Filly RA, Damato N. Sonographic diagnosis of ectopic pregnancy with endovaginal probes: what really has changed? J Ultrasound Med 1993;12(3):145–151.

34 Burry KA, Thurmond AS, Suby-Long TD, et al. Transvaginal ultrasonographic findings in surgically verified ectopic pregnancy. Am J Obstet Gynecol 1993;168(6):1796–1800.

35 Parvey HR, Maklad N. Pitfalls in the transvaginal sonographic diagnosis of ectopic pregnancy. J Ultrasound Med 1993;12(3):139–144.

36 Penzias AS, Huang P-L. Imaging in ectopic pregnancy. J Reprod Med 1992;37(1):47–53.

37 Emerson DS, Cartier MS, Altieri LA, et al. Diagnostic efficacy of endovaginal color Doppler flow imaging in an ectopic pregnancy screening program. Radiology 1992;183(2):413–420.

38 Kirchler HC, Seebacher S, Alge AA, Muller-Holzner E, Fessler S, Kolle D. Early diagnosis of tubal pregnancy: change in tubal blood flow evaluated by endovaginal color Doppler sonography. Obstet Gynecol 1993;82(4):561–565.

39 Carson SA, Buster JE. Ectopic pregnancy, review article. N Engl J Med 1993;329(16):1174–1181.

40 Hochner-Celnikier D, Ron M, Goshen R, Zacut D. Amir G, Yagel S. Rupture of ectopic pregnancy following disappearance of serum beta subunit of hCG. Obstet Gynecol 1992;79(5):826–827.

41 Weissman A, Hakim M. Diagnosis and treatment of cervical pregnancy. J Reprod Med 1993;38(8):656–658.

42 Grimes DA. Frontiers of operative laparoscopy: a review and critique of the evidence. Am J Obstet Gynecol 1992;166(4):1062–1071.

43 Bruhat MA, Pouly JL. Endoscopic treatment of ectopic pregnancies. Curr Opin Obstet Gynecol 1993;5(2):260–266.

44 Wagner J, Droesch J, Mann WJ. Laparoscopic management of ectopic pregnancy in a resident training program. South Med J 1993;86(6):619–622.

45 Shwayder JM, Mahoney V, Bersinger DE. Unilateral twin ectopic pregnancy managed by laparoscopy. A case report. J Reprod Med 1993;38(4):314–316.

46 Stovall TG. Medical management. Extrauterine pregnancy, clinical diagnosis and management. New York: McGraw-Hill, 1993:249–269.

47 Paulson JD. The use of carbon dioxide laser laparoscopy in the treatment of tubal ectopic pregnancies. Am J Obstet Gynecol 1992;167(2):382–385.

48 Seifer DB, Gutmann JN, Grant WD, Kamps CA, DeCherney AH. Comparison of persistent ectopic pregnancy after laparoscopic salpingostomy versus salpingostomy at laparotomy for ectopic pregnancy. Obstet Gynecol 1993;81:378–382.

49 Bengtsson G, Bryman I, Thorburn J, Lindblom B. Low-dose oral methotrexate as second-line therapy for persistent trophoblast after conservative treatment of ectopic pregnancy. Obstet Gynecol 1992;79(4):589–591.

50 Hoppe DE, Bekkar BE, Nager CW. Single-dose systemic methotrexate for the treatment of persistent ectopic pregnancy after conservative surgery. Obstet Gynecol 1994;83(1):51–54.

51 Johnson N. Simplifying laparoscopic surgery for ectopic pregnancies. Br J Obstet Gynaecol 1993;100:286–287.

52 Ory S, O'Brien PS, Nnadi E, Melton LJ, Herrmann R. Fertility after ectopic pregnancy. Fertil Steril 1993;60(2):231–235.

53 Sultana CJ, Easley K, Collins RL. Outcome of laparoscopic versus traditional surgery for ectopic pregnancies. Fertil Steril 1992;57(2):285–289.

54 Pouly JL, Chapron C, Manhes H, Canis M, Wattiez A, Bruhat MA. Multifactorial analysis of fertility after conservative laparoscopic treatment of ectopic pregnancy in a series of 223 patients. Fertil Steril 1991;56(3):453–460.

55 Silva PD, Schaper AM, Rooney B. Reproductive outcome after 143 laparoscopic procedures for ectopic pregnancy. Obstet Gynecol 1993;81(5):710–715.

56 Guirgis R, Craft I. Gamete intrafallopian transfer in women who had ectopic pregnancy previously. Obstet Gynecol 1992;79(4):586–588.

57 Fernandez H, Lelaidier C, Thouvenez V, Frydman R. The use of a pretherapeutic, predictive score to determine inclusion criteria for the non-surgical treatment of ectopic pregnancy. Hum Reprod 1991;6(7):995–998.

58 Stovall TG, Ling FW. Single-dose methotrexate: an expanded clinical trial. Am J Obstet Gynecol 1993;1686(1):1759–1762.

59 Frishman GN, Seifer DB. Hematosalpinx after methotrexate treatment of unruptured ectopic pregnancy. Fertil Steril 1993;60(3):571–572.

60 Brown DL, Felker RE, Stovall TG, Emerson DS, Ling FW. Serial endovaginal sonography of ectopic pregnancies treated with methotrexate. Obstet Gynecol 1991;77(3):406–409.

61 Pansky M, Bukovsky J, Golan A, et al. Reproductive outcome after laparoscopic local methotrexate injection for tubal pregnancy. Fertil Steril 1993;60(1):85–87.

62 Groutz A, Luxman D, Cohen JR, David MP. Rising β-hCG titres following laparoscopic injection of methotrexate into unruptured, viable tubal pregnancies. Br J Obstet Gynaecol 1993;100:287–288.

63 Fernandez H, Benifla JL, Lelaidier C, Baton C, Frydman R. Methotrexate treatment of ectopic pregnancy: 100 cases treated by primary transvaginal injection under sonographic control. Fertil Steril 1993;59(4):773–777.

64 Risquez F, Forman R, Maleika F, et al. Transcervical cannulation of the fallopian tube for the management of ectopic pregnancy: prospective multicenter study. Fertil Steril 1992;58(6):1131–1135.

65 Tulandi T, Atri M, Bret P, Falcone T, Khalife S. Transvaginal intratubal methotrexate treatment of ectopic pregnancy. Fertil Steril 1992;58(1):98–100.

66 Timor-Tritsch IE, Monteagudo A, Matera CR, Veit C. Sonographic evolution of cornual pregnancies treated without surgery. Obstet Gynecol 1992;79(6):1044–1049.

67 Goldenberg M, Bider D, Oelsner G, Admon D, Mashiach S. Treatment of interstitial pregnancy with methotrexate via hysteroscopy. Fertil Steril 1992;58(6):1234–1236.

68 Fernandez H, De-Ziegler D, Bourget P, Feltain P, Frydman R. The place of methotrexate in the management of interstitial pregnancy. Hum Reprod 1991;6(2):302–306.

69 Perez JA, Sadek MM, Savale M, Boyer P, Zorn JR. Local medical treatment of interstitial pregnancy after in vitro fertilization and embryo transfer: two case reports. Hum Reprod 1993;8(4):631–634.

70 Fernandez H, Fournet P, Lelaidier C, Olivennes F, Doumerc S, Frydman R. Nonsurgical treatment of heterotopic pregnancy: a report of six cases. Fertil Steril 1993;60(3):428–432.

71 Leach RE, Ney JA, Ory SJ. Selective embryo reduction of an interstitial heterotopic gestation. Fetal Diagn Ther 1992;7(1):41–45.

72 Roussis P, Ball RH, Fleischer AC, Herbert CM III. Cervical pregnancy: a case report. J Reprod Med 1992;37(5):479–481.

73 Brand E, Gibbs RS, Davidson SA. Advanced cervical pregnancy treated with actinomycin-D. Br J Obstet Gynaecol 1993;100(5):491–492.

74 Schwartz LB, Carcangiu ML, DeCherney AH. Primary ovarian pregnancy: a case report. J Reprod Med 1993;38(2):155–158.

75 Carter JE, Ekuan J, Kallins GJ. Laparoscopic diagnosis and excision of an intact ovarian pregnancy: a case report. J Reprod Med 1993;38(12):962–963.

76 Shamma FN, Schwartz LB. Primary ovarian pregnancy successfully treated with methotrexate. Am J Obstet Gynecol 1992;167(5):1307–1308.

77 Laatikainen T, Tuomivaara L, Kaar K. Comparison of a local injection of hyperosmolar glucose solution with salpingostomy for the conservative treatment of tubal pregnancy. Fertil Steril 1993;60(1):80 84.

78 Fernandez H, Baton C, Lelaidier C, Frydman R. Conservative management of ectopic pregnancy: prospective randomized clinical trial of methotrexate versus prostaglandin sulprostone by combined transvaginal and systemic administration. Fertil Steril 1991;55(4):746–750.

79 Deckardt R, Saks M, Graff H. Laparoscopic therapy for tubal pregnancy using prostaglandins. J Reprod Med 1993;38(8):587–591.

80 Carson S. Expectant management: its role in the treatment of ectopic pregnancy. In: Stovall TG, Ling FW. Extrauterine pregnancy, clinical diagnosis and management. New York: McGraw-Hill, 1993:271–278.

81 Atri M, Bret PM, Tulandi T. Spontaneous resolution of ectopic pregnancy: initial appearance and evolution at transvaginal US. Radiology 1993;186(1):83–86.

82 Ylostalo P, Cacciatore B, Sjoberg J, Kaariainen M, Tenhunen A, Stenman UH. Expectant management of ectopic pregnancy. Obstet Gynecol 1992;80(3):345–348.

83 Fernandez H, Lelaidier C, Baton C, Bourget P, Frydman R. Return of reproductive performance after expectant management and local treatment for ectopic pregnancy. Hum Reprod 1991;6(10):1474–1477.

Suggested readings

Bruhat, MA, Poula JL. Endoscopic treatment of ectopic pregnancies. Curr Opin Obstet Gynecol 1993;5:260–266.

Carson SA, Buster JE. Ectopic pregnancy [review article]. N Engl J Med 1993;329(16):1174–1181.

DeCherney AH, ed. Ectopic pregnancy. Rockville, Md: Aspen Publications, 1986.

DeCherney AH, Penzias AS. Ectopic pregnancy. In: Rock JA, Murphy AA, Jones HW Jr, eds. Female reproductive surgery. Baltimore: Williams & Wilkins, 1992:170–189.

Doyle MB, DeCherney AH, Diamond MP. Epidemiology and etiology of ectopic pregnancy. Obstet Gynecol Clin North Am, 1991;8(1): 1–17.

Kadar N. Diagnosis and treatment of extrauterine pregnancies. New York: Raven Press, 1990.

Shamma FN, Penzias AS, DeCherney AH. Ectopic pregnancy: evaluation and management. Semin Reprod Endocrinol 1991;9: 118–126.

Stovall TG, Ling FW, eds. Extrauterine pregnancy, clinical diagnosis and management. New York: McGraw-Hill, 1993.

Stovall TG, Ling FW. Single-dose methotrexate: an expanded clinical trial. Am J Obstet Gynecol 1993;168(6):1759–1765.

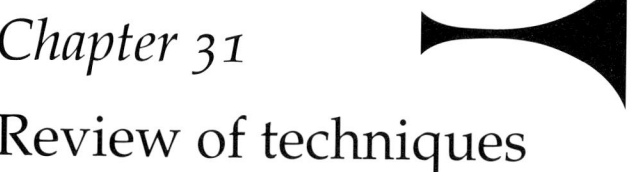

Chapter 31

Review of techniques for tubal sterilization

Jacques-E. Rioux and Richard Soderstrom

Sterilization remains the preferred method of birth control for couples who have completed their families or wish to have no children. The practicing gynecologist is confronted with a wide array of available techniques to recommend. Which technique is best: the easiest to perform? the most readily reversible, especially for young couples? or simply the most effective overall? Even better, is any technique highly efficacious *and* readily reversible?

Numerous approaches

The tubes may be approached by conventional laparotomy, minilaparotomy, colpotomy, laparoscopy, or hysteroscopically, through the natural passages.

Practicing obstetrician-gynecologists are reluctant to perform a laparotomy solely for a tubal ligation. However, if a laparotomy is indicated either for a cesarean section or for a gynecologic or a surgical indication, any of several techniques can be used.

Irving technique

In 1924, Irving described a method to be used exclusively for sterilization coincidental with cesarean section (1). By burying the proximal stump within the myometrium and the distal portion between the leaves of the broad ligament, he was able to keep the ends of the severed tube away from each other. Faultless sterilization ensued (Fig. 31-1).

Pomeroy technique

Although Pomeroy never published a description of his technique, it is probably used more than any other method of tubal ligation. In 1930, Pomeroy's associates, Bishop and Nelms, reported 60 sterilizations performed following his principles (2):
• Do not crush the tube; doing so may cause tubal fistula formation.
• Use absorbable suture material (plain catgut). As soon as the suture dissolves, the proximal and distal segments separate, making recanalization unlikely (Fig. 31-2).

Kroener technique

In 1935, Kroener proposed occluding the tubes by distal salpingectomy or fimbriectomy. The tube is double-ligated at the ampulla, and the fimbria is excised (Fig. 31-3). If a fimbria ovarica is present, it should be ligated as well (3). The Kroener technique is simple to perform when the distal portion of the tube is free. Its popularity has waned, however, with reports of an unacceptable failure rate (4). Another disadvantage is that hydrosalpinx is a frequently encountered late complication.

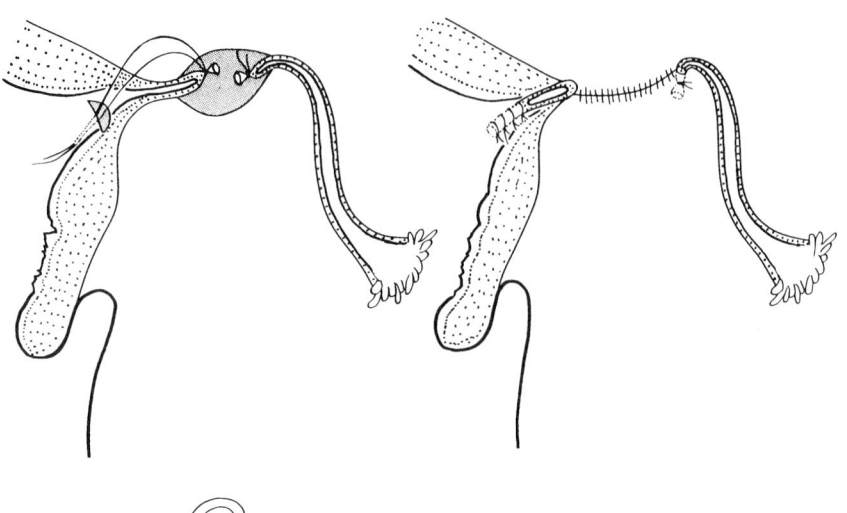

Fig. 31-1 Irving technique. At the time of cesarean section, both proximal tubal stumps are buried.

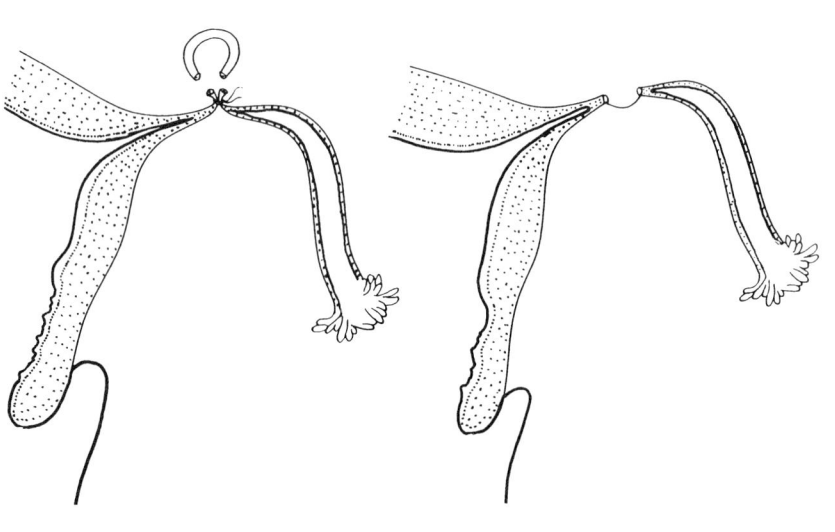

Fig. 31-2 Pomeroy technique. Caveats are to avoid crushing the tube, to tie with absorbable suture material (plain catgut), and to excise the loop of tube.

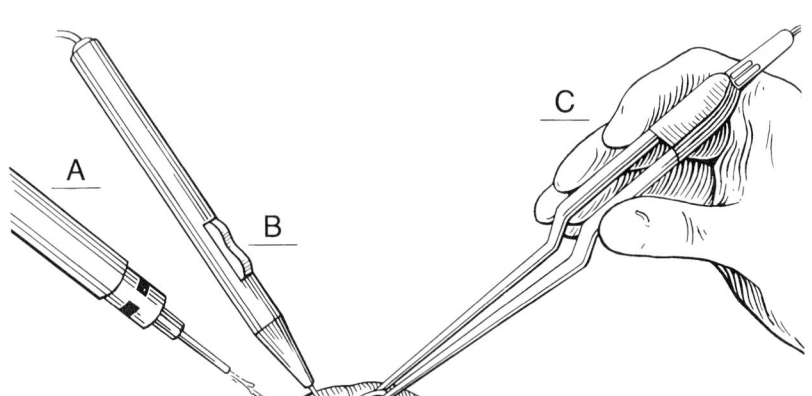

Fig. 31-3 Kroener technique. The tubes are occluded by distal salpingectomy or fimbriectomy.

Total salpingectomy

This procedure is indicated if the tubes are found to be diseased.

Partial salpingectomy

In this technique, often referred to as a modified Pomeroy, a midsegment of tube is removed. Both cut ends are ligated separately with absorbable suture material.

Cornual resection

The intramural portion of the tube is removed. Large mattress sutures are placed in the myometrium to achieve hemostasis.

Uchida technique

Since 1945, Uchida himself has reportedly used this technique to perform more than 25,000 sterilizations without a single failure (5). A saline-epinephrine solution is injected into the subserosa to separate the serosa from the muscular layer. When this edematous bleb is opened, the tube is easily seen and severed. The proximal portion is ligated and buried beneath the serosa. The distal end is ligated with the open fringe of the serosa. Of all the techniques described here, this is one of the most efficacious, but it does remove 3 to 5 cm of tube (Fig. 31-4).

Minilaparotomy

In the hands of experienced surgeons, minilaparotomy is probably the safest method of female sterilization. It is also the least expensive and the most adaptable for use in developing countries.

Minilaparotomies can be done after abortion or delivery or as an interval procedure—that is, unrelated to a pregnancy or termination. Contraindications are obesity, which prevents palpation of the uterine fundus through the lower abdominal wall, and fixed uterine retroversion. Many techniques of tubal occlusion are available. The most popular is the Pomeroy.

Colpotomy

Theoretically, the vaginal route seems ideal for safe, rapid tubal sterilization, as it obviates an abdominal incision. In practice, this is far from true. The severe complications associated with vaginal tubal sterilization—cellulitis or pelvic abscess, hemorrhage, proctotomy, cystotomy—may place too high a price on avoiding a small abdominal scar (6). Shepard concluded in her extensive review: "At the moment, the serious nature of complications encountered after vaginal tubal sterilization would appear to prohibit wholehearted endorsement of this procedure as a quick, effective means of performing female sterilization" (7).

Endoscopic methods

Fiberoptic transmission of light from an external source, available to clinicians in the early 1960s, opened new horizons in endoscopic surgery. In gynecology, the laparoscope and hysteroscope provided tools with which to accomplish and explore new methods of tubal sterilization procedures.

Laparoscopy

The popularity of laparoscopic sterilization has increased during the past decade. This procedure provides superb visualization of not only the entire pelvic cavity, but also much of the intra-abdominal contents. Few situations make laparoscopy impossible to perform. It is a sophisticated procedure requiring an array of highly technical, expensive instruments.

The introduction of laparoscopic techniques has given women access to a safe, effective, dependable method of tubal sterilization. In well-trained hands, laparoscopic tubal sterilization may be performed with local anesthesia. The procedure is then comparable to vasectomy in safety, efficacy, and ease of performance. However, laparoscopic sterilization is not altogether innocuous; any decision to undergo sterilization must be considered with great care. The assumption must be that the procedure will be irreversible.

Electrocoagulation

The delivery of high-frequency sinusoidal waves of electric energy through the living cell creates heat. When that heat is concentrated (high current density), cellular heat exceeds 100°C. The result is cell disruption, desiccation, and collapse: electrocoagulation.

Unipolar method

The first instrument used for laparoscopic tubal electrocoagulation was the Palmer biopsy forceps, adapted for electrosurgical capabilities (8). Powerful, high-voltage generators that produced unipolar electrical current were used 30 years ago. Electrical energy was concentrated at the site where the jaws of the forceps grasped the fallopian tube. When the current began to flow, it traveled through the pa-

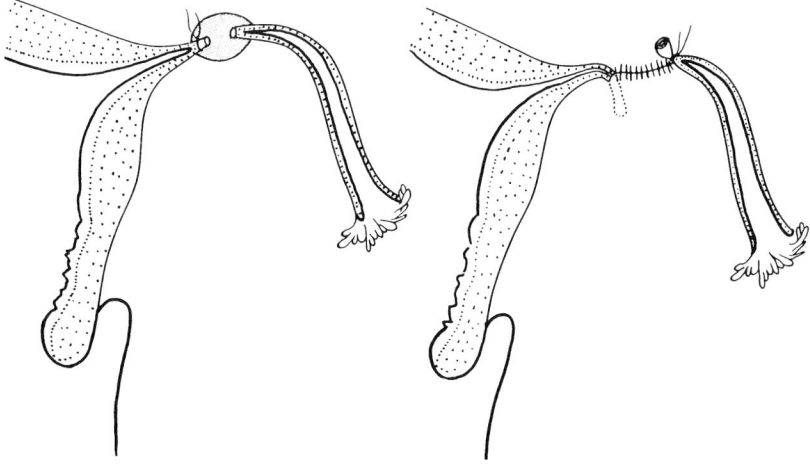

Fig. 31-4 Uchida technique. This method calls for burying the ligated proximal portion of the tube beneath the serosa and tying the distal end outside. No part of the tube is removed.

tient's body from the tube to a ground plate or return electrode, completing the electrical circuit.

The original technique involved electrocoagulation of the tubal isthmus, followed by tubal transection and recoagulation of the cut edges. Some authors subsequently indicated that coagulation is equally effective without tubal transection, provided the surgeon is experienced and confident that coagulation is complete (9). Other investigators recommend that a specimen of the tube be excised for pathologic confirmation. This step appears to have evolved as much for medicolegal reasons as for scientific ones (10). Unfortunately, the tube is frequently charred and unrecognizable, thus defeating the primary purpose of the biopsy.

The unipolar electrical system became associated with certain inherent dangers. In 1973, Thompson and Wheeless reported 11 cases of bowel burns from accidental electrical injury incurred during tubal electrocoagulation (11). Later reports emphasized the potential dangers of unipolar current. But because there was no rational explanation for such accidents, they were difficult or impossible to avoid.

We now know that although a few mishaps were caused by faulty technique, most were related to the inherent dangers associated with high-voltage grounded generators. Some of these units, when set in the coagulation mode, could produce thousands of volts and hundreds of amps of current. As tubal tissue was being dehydrated, tissue resistance increased. To overcome this resistance, the generator sent the electrons down aberrant pathways.

By the late 1970s, more sophisticated generators, generally of solid-state construction, produced low-voltage, high-frequency current. They were not grounded, but isolated from ground (12). Although these machines were much safer, bowel burns continued to occur (13). A study using an animal model suggests those injuries were traumatic, and usually beyond the control of the surgeon (14).

Bipolar method

In 1973, after reading the reports of such accidents, one of us (J-E.R.) devised the first bipolar technique for tubal electrocoagulation (15,16). This method differs from the conventional unipolar system by using operating forceps that contain both the active and the return electrode. Isolating the jaws of the forceps permits low-voltage, high-frequency current to be passed through one jaw, then retrieved and returned to the generator through the other. Thus, the current passes through only the tissue grasped between the jaws of the forceps.

Although high-frequency current is used, it travels only a very short distance—the thickness of the tube grasped within the jaws. The bipolar procedure appears to be safer than the unipolar system because no aberrant pathways pose a danger. Inadvertent electrosurgical injury to the bowel with bipolar forceps can therefore occur only if the bowel is grasped directly with the activated forceps, usually as a result of surgical error. A further advantage of bipolar electrocoagulation is that the burn it creates is discrete and localized, selectively destroying only the tube in the grasp of the forceps' jaws and leaving the mesosalpinx unaffected (Fig. 31-5).

A word of caution: Bipolar instruments should be used only with compatible electrosurgical units as recommended by the manufacturer. Recent studies indicate that a cutting waveform, rather than a coagulation waveform, should be used.

Tubal electrocoagulation techniques fail at a rate of about one per 1000 per year. The complication rate for laparoscopy is directly proportional to the operator's experience and attention to safety guidelines. Electrosurgical complications should be less frequent with the advent of the bipolar technique and with the use of low-voltage, high-frequency generators. Education of physicians and operating room personnel about electrosurgical instruments has reduced complications.

Electrocautery

Another approach that uses local heat to produce coagulation as well as transection of the tube is the Gyneco Thermal Cautery System (Gyneco, Branchburg, NJ). The apparatus

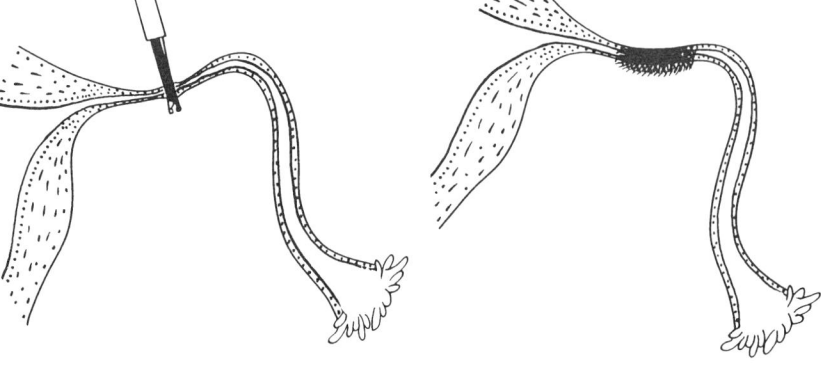

Fig. 31-5 Bipolar forceps. The first bipolar instrument for laparoscopic tubal electrocoagulation was devised in 1973.

includes a small metallic hook that is heated by electric current produced from a battery-operated power source. The tube is grasped with the hook and pulled inside an insulated outer sheath. The tube is coagulated and transected; hemostasis is achieved by cauterization. Because the sectioned ends of the tube remain in close proximity, recanalization may occur more easily than with some of the other techniques—at least in theory. Data for evaluating the true failure rate of this method are not currently available (see below, "Sterilization failures").

Mechanical techniques

Mechanical devices to obstruct the fallopian tubes were designed to eliminate the risks entailed in electrocoagulation. With these devices, as with any other mechanical tool, meticulous attention to proper care and application make the difference between success and failure.

Clips

Hulka was aware of the high failure rate associated with the use of the tantalum clip—up to 27%, according to Wheeless—yet was still fascinated by the simplicity of the concept. He then spent years developing a spring-loaded clip of Lexan plastic (17). The clip, applied to the fallopian tube using a specifically designed instrument, is held in the closed position by a stainless steel spring that has been gold-plated to diminish peritoneal reaction. The plastic jaws, which have interlocking teeth, leave no room for recanalization. Maximal pressure is applied to the tube for 3 days to reduce the acute crushing effect that could result in fistula formation.

The Filshie clip, not yet available in the United States, is rapidly becoming the most popular method of female sterilization in Canada (18). The clip is made of titanium lined with Silastic. The locking device is mechanical. When fully closed, it leaves no space at all, thus achieving complete closure (Fig. 31-6). The grasping effect provided by the curve on the upper part of the clip makes it easy to place. It is small enough to place on almost any size and shape of tube, even postpartum.

Falope ring

This device, created by Yoon and King, is ingeniously simple (19). A loop of tube is drawn within the central hollow cylinder of the ring applicator forceps, which itself can be inserted by either a single- or a double-puncture technique. The loaded Silastic band is then forced down over the loop of tube by the forward action of an outer cylinder, resulting in a release of the band from the applicator and, thus, tubal occlusion. The loop portion of the tube encircled by the ring gradually atrophies (Fig. 31-7).

Hysteroscopy

Like laparoscopy, this apparently simple procedure uses sophisticated equipment and appeals to the enthusiastic endoscopist. However, it is tricky and fraught with pitfalls that demand a great deal of patience. Hysteroscopic tubal occlusion may become more popular as instruments are simplified and reversibility is improved (20). Indeed, with the smaller instruments, hysteroscopy is becoming an office procedure that can be performed in minutes using local anesthesia.

Three investigational approaches have not yet been approved by the Food and Drug Administration:
• electrical current to coagulate the tube from inside;
• chemical agents, which initiate sclerosis of the endosalpinx; and
• a plug, already shaped or formed in place, to obstruct the tubal lumen with an option for removal and theoretically a degree of reversibility.

Electrical current

As with laparoscopy, electricity can be used to electrocoagulate (diathermy) or to thermocoagulate (using heat). Electrocoagulation, whether unipolar or bipolar, is achieved by

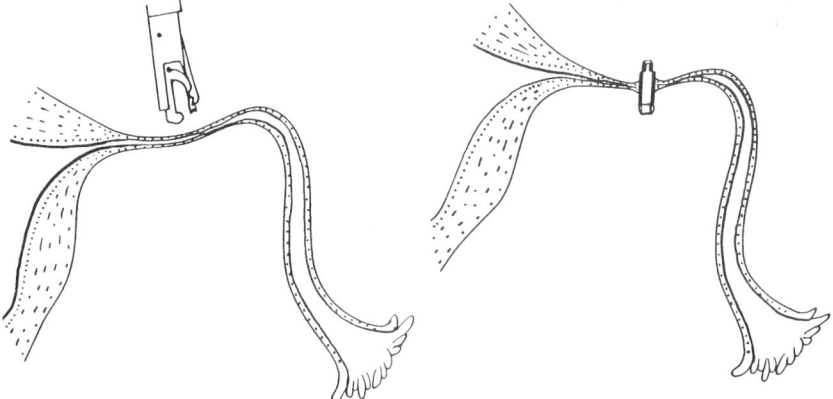

Fig. 31-6 The Filshie clip, popular in Canada but not yet available in the United States, achieves complete closure with a mechanical locking device.

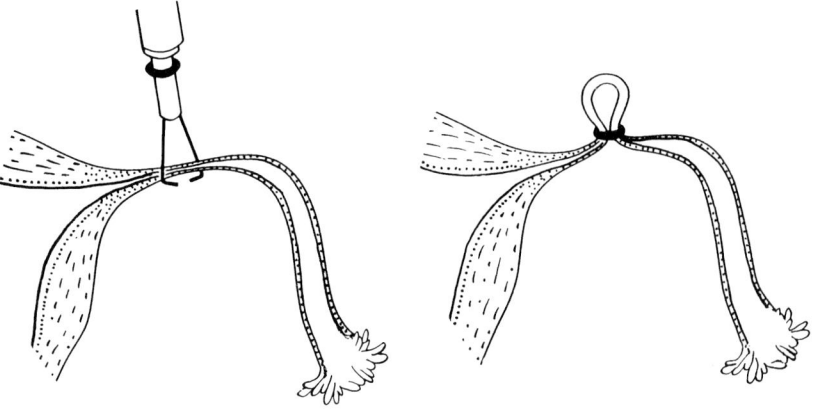

Fig. 31-7 The falope ring. A loop of tube is drawn within the central hollow cylinder of the applicator forceps. Forward action of an outer cylinder forces a loaded Silastic band down over the loop of tube.

introducing an electrode with a conductive tip via the tubal ostium into the proximal portion of the tube.

Identification of the ostia may, however, be difficult; in fact, these openings can be identified with absolute certainly in only 80% of cases. Once the electrode has been introduced into the intramural portion of the tube, electric current is applied. Permanent occlusion should result from electrocoagulation of the endosalpinx and proximal layer of muscularis. Thermocoagulation is achieved by heating the probe itself, using low-voltage current. The tissue surrounding the probe is "cooked."

Chemical agents

Chemical agents cause sclerosis of the endosalpinx. The agents can be instilled into the tubes either under hysteroscopic control or blindly, by means of a special injecting apparatus. Many different substances have been used. Those that have met some success in human trials include the following (21):
• strong caustic agents (silver nitrate, zinc chloride, formaldehyde, or ethanol-formalin);
• a strong base (phenol);
• a sclerosing agent (sodium morrhuate);
• a granuloma-producing agent (talc);
• a cytotoxic agent (quinacrine); and,
• a tissue adhesive (methylcyanoacrylate).

The mode of delivery varies. Direct tubal instillation can be done under hysteroscopic control by catheterizing the tubal ostia. Alternatively, the ostia can be catheterized indirectly under fluoroscopic control with a test dose of radiopaque material. The agent may also be loaded into the long arm of a T-shaped intrauterine device and diffused slowly into the fallopian tubes.

Plugs

Three preshaped plugs have reached human clinical trials:
• the uterotubal junction-blocking devices, developed by Hosseinian and coworkers (22);

• the P-Block, a hydrogel tubal blocking device, being developed by Brundin (23); and
• the Hamou intratubal device, made of nylon, and the simplest of the three (24).

The diameter of the Hamou device, which exceeds 1 mm if the anchoring system is included, fits most ostia. An intrauterine loop permits subsequent retrieval. The device does not attempt to fill the lumen of the tube but acts intratubally (Fig. 31-8).

Another approach is to tailor the plug to the tube. These formed-in-place silicone plugs, devised by Erb and Reed, involve a flow of catalyzed liquid silicone polymer into the fallopian tube through a silicone rubber obturator tip positioned at the tubal ostium (25). The formed-in-place plug becomes bonded to the tip. In the resulting flexible structure, the diameter is larger at both ends than in the isthmus. The shape of the plug keeps it in place, effecting tubal occlusion.

In theory, the four techniques that involve plugs are more readily reversible than methods using electricity or chemical agents, which destroy the tissue. However, the reversibility of plugs has not been proved and therefore should not be presumed. All methods should be discussed extensively during counseling with the patient about to make a decision.

Sterilization failures

Each technique has inherent problems, and nature has a remarkable propensity to reconstitute the integrity of the normal fallopian tube. Statistical reports on the failure of techniques are usually flawed because they reflect anecdotal experience, retrospective review, and short-term follow-up. Too frequently, surgeons modify the classic techniques, virtually inventing new methods independently. The following comments are summarized from reports in the literature, the authors' experiences, and anecdotal experiences of other practitioners.

The Irving technique is essentially faultless. Although one failure has been reported, the explanation is unclear.

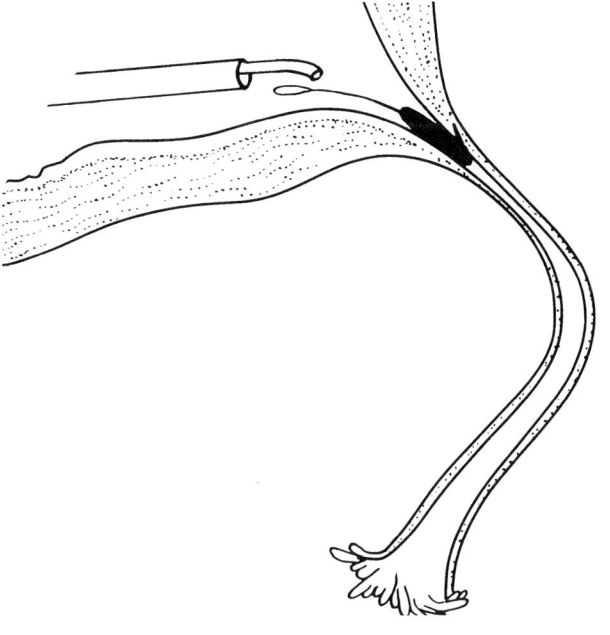

Fig. 31-8 The Hamou device. An intrauterine loop permits subsequent retrieval. The device does not attempt to fill the lumen of the tube, but acts within the tube.

All reports of failure for the widely used Pomeroy technique appear to have one explanation: fistula formation.

The increased failure rate associated with the Kroener technique is usually caused by a departure from the technique as originally described. A change from a double ligature to a single ligature is the typical cause of failure. When a repeat sterilization procedure is performed, a portion of the fimbria ovarica remains.

Although total salpingectomy should be foolproof, a few failures have been reported. Studies are inadequate—describing partial salpingectomy with ligation using a nonabsorbable suture. When suture material that is nonabsorbable or absorbs slowly is used—polyglactin 910 (Vicryl) or polyglycolic acid (Dexon), for example—pressure necrosis of the tube's muscular wall may eventually allow the encircled tissue to atrophy or recede until the endosalpinx contained within the ligature reopens. The modified Pomeroy method has yet to be studied and could open a medicolegal Pandora's box.

Uchida has documented a large personal series without a single failure. Other medical centers have not surveyed the technique.

Electrocoagulation failures

Of the various laparoscopic procedures, unipolar electrocoagulation without transection has boasted the lowest failure rate. The alleged risks have spurred practitioners to select techniques that are presumed to be safer. When unipolar failures occur, a fistula is always the culprit.

The literature has begun to discuss failures with bipolar electrocoagulation as well. Incompatible equipment and inadequate coagulation appear to play major roles in these disturbing reports. At present, bipolar techniques that coagulate less then 2 cm of tube and deliver less than 20 to 25 W of power seem to have an unacceptable failure rate. Research has shown *a cutting waveform* is therefore preferable (26,27).

When bipolar failures are examined, the endosalpinx is usually healthy. Scarred muscular tissue surrounds the patent salpinx. The probable cause is incomplete electrocoagulation. This finding suggests that the visual endpoint of electrocoagulation is insufficient to declare the tube coagulated. Using an ammeter or optical meter such as those manufactured by the Richard Wolf Medical Instruments Corp. (Rosemont, Ill.) seems to reduce the risk of incomplete coagulation.

Clips and rings

Failures associated with the Hulka clip frequently follow misplacement of the clip—too distal on the tube, at oblique angles to the axis of the tube, or accidentally applied to other structures. Furthermore, there is always the risk that a mechanical defect in the device being used will render the operation unsuccessful.

Failures with the Falope ring can usually be attributed to spontaneous reanastomosis. Once the loop contained above the applied loop has atrophied, the tube fails to separate, creating a propensity for spontaneous reanastomosis. In such cases, the ring is frequently found on top of or adjacent to the anastomosis on the mesosalpinx.

Documenting procedures

Too often repeat sterilization is performed by a physician who may or may not be expert at the technique used by the primary surgeon. It is that second surgeon's duty to approach the matter scientifically. The description of the anatomy should be clear and, when possible, photographs should be taken. Either at the operating table or in the pathology laboratory the tube suspected of patency should be instilled with chromotubation to pinpoint the failure. If necessary, multiple microscopic slides of the area should be obtained for scrutiny by a trained pathologist. To say "the tube looked normal to me" serves neither the physician nor the patient and may fail to remedy the situation.

Reversal of sterilization

Requests for reversal of sterilization procedures are increasing. The most common motivating factors are the so-called three D's: divorce, death, and disaster. Other factors include changes in lifestyle and economic status that may suddenly permit a couple to have a larger family (28).

All candidates for reversal should be thoroughly investigated psychologically and physically. The operative report of the sterilization procedure should be available. Before any kind of surgery is contemplated, the partner's sperm should be analyzed.

Some sterilization methods are not reversible—an injection of methylcyanoacrylate, for example, or a bilateral salpingectomy. In such cases, pregnancy can be achieved only with in vitro fertilization and embryo transfer.

End results of other forms of sterilization are frequently unpredictable. For example, a unipolar coagulation may destroy the whole tube, leaving barely a few fimbriae behind. The Kroener technique can remove the fimbria and the entire ampulla. Conversely, if only the fimbria was excised, a complete ampulla may remain, permitting an adequate salpingoneostomy. A bipolar burn or a Falope ring ligation can often be reversed by isthmic-ampullary anastomosis. This type of reversal, however, is more difficult than the isthmic-isthmic anastomosis performed in most cases of clip reversal.

In short, no method is 100% reversible. The clip and microsurgical technique is nearly 90% effective. Other approaches have less success, but are sufficient for many patients who request reversal (29).

Approximately 98% of women undergoing tubal sterilization want the procedure to be permanent and irreversible. Women who want a reversal may obtain it with microsurgery, in vitro fertilization, or embryo transfer.

Tubal sterilization should always be considered irreversible. The procedure of choice for each patient remains the method of sterilization that will maintain a high degree of efficacy while providing adequate, yet minimal, overall tissue destruction.

References

1 Irving FC. A new method of insuring sterility following cesarean section. Am J Obstet Gynecol 1924;8:335.

2 Bishop E, Nelms WF. A simple method of tubal sterilization. NY State J Med 1930;30:214.

3 Kroener WF Jr. Surgical sterilization by fimbriectomy. Am J Obstet Gynecol 1969;104:247.

4 Metz KGP. Failures following fimbriectomy. Fertil Steril 1977;28:66.

5 Uchida H. Uchida tubal sterilization. Am J Obstet Gynecol 1975;121:153.

6 Miesfeld RR, Giarratano RC, Mayers TG. Vaginal tubal ligation: is infection a significant risk? Am J Obstet Gynecol 1980;137:183.

7 Shepard MK. Female contraceptive sterilization. Obstet Gynecol Surg 1974;29:739.

8 Palmer MR. Essais de sterilisation tubaire coelioscopique par electrocoagulation isthmique. Bull Fed Soc Gynecol Obstet Lang Fr 1962;14:298.

9 Yuzpe AA, Rioux J-E, Loffer FD, et al. Laparoscopic tubal sterilization by the "burn only" technique. Obstet Gynecol 1977;49:106.

10 Soderstrom RM. Legal aspects of female sterilization: a comparison of methods. In: Phillips JM, ed. Endoscopic female sterilization: a comparison of methods. Downey, Calif: American Association of Gynecologic Laparoscopists, 1983:199–201.

11 Thompson BH, Wheeless CR Jr. Gastrointestinal complications of laparoscopic sterilization. Obstet Gynecol 1973;41:669.

12 Rioux J-E, Yuzpe AA. Know thy generator! Contemp Obstet Gynecol 1975;6(October):52.

13 Peterson HB, Ory HW, Greenspan JR, et al. Deaths associated with laparoscopic sterilization by unipolar electrocoagulating devices, 1978 and 1979. Am J Obstet Gynecol 1981;139:141.

14 Soderstrom RM, Levy BS. Bowel injuries during laparoscopy: causes and medicolegal questions. Contemp Obstet Gynecol 1986;27(March):41.

15 Rioux J-E, Cloutier D. Laparoscopic tubal sterilization: sparking and its control. Vie Med Canada Franc 1973;2:760.

16 Rioux J-E, Cloutier D. A new bipolar instrument for laparoscopic tubal sterilization. Am J Obstet Gynecol 1974;119:737.

17 Hulka JF, Fishburne JI, Mercer JP, et al. Laparoscopic sterilization with a spring-clip: a report of the first fifty cases. Am J Obstet Gynecol 1973;116:715.

18 Filshie GM. The Filshie clip. In: Van Lith DAF, Keith LG, Van Hall EV, eds. New trends in female sterilization. Chicago: Year Book Medical Publishers, 1983:115–123.

19 Yoon IB, King TM. A preliminary and intermediate report on a new laparoscopic tubal ring procedure. J Reprod Med 1975;15:54.

20 Siegler AM. The rise and fall of hysteroscopic tubal sterilization. In: Phillips JM, ed. Endoscopic female sterilization: a comparison of methods. Downey, Calif: American Association of Gynecologic Laparoscopists, 1983:185–190.

21 Richart RM. The use of chemical agents in female sterilization. In: Zatuchni GI, Shelton JD, Goldsmith A, et al, eds. Female transcervical sterilization. New York: Harper & Row, 1983:24–35.

22 Hosseinian AH, Lucero S, Kim MH. Hysteroscopic implantation of uterotubal junction blocking devices. In: Sciarra JJ, ed. Advances in female sterilization techniques. New York: Harper & Row, 1976:169–175.

23 Brundin JO. Experiences with the P block, a hydrogelic tubal blocking device. In: Siegler AM, Lindemann HJ, eds. Hysteroscopy principles and practice. Philadelphia: JB Lippincott, 1983:251–256.

24 Hamou J, Taylor PJ. Panoramic, contact, and microcolpohysteroscopy. In: Current problems in obstetrics and gynecology: VI. Gynecologic practice. Chicago: Year Book Medical Publishers, 1982:61–64.

25 Erb RA, Reed TP. Hysteroscopic oviductal blocking with formed-in-place silicone rubber plugs: method and apparatus. J Reprod Med 1979;23:65.

26 Soderstrom RM, Levy BS. Bipolar systems—do they perform? Obstet Gynecol 1987;69(3):425–426.

27 Soderstrom RM, Levy BS, Engel T. Reducing bipolar sterilization failures. Obstet Gynecol 1989;74(1):60–63.

28 Gomel V. Profile of women requesting reversal of sterilization. Fertil Steril 1978;30:39.

29 Gomel V. Microsurgical reversal of female sterilization: a reappraisal. Fertil Steril 1980;33:587.

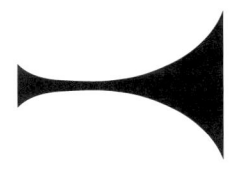

Chapter 32

Metroplasty

Preston C. Sacks

Most women with congenital uterine malformations have no reproductive difficulties. Consequently, the true incidence of uterine malformations is unknown, and their clinical significance is poorly studied. This has led to confusion regarding the indications and benefits of metroplasty. This chapter, after reviewing developmental defects that may lead to lateral fusion defects in the uterus, will discuss how to evaluate candidates for metroplasty and perform two of the more common surgical procedures.

Normal embryology of the müllerian ducts

The internal reproductive ducts originate near the base of the dorsal mesentery in intimate association with the urinary tract, which develops in three stages. This close relation explains the high frequency of urinary tract anomalies in association with abnormalities of the müllerian system.

The first stage of development of the urinary system is the extremely short-lived anterior pronephros, which has ducts that lead to the cloaca. The more advanced mesonephros develops in the fourth week of embryonic life, caudad to the already degenerating pronephros. Its tubules drain into the pronephric ducts, which are thereafter called the mesonephric or wolffian ducts. The mesonephric ducts, under the influence of testosterone, become the internal ducts of the male reproductive system. In the absence of testosterone, the ducts regress. The final renal system, the metanephros, develops still more caudally, with its own distinct duct system.

At 5 to 6 developmental weeks, new reproductive ducts, the paramesonephric or müllerian ducts, appear lateral to the mesonephric ducts. In the female embryo, these are the precursors of the fallopian tubes, uterus, and upper vagina. They are open, where they originate, to eventually form the fimbriated ends of the fallopian tubes. The paramesonephric ducts extend caudally by progressive development of a solid bud. As they approach the lower abdomen, they course toward the midline and fuse where they make contact with the primitive vagina. The septum between the two ducts is then reabsorbed, yielding a single uterine cavity. Toward the end of the third month of embryonic life, distinct muscular and connective tissue layers can be seen in the uterus, and by the end of the sixth month the endometrium appears (1). In males, the müllerian ducts disappear, under the influence of the müllerian inhibiting factor produced by the testes.

Defects in müllerian fusion

A deviation in the normal fusion pattern of the solid müllerian duct buds can result in duplication of the uterus, cervix, and upper vagina. There are many degrees of fusion failure, ranging from complete duplication (two uteri, cervixes, and a longitudinal vaginal septum) to a bicornuate uterus. When evaluating a patient with a müllerian fusion defect, it is helpful to remember that fusion of the müllerian ducts begins in the most caudal portion and extends upward. Therefore incomplete or partial fusion always results in duplication of the upper uterus, and never in a normal single uterus together with a double cervix and vagina. If a double cervix is present, there are always two uterine horns.

Following fusion, the septum separating the two ducts is reabsorbed in a caudad-to-cranial direction to produce a single uterine cavity. Incomplete reabsorption leads to a persistent uterine septum, which is relatively avascular, and may extend the entire length of the uterine cavity.

Incidence

Because most patients are asymptomatic, the true incidence of müllerian fusion defects is difficult to determine. Estimates have ranged from one in 100 to one in 700 women (2–4). Although müllerian fusion defects commonly do not cause reproductive loss, they are disproportionately represented in women with repeated pregnancy loss. Makino and associates studied a group of 1200 women with a history of repeated pregnancy loss. On hysterosalpingography, 188 cases of uterine anomalies were seen, yielding an incidence of 15.7% (5). These authors performed metroplasty in these patients and reported a continuing pregnancy rate of 84%.

Jones and Wheeless reported that 173 patients with duplication of the müllerian system were seen at Johns Hopkins Hospital from 1936 to 1963, but that only in 22 (13%) was the duplication felt to warrant corrective surgery (6). More recently at Johns Hopkins, Rock stated that only 20% of patients with fusion defects have related reproductive failure (7).

A report from a different institution discusses 102 women with bicornuate or septate uteri treated with laparotomy and metroplasty from 1970 to 1990 (8). This strikingly large number of patients seen over such a short time can be explained by an increase in the incidence of fusion defects, improved diagnostic procedures, and/or more liberal diagnostic criteria. It remains true, however, that the decision to perform metroplasty should be based on both the clinical history and the extent of the uterine defect, as an estimated 80% of women with uterine defects will not require surgical intervention.

Fusion defects and reproductive failure

Complete uterine duplication has been described as a medical curiosity for centuries. In 1773, a Dr. Purcell of Dublin opened the body of a woman who had died in the ninth month of pregnancy and described the uterus to be "of ordinary size and form . . . but with only one ovary attached to single fallopian tube. On the left side [was] a second uterus, unimpregnated, and of usual size, to which another ovary and tube were attached" (9). Perhaps because of the frequency of maternal death in that era, no mention was made of the cause of death, nor was any clinical significance attached to the duplication.

In 1859, Kussmaul stated that "most women (with a double uterus) who become pregnant have only a slightly higher morbidity than women with a single uterus. Twenty percent . . . who conceive abort . . . [but] generally . . . a double uterus doesn't impede maturation of the fetus."

It is now agreed that complete fusion failure is a fairly benign condition. Any temptation to unite the uteri surgically should therefore be avoided. A defect falling between the completely duplicated and the septate uterus is the bicornuate uterus, with two horns and one cervix. Proper diagnosis is important because surgical correction of a bicornuate uterus is very seldom necessary (10).

Of all of the disorders produced by fusion defects, it is the septate uterus that is most likely to result in pregnancy wastage. A septate uterus is created by incomplete or absent resorption of the septum produced by fusion of the two müllerian ducts. Because it is the defect most likely to result in pregnancy wastage, it is also most likely to require surgical correction.

Diagnosis of fusion defects

There are many ways in which a müllerian fusion defect may come to medical attention. A double uterus may be discovered during a routine pelvic examination, when a longitudinal vaginal septum or double cervix is visualized. Pubertal girls may come to medical attention when there is dysmenorrhea or a pelvic mass secondary to obstruction of one of the outflow tracts. A müllerian fusion defect may be suspected when there is a uterine perforation while attempting a pregnancy termination. The characteristic reproductive problem leading to the diagnosis of a uterine fusion defect, however, is a second-trimester pregnancy loss. This is true despite the fact that 80% of patients with fusion defects have no reproductive problems. Furthermore, it is impossible to determine prospectively which cases will lead to pregnancy loss. In cases of pregnancy loss secondary to a fusion defect, typically there is pain, bleeding, and passage of a well-formed fetus. Blighted ovum is *not* a frequent finding.

Whether a septate uterus can impede conception is uncertain. In a study of 2240 patients with infertility, a 1% incidence of müllerian fusion defects was reported, which is about the same as or less than the incidence in all gynecologic patients (11). Therefore, when infertility and a müllerian fusion defect coexist, the clinician must be careful to evaluate all other possible causes of infertility before performing metroplasty.

Hysterosalpingography (HSG) is the most frequent method of detecting a uterine fusion defect. We prefer to use an aqueous contrast medium, as it is less radiopaque than the oil-based dye, which may obscure a thin septum. The procedure is performd under fluoroscopy, and the patient is manipulated to provide a complete view of the uterus. Differentiation between a septate and bicornuate uterus is difficult by HSG alone. Therefore, if a fusion defect is diagnosed by HSG, the uterus should further be evaluated with sonography or magnetic resonance imaging. This is important when selecting patients for metroplasty. The septate uterus is more likely to result in pregnancy wastage and is easily repaired at hysteroscopy, while the bicornuate uterus is a less common cause of reproductive loss and requires laparotomy and uterine reunification for correction. In some cases, it is difficult to differentiate between a septate and bicornuate uterus without performing a laparoscopy to visualize the fundus and uterine contour. Before performing metroplasty, it is necessary to rule out other causes of pregnancy wastage. These include genetic defects, ovulatory deficiencies, endocrinopathies (such as thyroid and adrenal disorders), infections (chlamydia, gonorrhea, and streptococcus), and cervical incompetence. Because of the close association of the developing reproductive and urinary tracts, approximately 40% of women with uterine abnormalities have an abnormality of the urinary tract. Intravenous pyelography is therefore recommended in patients with müllerian fusion defects.

Repair of müllerian fusion defects

When discussing repair of a müllerian fusion defect, it is helpful to consider bicornuate uteri and septate uteri separately. This is because a bicornuate uterus requires laparotomy for adequate repair, whereas a septum is typically repaired at hysteroscopy.

Repair of the bicornuate uterus

Surgery to repair a bicornuate uterus involves reuniting the two uterine horns to produce a single, capacious cavity. The technique most commonly used is the Strassmann procedure, developed in the 1900s by Paul Strassmann and popularized by his son Erwin (12).

At laparotomy, the bicornuate uterus is exposed. Often there will be a ligament extending between the two uterine horns from the bladder to the sigmoid colon. If present, this rectovesical ligament is excised. We then use a Kelly clamp to perforate the broad ligament of the uterus in an avascular area just above the level of the uterine arteries and place a medium-sized Penrose drain as a tourniquet, holding it in place with a large vascular "bulldog" clamp. When the tourniquet is tightened, the blood supply to the uterus is reduced, minimizing operative blood loss. In addition, we use a suction device that collects and processes the blood removed from the operative field to allow for autologous transfusion.

The two uterine horns are incised longitudinally on the medial side to expose the endometrial cavity (Fig. 32-1). At this point, the myometrial edges of the hemicorpora will retract to face the opposite side. The apposing edges are then approximated with 3-0 interrupted figure-of-eight sutures of a monofilament delayed absorbable suture, polydioxanone ([PDS], Ethicon, Somerville, NJ) or polyglyconate (Maxon, Davis and Geck, Manati, Puerto Rico). This layer approximates the endometrium and myometrium. If the uterine wall is too thick to achieve good approximation with one suture layer, then we use two layers; the first layer approximates the endometrium and inner half of myometrium, and the second layer the outer half of the myometrium. There should be very little tension on the suture line, to avoid later separation of the uterine incision and poor healing. A continuous suture of 5-0 monofilament delayed absorbable material is used to close the serosal layer of the uterus.

The tourniquet is then removed, and the suture site is inspected for hemostasis. It is reinforced as necessary, and the rents in the broad ligament are repaired with 5-0 suture. At this point, the uterus should be suspended anteriorly by placing a mattress suture of No. 1 delayed absorbable suture through the proximal portion of each round ligament. Bring both ends of each suture through the peritoneum, rectus abdominis muscles, and rectus fascia, and secure them to the underside of the rectus fascia. Prior to abdominal closure, we place 100 ml of high molecular weight dextran (Hyskon) in the peritoneal cavity.

To minimize adhesions, we administer 20 mg of dexamethasone sodium phosphate and 25 mg of promethazine hydrochloride intravenously every 4 hours for a total of nine doses. Although the effectiveness of these two agents in fertility therapy has been questioned, we have had no complications attributable to their use, and adhesions, either intrauterine or extrauterine, have not been a major postoperative problem. Follow-up should include HSG at 6 months and a laparoscopy and hysteroscopy at one year should the woman fail to conceive.

Repair of the septate uterus

Before the advancement of operative hysteroscopy in the 1980s, repair of a septate uterus required laparotomy and incision (Tompkins procedure) or excision (Jones procedure) of the septum. Now laparotomy is reserved for only very broad septa that may be technically difficult to remove via hysteroscopy. Our group prefers a modified Tompkins procedure to excise broad uterine septum, though this has not been necessary in the past 5 years. A description of this technique can be found in the first edition of this text.

Most septa are easily resected at hysteroscopy using either hysteroscopic scissors or a resectoscope. The smaller, more narrow septa are typically resected with scissors, while the resectoscope works well for broad septa. Our group always performs concomitant laparoscopy to both evaluate the fundal contour and guide in determining the

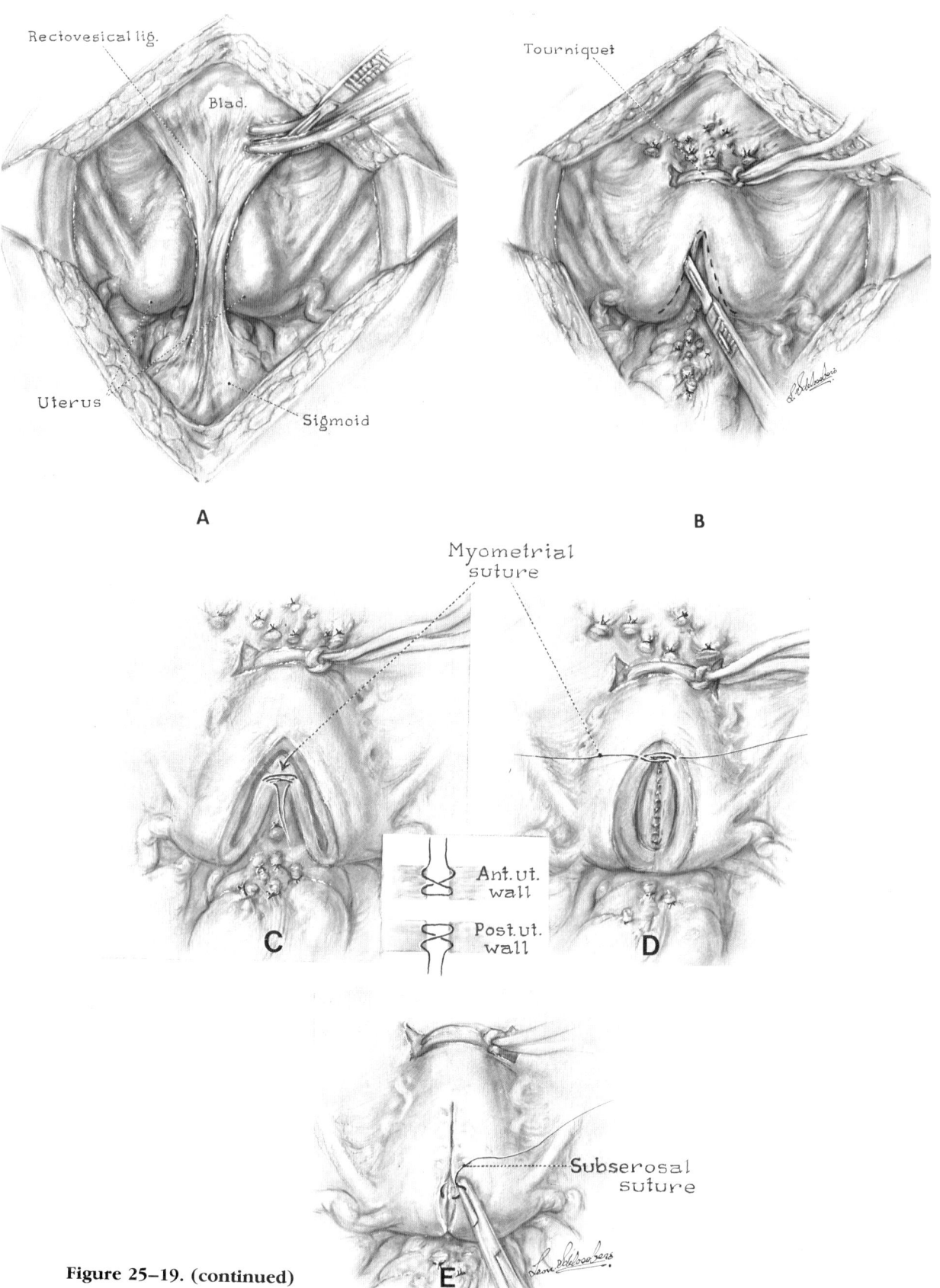

Figure 25–19. (continued)

Fig. 32-1 The Strassmann metroplasty with modifications. (A) If a rectovesical ligament is found, it should be removed. (B) An incision is made on the medial side of each hemicorpus and carried deep enough to enter the uterine cavity. The edges of the myometrium will evert to face the opposite side. (C and D) The myometrium is approximated using interrupted vertical figure-of-eight No. 3-0 polyglycolic acid sutures. Avoid placing sutures too close to the interstitial por-

tion of the fallopian tubes. (E) A continuous No. 5-0 polyglycolic acid subserosal suture is used as a final layer. Tourniquets are removed, and defects in the broad ligament are closed. (Reproduced by permission from Thompson JD, Rock JA, eds. Surgery for anomalies of the müllerian ducts. In: Thompson JD, Rock JA, eds. TeLinde's operative gynecology, ed 7. Philadelphia: JB Lippincott, 1983:636.)

endpoints for resection. By reducing the light source to the laparoscope, the fundus can be visualized and septal resection halted when the hysteroscope light source begins to transilluminate the fundus.

Preoperative preparation

Adequate visualization of the septum is imperative for safe and effective surgical resection. A thick endometrium or blood will obscure the view through the hysteroscope; therefore hysteroscopic resection should be performed in the early to midfollicular phase of the cycle. Many surgeons prefer to pretreat patients with a gonadotropin-releasing-hormone agonist such as leuprolide acetate (Lupron; TAP Pharmaceutical, North Chicago, Ill.) or nafarelin acetate (Synarel, Syntex, Palo Alto, Calif.) for 1 to 2 months to suppress endometrial growth. Our group has not routinely pretreated patients with such agonists, and we have been pleased with the visualization of the septum at resection.

Septal incision with scissors

When incising a thin uterine septum with scissors, we prefer to use an operative hysteroscope with a 3-mm straight operating port and 45-degree offset optics with a 0-degree angle of vision (Fig. 32-2) (Cohen-Eder hysteroscope No. 150331, Eder, Chicago, Ill.). Rigid scissors (3 mm) can be placed through the operative port and the septum incised beginning at its base. We prefer this instrumentation to the flexible scissors used with other hysteroscopes, as there is greater control and stability. When the septum is incised, the uterine walls retract, and the septum is pulled apart. Because of the relative avascularity of the septum, there is little bleeding. The septum is serially incised toward the fundus, until the light of the hysteroscope is seen transilluminating the fundus, or there is an increase in bleeding from the incision site, signifying that normal myometrium has been reached. The hysteroscope is then withdrawn to the internal cervical os, and a panoramic view of the uterine cavity should reveal absence of a midline division, and both tubal ostia should be visible.

Septal resection with the resectoscope

When the septum is broad, it is technically difficult to incise using the relatively small operative scissors. In these cases,

the resectoscope is ideal. The uterine cavity is distended with a 1.5% glycine solution delivered through the infusion port of the resectoscope. The septum is then electrosurgically incised from base to fundus using the cutting loop (Fig. 32-3). The progress is monitored by laparoscopy, and resection is terminated when the fundus is reached. Again, this will be evident when either the hysteroscope light is seen through the fundus by laparoscopy, or both tubal ostia are visible on a panoramic view of the uterus. Because the resectoscope uses electrosurgical current to remove the septum, there may not be an increase in bleeding when the base of the septum is reached. Consequently, perforation of the fundus may occur more readily, and the surgeon should carefully monitor the resection with concomitant laparoscopy.

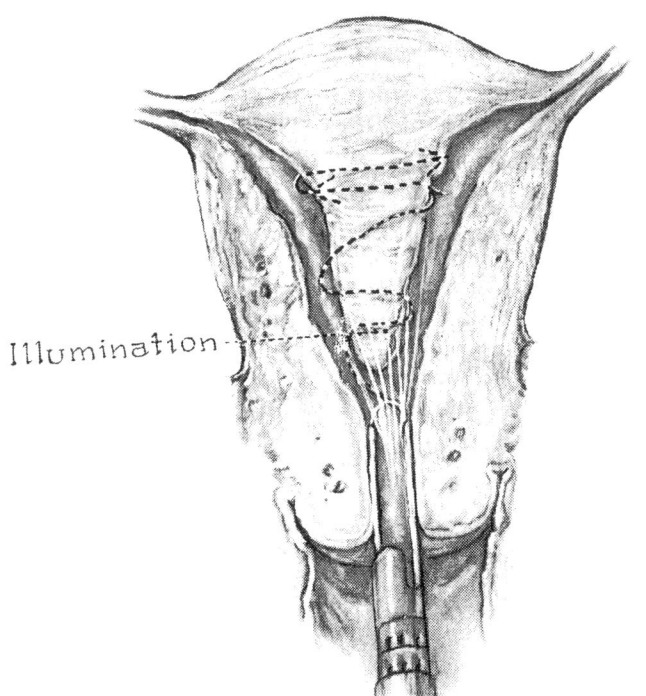

Fig. 32-3 Resectoscopic metroplasty. The septum is inased with the straight loop of the resectoscope, until both internal ossa are visualized. (Reproduced with permission from Rock JA. Surgery for anomalies of the müllerian ducts. In: Thompson JD, Rock JA, eds. TeLindés operative gynecology, ed 7. Philadelphia: JB Lippencott, 1988:632.)

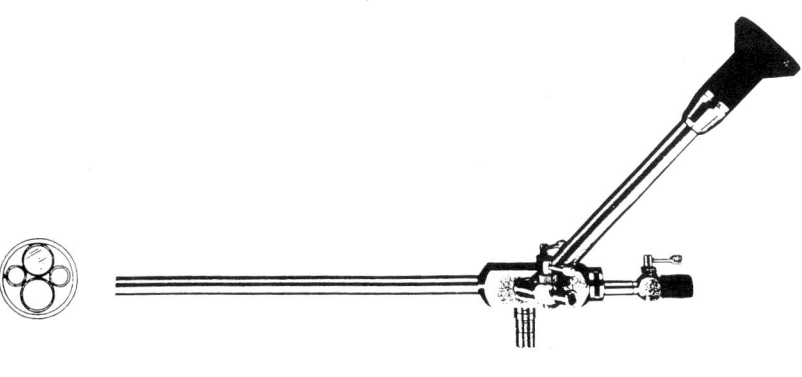

Fig. 32-2 Cohen-Eder hysteroscope with two flow channels and a 3-mm instrument channel, 18-cm working length, 45-degree eyepiece. No. 150331 8-mm diameter, 0-degree direction of view.

Postoperative management

Typically there is minimal bleeding following incision or resection of a uterine septum. If bleeding is encountered, the uterus can be tamponaded with a Foley catheter having a 30-cc balloon. The catheter is placed into the uterine cavity, and the balloon is inflated with saline. As the balloon expands, pressure is placed on the bleeding sites, and hemostasis should be achieved within minutes. The balloon is removed 4 to 6 hours postoperatively, before the patient is discharged.

We place our patients on supplemental estrogen (conjugated equine estrogens 1.25 mg/day) for 2 months following the surgery to assist in endometrial healing and decrease the formation of intrauterine synechiae. Pregnancy should be deferred during this period of time to allow for regeneration of the endometrium. If conception has not occurred in 6 to 12 months following septal repair, or there is a marked decrease in menstrual flow, a hysterogram should be performed to evaluate the adequacy of resection and screen for intrauterine synechiae.

References

1 Patten BM. Human embryology. New York: McGraw-Hill, 1953:579–587.

2 Jarcho J. Malformation of the uterus. Am J Surg 1946;71:106.

3 Moore O. Congenital abnormalities of the female genitalia. South Med J 1941;34:610.

4 Jones GS. Obstetrical significance of female genital anomalies. Obstet Gynecol 1957;10:113.

5 Makino T, Umeuchi M, Nakada K, et al. Incidence of congenital uterine anomalies in repeated reproductive wastage and prognosis for pregnancy after metroplasty. Int J Fertil 1992;37:167.

6 Jones HW, Wheeless CR. Salvage of the reproductive potential of women with anomalous development of the müllerian ducts: 1868–1968–2068. Am J Obstet Gynecol 1969;104:348.

7 Rock JA. Diagnosing and repairing uterine anomalies. Contemp Ob/Gynecol 1981;17(June):43.

8 Ayhan A, Yücel I, Tuncer ZS, Kisnisci HA. Reproductive performance after conventional metroplasty: an evaluation of 102 cases. Fertil Steril 1992;57:1194.

9 Purcell. Philosophical transactions of the Royal Society of London, 629 LXIV. In: Gould GM, Pyle WL. Anomalies and curiosities of medicine. Philadelphia: WB Saunders, 1896:311.

10 Jones HW, Rock JA. Reparative and constructive surgery of the female generative tract. Baltimore: Williams & Wilkins, 1983: 146–185.

11 Tulandi T, Arronet GH, McInnes RA. Arcuate and bicornuate uterine anomalies and infertility. Fertil Steril 1980;34:362.

12 Strassmann E. Plastic unification of double uterus: a study of 123 collected and five personal cases. Am J Obstet Gynecol 1952;64:25.

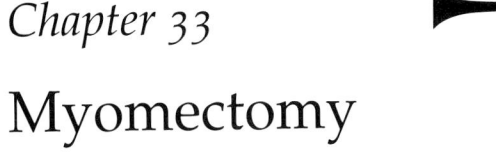

Chapter 33
Myomectomy

Luis E. Sanz and Patricia M. Hoyne

It has been estimated that approximately 25% of women of childbearing age have uterine leiomyomata. The most common solid tumor of the pelvis, it is much more common in black females than in white. As such, it is a commonly encountered problem in the gynecology practice. A plan for management of these patients as well as the techniques for myomectomy will be discussed.

The origin of leiomyomata is unknown. The cell line is thought to be from immature, smooth muscle cells of the myometrium and unicellular in origin. It is not clearly understood what affects the growth of leiomyomata, but three factors are commonly implicated: estrogen, growth hormone, and progesterone (1). Estrogen has long been associated with leiomyoma growth. Leiomyomata arise in reproductive years, grow during pregnancy, and tend to get smaller after menopause. Recent studies have looked at estrogen receptors in leiomyomata and in the endometrium in an attempt to show why there seems to be an estrogen response. The results are varied. Wilson et al. showed an increased concentration of estrogen receptors in leiomyomata (2). Other investigators have not substantiated these findings. Growth hormone is the second factor that studies have associated with leiomyomata growth. It is synergistic with estradiol in increasing uterine weight in hypophysectomized-ovariectomized rats (3).

There is also a higher growth hormone response in black women, who have a higher rate of leiomyomata (4). Growth hormone decreases in pregnancy, but it is similar in structure to human placental lactogen, which does achieve high levels in pregnancy (5). Progesterone is the third factor associated with leiomyoma growth. Large doses of progesterone given to patients for 2 to 3 weeks before hysterectomy caused generation of myomas in a study by Goldzieher and colleagues (6). Other studies have also shown inhibition of leiomyomata growth by progesterone.

Leiomyomata are classified according to location. Submucous myomata are located inferior to the endometrium and project into the endometrial cavity by varying degrees. They may also be pedunculated and occasionally may prolapse through the cervix. Intramural leiomyomata occur within the myometrium. Subserosal myomata can be located in the ligaments of the uterus or in the body of the uterus. They are often pedunculated and occasionally parasitic. They range in size from microscopic to immense, and may occur singly or in groups.

Signs and symptoms

The clinical presentation of uterine myomata varies considerably. Many are asymptomatic and are discovered on routine pelvic examination. Occasionally they are discovered at exploratory laparotomy or when a patient is undergoing diagnostic tests for another reason. Approximately one fourth of patients with this condition are symptomatic. The symptoms include excessive bleeding, pain, pressure, infertility, or fetal wastage. Most women who have bleeding problems related to myomata have unusually long and heavy periods. Theories to explain this include increased endometrial surface area because of cavity distortion, interference with the ability of the uterus to contract, or compression and obstruction of venous plexi in the uterus. Submucosal leiomyomata can cause bleeding because of location.

Pain is another symptom experienced by women with myoma. It is the result of degenerative changes within the tumor, torsion of a pedunculated myoma, or contractile activity of the uterus against the myoma. If a myoma is very large, it may press on pelvic nerves and cause radiating pain. Some women will describe a feeling of pelvic fullness or pressure.

More rarely, women with a large tumor may suffer obstructive effects from it. It may cause ureteral compression or displacement, resulting in hydroureter or hydronephrosis. Compression of the bladder may lead to frequent voiding or even urinary retention if a myoma exerts pressure on the urethra. Dependent upon location, a leiomyoma may cause leg edema, constipation, and rarely intestinal obstruction.

With the recent trend toward childbearing in the later reproductive years, leiomyomata are being seen more often in pregnancy, and they are sometimes present in women with infertility. Leiomyomata are not usually the cause of infertility, but there are instances that can be directly attributed to them. Sometimes a large pedunculated submucous fibroid may act as an intrauterine device and prevent implantation. If a myoma is situated in a position that impinges upon the endocervical canal or tubal lumina, infertility may result. They may interfere with sperm transport by increasing the distance sperm have to travel or by interfering with uterine contractility. They may also be associated with a higher rate of abortion. This may be due to uterine irritability, or to alterations in the endometrium. During the third trimester, myomata may be associated with premature labor and delivery or may cause obstruction in labor. Hemorrhage may also be associated with a uterine leiomyoma in the postpartum period.

Many myomata are easily diagnosed on pelvic examination. However, there is other pelvic pathology that may be difficult to distinguish from uterine fibroids. Sounding the uterus is often mentioned as an easy test to help differentiate between myomata and other pelvic neoplasms. Incidental abdominal x-ray may demonstrate calcification within a myoma, but it is not required for preoperative evaluation. An intravenous pyelogram is essential in the workup of a woman with a very large leiomyoma. It may reveal ureteral compression or deviation and will assist in identification of the ureter during surgery. Laparoscopy can be done to differentiate a pedunculated fibroid from an ovarian tumor if the patient refuses laparotomy. Ultrasonography helps to distinguish a leiomyoma from other pelvic pathology, or to reveal an unsuspected pregnancy. It also gives an idea on the size and position of the fibroids.

The use of endovaginal sonography is critical in the identification of submucous fibroids.

Hysterosalpingography and hysteroscopy are important tools in the evaluation of infertility or abnormal uterine bleeding associated with myomata. Submucous myomata that are not palpable on pelvic examination may be easily demonstrated by these techniques. Encroachment on a tubal lumen or the endocervical canal may also be demonstrated.

Preoperative evaluation

Preoperative evaluation includes a pregnancy test, complete blood count, type, and screen, autologous donation of the patient's blood, and other blood work as indicated by the patient's history. Anemia is often present in the woman with menorrhagia, and an attempt should be made to correct this with iron before any surgical intervention. Polycythemia is also seen in association with myomata. The etiology of this is unknown, and it resolves after removal of the fibroid. An endometrial sample should be obtained for all women with abnormal bleeding before surgical intervention to rule out endometrial cancer. All women should have a pap smear to rule out concurrent cervical intraepithelial neoplasia. The surgery should be performed during the early proliferative phase of the cycle to decrease blood loss. Intravenous antibiotic is given at the time of surgery, and 12 hours later.

The decision to perform myomectomy is based on many factors, the most important of which is the patient's desire for future fertility. Most women who are asymptomatic can be followed conservatively with pelvic examinations every 6 to 12 months. If no significant growth is occurring, no intervention is necessary. Many feel that a uterine size comparable to approximately 12 to 14 weeks' gestation requires treatment, regardless of symptoms, especially if the ovaries cannot be palpated.

In a woman with an enlarged uterus desirous of pregnancy, a trial of conception is advisable. Many women with uteri of 12 to 14 weeks' size conceive without difficulty. If conception is not obtained in a reasonable length of time and there is no other cause of infertility, myomectomy is advisable. If significant growth is noted, or if someone with a rather large uterus wishes to delay fertility for more than one year, myomectomy is advised. Many feel that myomectomy is more successful if the surgery is performed before the myoma reaches an excessive size. Early myomectomy may mean that subsequent surgery is necessary, as 30% may recur. Therefore, the choices for a patient with fibroids depend on her symptoms and her desire for fertility. The choices are as follows: monitoring the fibroids, hysteroscopic resection, myomectomy (laparoscopically or by laparotomy), or hysterectomy (vaginal or abdominally).

One of the newest developments is the use of gonadotropin-releasing hormone (GnRH) analogues, such as leuprolide acetate (Lupron Depot) intramuscularly or nafarelin acetate by nasal spray (Synarel), which produce a menopausal state with marked decrease in ovarian function and uterine atrophy. I use Lupron Depot (3.75 mg, IM) (7) every month for 2 to 3 months before planned surgery to decrease the blood supply and cause atrophy of the myoma. This can result in a less difficult case, with less blood loss and a shorter operating time. This treatment may also be applicable to the patient who is a poor surgical risk. To use it beyond that time may make it more difficult to identify the proper surgical plane between the myoma and the myometrium. The most common side effects are those associated with a hypoestrogenic state such as hot flashes, headaches, vaginitis, and reversible osteoporosis, especially if used for more than 6 months.

Certain conditions preclude any attempt at myomectomy as therapy. Pelvic malignancy is an absolute contraindication to myomectomy, as is active pelvic infection. Certain pelvic conditions make the likelihood of success doubtful, including extensive endometriosis, pelvic inflammatory disease, and adenomyosis. Pregnancy is a relative contraindication to myomectomy because of the high probability of losing the pregnancy or excessive blood loss. If a patient does not desire fertility, then hysterectomy is the treatment of choice.

Surgical techniques

The key to successful outcome after myomectomy is meticulous surgical technique. Decreasing blood loss and preventing postoperative adhesion formation are extremely important. Adequate exposure is necessary for successful myomectomy. A Pfannenstiel or a Maylard skin incision offers adequate exposure of pelvic organs. Only if the uterus is very large is a vertical skin incision required. After placing the patient in Trendelenburg's position and packing away the bowel, steps are taken to reduce blood loss.

Bonney designed a special clamp that grips the round ligament and uterine arteries. Lock used rubber-shod sponge forceps across the uterine and ovarian vessels. We advocate the use of vascular clamps (DeBakey's) across the utero-ovarian ligament to stop blood flow from the ovarian artery. A 2-cm incision is then made on the anterior and posterior leaf of the broad ligament by the area of the internal os to expose the uterine vessels. A quarter-inch Penrose drain is then inserted through the opening of the broad ligaments, and the Penrose is tied posteriorly to decrease the blood flow from the uterine vessels. However, with any of the above techniques, care must be taken to avoid ischemia and necrosis. This can be done by periodically releasing clamps for short periods. Care must be taken to put enough pressure to stop both arterial and venous flow.

The injection of vasopressin, neosynephrine, or oxytocin (Pitocin) has been used to minimize blood loss. This is not as effective with multiple large fibroids, and the patient must be carefully monitored.

A single elliptical incision is made on top of the fibroid either with the scalpel or the carbon dioxide or neodymium-yttrium-aluminum-garnet (Nd-YAG) laser (Fig. 33-1). The Nd-YAG laser has more penetrating and coagulating power than the carbon dioxide laser. We prefer to use the laser for its hemostatic capabilities and its precision. There is minimal thermal damage to peripheral tissues. The ability to seal blood vessels of up to 1 mm is of benefit. It can also be used to destroy small leiomyomata at laparotomy. We use the carbon dioxide laser with a continuous mode at a setting of 40 W. This lowers the average blood loss by 300 to 450 cc. The incision on the uterus should be vertical and on the midline to avoid the lateral uterine vascular supply and the fal-

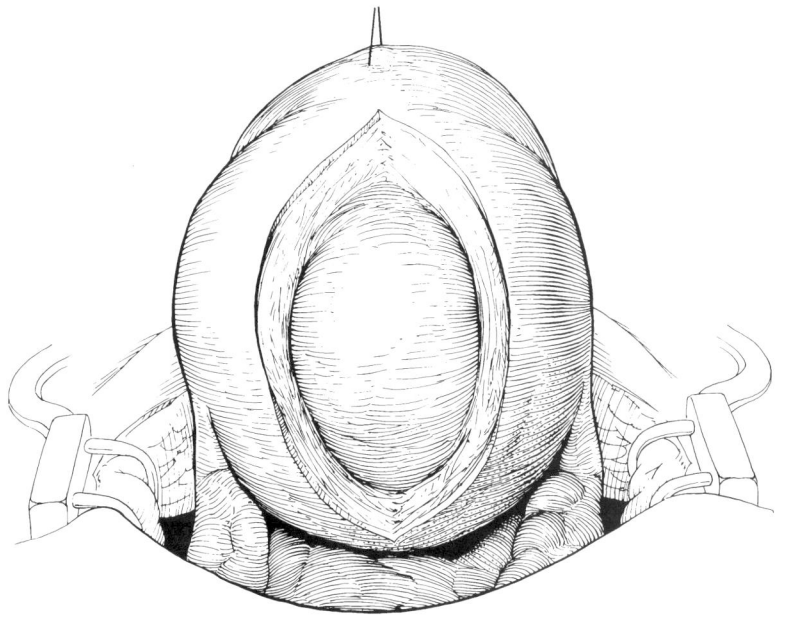

Fig. 33-1 A single elliptical vertical incision is made as low as possible on the area of the fibroid. Care must be taken to ligate any major arterial bleeding.

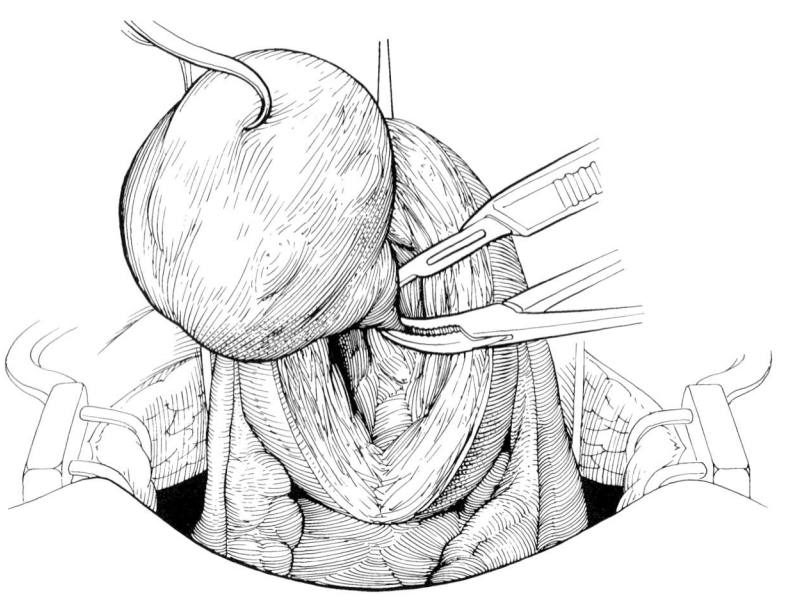

Fig. 33-2 The posterior wall of the fibroid is carefully dissected to avoid entering the endometrial cavity.

lopian tubes. The incision should be on the low anterior uterine wall whenever possible. If the fibroid is in the posterior wall, we prefer to make a low posterior midline vertical incision rather than going anteriorly through the endometrial cavity. Then the myoma is quickly dissected from the myometrium trying not to penetrate the endometrial cavity. Most of the time this can be accomplished with blunt dissection. If there is a cluster of fibroids, it is better to make a single incision to remove all the fibroids to avoid adhesions. Incisions in the area of the cornua or lateral uterine wall should be avoided. Surgical speed is very important to minimize blood loss. Many times one is able to identify the vascular supply to the myoma; the pedicle should then be clamped, cut, and ligated to prevent unnecessary blood loss.

After enucleating the fibroid by blunt dissection, a single artery is often noted. This should be clamped and ligated with 2-0 poliglecaprone 25 (Monocryl) suture (Fig. 33-2). Monocryl is a new synthetic monofilament suture with a great tensile strength, which is quite inert, and it is absorbed in 14 to 21 days, therefore quickly eliminating foreign tissue. The dead space created should then be closed in multiple layers by interrupted hemostatic figure-of-eight sutures of 3-0 Monocryl or 3-0 polyglactin (Vicryl) (Figs. 33-3A and 33-3B). Care should be taken to avoid hematoma formation. Traumatizing tissue should be avoided because myometrial specimens from myomatous uteri have been shown to contain large amounts of plasminogen activator, which has anticoagulant activity. Therefore, the larger the surface area or the greater the number of fibroids, the greater the chance of bleeding (8). Too tightly placed sutures will lead to tissue necrosis. Excessive myometrium and serosa should be trimmed. The serosa is closed with a continuous inverting suture of 5-0 Monocryl (Fig. 33-4). This is done to minimize a raw surface on the uterus. The

pelvic organs are kept moist throughout surgery with a continuous irrigation of lactated Ringer's solution or normal saline.

Careful consideration must be made to the patency of the fallopian tubes and the integrity of the uterine blood supply. The bladder flap is used to cover low anterior incisions whenever possible. The removal of large fibroids or of numerous fibroids usually causes postoperative bleeding. In that case, or if there is oozing from the uterus, it is better to tie both uterine arteries to decrease blood flow to the uterus. This can be accomplished easily by placing a suture ligature of 0 Monocryl or Vicryl around the uterine artery at the level of the internal os. This will not compromise the blood supply to the uterus.

In an effort to decrease postoperative adhesions, various techniques have been advocated. The use of interceed (TC7), a fabric of oxidized, regenerated cellulose, is very popular currently because it is easy to use and very good in preventing adhesion formation. Another material to prevent adhesions is Goretex surgical membrane.

The placement of 50 cc of Hyskon (32% in dextran, 70% in dextrose) solution in the pelvis at the completion of surgery is another popular method of decreasing adhesion formation. This creates a medium to decrease the formation of fibrin adhesions of the pelvic organs and to draw fluid into the pelvic cavity. Care should be taken, as cases of anaphylaxis and fluid overload have been reported with dextran.

Recurrent myoma is a complication that is more common in the patient with multiple myomata and could be the result of small tumors that were left behind at the original surgery. In carefully selected patients, a subsequent myomectomy can be performed. Malone had a series in which four out of five patients who underwent a repeat myomectomy conceived and carried the pregnancy successfully (9).

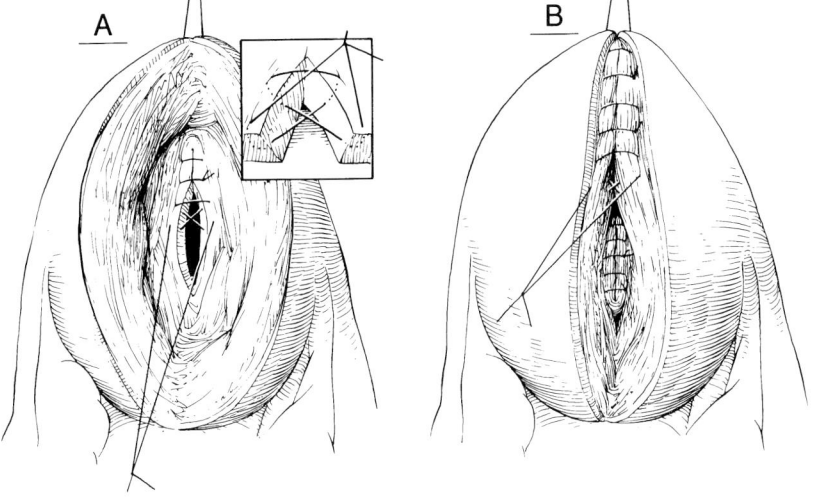

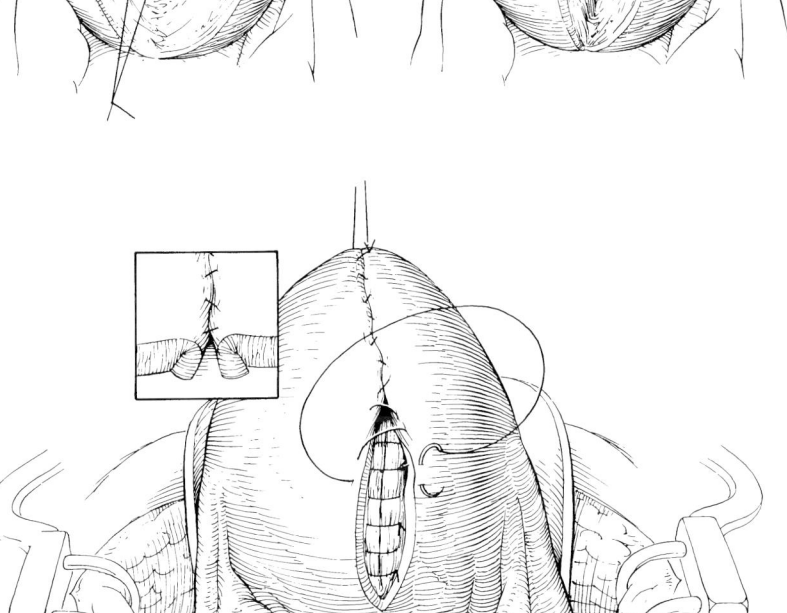

Fig. 33-3 (A) The myometrium is closed in multiple layers with hemostatic figure-of-eight sutures of 4-0 Dexon or Vicryl. (B) Coaptation of last myometrial layer should be close to the peritoneal surface of the uterus.

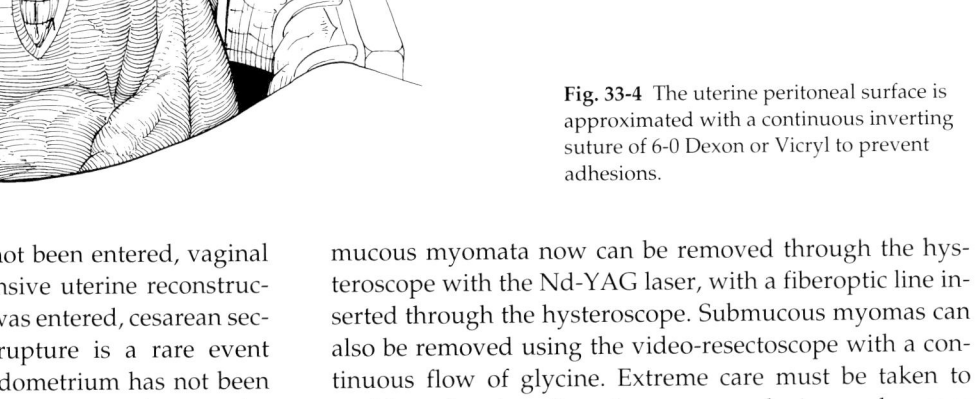

Fig. 33-4 The uterine peritoneal surface is approximated with a continuous inverting suture of 6-0 Dexon or Vicryl to prevent adhesions.

If the endometrial cavity has not been entered, vaginal delivery is advisable unless extensive uterine reconstruction was performed. If the cavity was entered, cesarean section is recommended. Uterine rupture is a rare event following myomectomy if the endometrium has not been entered. As with any surgical procedure, complications include hemorrhage, infection, adhesions, and injury to the surrounding structures. All of these can be decreased by practicing good surgical technique. Rarely, sarcoma may be discovered in the specimen, requiring further surgery.

Aborting cervical myomata should be removed vaginally (10). This is accomplished by doing a cervical myomectomy and placing a figure-of-eight suture by the base with 0 polyglycolic acid (Dexon) or Vicryl. If the hysterectomy is done to remove the cervical myoma, infection will complicate the hysterectomy. It is necessary to wait 6 to 8 weeks before performing subsequent surgery. Small sub-mucous myomata now can be removed through the hysteroscope with the Nd-YAG laser, with a fiberoptic line inserted through the hysteroscope. Submucous myomas can also be removed using the video-resectoscope with a continuous flow of glycine. Extreme care must be taken to avoid perforating the uterus or producing pulmonary edema by the excessive use of fluids. The patient has to be aware that blood loss can be significant.

Laparoscope-assisted myomectomy is another alternative in selected cases (11,12).

Summary

It has been shown that the pregnancy rate after myomectomy is approximately 50%. Given this figure, we consider myomectomy an acceptable therapy for women with leiomyoma. When careful surgical technique is followed, the outcome is optimized and the complication rate is acceptable. The procedure should be offered to women who want to maintain their fertility or to women who want another alternative to hysterectomy. Careful counseling of the patient with regard to the risks, including the possibility of hysterectomy, and the benefits must be given. Myomectomy is not a procedure that will benefit everyone, but in selected cases it is clearly the surgery of choice.

References

1 Buttram VC, Reiter RC. Uterine leiomyomata: etiology, symptomatology, and management. Fertil Steril 1981;36:433.

2 Wilson EA, Yang F, Rees ED. Estradiol and progesterone binding in uterine leiomyomata and in normal uterine tissues. Obstet Gynecol 1980;55:20.

3 Grattorola R, Lich A. Effect of growth hormone and its combination with estradiol-17-beta on the uterus at hypophysectomized and hypophysectomized-ovariectomized rats. Clin Endocrinol 1959; 65:802.

4 Rubenstein AH, Seftel HC, Milterk BI, et al. Metabolic response to oral glucose in healthy South African white, Indian, and African subjects. Br Med J 1969;1:748.

5 Spellacy WN, Buhi WC. Pituitary growth hormone and placental lactogen measured in normal term pregnancy and at the early and late postpartum periods. Am J Obstet Gynecol 1969;105:888.

6 Goldzieher JW, Magueo M, Ricaud L, et al. Induction of degenerative changes in uterine myomas by high-dose progestin therapy. Am J Obstet Gynecol 1966;96:1078.

7 Hutchins FL. Myomectomy after selective preoperative treatment with a gonadotropin releasing hormone analog. Reprod Med 1992;37:699.

8 Sacks PC, Hoyne PM. Disseminated intravascular coagulation, hemolytic anemia, and acute renal failure associated with extensive multiple myomectomy. Obstet Gynecol 1992;79:835.

9 Malone LJ. Myomectomy: recurrence after removal of solitary and multiple myomas. Obstet Gynecol 1969;34:200.

10 Goldrath MH. Vaginal removal of the pedunculated submucous myoma. J Reprod Med 1990;35:921.

11 Harris WJ. Uterine dehiscence following laparoscopic myomectomy. Obstet Gynecol 1992;80:545.

12 Hasson HM, Rotman C, Rana N, et al. Laparoscopic myomectomy. Obstet Gynecol 1992;80:884.

Suggested readings

Sciarra JJ, Droegemueller W, eds. Myomectomy in gynecology and obstetrics, revised ed. Philadelphia: Harper & Row, 1984:chapter 58.

Part 5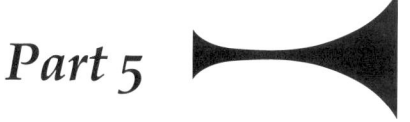

Endoscopic and Laser Surgery

Chapter 34

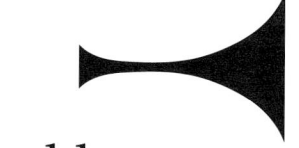

Intra-abdominal laser applications

Michael S. Baggish

To date, most intra-abdominal applications of carbon dioxide (CO_2) lasers have been for infertility surgery (1–4). Specific procedures include neosalpingostomy, myomectomy, cornual shaves, adhesiolysis, tubal incision to remove products of ectopic pregnancy, and vaporization of endometrial lesions.

Advantages of the CO_2 over the argon and other lasers are its high power and ability to make precise knifelike wounds, effect reasonable hemostasis without color dependency, and allow careful depth control. As a result, it can reach otherwise inaccessible locations with consistently excellent visualization, unobscured by blood in the operating field.

Laser basics

Power density (W/cm²) is the laser energy absorbed by tissue or actual power delivered at the target. The *focal length* of the laser beam is the distance between the focusing lens and the beam's focal point. *Spot size* is the diameter of the focal point. Generally, shorter focal lengths produce smaller spot sizes and, with constant power, deeper craters. Longer focal lengths give larger spot sizes and shallower craters.

Continuous wave exposure delivers laser energy for as long as the shutter remains open. By contrast, a *pulsed beam* delivers laser energy in short bursts, with interspersed refractory periods. In *superpulsing,* power is very high, and both delivery and interspersed refractory periods are measured in fractions of milliseconds. *Pulsing* must not be confused with *time gating,* which does not alter the mode of delivery. Gating the shutter permits delivering the beam (continuous wave) over a preselected short time interval regardless of how long the foot pedal is depressed.

Superpulsing is used when it is advantageous to minimize thermal effects on tissue. The short refractory periods allow the tissue to cool down between pulses and reduce peripheral heat conduction.

Typical focal length for *handpiece* delivery is between 50 and 100 mm, and for *micromanipulator* delivery 250, 300, or 400 mm. Typical *fine* spot size is between 0.2 and 0.5 mm, *medium* spot size between 1 and 1.5 mm, and *large* spot size between 2 and 3 mm. Typical *low* power settings are between 10 and 15 W, *high* settings between 20 and 30 W, and *very high* power settings more than 50 W.

High power is preferable

To minimize damage to surrounding tissue by operating with higher power for a shorter time, it is advisable to use a system with a power output of more than 30 W. Use of superpulsing, in which very high wattages are released in very brief surges, further controls heating by allowing time for tissue to cool between pulses.

The beam can be directed to the tissue site either by an articulated arm and handpiece or by a micromanipulator connected to an operating microscope and guided by a joystick. Handpiece delivery offers short focal distance and ablation craters, or spots, 0.2 mm or less in diameter. By contrast, micromanipulator delivery, which produces 0.5-mm spots at focal distances of 250 to 300 mm, offers more precise movement and positioning of the beam and absence of tremor. Fixing special lenses to tubular metal light guides allows delivery of the fine micromanipulator-directed beams to tissue via single- or double-puncture laparoscopy (5). Flexible, hollow fibers measuring 2 mm in diameter have further facilitated laser laparoscopy.

Works through cell water

Without actually making direct contact with tissue, the laser beam is absorbed by cell water. Almost instantly, it heats to 100°C, forming steam that expands to explode cellular contents into vapor. Temperatures approaching 800°C within the laser wound eliminate virtually every microorganism and sterilize the wound.

The resulting wound, devoid of debris, contains only a small band of necrotic tissue and is hemostatic. Thus laser wounds are more akin to knife wounds than to microcautery injuries. Because the beam is invisible and there is no blood, a continuous clear view of abnormal tissue is possible, provided smoke is removed.

Preparing the patient

Obtain informed consent. Explain that although heat-induced tissue desiccation and necrosis are major disadvantages of laser surgery, rapidity of heating restricts such effects to a tiny area (Fig. 34-1). Note that an early study showing heat damage limited to less than 500 μm from the impact point was made when maximum power densities of such lasers were only 8000 W/cm² (6). Point out that contemporary instruments, which can deliver more than 100,000 W/cm², can reduce thermal damage to surrounding tissue even more by operating for shorter times.

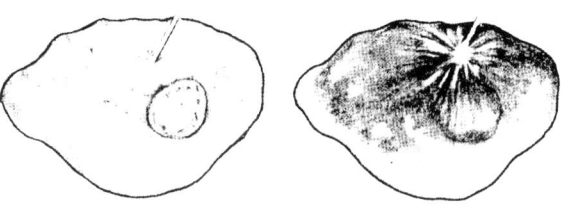

Tissue temperature 100°C   Tissue temperature 1,000°C

Fig. 34-1 Laser-induced tissue damage. At high power densities, the laser beam superheats cells instantaneously to 100°C, vaporizing them with little damage to surrounding tissue. However, when low power densities are delivered over a relatively longer time, carbon forms and superheats surrounding tissue as it is itself vaporized.

Exclude flammable materials from the operative field and drape the immediate incision area with cloth towels moistened with sterile water. After opening the abdomen and completing exploration, thoroughly soak all packing material with lactated Ringer's solution and flood the abdominal cavity to protect surrounding viscera.

Before operating, calibrate the beam on a wooden tongue blade. Make imprints of various spot sizes using different power settings. *Baggish's rule* observes that a 0.5-mm spot delivered at 10 W for 0.1 second will penetrate a standard wooden tongue blade.

Then set laser power and spot size, and select either a continuous wave or pulsed mode of operation. Several contemporary machines incorporate microprocessors that can store two or three setting combinations. For cutting, I use either 40 to 50 W, spots between 0.2 and 0.5 mm, and continuous wave exposure, or between 300 and 400 superpulses per second at intervals of 0.2 to 0.4 msec.

Manipulatory rods, spatulas, and grasping tools should be spherical, irregularly surfaced, and heat-dissipating to avoid accidentally reflecting the beam. Whereas titanium and anodized aluminum are appropriate materials, Pyrex or quartz glass have tended to superheat, melt, and break. To guide the beam deliberately to a hard-to-reach site, use of a long-handled mirror coated with gold or another highly reflective material is recommended.

For clearing smoke from the operating field, use a high-flow-volume vacuum pump equipped with a filter to absorb the odor of vaporized tissue as well as trapping particles 0.5 μm in size. Using operating room wall suction is inadvisable, because equipment can be clogged by particulate material in the laser plume.

Making the anterior abdominal wall incision

To make an incision, sweep the beam's focal point across the lower abdomen, determining incision depth by velocity of hand movement (Fig. 34-2). Generally, this motion will seal vessels smaller than 0.5 mm in diameter. For larger vessels, raise the focal point above the abdomen to effect hemostasis by creating a larger spot with greater thermal action (defocusing) (Fig. 34-2).

After cutting the skin, one will need to raise power to pierce the fatty layer, as it contains greater amounts of water that will absorb the beam and so retard penetration. Then cut the rectus fascia. If the muscles are to be divided, place a "laser" spatula beneath them to permit severing the belly of the rectus close to the symphysis pubis.

Neosalpingostomy to open the hydrosalpinx

Fill the obstructed tube with methylene blue via a uterine cannula, free it of adhesions, mobilize it, and stabilize it with two or three 6-0 polyglactin (Vicryl) stay sutures. Then

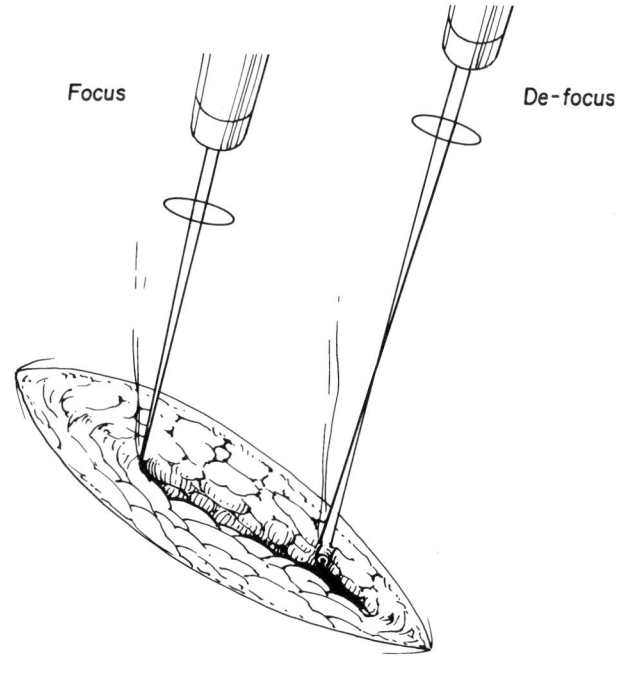

Fig. 34-2 Performing the incision. A highly focused laser beam concentrates intensity at a fine point, cutting tissue like a sharp knife (*left*), while a defocused beam coagulates blood vessels by delivering a large spot with correspondingly greater thermal action (*right*).

locate the central point of fimbrial closure (umbilicated) and, using a laser handpiece with a 125-mm focal lens, aim a 0.2-mm spot at it to drill an opening (Fig. 34-3). I suggest using a minimum power density of 32,000 W/cm². Select eyeglass-mounted microscopes with a coaxial headlight for magnification and lighting.

Once methylene blue flows freely from the opening, enlarge the opening to permit insertion of the 1-mm tip of an angulated laser rod into the lumen. Absorption by methylene blue will prevent spare laser energy from inadvertently striking the endosalpinx.

Using the inserted rod as a backstop, make four 1-cm incisions radiating from the central opening to create flaps and form a pseudofimbriated end. If the hydrosalpinx is very vascular, inject 1 to 2 ml of 1:30 vasopressin (Pitressin) into the muscularis, using a tuberculin syringe with a 25-gauge needle. The vascular spasm produced will reduce vessel diameters to 0.5 mm or less, allowing laser sealing.

One may either suture the flaps back with 6-0 coated polyglactin or play the laser over their serosal surfaces at a power density of less than 300 W/cm² to effect retraction (Fig. 34-5; 1). After completing surgery and thoroughly irrigating the operative site, place 200 ml of dextran 70 (Hyskon) into the cul-de-sac.

Linear salpingostomy for ectopic pregnancy

A high index of suspicion, liberal β-subunit human chorionic gonadotropin pregnancy testing, and early laparoscopy in-

crease chances of diagnosing tubal ectopic pregnancy before rupture and therefore of saving the oviduct during treatment.

Using a handpiece, whose shorter focal length permits finer cutting, focus the beam on the tube and infiltrate 3 ml of 1:30 vasopressin into the superficial tubal muscularis. Then set power at 400 pulses per second, pulse width at 0.3-msec intervals, focus to a 0.2-mm spot, and make a linear incision 3 to 4 cm long through the tube's full thickness.

On encountering the products of conception, use fine laser hooks to spread incision edges, place a hook on the products, and wash them out by irrigating the tube vigorously through the fimbriated end. Once the tube is empty, close the incision with a single layer of interrupted 6-0 coated polyglactin sutures. Irrigate the operative field with lactated Ringer's solution and add 200 ml of dextran 70 over it.

Cornual shave

When there is an interstitial obstruction, it is necessary to locate an open portion of oviduct before attempting reimplantation. Begin by injecting 5 ml of 1:30 vasopressin into the cornu. Set power either at 30 to 40 W or at 300 to 400 pulses per second released at 0.3-msec intervals, and focus to a 0.2-mm spot. Then make small serial cuts in the highly vascular cornual portion of the uterus, proceeding toward the endometrial cavity, until a supple, open portion of interstitial tube can be identified.

One may inject methylene blue from below to help establish patency. When dye spill indicates an open tube, take a final section with the sharp scalpel, and coagulate bleeding points by defocusing and reducing the power to 15 W.

Adhesiolysis

For separating small adhesions that are between the tube and ovary or between the adnexa and uterus, use a micromanipulator and a power density of less than 1000 W/cm². Ovarian investment adhesions—thin, extensive collagenous envelopes—often contain many fragile blood vessels. Attempts to dissect them away usually cause profuse bleeding and injury to the underlying ovarian cortex.

To bloodlessly vaporize adhesions that entirely envelope the ovary, use a spot size of 1.5 to 2.0 mm and a power setting of 10 to 15 W. With a circular motion, play the laser rapidly over the ovarian surface, and remove char with irrigation and moistened cotton-tipped applicator swabs.

One can lyse tubo-ovarian adhesions at the point of formation by chipping away successive layers with a tightly focused 0.5-mm spot at 2- to 5-W power with intermittent time exposure of 0.2 sec to prevent excessively deep penetration. When one can slip a 1-mm rod behind adhesions, increase power to between 20 and 30 W, set for continuous time exposure and a spot between 0.2 and 0.5 mm, and rapidly cut the adhesion over the backstop (Fig. 34-4).

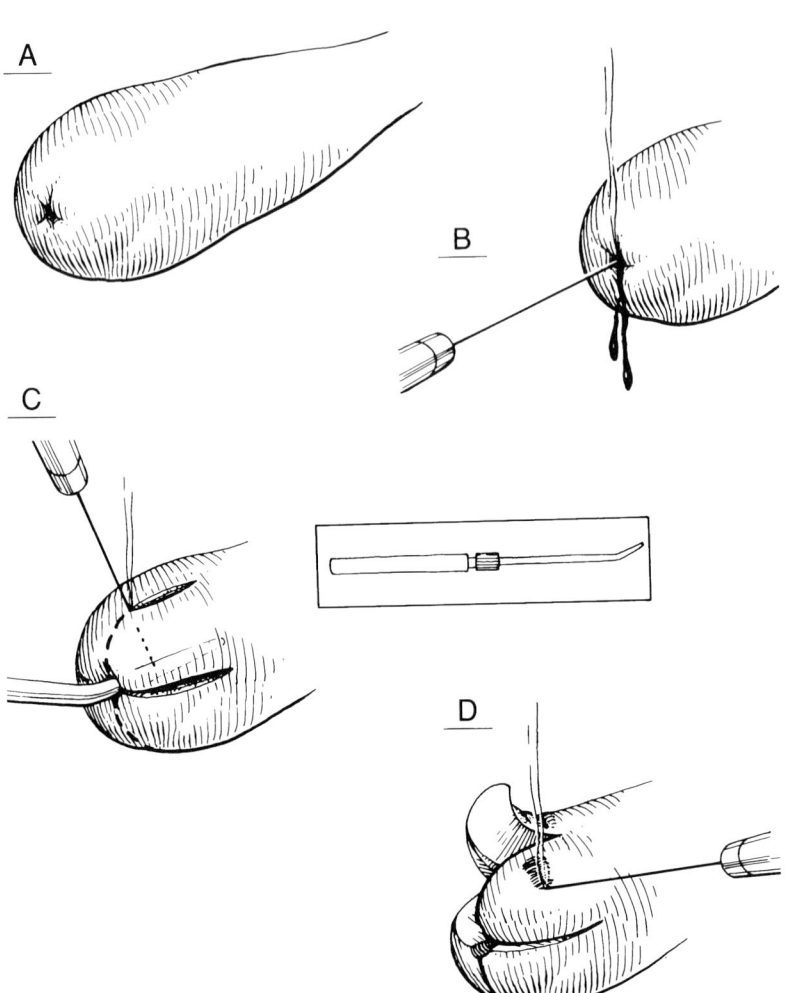

Fig. 34-3 Opening the fimbrial closure. (A) Locate the central point of fimbrial closure. (B) Using high power densities, drill a hole with the laser into the hydrosalpinx. (C) Insert a laser rod (*inset*) into the initial drill-hole and cut flaps sharply into the tube. (D) Finally, using low power settings and a 1- to 1.5-mm spot, play the laser over the serosal surface, causing retraction of tissue protein and eversion of flaps.

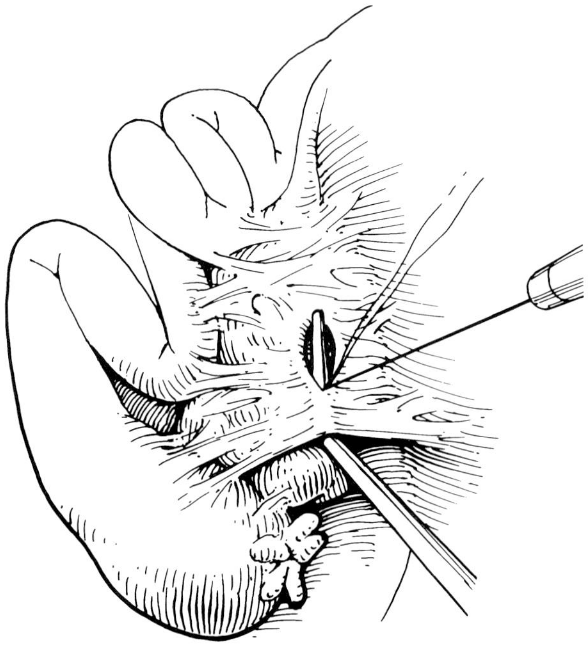

Vaporizing endometriosis

Lesions of endometriosis may consist of single or multiple implants, cystomas, or scarring. Handpiece use is appropriate for superficial lesions, a micromanipulator for deeper, pelvic ones.

For vaporizing of strategically located implants within the large bowel, bladder, or iliac vessels, use power densities below 1000 W/cm^2 and intermittent time gating to control ablation depth. When the implant is unroofed, hemosiderin-laden fluid will flow out of it. At this point, one or two 0.2-second bursts will complete vaporization.

One can devascularize fine adhesions by brushing them with a 2-mm low-power spot with a power density of 250 W/cm^2 to blanch tissue and thrombose small vessels. Wash away char material.

Uncap an ovary with an endometrial cyst by making an incision into the cyst wall at 50,000 W/cm^2 and removing a disk of tissue. Evacuate the dark brown hemosiderin liquid, thoroughly irrigate the cyst's interior with lactated Ringer's solution, using fine iris hooks or 6-0 polyglactin for wide exposure, and vaporize the entire cyst lining at 500 W/cm^2. Wash away char and close the cavity in two layers.

Fig. 34-4 Lyse tubo-ovarian adhesions at high power density over a light-absorbing laser backstop rod.

Before vaporizing implants on the sigmoid colon, inject 1 ml of 1:30 vasopressin beneath the implant's serosa to create a liquid cushion that will protect the underlying bowel. Do partial ovarian excision over an energy-absorbing spatula, using a handpiece and a power setting of either 150,000 W/cm^2 or 400 pulses per second at 0.4-msec intervals with a 0.2-mm spot.

Myomectomy

Vaporize small seedling myomata by using a handpiece-directed spot of 1.0 to 1.5 mm with power set at 10 to 20 W/cm^2. Wash the wound thoroughly with lactated Ringer's and remove all char with moist cotton-tipped applicators. Do not place any sutures.

The procedure for removing large myomata is virtually bloodless and minimally traumatic to surrounding musculature. Trace the initial incision with a series of 1.0- to 1.5-mm spots and power set at 300 to 400 W/cm^2. Coagulate surface vessels by defocusing to 2.0 mm, keeping power at 300 W/cm^2. Then make an incision into the tumor's serosal surface, connecting the trace spots, at 30,000 to 50,000 W/cm^2, using a spot size of 0.5 mm.

Next turn power down, enlarge the spot to 1.5 cm, and vaporize the capsule. Apply traction to the myoma with fine skin hooks as vaporization progresses. As the capsule disappears, the myoma will rise out of the uterus. Cut its base across, remove it, and cut away remaining excess tissue at high power density. Irrigate the tumor bed and close the defect in layers.

Summary

The CO_2 laser is a splendid tool for carrying out specialized surgical procedures. I have discussed only those intra-abdominal procedures experience has already shown to be well suited for CO_2 laser surgery, compared with conventional techniques. Advances most likely to emerge in the near future include the use of multiple lasers, such as neodymium-yttrium-aluminum-garnet (Nd-YAG); frequency-doubled YAG, argon, dye, and CO_2 lasers; CO_2 laser fibers; and voice-controlled micromanipulators. As technology allows the surgeon to perform more delicate operations, indications for using the laser will increase.

References

1 Mage G, Bruhat MA. Pregnancy following salpingostomy: comparison between CO_2 laser and electrosurgery procedures. Fertil Steril 1983;40:472.

2 Chong AP, Baggish MS. Management of pelvic endometriosis by means of intra-abdominal carbon-dioxide laser. Fertil Steril 1984;41:14.

3 Kelly RW, Roberts DK. Experience with the carbon dioxide laser in gynecologic microsurgery. Am J Obstet Gynecol 1983;146:585.

4 McLaughlin D. Advanced surgical instrumentation for intra-abdominal application of CO_2 laser in reproductive biology. Laser Med Surg 1983;2:241.

5 Daniell JF, Pittaway DE. Use of the CO_2 laser in laparoscopic surgery: initial experience with the second puncture technique. Infertility 1982;5:15.

6 Baggish MS, Chong AP. Carbon dioxide laser microsurgery of the uterine tube. Obstet Gynecol 1981;58:111.

Chapter 35

Laser laparoscopy

Dan C. Martin

Lasers have been features of intra-abdominal laser surgery since 1969 (1) and have been combined with laparoscopy since 1979 (2). This coupling of laser laparoscopy (3) has been accompanied by the development of videoendoscopy techniques (4) and other forms of operative endoscopy (5). This combination has many names, but all fit within the concepts of minimally invasive surgery. These concepts include not only laparoscopy but also outpatient laparotomy and combined laparoscopy, laparotomy, and colpotomy techniques.

Although certain of these techniques may have decreased the operating time, blood loss, and cost (6,7), others such as laparoscopically assisted vaginal hysterectomy may actually increase the cost, pain, and blood loss (8,9). Although some of these techniques may be clinically effective, they may be so cost-ineffective that they are not affordable. Physicians involved in assessing clinical utilization must take care to distinguish the differences in both clinical effectiveness and cost-effectiveness for specific techniques. This appears particularly true in light of ongoing attempts to create uniform standards for care and for reimbursement (10–12).

Basic tissue interaction

The laser is named for the molecules used to generate the beam. These molecules may be gas such as carbon dioxide (CO_2), argon, and helium neon (HeNe), or crystals such as potassium-titanyl-phosphate (KTP) and neodymium-yttrium-aluminum-garnet (Nd-YAG) (3,13). These lasers each have their own characteristics. A review of these is beyond the scope of this article. Surgeons who are going to use a specific laser must be educated in the characteristics of that laser (4,14–20).

Techniques and procedures

Lasers are capable of desiccating, vaporizing, or excising tissue (Fig. 35-1). Excision is performed using small focal point vaporization and can be performed with CO_2 lasers, small fibers with fiber lasers, or artificial (commonly sapphire) tips on fiber lasers. All of these can produce power densities in excess of 5000 W/cm². This power density appears necessary for adequate excision (13,21).

Vaporization occurs when water-containing tissue is raised to 100°C. This vaporization can be a thin zone as is used in excision or can be a wide zone, in which case the entire lesion is vaporized. It is generally easier and more time-efficient to vaporize small lesions and to excise large lesions. Small lesions are difficult to excise because control is difficult, whereas large lesions are difficult to vaporize because of the amount of smoke produced.

In addition, temperatures higher than 100°C are created when vaporizing fat or sublimating carbon. Fat vaporizes at a temperature of 200°C, and carbon sublimates at 3653°C (13).

Surgical Technique

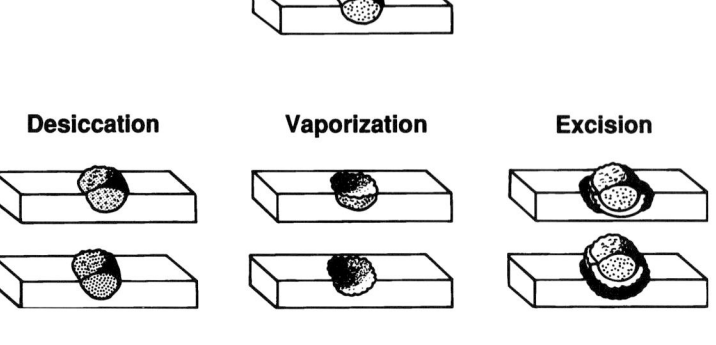

Fig. 35-1 Various combinations of lasers, bipolar electrosurgery, mechanical dissection techniques, and thermal cautery can be used to desiccate, vaporize, or excise tissue. Desiccation (coagulation) of tissue is drying and denaturing of tissue without removal. Vaporization is flash boiling of water-containing tissues so that the tissue is taken away in a vapor. Vaporization is generally performed using either high-power-density laser or high-power-density electrosurgery. Excision can be performed with scissors, laser, or electrosurgery. When scissors are used, desiccation with bipolar electrosurgery or thermal cautery may be needed. (Adapted with permission from Martin DC, Absten GT, Levinson CJ, Photopulos GJ, eds. Intraabdominal laser surgery. Memphis: Resurge Press, 1986:124.)

Small lesions can also be desiccated or cauterized using fiber lasers. The argon laser is effective as a desiccator to a depth of 0.3 to 0.8 mm using laser penetration and conversion of laser energy into heat. With long exposure, secondary thermal cauterization and desiccation occur as heat is conducted away from the penetrated area (Fig. 35-2). This secondary cautery can generally be used to a depth of 2 to 3 mm. On the other hand, the Nd-YAG laser can penetrate to a depth of 4.2 mm. This has been more useful in the treatment of gastrointestinal hemorrhage from ulcers than it has been in gynecology (22).

Controlling laser effects

Lasers are controlled by a combination of mechanical and electronic techniques. Mechanical techniques include use of fibers, shutters, lens, and backstops. Electronic controls include wave generation, power settings, and duration of exposure. These controls are modified for the specific laser used (Table 35-1). Power density settings and actions are covered in Table 35-2. As a general concept, the tissue effects for a given power density appear similar at high power densities for all lasers and electrosurgical equipment (13,22,23).

Inasmuch as the combination of controls used is specific to each laser and often to a particular company, these will not be covered in this chapter. Those physicians who are to use the laser must understand the specific characteristics of their laser type and laser unit.

Certain generalities, however, are worth mentioning. Superpulse, ultrapulse, and chopped wave laser output are used to increase the peak power density but to decrease the average power density. This technique has the advantages of a clean cut and decreased carbon associated with the in-

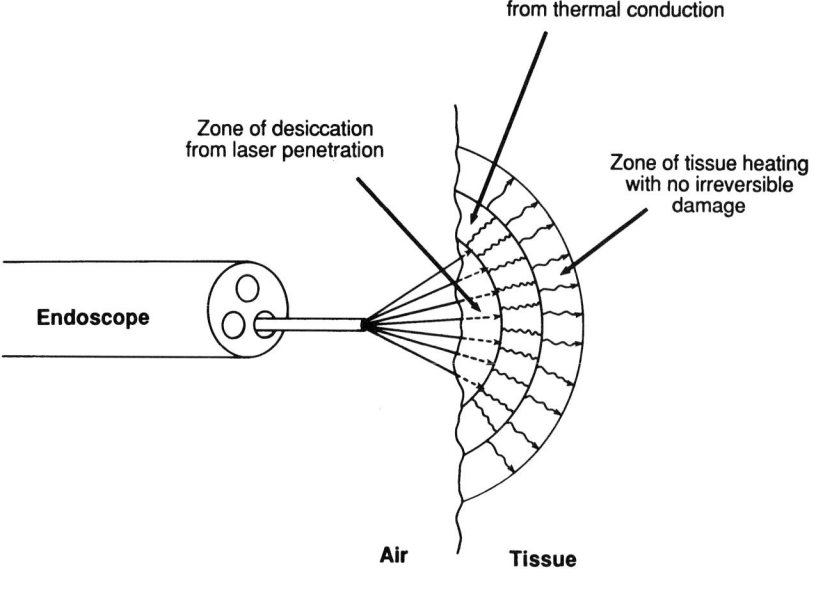

Fig. 35-2 Argon and KTP lasers have an effective penetration of 0.3 to 0.8 mm. Tissue absorption of the laser penetrating to this depth has a direct conversion of laser into heat energy. Tissue damaged past that point is related to thermal conduction. This results in three thermal zones. The first is desiccation from direct conversion of laser to heat energy, the second is denatured tissue as sufficient heat is conducted into this zone. The third is tissue that is heated but undergoes no irreversible damage and is not desiccated. (Adapted with permission from Martin DC, Absten GT, Levinson CJ, Photopulos GJ, eds. Intra-abdominal laser surgery. Memphis: Resurge Press, 1986:121.)

Table 35-1 Laser control terminology

Photocoagulation: desiccation (coagulation) of the tissue in the field without removing it.

Photovaporization: vaporization of tissue in the absorption zone.

Transverse electromagnetic mode (TEM): the spatial distribution of the energy in impact zone. A TEM 00 mode has a Gaussian distribution and is hottest at the center. A TEM 01 mode has a donut distribution and is cool at the center and hotter at the edges.

Spot size: the calculated theoretical size of the laser beam at a plane in space. The minimum spot size is calculated at the focal length of the laser.

Power density: the calculated concentration of power at laser impact.

Continuous wave laser: a continuous output of the laser beam.

Pulsed laser: a laser that stores its energy to be released at one instant.

Pulsed mode: mechanical pulses of a continuous wave laser that can be used to decrease the thermal spread.

Superpulse: electronic pulsing of a continuous wave laser designed to decrease thermal spread and decrease tissue damage.

Ultrapulse: electronic pulsing similar to superpulse but with a more rapid onset and decline of the waveform.

Table 35-2 Tissue effects of different power densities

Power (W/cm^2)	Action
0–25	Warming
5–400	Superficial contraction/desiccation
200–1200	Gross vaporization
800–4700	Fine vaporization/incision
1200–65,000	Rapid incision/vaporization

creased peak power density while slowing the operating speed with the low average power density. Other techniques that allow the use of high power density include the use of artificial tips and backstops. High peak power densities with artificial tips result in rapid defocus of the laser past the operating tip itself. This generally limits unintended damage to the immediate vicinity of the tip and appears to be limited to depths no greater than 400 μm (22). For the CO_2 laser, placing water behind peritoneal lesions appears useful although this may interfere with surgery and recognition of tissue. An alternative approach is to flood the pelvis and hold the lesion directly above the solution surfaces. The lesion is then amputated as the laser is stopped by the deep peritoneal fluid.

Smoke and carbon

Smoke and carbon are two problems associated with surgery itself and may be associated with long-term side effects. As an acute problem, smoke can interfere with the ability to see at the time of surgery. Although recirculators have been used to decrease this problem, rapid flow insufflators make it easy to deflate the entire abdomen and reinsufflate it intermittently. Smoke has been anecdotally associated with acute bronchitis following instruction in the laboratory setting (24). There appears to be greater concern for the chronic possibility of pulmonary disease, carcinogenic potential, and potential for spreading viruses such as the human immunodeficiency virus. All of these concerns suggest that adequate filtration and pulmonary plume control are necessary (14).

Carbon particles interfere with the performance of surgery and with second-look laparoscopy. Endometriosis can be hidden (25). Carbon accumulation is decreased by using high power density, rapid speed, brushing after vaporization, and irrigation. Using these techniques, close carbon deposition can be avoided. Fine carbon particles are more difficult to remove and frequently remain. Observations at second-look laparoscopy of carbon particles has demonstrated only foreign body giant cell reaction. However, observations looking for other types of reaction have yielded serendipitous findings regarding endometriosis and chlamydia, as discussed later in this chapter. In the process of performing these studies, carbon itself has been associated with foreign body giant cell reactions (3,25) and adhesions (26,27) but no other histologic response.

The learning curve

Mastery of any new technique requires experience and time. This appears particularly true of operative endoscopy in which previously tried and true techniques have to be replaced or relearned. Re-education can be dangerous to patients (7,28). Personal experience with changing to videoendoscopy suggests that 3 to 5 years of videoendoscopy experience was necessary to reach a level of expertise similar to that using the eyepiece directly. At 7 years of experience with videoendoscopy, delicate small tissue techniques are still easier with direct visualization. New techniques do not come easily or without time and financial expense.

As an added concern, current development of electrosurgical monopolar equipment may make it possible to replace most, if not all, laser equipment. Ongoing refinement of electrosurgical equipment and electrosurgical safety monitoring has produced safer equipment than was previously available. Innovations such as dual pad return electrodes and active electrode shielding are among the changes increasing safety in electrosurgery (29,30).

It is possible that although laser technology may be one of the driving forces in the development of minimally invasive surgery, it may have been more necessary for development than for ongoing utilization. Electrosurgical and mechanical techniques may replace laser use.

Clinical procedures

Most publications on laser laparoscopy relate to endometriosis. More than 2400 patients have been reported as summarized in Tables 35-3, 35-4, and 35-5 (31–50). A statistical analysis by Gant of the literature on endometriosis concluded that although there was inadequate evidence to suggest abandoning laparotomy, there are recommendations relating laparoscopy to cost savings and decreased recovery times (51). More substantial data are needed before declaring laparotomy detrimental to patients' health. Table 35-6 summarizes the findings of the operative laparoscopy panel from the American Gynecological and Obstetrical Society in 1991. In this panel, for any indication studied, laparoscopy was either preferred or was equal to laparotomy. At present, there are sufficient reports to suggest that operation for the treatment of ectopic pregnancy, ovarian pregnancy, ovarian biopsy, and polycystic ovarian disease is superior to laparotomy. For all other indications studied, laparoscopy was equivalent to laparotomy, but recommendations were made on other grounds such as cost, acute morbidity, chronic morbidity, patient preference, and physician preference (51–54).

Furthermore, the development of excisional techniques for the removal and confirmation of tumor (55) have given gynecologists the ability to dissect out the cul-de-sac (44,56–58) while at the same time increasing the recognition not only of endometriosis (59,60), but also of psammoma bodies associated with chlamydia (61). Excisional techniques have also produced a correlation of focal pelvic tenderness with implant volume (62). Moreover, studies on the histogenesis and collagen type for endometriosis and infiltrating endometriosis suggest that infiltrating endometriosis predates ovarian endometrioma (63). This implies that ovarian endometriosis may be an infiltration from pelvic wall endometriosis rather than the contrary. However, either of those possibilities and coexistent development of independent foci are all possible.

A complete analysis of each of the operations covered in the reports by Gant (51) and Grimes (52) is outside the scope of this chapter. These are summarized in Table 35-6. The use of uterine nerve ablation at laparoscopy has been followed in both short-term and long-term studies (16,64). Of note, although studies suggest that there is good short-term relief, only 45% of patients appear to have relief at one year (Table 35-7).

The use of laparoscopy and lasers for neosalpingostomies in Daniell's series is covered in Table 35-8 and is representative of that described in other publications (16). In these reports, there appears to be no difference in the results of laparoscopy and microsurgery (52). Therefore, we must remember that the results of salpingostomy appeared to be

Table 35-3 CO_2 laser laparoscopy: endometriosis in all patients

Author	(Ref.)	All patients		Minimal/mild		Moderate		Severe/extensive	
		No.	No. pregnant	No.	No. pregnant	No.	No. pregnant	No.	No. pregnant
Kelly, 1983	(31)	10	6 (60%)	3	3 (100%)	7	3 (43%)	0	0 (NA)
Feste, 1985	(32)	140	82 (59%)	106	62 (58%)	31	18 (58%)	3	2 (67%)
Daniell, 1985	(33)	48	26 (54%)	24	16 (67%)	15	7 (47%)	9	3 (33%)
Martin, 1986	(34)	115	54 (47%)	56	23 (41%)	45	22 (49%)	14	9 (64%)
Davis, 1986	(35)	64	37 (58%)	31	20 (65%)	26	15 (58%)	7	2 (29%)
Nezhat, 1986	(36)	102	65 (64%)	24	18 (75%)	51	32 (63%)	27	15 (56%)
Bowman, 1986	(37)	35	18 (51%)	19	12 (63%)	13	4 (31%)	3	2 (67%)
Donnez, 1987	(38)	70	40 (57%)	42	26 (62%)	21	11 (52%)	7	3 (43%)
Paulson, 1987	(39)	431	225 (52%)	257	144 (56%)	174	81 (47%)	0	0 (NA)
Gast, 1988	(40)	122	57 (47%)	105	49 (47%)	17	8 (47%)	0	0 (NA)
Adamson, 1988	(41)	156	85 (55%)	133	78 (58%)	20	7 (33%)	3	0 (0%)
Nezhat, 1989	(42)	243	168 (69%)	39	28 (72%)	86	60 (70%)	118	80 (68%)
Paulson, 1991	(43)	556	300 (54%)	331	188 (57%)	225	112 (49%)	0	0 (NA)
Reich, 1991	(44)	46	34 (74%)	0	0 (NA)	21	16 (76%)	25	18 (72%)
Total		2138	1197 (56%)	1170	667 (57%)	752	396 (51%)	216	134 (62%)

NA, not available.

Adapted from Martin DC, Diamond MP. Operative laparoscopy: comparison of lasers with other techniques. Curr Probl Obstet Gynecol Fertil 1986;9:563–601.

Table 35-4 CO$_2$ laser laparoscopy: endometriosis as an isolated factor

Author	(Ref.)	All patients		Minimal/mild		Moderate		Severe/extensive	
		No.	No. pregnant	No.	No. pregnant	No.	No. pregnant	No.	No. pregnant
Feste, 1985	(32)	60	42 (70%)	44	31 (70%)	14	10 (71%)	2	1 (50%)
Martin, 1986	(34)	34	23 (67%)	13	9 (69%)	11	6 (55%)	10	8 (80%)
Nezhat, 1986	(36)	102	65 (64%)	24	18 (75%)	51	32 (63%)	27	15 (56%)
Paulson, 1987	(39)	228	169 (74%)	140	109 (78%)	88	60 (68%)	0	0 (NA)
Gast, 1988	(40)	27	7 (26%)		NA		NA	0	0 (NA)
Adamson, 1988	(41)	60	39 (65%)	47	32 (66%)	11	7 (61%)	2	0 (0%)
Nezhat, 1989	(42)	243	168 (69%)	39	28 (72%)	86	60 (70%)	118	80 (68%)
Sutton, 1990	(45)	56	45 (80%)	41	32 (78%)	13	11 (85%)	2	2 (100%)
Chong, 1990	(46)	11	6 (55%)	0	0 (NA)	0	0 (NA)	11	6 (55%)
Paulson, 1991	(43)	296	227 (77%)	181	147 (81%)	115	80 (70%)	0	0 (NA)
Reich, 1991	(44)	40	34 (85%)	0	0 (NA)	19	16 (84%)	21	18 (86%)
Luciano, 1992	(47)	60	36 (60%)	0	0 (NA)	36	22 (61%)	24	14 (58%)
Total		1217	861 (71%)	529	406 (77%)	444	304 (68%)	217	144 (66%)

NA, not available.
Adapted from Martin DC, Diamond MP. Operative laparoscopy: comparison of lasers with other techniques. Curr Probl Obstet Gynecol Fertil 1986;9:563–601.

Table 35-5 Fiber laser laparoscopy

Author	(Ref.)	All patients		Minimal/mild		Moderate		Severe	
		No.	No. pregnant	No.	No. pregnant	No.	No. pregnant	No.	No. pregnant
Keye, 1987	(48)	56	19 (34%)	41	15 (37%)	10	3 (30%)	5	1 (20%)
Kojima, 1988	(49)	29	15 (52%)	NA	NA	NA	NA	NA	NA
Corson, 1991	(19)	126	73 (58%)	55	35 (64%)	36	29 (81%)	35	9 (26%)
Dlugi, 1992	(50)	74	28 (38%)	49	20 (41%)	21	8 (30%)	4	0 (0%)
Total		285	135 (47%)	145	70 (48%)	67	40 (59%)	44	10 (23%)

NA, not available.

more related to the prognostic class of hydrosalpinges than to the equipment used (65,66; Tables 35-9 and 35-10).

Laser safety

Safety is a major concern for any type of surgery. One of the major worries is that lasers can be aimed at unintended targets. This is dangerous to the patient, to the surgeon, and to operating room personnel. Laser safety and laparoscopic safety are covered in several publications that are worth review (13,14,67,68).

Diligence, education, and care are needed to decrease the occurrence of complications, which include hypothermia, emphysema, hemorrhage from hilar vessels, amputation of tubes, transection of tubes, transfusions, urinary cystotomy, bowel laceration, ureteral fistula, uterine perforation, ureteral transection, periappendiceal abscess, sterile peritonitis, aortic laceration, common iliac artery laceration, cardiac arrest, and air embolus. These complications can be associated with significant morbidity including death (3,67,68).

Summary

Lasers have greater functional precision than other techniques, but this precision may have been more useful for the development of techniques than for the ongoing utilization of these techniques. Ongoing development of laser, electrosurgical, and mechanical techniques is expected to demonstrate which of these is the most cost-effective, the

Table 35-6 Strength of recommendations for laparoscopy over laparotomy

A. There is good evidence to support the recommendation that operative laparoscopy be used for this indication.	(None)
B. There is fair evidence to support the recommendation that operative laparoscopy be used for this indication.	Ectopic pregnancy, ovarian biopsy, and Stein-Leventhal syndrome
C. There is inadequate evidence regarding the use of operative laparoscopy, for this indication, but recommendations may be made on other grounds.	Salpingectomy, salpingostomy, oophorectomy, ovarian cystectomy, pelvic abscess, laparoscopic uterine nerve ablation, uterine suspension, myomectomy, hysterectomy, salpingo-ovariolysis, and endometriosis
D. There is fair evidence to support the recommendation that operative laparoscopy not be used for this indication.	(None)
E. There is good evidence to support the recommendation that operative laparoscopy not be used for this indication.	(None)

Recommendations are from Gant NF. Infertility and endometriosis: comparison of pregnancy outcomes with laparotomy versus laparoscopic techniques. Am J Obstet Gynecol 1992;166:1072–1081. Grimes DA. Frontiers of operative laparoscopy: a review and critique of the evidence. Am J Obstet Gynecol 1992;166:1062–1071. Adapted from United States Preventive Services Task Force. Guide to clinical preventive services. An assessment of the effectiveness of 169 interventions. Baltimore: Williams & Wilkins, 1989:387–388.

Table 35-7 Short-term and long-term pain relief following laparoscopic uterine nerve ablation

Indications	No. of patients	Improvement at		
		3 mo	6 mo	1 year
Primary dysmenorrhea*	11	9 (82%)	NR	5 (45%)
Primary dysmenorrhea[†]	20	NR	12 (60%)	NR
Endometriosis[†]	80	NR	60 (75%)	NR

NR, not reported.
*Lichten EM, Bombard J. Surgical treatment of primary dysmenorrhea with laparoscopic uterine nerve ablation. J Reprod Med 1987;32: 37–41.
[†]Daniell JF. Laparoscopic use of KTP/YAG laser. In: Soderstrom RM, ed. Operative laparoscopy. The master's techniques. New York: Raven Press, 1993:63–71.

Table 35-8 Results of laparoscopy neosalpingostomy with lasers

Type laser	Years	Total patients	Open tubes at 6 wks HSG	Attempting pregnancy	Pregnancy results		
					IUP	Abort	Ectopic
CO_2	1982–1985	104*	58/71 (82%)	88	22 (25%)	11 (13%)	11 (13%)
KTP	1985–1987	36[†]	24/28 (86%)	32	10 (31%)	3 (9%)	5 (16%)
Totals		140	82/99 (83%)	120	33 (28%)	14 (12%)	16 (13%)

There was an 18-month minimum follow-up. HSG, hysterosalpingogram; IUP, intrauterine pregnancy.
*Sixty procedures were in recurrent hydrosalpinges with at least 2-year follow-up.
[†]Only three procedures were recurrent hydrosalpinges.
Reproduced by permission from Daniell JF. Laparoscopic use of the KTP/YAG laser. In: Soderstrom RM, ed. Operative laparoscopy. The master's techniques. New York: Raven Press, 1993:63–71.

Table 35-9 Prognostic value of tuboscopy

Appearance	No. of patients	Term	Abortion	Ectopic
Normal	80	43%	4%	4%
Synechiae	12	0%	25%	25%
Flat areas	21	0%	10%	10%
Folds, 1–2	9	0%	0%	10%
Flat	14	0%	0%	0%

Reproduced by permission from Henry-Suchet J, Loffredo V, Tequier L, Pez JP. Endoscopy of the tube (= tuboscopy): its prognostic value for tuboplasties. Acta Eur Fertil 1985;16:139–145.

Table 35-10 Pregnancy outcome in relation to the prognostic class of hydrosalpinges following microsurgery

Class	Patients	Term	Abortion	Ectopic	If pregnant Abortion	Ectopic
I	27	16 (59%)	5 (18%)	1 (4%)	23%	5%
II	44	7 (17%)	2 (5%)	12 (27%)	10%	57%
III	37	1 (3%)	0 (0%)	6 (16%)	0%	86%

Classification system based on nature and extent of adhesions, macroscopic appearance, thickness, and diameter of tubes. Reproduced by permission from Boer-Meisel ME, te Velde ER, Habbema JDF, Kardaun JWPF. Predicting the pregnancy outcome in patients treated for hydrosalpinx: a prospective study. Fertil Steril 1986;45:23–29.

most clinically effective, the easiest to learn, and ultimately the optimal technique. However, at present, these conclusions are based on personal preference and experience more than on published data.

References

1 Fox JL. The use of laser radiation as a surgical "light knife." J Surg Res 1969;9:199–205.
2 Bruhat MA, Mage G, Manhes M. Use of the CO_2 laser via laparoscopy. In: Kaplan I, ed. Laser surgery. III. Proceedings of the 3rd International Congress for Laser Surgery. Graz: OT-PAZ, 1979:274–276.
3 Martin DC, Diamond MP. Operative laparoscopy: comparison of lasers with other techniques. Curr Probl Obstet Gynecol Fertil 1986;9:563–601.
4 Nezhat CR, Nezhat FR, Silfen SL. Videolaseroscopy. Obstet Gynecol Clin North Am 1991;18:585–604.
5 Semm K, Friedrich ER, eds. Operative manual for endoscopic abdominal surgery. Chicago: Year Book Medical Publishers, 1987.
6 Levine RL. Economic impact of pelviscopic surgery. J Reprod Med 1985;30:655–659.
7 NIH Consensus Development Panel on Gallstones and Laparoscopic Cholecystectomy. Gallstones and laparoscopic cholecystectomy. JAMA 1993;269:1018–1024.
8 Nezhat C, Nezhat F, Bess O. Hospital cost comparison between abdominal, vaginal and laparoscopically assisted vaginal hysterectomies. Washington, DC: ACOG Abstracts, 41st Annual Clinical Meeting, 1993.
9 Summitt RL, Stovall TG, Lipscomb GH, Ling FW. Randomized comparison of laparoscopy-assisted vaginal hysterectomy with standard vaginal hysterectomy in an outpatient setting. Obstet Gynecol 1992;80:895–901.
10 Federal Register, 1992;57(228):55895–56230.
11 Martin DC. CPT codes and RV. Thorofare, NJ: Membership newsletter, Gynecologic Laser and Advanced Technology Society, Summer 1993;1(1):3.
12 Martin DC. Cost of minimally invasive surgery. Thorofare, NJ: Membership newsletter, Gynecologic Laser and Advanced Technology Society, Summer 1993;1(1):3–4.
13 Martin DC. Tissue effects of lasers. Semin Reprod Endocrinol 1991;9(2):127–137.
14 Martin DC. Laser safety. In: Keye WR Jr, ed. Laser surgery in gynecology and obstetrics, ed. 2. Chicago: Year Book Medical Publishers, 1990:35–45.
15 Martin DC. Carbon dioxide laser laparoscopy for endometriosis. Obstet Gynecol Clin North Am 1991;18(3):575–583.
16 Daniell JF. Laparoscopic use of the KTP/YAG laser. In: Soderstrom RM, ed. Operative laparoscopy. The masters' techniques. New York: Raven Press, 1993:63–71.
17 Keye WR Jr. KTP and argon laser laparoscopy. Obstet Gynecol Clin North Am 1991;18(3):605–611.
18 Osher SS. The argon laser in gynecologic op lap. In: Soderstrom RM, ed. Operative laparoscopy. The masters' techniques. New York: Raven Press, 1993:73–80.
19 Corson SL. Use of the YAG laser in laparoscopic gynecologic procedures. Obstet Gynecol Clin North Am 1991;18(3):619–636.
20 Martin DC. Complications of gynecologic endoscopic surgery. Infertil Reprod Med Clin North Am 1992;3(4):829–838.
21 Taylor MV, Martin DC, Poston W, Dean PJ, Vander Zwaag R. Effect of power density and carbonization on residual tissue coagulation using the continuous wave carbon dioxide laser. Colposc Gynecol Laser Surg 1986;2:169–175.
22 Joffe SN, Brackett KA, Sankar MY, Daikuzono N. Resection of the liver with the Nd:YAG laser. Surg Gynecol Obstet 1986;163:437–442.
23 Luciano AA, Whitman G, Maier DB, Randolph J, Maenza R. A comparison of thermal injury, healing patterns, and postoperative adhesion formation following CO_2 laser and electromicrosurgery. Fertil Steril 1987;48:1025–1029.
24 Davis GD, Martin DC. Carbon dioxide laser laparoscopy. In: McLaughlin DS, ed. Lasers in gynecology. Philadelphia: JB Lippincott, 1991:199–214.
25 Martin DC, Absten GT, Levinson CJ, Photopulos GJ, eds. Intraabdominal laser surgery. Memphis: Resurge Press, 1986:28–29.
26 Diamond MP, Daniell JF, Feste J, et al. Adhesion reformation and de novo adhesion formation after reproductive pelvic surgery. Fertil Steril 1987;47:864–866.
27 Diamond MP, Daniell JF, Johns DA, et al. Postoperative adhesion development after operative laparoscopy: evaluation at early second-look procedures. Fertil Steril 1991;55:700–704.
28 Phillips JM. Complications in laparoscopy. Int J Gynaecol Obstet 1977;15:157–162.
29 Tucker RD, Voyles CR, Salvis SE. Capacitive coupled stray currents during laparoscopic and endoscopic electrosurgical procedures. Biomed Instrum Technol 1992;26:303–311.
30 Voyles CR, Tucker RD. Education and engineering solutions for potential problems with laparoscopic monopolar electrosurgery. Am J Surg 1992;164:57–62.
31 Kelly RW, Roberts DK. CO_2 laser laparoscopy: a potential alternative to danazol in the treatment of stage I and II endometriosis. J Reprod Med 1983;28:638–640.
32 Feste JR. Endoscopic laser surgery in gynecology. In: Reproductive surgery. Course IV. Eighteenth Annual Postgraduate Course. Chicago: American Fertility Society, 1985:51–69.

33 Daniell JF. Management of severe endometriosis. Presented at the Fourth Annual Gynecologic Surgery Seminar, Baptist Memorial Hospital, Memphis, 1985.

34 Martin DC. CO_2 laser laparoscopy for endometriosis associated with infertility. J Reprod Med 1986;31:1089–1094.

35 David GD. Management of endometriosis and its associated adhesions with the CO_2 laser laparoscope. Obstet Gynecol 1986;68: 422–425.

36 Nezhat C, Crowgey SR, Garrison CP. Surgical treatment of endometriosis via laser laparoscopy. Fertil Steril 1986;45:778–783.

37 Martin DC, Diamond MP. Operative laparoscopy: comparison of lasers with other techniques. Curr Probl Obstet Gynecol Fertil 1986;9:563–601.

38 Donnez J. CO_2 laser laparoscopy in infertile women with endometriosis and women with adnexal adhesions. Fertil Steril 1987;48:390–394.

39 Paulson JD, Asmar P. The use of CO_2 laser laparoscopy for treating endometriosis. Int J Fertil 1987;32:237–239.

40 Gast MJ, Tobler R, Strickler RC, Odem R, Pineda J. Laser vaporization of endometriosis in an infertile population: the role of complicating infertility factors. Fertil Steril 1988;49:32–36.

41 Adamson GD, Lu J, Subak LL. Laparoscopic CO_2 laser vaporization of endometriosis compared with traditional treatments. Fertil Steril 1988;50:704–710.

42 Nezhat C, Crowgey SR, Nezhat F. Videolaseroscopy for the treatment of endometriosis associated with infertility. Fertil Steril 1989;51:237–240.

43 Paulson JD, Asmar P, Saffan DS. Mild and moderate endometriosis. Comparison of treatment modalities for infertile couples. J Reprod Med 1991;36:151–155.

44 Reich H, McGlynn F, Salvat J. Laparoscopic treatment of cul-de-sac obliteration secondary to retrocervical deep fibrotic endometriosis. J Reprod Med 1991;36:516–522.

45 Sutton C, Hill D. Laser laparoscopy in the treatment of endometriosis. A 5-year study. Br J Obstet Gynaecol 1990;97:181–185.

46 Chong AP, Luciano A, O'Shaughnessy AM. Laser laparoscopy versus laparotomy in the treatment of infertility patients with severe endometriosis. J Gynecol Surg 1990;6:179–183.

47 Luciano AA, Lowney J, Jacobs SL. Endometriosis treatment of endometriosis-associated infertility: therapeutic, economic and social benefit. J Reprod Med 1992;37:573–576.

48 Keye WR, Hansen LW, Astin M, Poulson AM. Argon laser therapy of endometriosis: a review of 92 consecutive patients. Fertil Steril 1987;47:208–212.

49 Kojima E, Yanagibori A, Yuda K, Hirakawa S. Nd:YAG laser endoscopy. J Reprod Med 1988;33:907–911.

50 Dlugi AM, Saleh WA, Jacobsen G. KTP/532* laser laparoscopy in the treatment of endometriosis-associated infertility. Fertil Steril 1992;57:1186–1193.

51 Gant NF. Infertility and endometriosis: comparison of pregnancy outcomes with laparotomy versus laparoscopic techniques. Am J Obstet Gynecol 1992;166:1072–1081.

52 Grimes DA. Frontiers of operative laparoscopy: a review and critique of the evidence. Am J Obstet Gynecol 1992;166:1062–1071.

53 United States Preventive Services Task Force. Guide to clinical preventive services. An assessment of the effectiveness of 169 interventions. Baltimore: Williams & Wilkins, 1989:387–388.

54 McDonough PG. The need for technology assessment in the reproductive sciences. Am J Obstet Gynecol 1992;166:1082–1090.

55 Martin DC, Vander Zwaag R. Excisional techniques for endometriosis with the CO_2 laser laparoscope. J Reprod Med 1987; 32:753–758.

56 Martin DC. Laparoscopic and vaginal colpotomy for the excision of infiltrating cul-de-sac endometriosis. J Reprod Med 1988;33: 806–808.

57 Reich H. Pelvic sidewall dissection. Clin Obstet Gynecol 1991;34: 412–422.

58 Nezhat C, Nezhat F, Pennington E. Laparoscopic treatment of infiltrative rectosigmoid colon and rectovaginal septum endometriosis by the technique of videolaparoscopy and the CO_2 laser. Br J Obstet Gynaecol 1992;99:664–667.

59 Martin DC, Hubert GD, Vander Zwaag R, El-Zeky FA. Laparoscopic appearances of peritoneal endometriosis. Fertil Steril 1989;51:63–67.

60 Martin DC, Ahmic R, El-Zeky FA, Vander Zwaag R, Pickens MT, Cherry K. Increased histologic confirmation of endometriosis. J Gynecol Surg 1990;6:275–279.

61 Martin DC, Khare VK, Miller BE. Association of chlamydia trachomatis immunoglobin gamma titers with dystrophic peritoneal calcification, γ psammona bodies and hydrosalpinges. Fertil Steril 1994 (in press).

62 Ripps BA, Martin DC. Correlation of focal pelvic tenderness with implant dimension and stage of endometriosis. J Reprod Med 1992;37:620–624.

63 Khare VK, Martin DC, Eltorky M. The histogenesis of ovarian and pelvic wall infiltrating endometriosis. J Gynecol Surg (in press).

64 Lichten EM, Bombard J. Surgical treatment of primary dysmenorrhea with laparoscopic uterine nerve ablation. J Reprod Med 1987;32:37–41.

65 Henry-Suchet J, Loffredo V, Tequier L, Pez JP. Endoscopy of the tube (= tuboscopy): its prognostic value for tuboplasties. Acta Eur Fertil 1985;16:139–145.

66 Boer-Meisel ME, te Velde ER, Habbema JDF, Kardaun JWPF. Predicting the pregnancy outcome in patients treated for hydrosalpinx: a prospective study. Fertil Steril 1986;45:23–29.

67 Borten M, Freidman EA, eds. Laparoscopic complications. Prevention and management. Philadelphia: BC Decker, 1986.

68 Corfman RS, Diamond MP, DeCherney A, eds. Complications of laparoscopy and hysteroscopy. Cambridge, Mass: Blackwell Scientific Publications, 1993.

Chapter 36

Laparoscopic assisted vaginal hysterectomy

Luis E. Sanz and James F. Barter

Laparoscopic assisted vaginal hysterectomy (LAVH) is a step forward in gynecologic surgery. Certainly there are situations in which laparoscopic skills may convert an abdominal procedure to one with a vaginal approach. Patients with severe endometriosis, pelvic adhesions, select kinds of ovarian pathology, or lack of descensus may benefit from an LAVH. The first report of an LAVH was in 1989 by H. Reich and associates (1); therefore there is a not a long history of this procedure. However, many reported series illustrate that the technique is feasible (2–5). Many patients may merely need a vaginal hysterectomy rather than an LAVH. Therefore, these patients may be spared the prolonged anesthesia time, cost, and potential morbidity and mortality associated with laparoscopic surgery. There are even reported cases of LAVH and anterior and posterior repair for prolapse. This is not the correct use of the LAVH approach and available technology. Other problems with the laparoscopic approach include the steep learning curve (6). Didactic instruction, experience with pelvic trainer sets, then extensive training in the laboratory are essential. Then only the easiest cases should be attempted, first with a preceptor. With present technology LAVH can be easily performed by a well-trained surgeon and trained operating room personnel. Many reports do not mention the cost of the surgery (2–4) because they are essentially feasibility studies. Summitt and colleagues reported, in a randomized series of vaginal hysterectomies, that the LAVH approach increased expenditures relative to vaginal hysterectomy (7). However, LAVH may be cost-effective as it allows patients to leave the hospital earlier and return to work sooner (8).

Interestingly, the abdominal approach may be avoided by the use of laparoscopic surgery in cases of early-stage endometrial cancer (9). In this procedure nodes are obtained laparoscopically, then an LAVH with bilateral salpingo-oophorectomy is done. Essential staging information (10) is still obtained, and laparotomy is avoided. Ongoing studies from gynecologic oncologists are further investigating this approach (11–15).

Indications

The indications for LAVH are those in which a vaginal approach cannot be used, as in patients with a history of endometriosis, history of pelvic inflammatory disease, history of uterine suspension, nulliparity with no descensus, large fibroid, and ovarian cysts. In the majority of these cases a vaginal hysterectomy is contraindicated because of the risks involved in penetrating the peritoneal cavity blindly and, as a result, causing damage to bowel or bladder (16). In these particular cases, the LAVH is a perfect procedure to evaluate pathology in the pelvic cavity and to lyse adhesions (17–19). Eventually, total abdominal hysterectomy will be done only on patients with very large ovarian tumors, uterine fibroids larger than 16 weeks' gestational size, cancers of the ovaries, advanced endometrial cancer, and invasive cancer of the cervix.

At present approximately 600,000 hysterectomies are performed yearly in the United States. Of those, 437,000 are total abdominal hysterectomies and 133,000 are total vaginal hysterectomies. Within the next 10 years probably 60% of the abdominal hysterectomies performed will be by laparoscopy, as gynecologic surgeons become better trained in their residency programs and the endoscopic instruments become better. Therefore, the gynecologic surgeon is faced with three modalities to perform a hysterectomy: the abdominal hysterectomy, the vaginal hysterectomy, and the LAVH. Strict criteria regarding when each one can be performed must be followed very carefully (20,21). Current instruments are of higher quality because they have laparoscopes that include better fiberoptic light bundles that use high-quality lenses with improved resolution. The new three-chip cameras, with their improved resolution, and television monitors are also much better today.

Preparation

Preoperative preparation, which includes the proper patient selection as mentioned above, is very important. The patient must be instructed on bowel cleansing before this surgery, on the complications and benefits of this operation, and on the alternatives to the surgery. The patient is instructed to take nothing by mouth after midnight the day before the surgery. In addition, a bowel preparation is performed before the surgery. If a complete bowel preparation is required, as with severe cases of endometriosis, a complete bowel preparation using oral polyethylene glycol solution (GoLytely) is preferable. The day before the surgery we usually tell the patient to use the GoLytely beginning at noontime because it takes 2 or 3 hours to drink the 4 L of fluid. The stomach should be empty, with the last meal at least 3 hours before drinking the GoLytely. This will induce diarrhea within 3 to 4 hours; therefore, it is better to do the cleansing during the day so the patient can have a good night's sleep. We also tell the patient to take an enema the night before the surgery. If the patient does not need a complete bowel preparation, then we give two tablets of laxative (Colace) at noontime and a Fleet's enema the night before the surgery and again early in the morning. The patient should not take any aspirin before the surgery and should take 1000 mg of vitamin C daily. On the day of the surgery prophylactic antibiotics are given. We usually use 1 g of cephalosporin (Cefotetan) one hour before the surgery and 1 g 12 hours after the surgery.

Video equipment

The use of video systems in the operating room allows the entire staff to watch the surgical procedure, enabling them to properly assist the laparoscopic surgeon. The videocamera system has several components: the laparoscope, the light source and fiberoptic light cable, the camera and camera control unit, the video monitors, cables, and video printers, and the videocassette recorder. The new three-chip cameras (Dionics, Stryker, and Storz) produce better resolution and more natural colors. A three-chip camera has between 750 and 800 lines of horizontal resolution. It is important to white-balance the camera before using it to achieve the proper colors. Cameras also have orienting features, focus, and autoexposure. There are two types of scopes: eyepiece endoscopes and videoendoscopes. Eyepiece endoscopes require the attachment of a videocamera, which has a greater chance of fogging. Both endoscopes have different diameters ranging from 4 to 10 mm and different angles of view ranging from 0 to 90 degrees. In gynecology the 0-degree angle and 10-mm diameter are most commonly used. There is also an operative laparoscope, but light and resolution are lost.

The light sources are metal halide and xenon. Xenon has the problem of pulsating and, therefore, interferes with autofocus and recording with super VHS signals. A 6.5-mm cable should be used for a 10-mm scope. There are several ways to record the operation: a videocassette recorder, video printers, and a videodisc system. Video monitors are 19 inches, with high resolutions that are capable of registering up to 800 horizontal lines.

The other instruments required for laparoscopic procedures are as follows: suction irrigators, laser, electrocoagulator, and special endoscopic instruments such as Endo Shears, an endoscopic gastrointestinal anastomosis stapler (Endo GIA), etc.

Operation

It is important in this type of high-technology surgery to do the operation as early in the day as possible with nursing personnel that is well trained in this type of surgery. One must check with the nursing personnel to make sure that all of the instruments are available, and that the monitors are working well before beginning the operation. If one of these instruments is not working, the operation cannot be carried out, and it would not be fair to anesthetize the patient. The patient must be aware that at any time, for whatever reason, one may have to do a laparotomy.

After one has checked with the nurses and checked the equipment, the patient is brought to the room and put to sleep in the usual fashion. Usually, ask the anesthesiologist to empty the stomach with a nasogastric tube to avoid perforation of the stomach while inserting the trocar, and to keep the intravenous lines on the right hand of the patient, so that the left hand can be at the side of the patient and the surgeon will have more room to move. At this point the patient is shaved as needed and is placed in Allen stirrups with care not to give undue traction to either of the legs. Embolization stockings are always used on all patients. After checking the position of the patient to ensure that it is correct and there are no pressures on any of the nerves, the patient is prepared and draped in the usual sterile fashion.

A Foley catheter is inserted into the bladder, and the bladder is distended with 150 cc of saline and methylene blue. The purpose of this is to identify the bladder, which is much easier to identify when it is distended, and to make it easier to identify and correct any perforation that is made while performing the bladder dissection. At this point a solution of bupivacaine (Marcaine) 0.25% with epinephrine is injected in the four abdominal skin port areas. This is done to minimize postoperative pain. The four port areas are as follows: the umbilical area, 2 cm above the symphysis pubis, and two that are located 3 cm lateral from the anterior superior iliac spine on each side. The purpose of making these lateral incisions lower than described elsewhere is that sometimes the instruments are not long enough to reach deep into the pelvis. At this point we also try to identify the rectus muscles so that the surgeon can remain lateral to them and avoid injury to the epigastric artery. If an injury to the epigastric artery occurs while inserting the trocar, it is better to remove the trocar, tie the vessel, and reinsert the trocar. Patients can have severe bleeding from these areas. However, sometimes if one inserts the trocar lateral to the rectus muscle, one may still perforate one of the lateral branches of the inferior epigastric artery.

Use 12-mm trocars with a Surgigrip on both lateral abdominal incisions and in the periumbilical area, and a 5-mm trocar on the suprapubic area. This allows the surgeon to move the laparoscope from the periumbilical area to the right and the left ports. It also allows the surgeon to use instruments according to the angles that may become necessary during the surgery. With the reducers one can reduce any of the ports so one can use the Endo Grasp instrument or Endo Shears as needed. A new trocar (Premium Surgiport, US Surgical) has a safer trocar release mechanism, a new colostomy bag type of holder that can be used instead of Surgigrips, and a universal converter that avoids having to switch converters. One may use two television monitors at either side of the legs of the patient so that all the assistants can see the monitors. One can also have a single monitor placed by the legs of the patient, which also allows all the assistants to see the monitors. We perform a direct insertion of the trocar without using the Verres needle, because there seem to be fewer complications in this fashion. We have done more than 250 laparoscopies in this way and have never had any complications. Dr. Nezhat has reported on this technique, and he does not use the Verres needle either. The rationale for direct trocar insertion is that if there are any adhesions close to the umbilical area, regardless of whether one cuts the bowel with the trocar or the Verres, one will still have to open the patient to correct the problem. There is less chance of injury with a single insertion than

with a double sequential insertion. We use disposable trocars, which are sharper and easier to introduce and have a retractable safety shield to prevent abdominal injuries. As with any other laparoscopic procedure, care must be taken to aim the trocar centered toward the pelvis to avoid injuries to the aorta, vena cava, iliac arteries and veins, or ureters. Once the laparoscope is inserted, and the pneumoperitoneum is created at a high flow rate, an initial laparoscopic examination of the abdominal cavity is performed to check for vascular injuries. At this point the camera is attached to the laparoscope. We like to use the new three-chip camera, which has much improved resolution and color.

The Stryker camera is very light and easy to use. The Dionics camera has the advantage that one can take a picture right from the camera and also change the intensity of the light through the camera, but this makes the camera much heavier, and if there is a breakdown, it is much more difficult to repair. At this point the abdominal cavity is insufflated with carbon dioxide for good visualization. Then the other 12-mm trocars are inserted on either side. The 5-mm trocar is inserted suprapubically.

The assistant inserts the vaginal speculum, grasps the cervix, and inserts a sound inside the uterus for uterine mobilization. This helps in mobilizing the uterus especially for the vesicouterine dissection. One can also use the Pelosi uterine manipulator and operative transilluminator, which allows for better uterine mobilization.

After the appropriate visualization of all the pelvic structures (Fig. 36-1), begin the operation by dissecting the bladder (Color Plate 16). However, if there are particular difficulties in doing that, go to another area. One does not have to be committed to do the operation exactly the same way at all times. One should try to have a routine, but allow for modifying it according to the needs of each case. At this point one can easily see the bladder and begin to dissect it with the Endo Shears roticulators (with unipolar cautery) from the cervix. Then with the Endo Shears roticulator, one begins to cut the small vesicofascial cervical fibers to dissect the bladder away from the cervix. We do this until the cervix is easily visualized (Color Plate 17). Another way to dissect the bladder is to make the first incision in the vesicouterine peritoneum and insert a suction irrigator, then with hydropressure, the bladder can be easily dissected from the cervix. Usually, if one is on the right plane, there is minimal bleeding from small vessels, which can be electrocoagulated with a suction irrigator with a Bovie tip and a laser channel (Surgiwand, US Surgical). At this point one is easily able to see the uterine arteries. Take the vesicouterine fold all the way to the anterior leaf of the broad ligament bilaterally to the level of the round ligament. At this point, if there is no injury to the bladder, remove the Endo Shears and empty the bladder completely.

Then with the Endo Gauge (US Surgical) measure the thickness of the round ligament. One should always use the

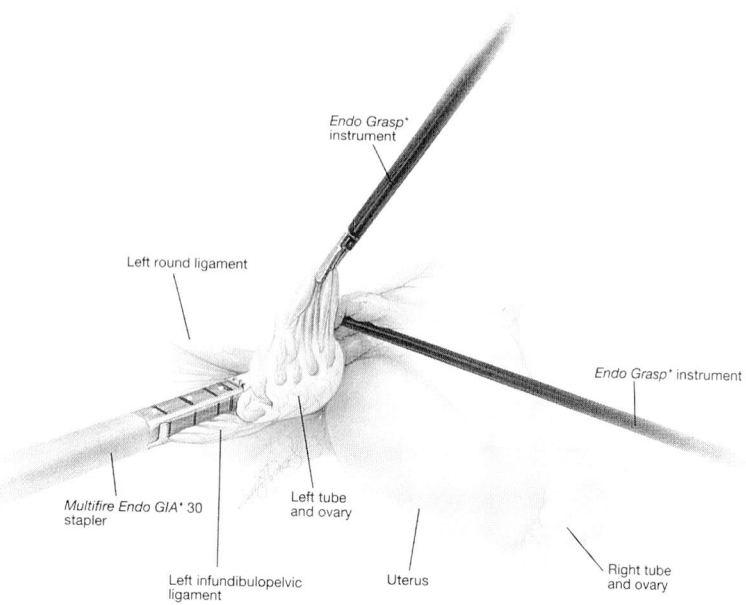

Fig. 36-1 The peritoneum is opened just over the point where the ureters course beneath the uterine vessels. Only a small window is opened, but it is large enough to tell at a glance the ureteral location, which is more difficult to determine once the dissection above has begun. (Courtesy of US Surgical Corporation.)

Endo Gauge so the appropriate multifire Endo GIA (US Surgical) can be used. Close the Endo GIA, but before cutting and stapling, always look on both sides to make sure that one has not grasped any other important structure (Color Plate 8). The assistant inserts the Endo Grasp through the lateral port and then pulls on one side of the uterus. After appropriate visualization is achieved, one cuts the round ligament on the right side and then repeats the same motion on the left side. At this point the bladder has been dissected, and the round ligament has been grasped (Color Plate 9). Then the question is whether to do a bilateral salpingo-oophorectomy or leave the ovaries in place. If leaving the ovaries in place, rather than grasping the round ligaments by themselves, we grasp both the round ligament and the uterine ovarian ligament with the Endo GIA, so in a single cut we have taken both of them, which is done bilaterally. This speeds up the operation.

If one needs to remove the ovaries and the fallopian tube, have the assistant grasp the ovary with Babcock clamps, pull medially, and with the Endo Shears open the parietal peritoneum superiorly away from the ureters (Fig. 36-2). By doing so one is able to get behind the infundibulopelvic ligament. Cut the parietal peritoneum medially and identify the ureters. This way, one has totally dissected the infundibulopelvic ligament. Then proceed to place an Endo GIA and cut and staple the infundibulopelvic ligaments. This is done on the other side also. If there are any adhesions, dissect them carefully after identifying all important structures such as the bowel, ureters, arteries, and veins. The only structures that are left are the cardinal ligaments, the uterosacral ligaments, and the uterine arteries. At this point one can decide to do a subtotal hysterectomy, as described by Pelosi and Pelosi (16). The endocervix is removed with the Bovie knife in a reverse conization technique, and the rest of the cervix is left in situ. The purpose of this V-shaped incision is to remove the endocervical canal and endometrial remnants. This prevents damage to the ureters and speeds up the operation. The uterus is then removed in sections through the umbilicus with the Endo Catch (US Surgical), or one may remove them through a posterior colpotomy. This is important for patients with medical complications. If the cervix is going to be removed, then we open the peritoneum and follow the ureter and ligate the uterine vessels with either the Endo GIA or a new thoracoabdominal instrument (Multifire Endo TA, US Surgical). The Endo TA staples do not cut, but are shorter and narrower to avoid damaging the ureters. We staple the uterine vessels bilaterally (Color Plates 20 and 21). At this point one has to be very careful. If one does not feel confident that the ureters are well isolated, do not take the cardinal ligaments. We very seldom do this anyway, because it is so easy to do vaginally. Most of the reported injuries to the ureters occur during attempts to staple the cardinal ligaments. Many injuries are also reported for the uterosacral ligaments. If one cannot identify them well and see where the ureters are, it is better to take the cardinal ligaments vaginally. At this point basically all of the adhesions have been removed. All the adnexal structures have been totally dissected, and the bladder has been dissected away from the cervix (Color Plate 22). The only procedure remaining is to vaginally cut the cardinal ligaments and remove the uterus. Again, we emphasize that one must be careful in this area. Because most of the injuries happen in this area, there is no need to be heroic in trying to reach the cardinal ligaments when one can easily reach them vaginally. At this point check for any bleeders and electrocoagulate the small ones. Sometimes one of the vessels will bleed more than usual; either electrocoagulate it or use Endo Clips.

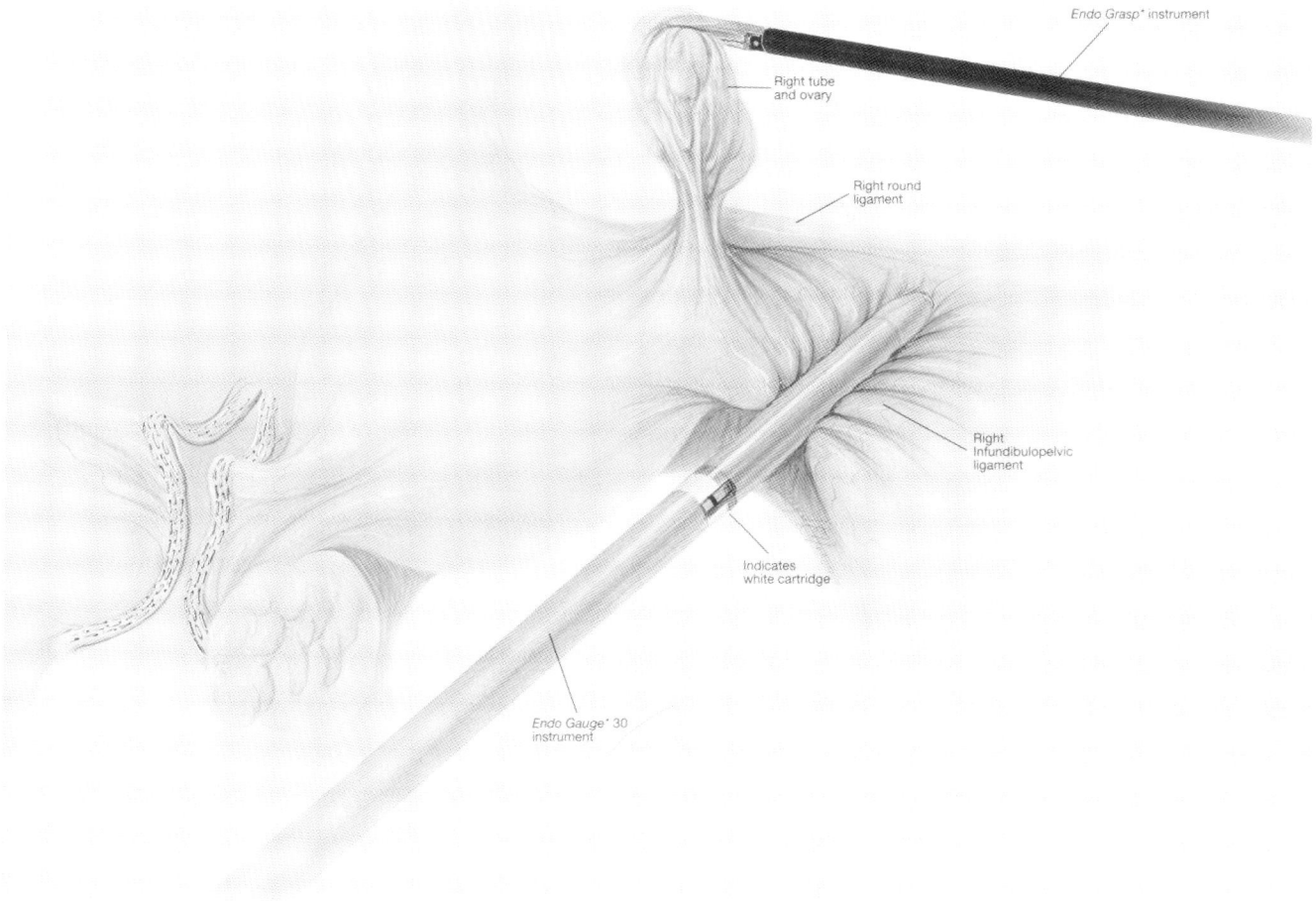

Fig. 36-2 After the round ligament is transected, the broad ligament is opened lateral to the adnexa to the level of the pelvic brim. This allows identification of the ureter, especially as it tunnels under the uterine artery. If the adnexae are to be removed, the infundibu- lopelvic ligament is transected with the Multifire Endo GIA 30 stapler. If the tube and ovary are to be conserved, the utero-ovarian ligament is transected. (Courtesy of U.S. Surgical Corporation.)

For the vaginal part of the hysterectomy, grasp the cervix with a Lahey clamp, pull down, and make a circumferential incision on the cervix. The bladder is easily dissected at this point because it was already dissected from above. The peritoneum is entered easily, and the insufflation is lost. We leave all the laparoscopic instruments inserted because we like to check for bleeders when the surgery is finished. Then, perform a colpotomy and dissect the posterior vaginal area from the cervix. If one has not grasped the uterosacral ligaments from above, grasp them at this time with a Heaney clamp and ligate them with a 0 poliglecaprone 25 (Monocryl) suture. At this point the cardinal ligaments are identified, and they are clamped bilaterally with Heaney clamps, cut, and ligated with 0 Monocryl suture. By then the uterus is totally free. If one has not been able to reach the uterine vessels from above, get them at this time.

At this point the uterus is removed in toto. A purse-string suture is used to close the peritoneum. The vaginal cuff is closed with a continuous suture of 0 Monocryl. One can do either a Heaney vaginal hysterectomy or a Doderlein vaginal hysterectomy. In a Doderlein vaginal hysterectomy, the fundus is delivered through an anterior colpotomy.

The whole operation should not take more than 2 1/2 to 3 hours unless there are extensive pelvic adhesions. Usually it should be accomplished in less than 2 hours. This would be the case with more experienced surgeons and nursing personnel. At this point we make sure there is no bleeding from the cuff. We change gloves and gowns and take a second look with the laparoscope to make sure there are no bleeders. One irrigates the cavity with 1000 cc of normal saline and examines the rest of the abdominal cavity (Color Plates 23 and 24).

All the trocars are removed and the laparoscope is removed. The laparoscope is removed last to make sure that there is no bleeding from any of the ports. The trocars have been held in place by the Endo Grasp instrument, which sometimes traumatizes the skin area. Therefore, we trim the skin areas and the port areas for better healing. However, with the new colostomy-type patch, there will be no need to use the Surgigrips. The fascia is closed with a single suture of 0 polyglactin (Vicryl). The trocar leaves a fairly large hole, so the fascia must be closed, or the patient may develop a hernia. The skin is closed with subcuticular closure of 5-0 Monocryl or Vicryl. At this point the patient's abdomen is cleaned, and the operation is finished. We like to videotape all the surgery and take different pictures throughout the operation to show the patient.

The patient is transported to the operating room, monitored for an hour, and then sent to her room. The patient can be discharged 24 to 48 hours later depending on her condition and the amount of time one spends during the surgery. Most of our patients go home within 48 hours and return to work within 2 weeks of the operation (22–24).

Results

One of us (Luis Sanz) has performed 32 LAVHs with excellent results. Two attempted LAVHs were turned into laparotomies: in one case because the patient was obese and in the other because of severe endometriosis and uterine fibroids that were hiding the anatomy of the pelvic organs on the left side. To avoid extensive unnecessary surgical time, I try to make the decision to perform the laparotomy as soon as possible. The only complications that I had were a small laceration of the bladder in a patient with previous surgery, which was easily identified and repaired laparoscopically, and also a perforation of a branch of the right epigastric artery with the trocar. The trocar was removed, the incision was extended, and the epigastric artery was tied. The operation was then continued by reinserting the trocar. The average time for the last seven cases has been 2 hours, with the patient going home in 48 hours.

Complications

The complications of this operation are perforations of arteries or bowel during the insertion of the trocars and perforation of bowel or stapling the ureters during the surgery. Thus it is important to know where the ureters are at all times during this operation. The bladder can be perforated when dissecting it.

Dr. Alan Johns (personal communication) from the University of Texas has several guidelines to minimize complications: in general, a laparoscopic procedure should not take more than twice as long as a laparotomy; a laparotomy is better when the procedure is complex or the surgeon or team is inexperienced; laparoscopic equipment failure should be a reason for laparotomy; and when complications occur and are difficult to handle endoscopically, a laparotomy should be performed.

Summary

Laparoscopically assisted vaginal hysterectomy will continue to be performed in the future by more and more surgeons as they become more adept at this type of surgery (25,26). We must remember that there is a very steep learning curve with this type of operation. Anyone who has taken courses in this procedure should have someone else who has done it before monitor them while learning to perform the procedure. We have a credentials committee at Georgetown University, and we are very careful to make sure the surgeons take hands-on courses before performing any surgery and then monitor them while doing the surgery to protect the surgeon and the patient.

References

1 Reich H, EdCaprio JR, McGlynn F. Laparoscopic hysterectomy. J Gynecol Surg 1991;5:213–215.
2 Maher PG, Wood EC, Hill DJ, Lolatgis NA. Laparoscopically assisted hysterectomy. Med J Aust 1992;155:316–318.
3 Langebrekke A, Skar OJ, Urnes A. Laparoscopic hysterectomy initial experience. Acta Obstet Gynecol Scand 1992;71:226–229.
4 Minelli L, Angiollo M, Caione C, Palmara V. Laparoscopically-assisted vaginal hysterectomy. Endoscopy 1991;23:64–66.
5 Daniell JF, Kurtz B, McTavish G, et al. Laparoscopically assisted vaginal hysterectomy. Reprod Endocrinol 1993;38:537–542.
6 Woodland M. Ureter injury during laparoscopy-assisted vaginal hysterectomy with the endoscopic stapler. Am J Obstet Gynecol 1992;167.
7 Summitt RL, Stovall TG, Lipscomb GH, Ling FW. Randomized comparison of laparoscopy-assisted vaginal hysterectomy with standard vaginal hysterectomy in an outpatient setting. Obstet Gynecol 1992;80.
8 Nezhat F, Nezhat C, Gordon S, Wilkins E. Laparoscopic versus abdominal hysterectomy. J Reprod Med 1992;37:247–250.
9 Childers JM, Survit EA. Case report: combined laparoscopic and vaginal surgery for the management of two cases of stage I endometrial cancer. Gynecol Oncol 1992;45:46–51.
10 Creaseman WT, Morrow CP, Bundy BN, Homesley HD, Graham JE, Heller PB. Surgical pathologic spread patterns of endometrial cancer: a Gynecologic Oncology Group study. Cancer 1987;60: 2035–2041.
11 Gitsch E, Vytiska-Binstorfer E, Skodler W. Various effects of abdominal and vaginal hysterectomy in benign disease. Eur J Obstet Gynecol Reprod Biol 1990;36:259.
12 Blass JD, Bermena ML, Blass LP, Bueller RE. Use of vaginal hysterectomy for the management of stage I for the medically compromised patient. Gynecol Oncol 1991;40:74–77.
13 Peters WA, Anderson WA, Thronton WN, Morley GW. The selective use of vaginal hysterectomy in the management of adenocarcinoma of the endometrium. Am J Obstet Gynecol 1983;146: 285–291.
14 Angriella W, Cosmi EV. Vaginal hysterectomy for the treatment of cancer of the corpus uteri. Am J Obstet Gynecol 1968;100: 541–543.
15 Candiani BG, Belloni C, Maggi R, Columbo G, Grigola A, Carinelli SG. Evaluation of different surgical approaches in the treatment of endometrial cancer at FIGO stage I. Gynecol Oncol 1982;14: 185–193.
16 Pelosi MA, Pelosi MA III. Laparoscopic supracervical hysterectomy using a single-umbilical puncture (mini laparoscopy). J Reprod Med 1992;37:777–784.
17 Mage G, Pouly JL, Canis M, et al. Laparoscopy hysterectomy. In: Proceedings of the First Advanced Laparoscopic Surgery Workshop; Royal Women's Hospital, Melbourne, 1990:248–249.

18 Kilkko PP. Total versus subtotal abdominal hysterectomy. In: Garcia CR, Mikuta JJ, Rosenblum NG, eds. Current therapy in surgical gynecology. Toronto: BC Decker, 1987:58.

19 Scrimgeour JB, Ng KB, Gaurdoin MR. Laparoscopy in vaginal hysterectomy. Lancet 1991;338:1465–1466.

20 Maher PJ, Hill DJ. Video-assisted laparoscopic vaginal hysterectomy. Med J Aust 1991;154:427.

21 Eisenberg DH. Video-assisted laparoscopic vaginal hysterectomy. Med J Aust 1991;154:550.

22 Magos AL, Broadbent MJ, Amso NN. Laparoscopically-assisted vaginal hysterectomy. Lancet 1991;338:1091–1092.

23 Fernandez H, LeLaider C, Frydman R. Laparoscopically-assisted vaginal hysterectomy. Lancet 1991;339:123.

24 Reiner IJ. Early discharge after vaginal hysterectomy. Obstet Gynecol 1991;71:416–418.

25 Childers J, Surwit E, Hatch K. Laparoscopically assisted surgical staging (LASS) and vaginal hysterectomy (LAVH) for endometrial cancer. Tucson: University of Arizona Health Sciences Center, 1992.

26 Parker W. Laparoscopic-assisted hysterectomy. Contemp Obstet Gynecol 1993;14:19–34.

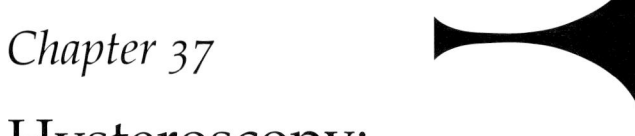

Chapter 37

Hysteroscopy: instrumentation and use of the resectoscope

Robert S. Neuwirth

Modern hysteroscopy is approximately 25 years old. Although the technique originated a century ago, it was still considered a curiosity as recently as 1970.

At that time, Lindeman developed a method for distending the uterus with carbon dioxide (CO_2) that, when used properly, gave a good image and was very safe (1). About the same time, Edstrom and Fernstrom devised a distention method using the high-viscosity liquid dextran 70 (Hyskon), and Quinnones and colleagues introduced a low-viscosity liquid distention approach making use of 5% dextrose and water (2,3).

The main reason behind revived interest in hysteroscopy was the desire to find a simple, effective method of transcervical sterilization. Although that objective has yet to be achieved, the hysteroscopic techniques developed promise to change traditional approaches to hysterectomy and diagnostic dilation and curettage (D & C). In addition, they have already proved superior for diagnosis and treatment of such uterine infertility factors as endometrial polyps, pedunculated submucous fibroids, intrauterine scarring, and subseptate anomalies.

Traditional methods inadequate

One traditional method of evaluating the uterine cavity is D & C, which involves examining the cavity tactilely plus sampling endometrial tissue. The other method is hysterography, or x-ray appraisal of a cavity that is filled with a radiopaque material.

A drawback of D & C is that it usually requires an anesthetic to permit careful probing of the endometrial cavity. It also tends to miss pedunculated lesions and protuberances from the top of the fundus, such as septa or submucous fibroids. Moreover, it is not therapeutic unless a polyp or remnants of a pregnancy are removed or the patient coincidently resumes ovulation, if anovulation has been the problem. In addition, D & C may produce a false impression of pathologic deformity when the endometrial cavity's natural configuration is not symmetric.

The hysterogram requires radiopaque dye, an x-ray machine, and exposure to radiation. Moreover, dye bubbles, uterine wall spasm, polypoid mucosa, or insufficient inflation of the uterine cavity—caused by poor cervical seal or low applied pressure—may produce a false impression of a lesion.

False-negative results, although rare, also occur. They are usually due to overfilling of the cavity or of the angle between the uterus and the x-ray beam, which should be perpendicular to the coronal or sagittal plane.

Combining approaches

Hysteroscopy avoids or reduces many of these problems. Although diagnostic hysteroscopy usually calls for a local anesthetic, it may be performed with mild analgesia only. I have found that when intrauterine scarring is suspected, it is preferable to obtain a hysterogram first to minimize risk that the hysteroscope will perforate the uterus.

If endometrial cancer is a possibility, a Pap smear is vital. Use endometrial biopsy for diagnosis, and the hysteroscope simply to evaluate the endocervical canal for involvement. Sometimes, too, the hysteroscope may show unsuspected focal endometrial cancers, alone or in association with fibroids.

In addition, hysteroscopy may reveal a polyp or submucous fibroid causing the bleeding. It is impossible to distinguish with certainty endometrial cancer from other mucosal or mass lesions. Always obtain tissue for microscopic examination.

Hysteroscopy is superior to a D & C or hysterogram alone for evaluating recurrent abortion or menometrorrhagia in women younger than 45. Use it also, together with traditional methods, when attempting to locate a uterine septum or foreign body, such as an intrauterine device (IUD).

Equipment and technique

Once one is familiar with the procedure, hysteroscopy can be done in the office if the woman is calm. To evaluate an abnormal Pap smear or determine length of a cone biopsy, a Hamou-type colpomicrohysteroscope is necessary. One must learn the in vivo cytologic findings possible with this instrument in order to take advantage of its specialized magnification equipment. Most ambulatory hysteroscopy I have done has been with standard infinity focus lens systems.

In the office, we begin with an endoscope 4 mm in diameter, including the sheath, and use CO_2 for distention. If the fit between the scope and the endocervical canal is so loose that gas leaks and the uterus will not distend, we fit a 6-mm cannula over the 4-mm cannula and switch to dextran 70. This alternative is more comfortable for the patient than a contracervical cap. If one uses the dextran 70 solution, wash the hysteroscope with hot running water immediately after dismantling it. Pay particular attention to cleaning the valve and lenses.

Office hysteroscopy takes about 5 minutes once the patient is in position on the table and the instruments are prepared. Caution her to take only liquids 4 hours before examination. If she is anxious, give her 5 mg of diazepam (Valium) orally 30 minutes before beginning the examination.

Either gas-sterilize the instruments or soak them in a glutaral disinfectant (Cidex) for 10 minutes and rinse them with sterile water. We also use sterile paper drapes and prepare the vulva and vagina with povidone-iodine (Betadine, PVP-iodine).

After bimanual examination to locate the uterine axis and rule out pelvic tenderness, insert a one-arm bivalve speculum into the vagina. If the cervix is open 4 mm, local anesthesia may not be necessary.

Grasp the cervix with a single-toothed tenaculum and insert the hysteroscope into the external os. Then turn the CO_2 gas on and advance the scope under direct view. We wear sterile gloves and introduce CO_2 using a control device that inflates up to 150 mm Hg pressure and delivers a maximum of 100 ml of CO_2 per minute at standard temperature and pressure.

Performing the examination

Explore in turn the endocervical canal, endometrial cavity, and tubes. CO_2 is preferable to dextran 70 for diagnostic viewing if blood or mucus is absent. If a local anesthetic is necessary, we use 2 ml of 1% lidocaine (Xylocaine) injected into the cervical stroma at the 2 and 4 o'clock, and 8 and 10 o'clock positions.

Do not dilate the cervix in the office unless the canal is too large for the 4-mm instrument and too small for the 6-mm instrument. Examine the uterus systematically, looking at the wall, tubal orifices, isthmus, and endocervix. When appropriate, one may use a flexible biopsy forceps in the office to perform directed biopsies or take endometrial samples with a Meigs or Vabra curette.

If it becomes necessary to switch to dextran 70 to remove debris, we withdraw the 4-mm instrument and lock the 6-mm sheath around the entire gas system, including the 4-mm sheath. We fill a 30- or 50-ml syringe and the male-female Luer-lok connector tubing (Becton-Dickinson & Co., Paramus, NJ) with dextran 70 and fasten one end of the tubing to the syringe and the other to the endoscope cannula. Prefilling the tubing drives out air and avoids bubbles in the uterus. We then reinsert the 6-mm scope into the cervix and repeat the examination, injecting the fluid through the scope to distend the uterus. Usually 50 to 150 ml of dextran 70 is needed.

Postexamination considerations

On completing the examination, we prepare a report with diagrams. Complications from examinations over the past 10 years have included only one anxiety attack and one vagal reaction. To date, we have seen neither infection nor serious bleeding.

An inconvenience of office hysteroscopy is the need for additional staff instruction. However, an assistant familiar with office pregnancy termination can easily learn to lay out equipment and participate in this procedure.

Advantages of the technique are its greater accuracy, lower cost, greater convenience for gynecologist and patient, and probable lessened risk. While the patient is in the office, one can discover what the endometrial cavity harbors, make a timely definitive diagnosis, and plan therapy. This alternative is greatly preferable to scheduling the premenopausal bleeding patient for a hysterogram or traditional hospital D & C to establish a merely presumptive diagnosis.

The hysteroscope as a surgical tool

Although considerable skill is required, the hysteroscope is ideally suited for treating Asherman's syndrome and septate uterus and for removing IUDs and other foreign bodies from the uterus. Scissors, clamps, biopsy forceps, or a scalpel can be fixed to its sheath or passed through or alongside it.

Fixing instruments to the scope's sheath makes it easy to insert and manipulate them (Fig. 37-1). Such an approach is suitable for endocervical biopsy or, possibly, resection of a septum. One drawback is that constant closeness of the instrument to the lens greatly restricts visualization.

Passing the instruments through the scope so that they can be manipulated independently overcomes these particular optical problems but creates others, because equipment permitting such passage has a smaller lens and fewer light bundles (Fig. 37-2). In addition, such special equipment is incompatible with use of dextran 70, which may be needed if the endometrial cavity fills with blood, mucus, or debris.

The third alternative, passage of instruments between the sheath and the endocervical canal, offers the greatest range for freehand surgery (Fig. 37-3). To accomplish insertion, withdraw the scope, insert the operating instrument just beyond the endocervix, reinsert the scope, and advance it and the operating instrument simultaneously, under visual control, into the uterine cavity to begin surgery.

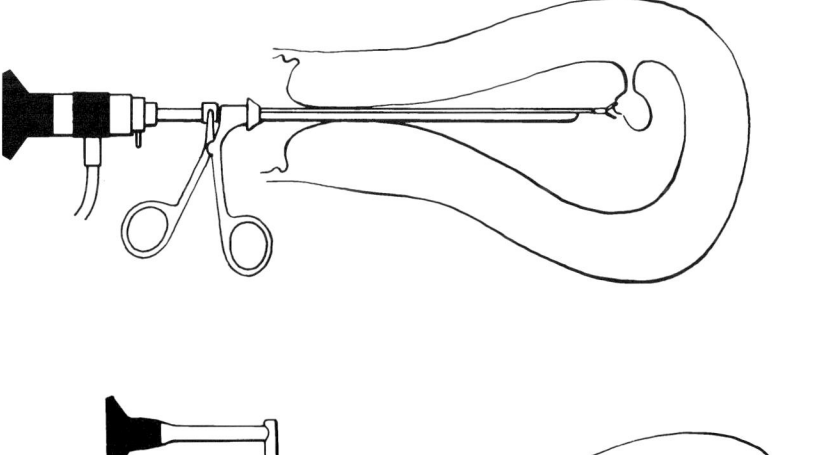

Fig. 37-1 Fixing the instrument to the scope's sheath makes insertion and manipulation easier but hinders visualization; it is most suitable for endocervical biopsy.

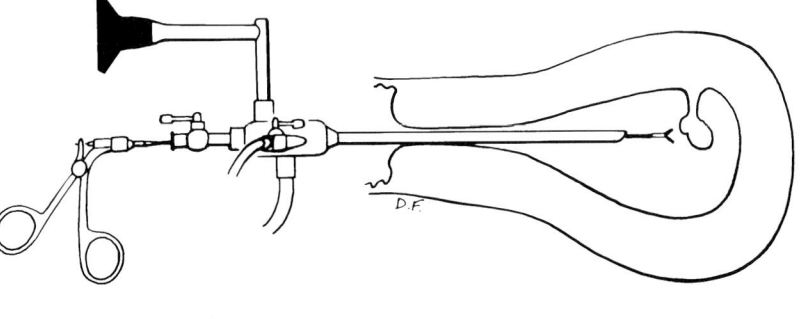

Fig. 37-2 Passing the instrument through the sheath allows the instrument to be manipulated independently and permits greater flexibility, but is incompatible with use of dextran 70.

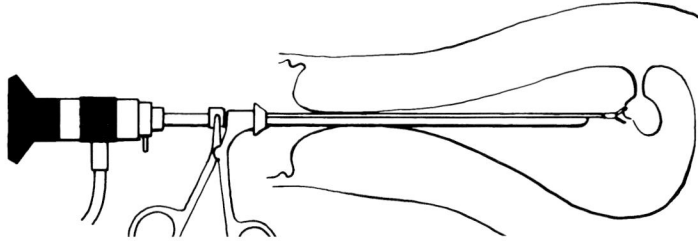

Fig. 37-3 Passing the instrument between the scope and the endocervical canal offers the greatest opportunity for freehand surgery.

Besides using freehand surgery, one can insert a modified resectoscope or surgical laser connected to a 2-mm fiberoptic cable through the endoscope. A further option is to pass an insulated malleable electrosurgical instrument through or around the scope, for cutting or coagulation.

Distention media

Procedures that produce smoke, heavy bleeding, or tissue debris require liquid systems to wash the scope's lens and keep the uterus well distended. Laser surgery permits choice of high- or low-viscosity conductive or nonconductive liquids, whereas electrocautery requires use of nonconductive liquids, such as glycine (component of Corilin) or dextran 70. If instruments are passed alongside the scope, which is our preference, dextran 70 is needed to maintain uterine pressure and ensure visibility, even during heavy bleeding, through good distention and lens-washing action. For procedures in which little bleeding is expected, such as septal transection, separation of mild intrauterine adhesions, or removal of a very small submucous fibroid, one may use CO_2.

Adjuncts

Hysterography before surgery is often useful. If risk of uterine perforation by the hysteroscope exists, simultaneous laparoscopy is important.

Unless maneuvers are to be very simple, we use regional or general anesthesia. Some recommend giving 2.5 mg of conjugated estrogens (Premarin) daily for 1 or 2 months before transecting either septa or intrauterine scars (4,5).

Permissible techniques

The marked ability of endometrium to migrate over raw surfaces and establish functional epithelium has led to good technical results with septum repair and many cases of Asherman's syndrome in which the scarred uterus contained modest amounts of normal endometrium. Some surgeons have used splinting with an IUD or special balloon for up to 2 months to aid such epithelial repair.

Semiblind techniques are also acceptable (Fig. 37-4). We do not hesitate to evacuate a pregnancy in a septate uterus or to use polyp or uterine dressing forceps to remove polyps or IUDs if we can locate this site hysteroscopically immediately before and after surgery.

Tubal sterilization

The Silastic plug method of tubal sterilization, which is currently being practiced in the Netherlands, incorporates hysteroscopic control (6). Dextran 70 is the distention medium. Ovabloc equipment (RSP Laboratories, Stamford, Conn.) is also necessary.

The procedure is done in the office under local anesthesia, with x-ray control after application of the plug to determine effectiveness. Success rates with repeated attempts are reported to be approximately 90%.

Silastic plug sterilization is apparently not so reversible as was once hoped. However, it seems to be an effective long-term contraceptive approach that could be an alternative to the IUD or Norplant (the Population Council's subdermal implant, manufactured in Finland) because it avoids transperitoneal surgery.

The resectoscope in hysteroscopy

The resectoscope was originally developed in the 1930s for urology primarily to resect the prostate in men with benign hypertrophy. It was a cystoscope with an internal mounting for control of a movable electrosurgical electrode which had cutting and coagulation wave current options. The resectoscope developed with a variety of electrodes including loop, hook, and ball tips. Leaf spring and rachet mechanisms were produced to control the to-and-fro motion of the active electrodes on the working element. The telescope and the light source were in the center of the cylindrical instrument package, and liquids were forced through the external cannula to fill the bladder so that the urologist could see to perform electrosurgery and wash the distal lens of blood and tissue fragments. The resectoscopic approach slowly gained favor, so that approximately 80% of transurethral prostatectomies currently are performed with this method.

In 1976 the resectoscope was used to morcellate submucous myomata to control menorrhagia and preserve fertility (7). Lasers and resectoscopic techniques were reported in the early 1980s to ablate the endometrium in the management of menorrhagia in the absence of malignancy (8,9). The operation is often best performed after the patient's menses or following ovarian suppression to reduce the thickness of the endometrium. The electrodes usually are 4 mm in width and have an excursion of 3 cm (Figs. 37-5, 37-6, 37-7). The electrode becomes magnified as it is drawn toward the objective lens of the hysteroscope, so the surgeon must develop comfort with this changing image or withdraw the hysteroscope with the electrode in a relatively fixed position to be comfortable with the view. The electrode can be moved back and forth to palpate tissue but should only be activated when being drawn toward the surgeon to avoid accidental perforation with the electrosurgical current on. The surgeon controls the wattage or power setting, the waveform (cutting or coagulation), the duration of the contact, and the precision of the electrode contact. Thermal penetrating burns can occur with the resectoscope if left in one place too long. This may lead to a bowel burn, perforation, and peritonitis several hours or days later. When cutting is performed, the pathologic anatomy of the uterine cavity must be understood by the surgeon, as it is possible to excavate through the uterus with a cutting loop.

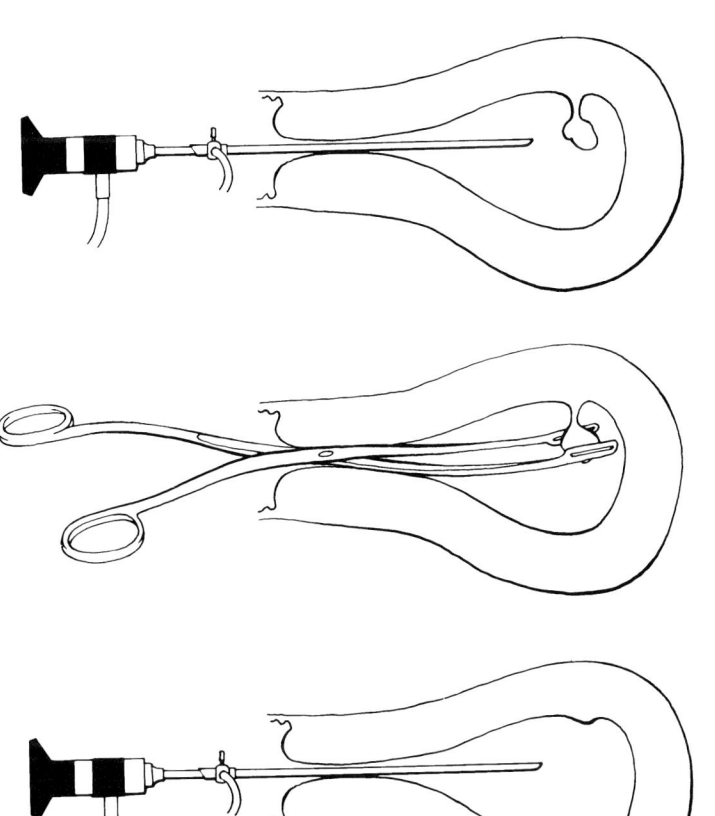

Fig. 37-4 Semiblind hysteroscopic surgery for an endometrial polyp involves indentification, removal, and checking.

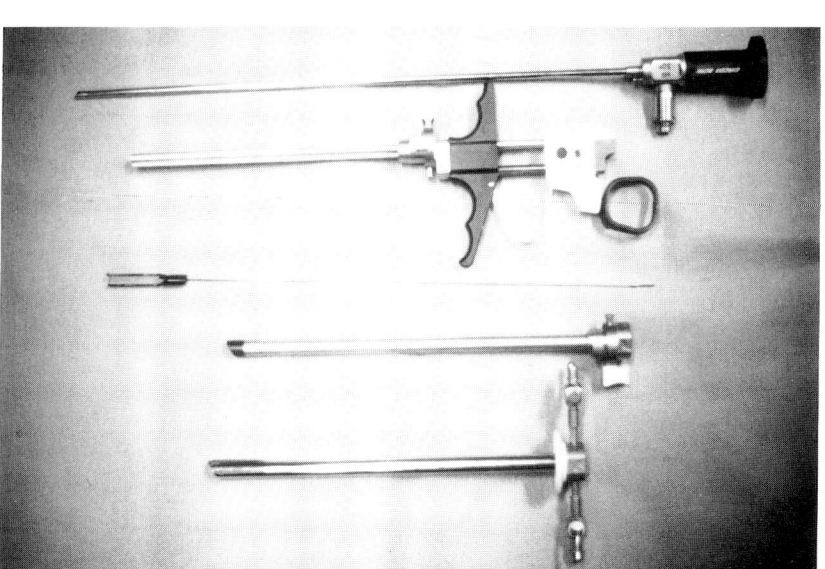

Fig. 37-5 Components of the resectoscope (top to bottom): endoscope, working element, loop electrode, inner sheath of continuous flow system, and outer insulated sheath of continuous flow system.

In resectoscopic surgery and some mechanical procedures under hysteroscopic control, the liquids used to distend the uterus can become a problem. As the pressure in the endometrial cavity must be about 80 mm Hg for good distention, the dextran 70, 5% dextrose in water, or glycine may be absorbed variably into the venous system, whose pressure is about 8 mm Hg. The hysteroscopist must track fluid balance to ascertain that overload and congestive fail-

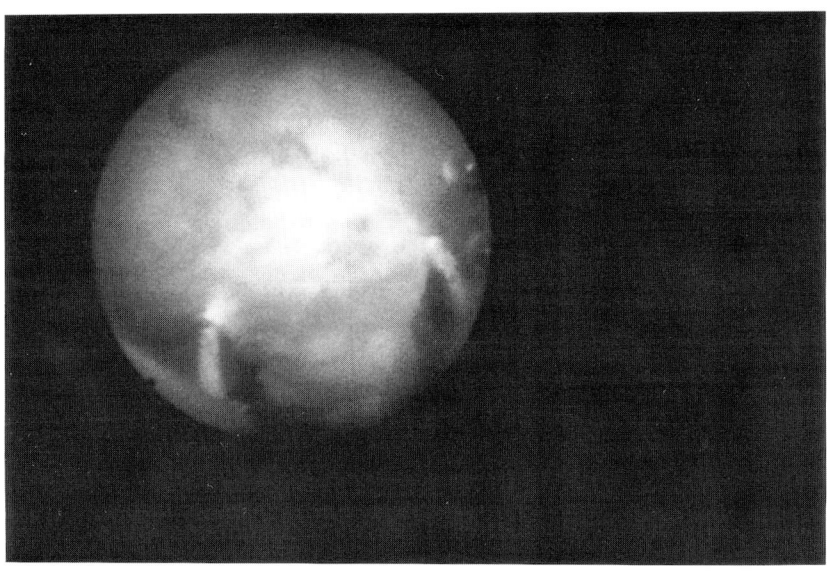

Fig. 37-6 Loop electrode during myomectomy.

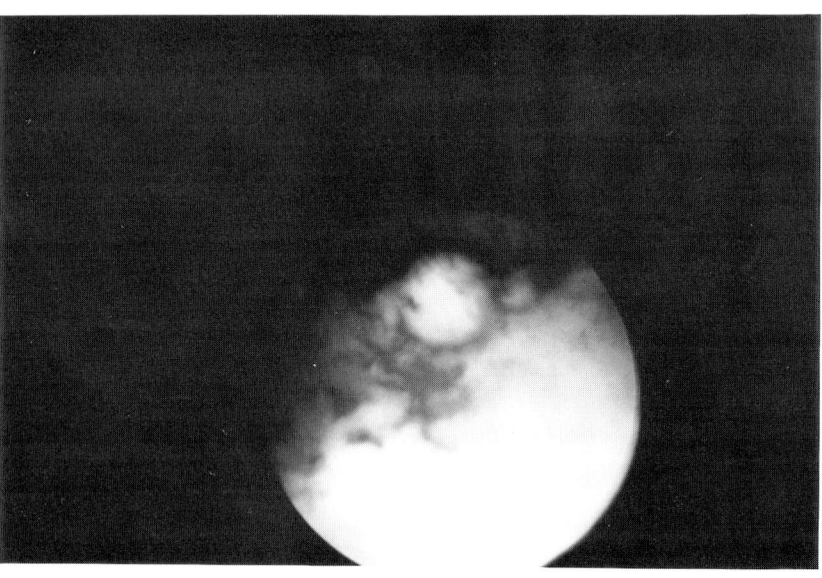

Fig. 37-7 Rollerball during endometrial ablation.

ure will not occur. For low-viscosity liquids about 3 L absorbed is the maximum tolerated. For Hyskon, which is hyperosmotic, 400 ml is the approximate limit of absorption. In addition, in prolonged cases with marked absorption, it is prudent to check the serum electrolytes as hyponatremia can occur.

Safety is always a primary consideration. The critical issues to follow are the fluid balance, good visual hysteroscopic control, and, if needed, simultaneous laparoscopy to avoid injury from a mechanical or thermal perforation of the uterus.

The resectoscope is being more widely used because it is a low-cost instrument and is technically easier to maneuver for myomectomy and ablation. The most advanced electrosurgical generators available can avoid accidental exit burns and can cut with almost no penetrating burn. The resectoscope is a most useful instrument but requires full fa-

miliarity with diagnostic hysteroscopy, electrosurgery, and fluid balances to be used properly.

Excising submucous fibroids

The method of removal will depend on the reproductive needs of the patient. When continued fertility is desired, it is feasible to remove submucous fibroids hysteroscopically if the uterus is small and the fibroids are small or pedunculated (7). With small, pedunculated fibroids, one method is to twist them off with a polyp forceps and extract them after hysteroscopically reviewing intrauterine pathology.

It is also worth trying to partially resect submucous components of intramural fibroids hysteroscopically if these components measure less than 2×2 cm. In such instances, epithelial healing should not be a problem. However, if the uterus is larger than 10 cm from exocervix to fundal tip or if fibroids are either essentially intramural or have a large submucous component, the abdominal route is preferable.

When performing hysteroscopic resection, locate the tubal orifices to avoid injuring them. Begin laparoscopy and shave the tumor down to the plane of the endometrial cavity by placing the resectoscope loop behind the tumor and drawing it toward the endoscope while simultaneously applying 30 to 40 W of cutting current.

The resectoscope will shave the tumor into slices measuring 4 mm × 3 cm that will float in the dextran 70. Continue resection until fragments block the objective lens or the procedure is completed.

To remove shavings, withdraw the resectoscope from the sheath, allowing the dextran 70 and fragments to run out, or remove the entire instrument and pull out the tissue pieces with ovum forceps. One can irrigate the uterus with saline or 5% dextrose and water, if necessary, to remove clots, bubbles, or debris. Then reinsert the resectoscope, redistend the uterus, and continue with the operation until the resection is complete.

Postoperative bleeding may be a problem. In such cases, we insert a Silastic rubber balloon with a slender stem and ball valve control that inflates up to 60 ml and stops bleeding by direct tamponade of the uterine cavity.

We inflate the balloon progressively. Pressure is felt to rise at the syringe plunger. Once balloon pressure equals arterial pressure, bleeding stops and we terminate laparoscopy.

We release balloon pressure after several hours, observe the patient overnight, remove the balloon the next morning, and discharge the patient home for ambulatory follow-up if there is no significant bleeding. Before discharge, we give her two doses of prophylactic antibiotics and prescribe a 10-day course of oral estrogen.

Coitus is not allowed for one month. Return to work or usual activities may commence one week after surgery. When weakening of the uterine wall is a possibility, we obtain a hysterogram after 2 months.

Thereafter, unprotected coitus is permitted, and pregnancy may follow. If the uterine wall is intact, we advise vaginal delivery with close observation. If it has been weakened by perforation or deep removal of part of an intramural tumor, we usually recommend cesarean section.

Removing fibroids when fertility is not a factor

If the patient does not wish to retain fertility and has significant uncontrollable bleeding, she may elect partial or total hysteroscopic ablation of submucous fibroids in preference to hysterectomy. Tumor size is less important than when fertility is a concern.

Before operating, rule out malignant and premalignant endometrium. It is also desirable to suppress the ovaries to keep the endometrium thin. Give danazol (Chronogyn, Danocrine) or norethindrone (Aygestin, Norlutate) for 3 or 4 weeks before surgery if contraindications are absent.

Destructive techniques are laser ablation or cautery (9,10). Perform ablation with a neodymium-yttrium-aluminum-garnet (Nd-YAG) laser set at 50 W. Use lactated Ringer's solution or dextran 70 as a medium. The recommended procedure is to come close enough to the endometrium without touching it to coagulate tissue to a depth of 4 mm. Tissue turns white as it is coagulated.

In a variant that is used by Goldrath and coworkers, one touches tissue, causing both carbonization and some damage to the laser's fiberoptic bundle (9). Goldrath's method probably produces a deeper burn. Clinically, it is easier and seems to be more effective in producing light menses or amenorrhea.

Regardless of which laser ablation procedure one uses, after inducing general or regional anesthesia, start at the fundus and work systematically toward the isthmus. Use simultaneous laparoscopy to ascertain absence of ovarian or major tubal pathology and control the hysteroscopic procedure.

Hospitalize the patient overnight and release her the next morning. Prescribe danazol for 2 weeks. Discharge and some bleeding will occur for several weeks or months thereafter. Sound the uterine cavity every 2 weeks to maintain a central tract that would otherwise be obliterated by scarring. Should significant bleeding occur, insert an intrauterine balloon for tamponade.

Electrocoagulation, which is somewhat faster than laser ablation because loop width is larger, takes about 15 minutes for a normal-sized uterus. Drag the resectoscope, set at 40 W, slowly over the endometrium to produce a white tissue coagulum. If charring occurs, reduce power or move the electrode more quickly. We have done electrocoagulation under laparoscopic control using dextran 70.

Long-term data on the outcome of hysteroscopic resection of myomata, endometrial ablation, and fertility following hysteroscopic myomectomy have recently been published by our group (11). Life table analysis shows an 85% chance of avoiding repeat surgery for 8 years following submucous myomectomy. There is a 91% chance of avoiding repeat surgery for 6 years following endometrial ablation. We have followed 25 women who have become pregnant after hysteroscopic myomectomy. The spontaneous abortion rate is 12%. Several patients have terminated pregnancy although they desired to retain the option of pregnancy. Eighteen women have had at least one term pregnancy. These data support the resectoscopic treatment of submucous myomectomy as well as endometrial ablation as a cost-effective approach to abdominal myomectomy or hysterectomy in selected cases.

Summary

In brief, hysteroscopy has a dual importance. Besides constituting a superior office diagnostic technique in conjunction with curettage, it is commonly used to remove IUDs and polyps, treat Asherman's syndrome and uterine septa, excise selected submucous myomata, and avoid hysterectomy for menorrhagia of benign origin.

References

1 Lindeman HJ. Eine new untersuchungsmethode für die Hysteroscopie. Endoscopy 1971;4:194.

2 Edstrom K, Fernstrom I. The diagnostic possibilities of a modified hysteroscopic technique. Acta Obstet Gynecol Scand 1970;49:307.

3 Quinnones RG, Alvarado DA, Aznar RA. Hysteroscopia una nueva technia. Genicol Obstet Mex 1972;32:237.

4 March CR, Isreal R. Hysteroscopic management of intrauterine adhesions. Am J Obstet Gynecol 1978;130:653.

5 Levine RU, Neuwirth RS. Simultaneous laparoscopy and hysteroscopy for intrauterine adhesions. Obstet Gynecol 1973;42:441.

6 Reed TP, Erb RA. Hysteroscopic oviductal bleeding with funnel in place. Silicone rubber plugs: II. Clinical studies. J Reprod Med 1979;23:69.

7 Neuwirth RS, Amin HK. Excision of submucous fibroids with hysteroscopic control. Am J Obstet Gynecol 1976;126:95–97.

8 DeCherney AH, Desmond MC, Lavy G, Dolan UL. Endometrial ablation for intractable uterine bleeding: hysteroscopic resection. Obstet Gynecol 1987;78:668–670.

9 Goldrath M, Fuller TA, Sepl S. Laser photovaporization of endometrium for the treatment of menorrhagia. Am J Obstet Gynecol 1981;140:14–19.

10 DeCherney A, Polan ML. Hysteroscopic management of intrauterine lesions and intractable uterine bleeding. Obstet Gynecol 1983;61:392.

11 Derman SG, Rehnstrom J, Neuwirth RS. The long term effectiveness of hysteroscopic treatment of menorrhagia and leiomyomas. Obstet Gynecol 1991;7:591–594.

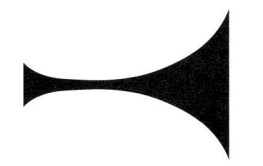

Chapter 38

Laparoscopic surgery for tubal pregnancy

Preston C. Sacks

For some decades after Lawson Tait reported the first surgical treatment of ectopic pregnancy in 1883, diagnosis commonly occurred after tubal rupture (1). These women were often hemodynamically unstable, and laparotomy with salpingectomy became the treatment of choice. When, as occasionally happened, an unruptured pregnancy was detected, surgeons did attempt to conserve the tube. This treatment was often discouraged, however, as there was a high incidence of repeat ectopic pregnancy with its attendant morbidity and mortality.

In the 1970s, the introduction of sensitive radioimmunoassays to measure the β-subunit of human chorionic gonadotropin (β-hCG) made the early diagnosis of pregnancy increasingly feasible. The widespread availability of ultrasonography (particularly transvaginal sonography) has made early diagnosis of an unruptured ectopic pregnancy the rule rather than the exception. This had reduced the morbidity and mortality related to ectopic pregnancies and increased the popularity of conservative surgery.

In patients suspected of having an ectopic pregnancy, laparoscopy is usually performed to confirm the diagnosis and surgically remove the products of conception. Recently, there have been several reports on the safety and efficacy of medical (nonsurgical) management of ectopic pregnancies (2,3). Women with unruptured ectopic pregnancies less than 3 cm in diameter have received the folic acid antagonist methotrexate. Success rates appear to be greater than 90%, and follow-up studies show pregnancy rates similar to those obtained with conservative surgery. Early data show the rate of adverse events to be low. Until more experience is obtained, however, surgery remains the mainstay for the diagnosis and treatment of ectopic pregnancies.

When is laparotomy indicated?

Laparotomy is appropriate in four instances: when the patient is hemodynamically unstable; when there is a contraindication to abdominal insufflation or laparoscopy; when the surgeon is inexperienced in laparoscopic surgical techniques; and when the anatomy of the pelvis is so distorted (i.e., by severe adhesions) that laparoscopic treatment is technically unwise. In most other cases, laparoscopy is the surgical approach of choice. Advantages to laparoscopy include a reduced length of hospital stay, shorter postoperative recovery time, and reduced overall health care cost. Virtually all surgical procedures that can be performed at laparotomy can be performed by an experienced operator during laparoscopy.

The most common procedures used to treat a pregnancy in the fallopian tube are salpingectomy, partial salpingectomy, linear salpingostomy, and fimbrial expression. Which procedure is most appropriate depends on the location of the pregnancy, the condition of the affected fallopian tube, and the condition of the contralateral fallopian tube.

Choosing the correct surgical procedure

It is difficult to decide in an individual case whether to perform conservative surgery (salpingostomy, fimbrial expression) or salpingectomy. Several large series have attempted to guide the surgeon in choosing the correct procedure, though to date there is no consensus. Summarizing several studies (4–8), one may draw the following conclusions:

1 Fertility following surgery for an ectopic pregnancy appears to be more closely related to fertility history than to the surgical procedure performed.

2 It is not clear whether conservative surgery (tubal conservation) yields a higher live birth rate than salpingectomy.

3 There is roughly a twofold greater incidence of repeat ectopic pregnancy following conservative surgery.

4 The incidence of persistent ectopic pregnancy requiring repeat surgery or chemotherapy following laparoscopic conservative surgery is roughly 15%.

With these facts in mind, the surgeon must evaluate each case in terms of fertility history, access to follow-up medical care, and status of the fallopian tubes (affected and contralateral) at the time of surgery. We discuss the benefits and risks of conservative surgery with each patient before surgery, then proceed at surgery on the basis of the history and status of the fallopian tubes.

Salpingectomy

Laparoscopic salpingectomy is the simplest procedure to perform and manage postoperatively. Most surgeons learning operative laparoscopic procedures will be able to perform salpingectomy, as the techniques are very similar to tubal sterilization. With laparoscopic salpingectomy there is minimal blood loss, and the pregnancy is removed in toto, eliminating the risk of persistent ectopic pregnancy. Intrauterine pregnancy rates following salpingectomy are equal to those following conservative surgery when one controls for fertility history and the status of the contralateral fallopian tube (7).

Instrumentation

- Two 5.5-mm accessory ports
- Bipolar forceps
- 5-mm self-locking grasping forceps
- 5-mm "hook" scissors
- Suction probe
- 10-mm grasping forceps (optional)
- One 10-mm accessory port (optional)

Procedure

Laparoscopic salpingectomy begins with three access ports: infraumbilical (10 mm), midline suprapubic accessory (5.5 mm), and ipsilateral suprapubic accessory (5.5 mm). Once the site of the tubal pregnancy has been identified and the entire pelvis inspected and rinsed of any blood, all adhesions surrounding the affected fallopian tube should be resected. This frees the tube from adjacent structures, such as bowel, pelvic blood vessels, and ureter, and ensures the safety of the procedure.

To begin the surgical procedure, the isthmic portion of fallopian tube is grasped with the bipolar forceps in an area well proximal to the pregnancy site (Fig. 38-1A). The tube is cauterized and transected with the scissors (Fig. 38-1B), gaining access to the mesosalpinx. The newly created distal stump is grasped with self-locking forceps placed through the ipsilateral accessory port, and the distal tubal segment containing the ectopic pregnancy is elevated to expose the mesosalpinx (Fig. 38-1C). The mesosalpinx is then serially cauterized and transected until the fallopian tube is completely free of its attachments (Fig. 38-1D).

Removing the specimen from the abdomen is often the most challenging and time-consuming portion of the procedure. Several methods have been devised to remove the specimen in its entirety. My preferred approach is to place a grasping forceps through the accessory port of the 10-mm right-angle laparoscope. The specimen and laparoscope are withdrawn together through the infraumbilical sheath under direct visualization (Fig. 38-2). When the laparoscope nears the trumpet valve on the sheath, one must remember to depress the valve to allow for unobstructed passage of the specimen.

An alternative approach is to replace the midline 5.5-mm suprapubic sheath with a 10-mm accessory port. Through this port one can place the 10-mm grasping forceps and remove the specimen. Again, care must be taken to depress the trumpet valve when the specimen is in the sheath. If the specimen is too large to fit through the 10-mm sheath (typically when the diameter is greater than 3 cm), either the specimen can be removed in pieces, or a posterior colpotomy can be created and the intact specimen can be removed through the vagina. If the specimen is removed in pieces, one should carefully inspect the pelvis to locate and remove all fragments of tissue, which could become explants and lead to persistent trophoblastic tissue.

Partial salpingectomy

Partial salpingectomy is appropriate when the portion of the tube containing the ectopic pregnancy has to be removed, yet future microsurgical tubal reconstruction remains a possibility. Partial salpingectomy may be used to remove isthmic and isthmicoampullary pregnancies. A prerequisite for success is the accessibility of the mesosalpinx. As with salpingectomy, before beginning partial salpingectomy, all adhesions surrounding the portion of tube being resected should be removed.

The instrumentation and surgical approach for partial salpingectomy are the same as for salpingectomy. The tube

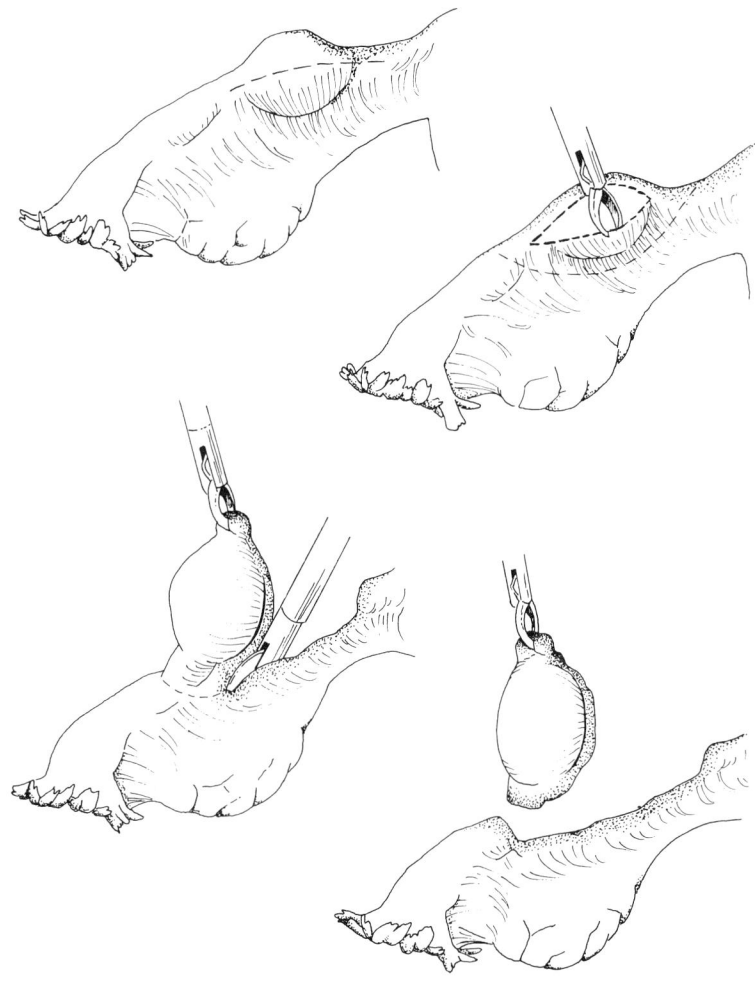

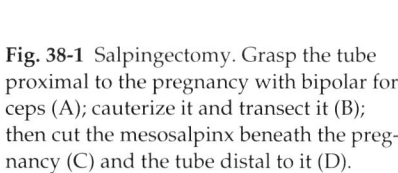

Fig. 38-1 Salpingectomy. Grasp the tube proximal to the pregnancy with bipolar forceps (A); cauterize it and transect it (B); then cut the mesosalpinx beneath the pregnancy (C) and the tube distal to it (D).

is cauterized at a site proximal to the pregnancy using the bipolar forceps. The tube is then transected and elevated, exposing the mesosalpinx. The mesosalpinx underlying the pregnancy is alternatively cauterized and transected to a distance just distal to the pregnancy site. The fallopian tube distal to the pregnancy is cauterized and transected, freeing the affected segment of tube. The specimen is then removed as described in the salpingectomy section.

With partial salpingectomy, the entire implantation site is removed, eliminating the risk of persistent trophoblastic tissue. One point of note is that with any tubal resection procedure, the extent of thermal damage and fibrosis often extends well past the area of resection. Therefore, prior to microsurgical repair, I perform a laparoscopy to assess the amount of remaining tube.

Linear salpingostomy

Linear salpingostomy is an effective method to remove an unruptured ectopic pregnancy in the ampullary portion of the fallopian tube. If the pregnancy is in the isthmic portion of the tube, partial or total salpingectomy is usually more appropriate, as there is increased bleeding and a high rate of persistent ectopic pregnancy with laparoscopic linear salpingostomy.

With linear salpingostomy, the fallopian tube is incised, the products of conception are removed, and the incision is allowed to heal by secondary intention. Tubal patency rates following salpingostomy are high, though repeat ectopic pregnancy rates in the affected tube point to the fact that patency does not ensure normal function.

At the time of diagnostic laparoscopy, the site of the tubal pregnancy can usually be identified as a distended area with a bluish hue. This appearance results from an increase in vascularity associated with the implantation site and localized hemorrhage in the fallopian tube. Typically the distention is distal to the implantation site, and often there is some leaking of blood from the fimbria. This fact is important when selecting the site for the tubal incision. There is a tendency to make the incision too far distal, not

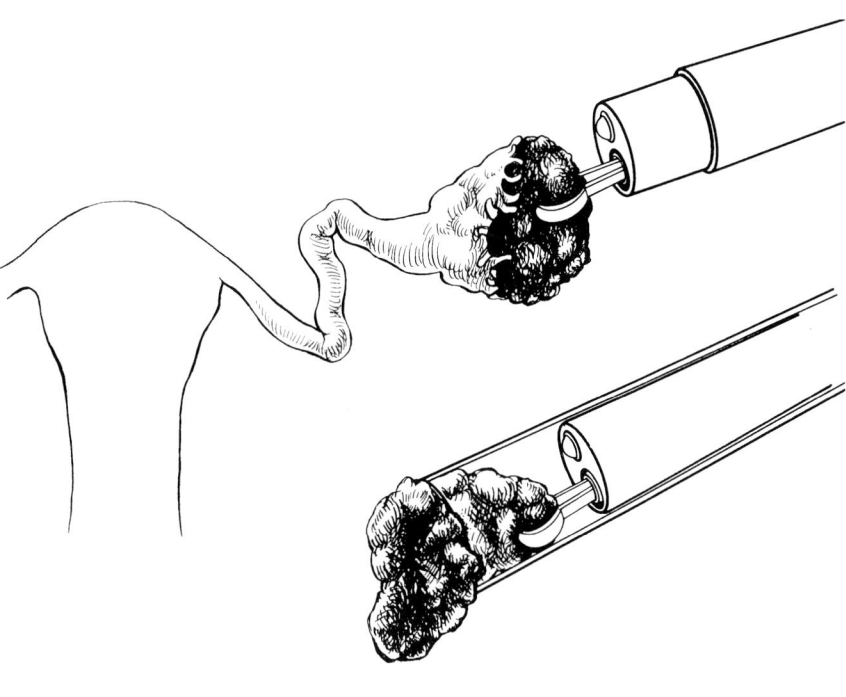

Fig. 38-2 Expression technique. Grasp the aborting tubal pregnancy through the operating laparoscope and remove the products of conception, along with the laparoscope, through the sheath.

exposing the implantation site. This can lead to incomplete removal of the products of conception and a higher rate of persistent ectopic pregnancy.

Because of the increased vasculature, many authors recommend injecting the mesosalpinx with a dilute vasopressin (Pitressin) solution before salpingostomy. Our group does not use Pitressin, and has performed more than 50 laparoscopic surgeries for ectopic pregnancy. No bleeding complications have occurred; however, there are so few complications related to Pitressin, that its routine use cannot be discouraged.

Instrumentation

Instrumentation is the same as for salpingectomy with the following additions:
- Suction irrigation probe
- 5-mm grasping forceps
- Instrument to make the tubal incision (either):
  - Knife or needle-tip electrocautery (3 mm)
  - Laser fiber (neodymium-yttrium-aluminum-garnet) or wave guide (carbon dioxide)

Procedure

When performing linear salpingostomy, I use the same three access ports as for salpingectomy. Once the site of the tubal pregnancy has been identified, the fallopian tube is stabilized by grasping the tubal serosa with the self-locking grasping forceps at a site distal to the pregnancy. The forceps typically are passed through the paramedian port, and the tube is stretched laterally to fully expose the anti-

mesenteric portion of the tube. The incision instrument is placed through the midline accessory port, and the tube is incised over the antimesenteric surface for a distance encompassing the implantation site (Fig. 38-3A). There is no evidence that laser energy is more effective than electrocautery when performing the tubal incision. Both provide cutting energy and will be helpful in achieving hemostasis. Because of its universal availability and ease of operation, I most frequently use electrocautery.

After incising the tube, the products of conception should begin to bulge out of the incision. If one waits a few seconds, the tube will often begin to contract, and the entire products will be expelled. If not, then grasping forceps can be inserted into the tubal incision, and the products can be gently teased from the tubal lumen (Fig. 38-3B). The products are removed through the infraumbilical sheath as described above for salpingectomy.

Following removal of the products of conception, the tube is irrigated and carefully inspected. The implantation site will typically have some areas of bleeding, which can be controlled by coagulation. This bleeding is not unexpected as the products of conception are not entirely intraluminal. As with any implantation site, the trophoblasts have invaded the mucosa to obtain vascular support. If one examines a tubal implantation site histologically, the muscularis of the fallopian tube is invaded by trophoblastic tissue (9). This fact is important when discussing linear salpingostomy. It explains why hemostasis is not usually achieved by simply removing the products of conception, and also why the incidence of persistent trophoblasic tissue is high.

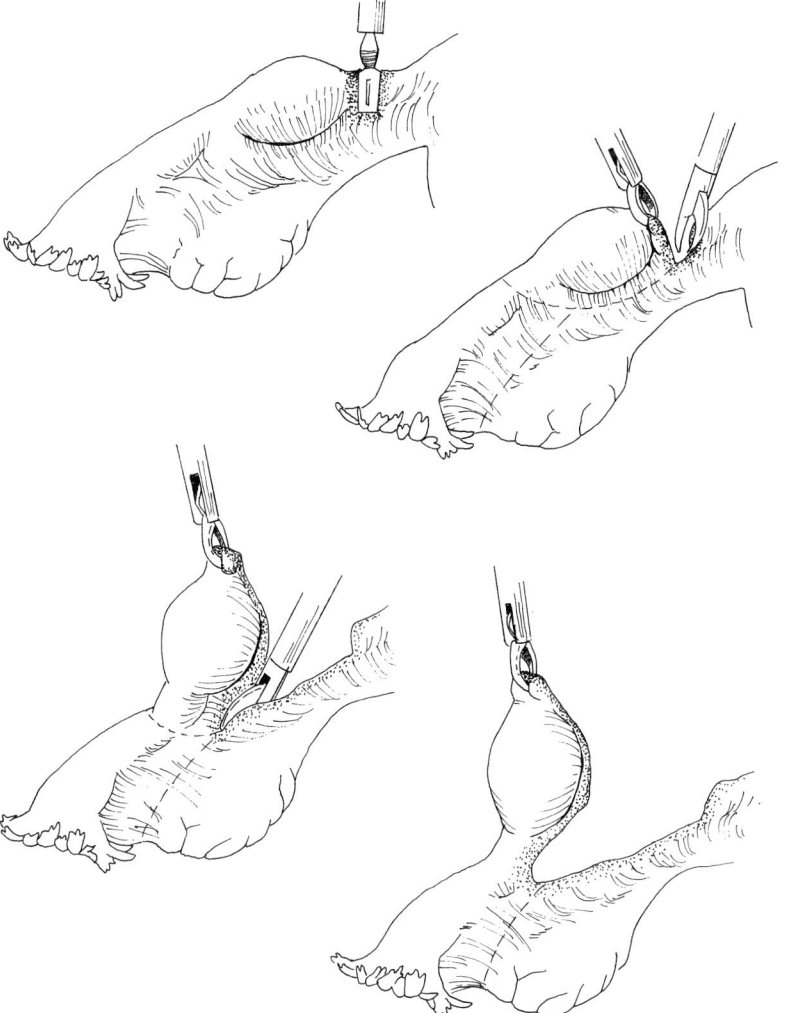

Fig. 38-3 Linear salpingostomy procedure. (A) Incise the anti-mesenteric portion of the fallopian tube overlying the ectopic pregnancy; (B) place grasping forceps inside incision to remove products of conception.

Fimbrial expression

This maneuver is most successful if the implantation is in the fimbriated end or the distal ampulla. To express an aborting ectopic pregnancy, grasp the products of conception with forceps placed through the operating port of the right-angle laparoscope. Gently tease the products from the tube, and withdraw them together with the laparoscope through the 10-mm sheath as described for salpingectomy.

If the pregnancy is in the distal ampulla, it may be expressed by squeezing the tube sequentially from proximal to distal end with two grasping forceps placed through the lower operating sheaths.

Seemingly atraumatic, expression has two major problems. First, fimbrial bleeding may occur. It can usually be controlled with electrocautery or laser coagulation; however, if the bleeding site is proximal, exposure is limited unless one radially incises the fallopian tube. This will lead to tubal damage, which may negate the benefits of retaining the tube. Second, there may be incomplete removal of the products of conception, increasing the likelihood for persistent trophoblastic tissue.

Postoperative care

The incidence of immediate postoperative morbidity is low and related mostly to the amount of blood lost before surgery. Most women will be able to be discharged within a few hours following surgery. If salpingectomy or partial salpingectomy was performed, then the patient returns to the office in 2 weeks for a postoperative examination.

Women undergoing conservative surgery (fimbrial expression or linear salpingostomy) require postoperative monitoring for persistent trophoblastic tissue. I follow the serum levels of the β-hCG on a weekly basis to ensure resolution of the pregnancy. Persistent trophoblastic tissue is detectable by an increase or plateauing of the serum levels of β-hCG. In this instance, repeat surgery or methotrexate administration is indicated. The β-hCG levels should be monitored until the level is no longer detectable, signifying the absence of any viable trophoblastic tissue.

References

1 Tait RL. Lectures on ectopic pregnancy and pelvic hematocele. Birmingham, England: Journal Printing Works, 1988.

2 Stovall TG, Ling FW, Gray LA. Single-dose methotrexate for treatment of ectopic pregnancy. Obstet Gynecol 1991;77:754–757.

3 Ory SJ. Chemotherapy for ectopic pregnancy. Obstet Gynecol Clin North Am 1991;18:123–134.

4 Abrams J, Farell DM. Salpingectomy and salpingoplasty for tubal pregnancy: survey of the literature. Obstet Gynecol 1964;24:281–285.

5 Tuomivaara L, Kauppila A. Radical or conservative surgery for ectopic pregnancy? A follow-up study of fertility of 323 patients. Fertil Steril 1988;50:580–583.

6 Uotila J, Heinonen PK, Punnonen R. Reproductive outcome after multiple ectopic pregnancies. Int J Fertil 1989;34:102–105.

7 Ory SJ, Nnadi E, Herrmann R, O'Brien PS, Melton LJ III. Fertility after ectopic pregnancy. Fertil Steril 1993;60:231–235.

8 Seifer DB, Gutmann JN, Grant WD, Kamps CA, DeCherney AH. Comparison of persistent ectopic pregnancy after laparoscopic salpingostomy versus salpingostomy at laparotomy for ectopic pregnancy. Obstet Gynecol 1993;81:378–382.

9 Budowick M, Johnson TRB, Genadry R, et al. The histopathology of the developing tubal ectopic pregnancy. Fertil Steril 1980;34:169.

Chapter 39

Laparoscopic management of gynecologic malignancies

Nicholas Kadar

Alice: There's no use trying—one can't believe impossible things.

The Queen: I dare say you haven't had much practice. Why, sometimes I've believed as many as six impossible things before breakfast.

(Alice's Adventures in Wonderland, Lewis Carroll)

In 1988, Harry Reich performed the first laparoscopically assisted hysterectomy in the world (1). What was then a highly controversial undertaking adumbrated the most remarkable development in surgery in recent times, the acme of which must surely be the ability to perform radical pelvic surgery laparoscopically. It is an astonishing fact that as techniques begin to mature, those of us who have been intimately involved in their development can already clearly foresee the day when almost all women with endometrial and cervical carcinoma who are surgical candidates will be treated laparoscopically rather than by traditional techniques. Indeed, laparoscopic surgery is potentially used to greatest advantage in gynecology in the treatment of gynecologic malignancies because the only reason to perform an operation laparoscopically is to reduce morbidity, and morbidity is generally higher after radical surgery than after operations for benign disease. Patients not only recover much faster, but if radiation therapy is required, it can usually be started sooner, and will probably be better tolerated, although this remains to be demonstrated.

Most physicians who can learn gynecologic surgery can learn to do it laparoscopically, for it is not difficult in the sense that playing Chopin's heroic polonaise is, and it does not take years to master. However, it depends for its success not so much on high technology as on strict adherence to the basic surgical principles of sharp scissor dissection and blunt development of tissue planes that are so elegantly described in the other chapters of this book. The challenges of laparoscopic surgery are far more intellectual than mechanical, for their solution requires a better understanding of the precise anatomic relation between pelvic structures, and the deployment of different strategies than are used at laparotomy, rather than the acquisition of a technical ability not already possessed by the surgeon.

In this chapter, the laparoscopic techniques I have developed for retroperitoneal dissection, pelvic and aortic lymphadenectomy, and simple and radical hysterectomy will be described (2–8). A detailed discussion of the malignancies treated and the role of surgery in their management is outside the scope of this chapter. Suffice it to say that the indications for surgery are the same regardless of whether it is performed laparoscopically or via laparotomy, and no patient has ever been treated differently as a consequence of having opted for a laparoscopic approach.

Role of laparoscopic surgery in gynecologic malignancies

Endometrial carcinoma

The laparoscopic treatment of women with endometrial carcinoma is outlined in Figures 39-1 and 39-2. The most noteworthy aspect of our management is that we restrict aortic lymphadenectomy to patients who have positive pelvic nodes. Although this strategy will result in two op-

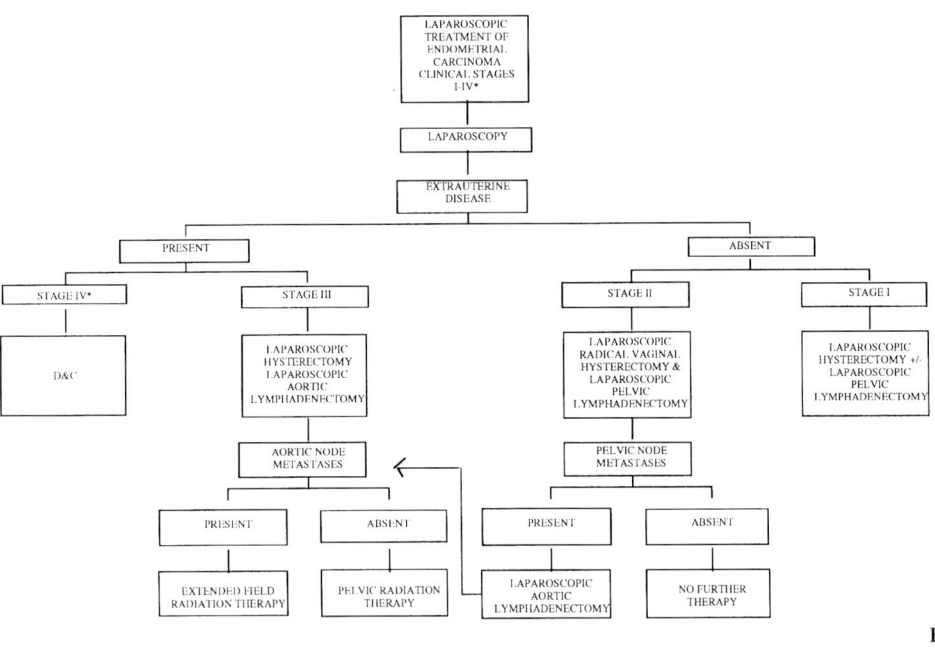

Fig. 39-1 Laparoscopic management of carcinoma of the endometrium.

* Some patients with Stage IV disease require hysterectomy for persistent bleeding.

erative procedures in a few patients, this drawback is minimized by the laparoscopic approach. Positive pelvic nodes are a more sensitive and specific criterion for aortic lymph node metastases than all the other criteria that could be used, including deep myometrial invasion. Thus, although the two-stage approach will result in two operations in approximately 7% of patients, it will identify 23% more patients with aortic lymph node metastases, and will require at least 35% fewer aortic lymphadenectomies than would be required if deep myometrial invasion were used as the criterion for aortic lymphadenectomy (9). It will also simplify therapy by avoiding the need for intraoperative frozen sections or expensive preoperative imaging studies to determine the depth of myometrial invasion.

Cervix cancer

The treatment of patients with cervix cancer is outlined in Figure 39-3. The contribution of laparoscopic surgery to the management of this malignancy is in its infancy, but it promises to be revolutionary. Laparoscopic aortic lymphadenectomy is arguably the most cost-effective laparoscopic procedure in gynecology. Patients go home in one to two days, they start radiation in 10 to 12 days, and they have virtually no pain or morbidity. What was once a questionable staging operation has been transformed into one with about the same morbidity as laparoscopic removal of a tubal pregnancy. The reduction in morbidity from laparoscopic radical vaginal hysterectomy is perhaps even more remarkable. (It is best expressed anecdotally by the patient who telephoned me a week after surgery to inquire if she could go swimming!) This is, of course, a com-

plicated operation to learn, and it will have to undergo the test of time. However, I predict that it will become the standard therapy for stage IA2-IIA cancer of the cervix within at most 10 years. Moreover, although complications are inevitably higher at first after inchoate procedures, it is inconceivable that morbidity will not be dramatically reduced by this approach.

Cancer of the ovary

The only truly controversial role for laparoscopic management of gynecologic malignancies is in the management of ovarian carcinoma, which is still evolving. That role is likely to be limited to stage I disease because it is difficult to foresee that the debulking of large pelvic or abdominal tumors will ever be feasible laparoscopically. There are, however, some exceptions. Approximately 10% of women with advanced ovarian cancer have normal-sized ovaries and no bulk disease and do not require debulking surgery. Laparoscopic surgery may be both feasible and preferable in these patients. Patients with stage III borderline tumors are also potential candidates for a laparoscopic approach, because the treatment of these indolent malignancies relies much more on repeated surgical resection than on adjunctive chemotherapy or radiation therapy, whose efficacy in borderline tumors has yet to be established. Clearly, the advantages of a laparoscopic approach compound if therapy involves multiple surgeries (10).

The greatest potential for laparoscopic surgery in the management of ovarian cancer is in stage I disease. Most oncologists have been reluctant to treat these patients laparoscopically until they have perfected their techniques

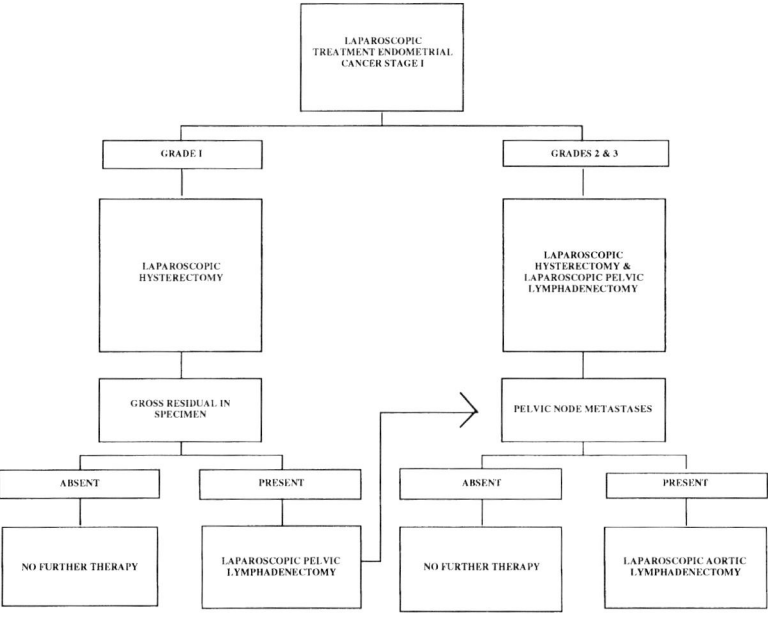

Fig. 39-2 Laparoscopic management of carcinoma of the endometrium grossly confined to the uterus.

for pelvic and aortic lymphadenectomy, but as techniques for these procedures have matured, the fear of rupturing a malignant cyst has become more important. Although the adverse effect of this has been overstated (11), the rarity of stage I disease and the inability to investigate the question in a prospective trial means that any claim that cyst rupture "makes no difference" must be made with some circumspection. Nonetheless, even if survival were to be marginally compromised by cyst rupture, this would not automatically contraindicate laparoscopic management of pelvic masses, because most masses are benign, and the increased morbidity and mortality from laparotomy in the majority of women who do not have malignancy may more than offset a slight decrease in survival of women who turn out to have ovarian carcinoma (12). Laparoscopic staging is, however, the treatment of choice in patients who are discovered to have ovarian carcinoma after ovarian cystectomy or simple oophorectomy, for the issue of cyst rupture does not arise.

Laparoscopic techniques

Deprived of the ability to palpate tissues, the laparoscopic surgeon must rely entirely on visual recognition to identify normal structures in the abdomen and pelvis. This requires detailed knowledge of pelvic anatomy and more extensive dissection of the retroperitoneum to display normal structure than is required with an open technique. However, the technique of pelvic dissection used during laparotomy does not easily lend itself to a laparoscopic approach, because if the same sequence of steps is followed as in an open case, the operator will find that tissues become progressively more slack and difficult to place on tension. This in turn

makes blunt dissection of the retroperitoneal spaces increasingly more difficult and, eventually, impossible. The strategy for laparoscopic retroperitoneal dissection I developed (2) allows all vital retroperitoneal structures to be freed and identified, but it depends for its success on executing the steps of the dissection in a precise sequence. It is also necessary for the operator to understand the logic of the dissection, and this requires a thorough knowledge of the relevant anatomy.

Preliminaries

Patients are positioned awake in Allen stirrups for all laparoscopic operations except laparoscopic aortic lymphadenectomy, for which they are placed flat on the operating table, with the knees flexed, and the thighs abducted but not flexed at the hips. Ureteric stents are also routinely passed because this makes the ureters much more prominent and aids in their identification and retraction. (The purpose of the stent is *not* to help "palpate" the ureter endoscopically with instruments.)

My current preference is to use Dexide trocars (Dexide Inc., Fort Worth, Tex) which have a built-in basketlike retention device that can be expanded once the trocars are in the abdomen, a rubber washer on the outside that prevents leakage of gas, and a nonflapper valve mechanism on which the instruments, particularly those with curved ends, do not snag. Three working ports are used in addition to the subumbilical port for the laparoscope. A 5-mm or a 10-mm port is placed suprapubically, and a 5-mm port is placed on either side of the rectus muscles just above a line joining the anterior superior iliac spines. A 10-mm trocar is inserted suprapubically for radical cases, but a 5-mm port is used for all other cases (Fig. 39-4).

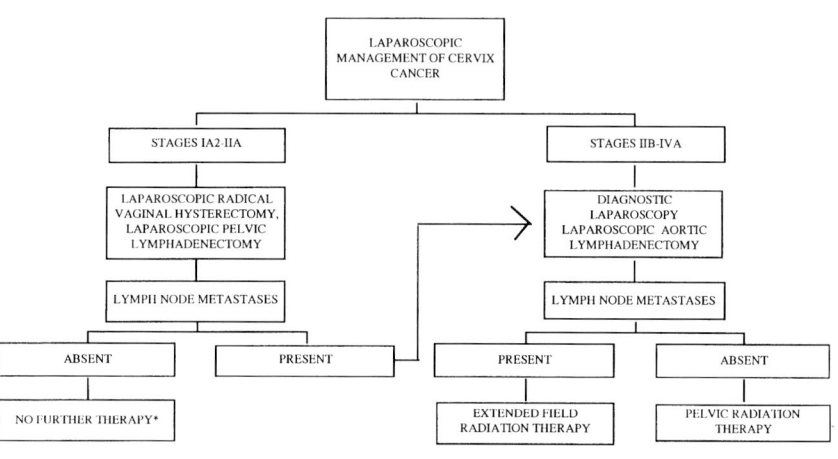

* Pelvic radiation is given for occult parametrial invasion or close surgical
techniques, but these are rare findings.

Fig. 39-3 Laparoscopic management of cervix cancer.

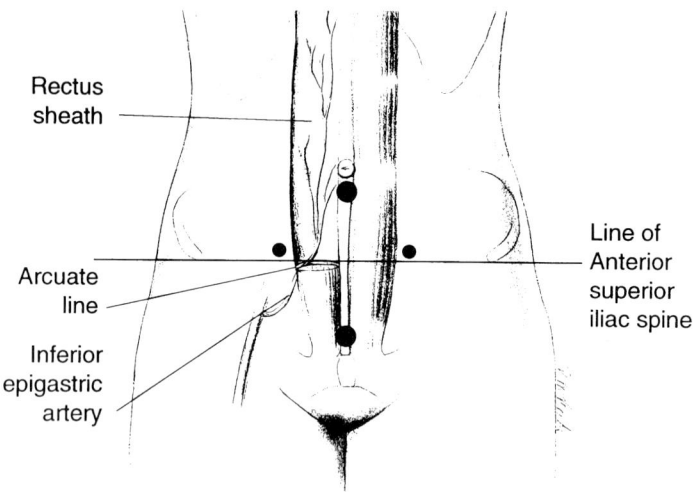

Fig. 39-4 Trocar placements used for laparoscopic radical pelvic surgery.

All trocars are inserted directly and a Veress needle is not used. After the infraumbilical trocar is inserted, its intraperitoneal location is checked with the laparoscope, and the abdomen is insufflated using a high flow rate (6–9 L per minute depending on the machine available). If there has been significant previous intraperitoneal surgery, open laparoscopy is performed.

Anatomy

Ureter

Halfway between the pelvic brim and the renal pelvis the ureters are crossed by the ovarian vessels, which come to lie lateral to the ureters. This is the relation at or just above the pelvic brim, where the ovarian vessels enter the infundibulopelvic ligament. The infundibulopelvic ligament runs medially from the pelvic brim to the ovary in the roof of the broad ligament. It crosses the ureter to lie at first above it, and then medial to it (Fig. 39-5). The important practical corollary is that,

• the ureter cannot be damaged as the incision in the pelvic sidewall peritoneum is extended proximally if the peritoneal incision is kept lateral to the anatomic position of the infundibulopelvic ligament (which must not, therefore, be displaced medially before the incision has been extended), and

• the infundibulopelvic ligament must be retracted medially before the ureter can be displayed at the pelvic brim.

Throughout their pelvic course the ureters lie in a connective tissue sheath attached to the medial leaf of the broad ligament. Upon crossing the pelvic brim, the ureters descend abruptly and follow the contours of the pelvis. This means that at first they actually bend laterally to run along

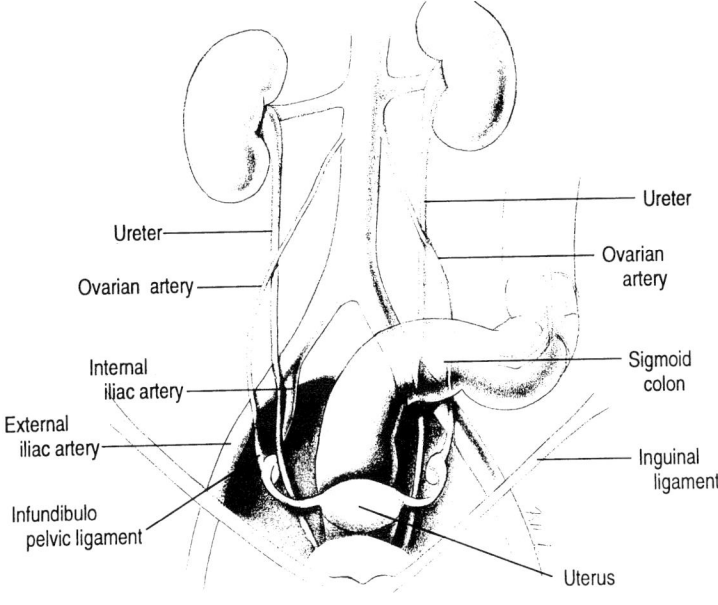

Ureter

Ovarian artery

Internal iliac artery

External iliac artery

Infundibulo pelvic ligament

Ureter

Ovarian artery

Sigmoid colon

Inguinal ligament

Uterus

Fig. 39-5 Relation between the ureter and the ovarian vessels in the abdomen and pelvis.

the pelvic sidewalls just above the internal iliac arteries. This is not appreciated surgically, however, because once the broad ligament is opened the ureters are displaced medially from their natural position on the pelvic sidewall and are seen as following a more or less straight course from the renal pelvis to the bladder, turning medially to join the bladder only after they have entered the ureteric tunnel in the vesicocervical ligaments or bladder pillars.

In the undisturbed state, at about the level of the ischial spines, the ureters run forward and medially in the base of the broad ligament, to pass under the uterine arteries approximately 1.5 cm lateral to the internal cervical os. (The left ureter is usually closer to the cervix than the right.) The ureters then turn abruptly medially to enter the bladder, passing over the anterior vaginal fornices as they do so. The terminal 1 to 2 cm of the ureter is called the genu or knee of the ureter. It lies in the vesicocervical ligament (also called the vesicouterine ligament or bladder pillar), the surgical anatomy of which can only be fully appreciated during radical vaginal hysterectomy or the Schauta-Amreich operation (see below).

Pelvic spaces

It is impossible to exaggerate the importance of being able to develop the paravesical and pararectal spaces reliably, for this is an absolute prerequisite for identifying vital structures in the retroperitoneum and dissecting them free.

The paravesical and pararectal spaces are potential spaces, which extend from the base of the broad ligament to the floor of the pelvis. At laparotomy, the broad ligament peritoneum can be opened in several ways, but most commonly the round ligament is first divided and the peritoneum is incised in a cephalad direction parallel and

lateral to the infundibulopelvic ligament up to the pelvic brim. The broad ligament is then opened bluntly by traction on its medial leaf. This maneuver will separate the loose areolar tissue between the leaves of the broad ligament, but an impasse will eventually be reached at about the level of the ureter and internal iliac artery where the areolar tissue is more condensed and will not separate any further. This point lies at the base of the broad ligament and marks the roof of the pararectal space. Once the broad ligament has been opened, the pararectal and paravesical spaces can be opened at laparotomy in the following way.

To begin, the bifurcation of the iliac artery is first identified by palpation, and the index finger is placed just medial to the internal iliac artery. (Identification of the bifurcation ensures that the dissection is medial to the internal, and not the external, iliac artery. Inadvertent dissection medial to the external iliac artery will risk injury to the external iliac vein as it lies between the internal and external iliac arteries.) The tissues medial to the dissecting finger are put on tension by traction in the direction of the patient's contralateral femoral head. A bloodless space will start to develop, and as it does, the plane of dissection should follow the curve of the pelvis, which, with the patient in a Trendelenburg position, is at first downward and forward, but then curves in an upward direction. The surgeon will find the ureter lying against the dissecting finger (still attached to the medial leaf of the broad ligament), for the ureter marks the medial border of the pararectal space, and its lateral border is formed by the internal iliac artery.

Frequently, especially in thin, young patients, the dense connective tissue forming the roof of the pararectal space cannot be disrupted bluntly, and a small opening must first be made in it with the point of a tonsil clamp or dissecting scissors as the tissue is held taut by medial traction with the dissecting finger. Once a small opening is made, the index finger is insinuated into the pararectal space, which will readily open if its medial wall is retracted in a medial direction as previously described.

After the pararectal space has been opened, the paravesical space is easily developed by running the index finger along the medial border of the external iliac artery in a caudad direction until the pubic ramus is reached. Upon reaching the pubic ramus the direction of the dissection changes abruptly through 90 degrees and is again directed medially toward the patient's contralateral femoral head. A large bloodless plane will again open up, which is the paravesical space, and a cordlike structure will be found in the dissecting finger, which is the lateral umbilical ligament or obliterated hypogastric artery.

The pararectal spaces cannot easily be developed laparoscopically in the same way as during laparotomy. First, the internal iliac artery is buried in areolar tissues and cannot be immediately visualized after opening the broad ligament, and obviously cannot be palpated. Second, the precise level (in a cephalad-caudad sense) at which to begin dissecting the pararectal space is also not at first obvious, and troublesome bleeding can occur if the dissection is begun over the cardinal ligament rather than proximal to it. Finally, with each successive step of the dissection—that is, division of the round ligament, opening of the broad ligament, and separation of the areolar tissues—the tissues become progressively more slack and difficult to work with.

A technique developed specifically to overcome these difficulties makes use of two strategies. First, the round ligaments are divided late in the course of the dissection, rather than at the beginning of it, which allows them to provide some countertraction on the broad ligament when the uterus is deviated to the contralateral side. Second, the obliterated hypogastric arteries (lateral umbilical ligaments) are used to identify the origin of the uterine arteries, which are then used as landmarks for the pararectal spaces and ureters.

Obliterated hypogastric arteries

The internal iliac artery arises from the bifurcation of the common iliac artery, at about the pelvic brim (and slightly higher on the left side). Although its anatomy is complicated (for the internal iliac artery has many visceral and parietal branches) its surgical anatomy is quite straightforward. The internal iliac arteries (or more properly their anterior divisions) descend steeply into the pelvis along the pelvic sidewalls to where the uterine arteries are given off at the lateral attachments of the cardinal ligaments. They then sweep sharply upward on either side of the bladder as the obliterated hypogastric arteries to cross the superior pubic rami, and run beneath the peritoneum of the anterior abdominal wall to the umbilicus.

The obliterated hypogastric arteries (lateral umbilical ligaments) are easily identified laparoscopically as promi-

nent peritoneal folds that hang laterally on either side of the anterior abdominal wall and are crossed by the distal portion of the round ligaments medial to the internal inguinal ring. They are also relatively fixed structures and are easily dissected free of the bladder and surrounding areolar tissues in the paravesical space. The corollary is that,
• once freed, the obliterated hypogastric arteries can easily be traced retrogradely to identify the uterine arteries, and
• because the uterine artery runs on top of the cardinal ligament at the caudal limit of the pararectal space, it provides an important landmark for the laparoscopic dissection of the pararectal space.

Laparoscopic dissection of the pelvic retroperitoneum

Step 1. The pelvic sidewall triangles are opened

The uterus is deviated to one side to delineate the triangle of the opposite pelvic sidewall. The base of this triangle is formed by the round ligament, the lateral border by the external iliac artery, the medial border by the infundibulopelvic ligament, and the apex by where the infundibulopelvic ligament crosses the common iliac artery (Fig. 39-6). The peritoneum in the middle of the triangle is desiccated with a bipolar current and incised with dissecting scissors, and the broad ligament is opened by bluntly separating the extraperitoneal areolar tissues. Even tiny vessels should be coagulated because the slightest bleeding can stain the extraperitoneal areolar tissues and obscure the view of the underlying structures.

The peritoneal incision is extended first to the round ligament, which is *not* divided at this time, and then to the apex of the triangle, lateral to the infundibulopelvic ligament (Fig. 39-7). It is important not to displace the infundibulopelvic ligament from its anatomic position before

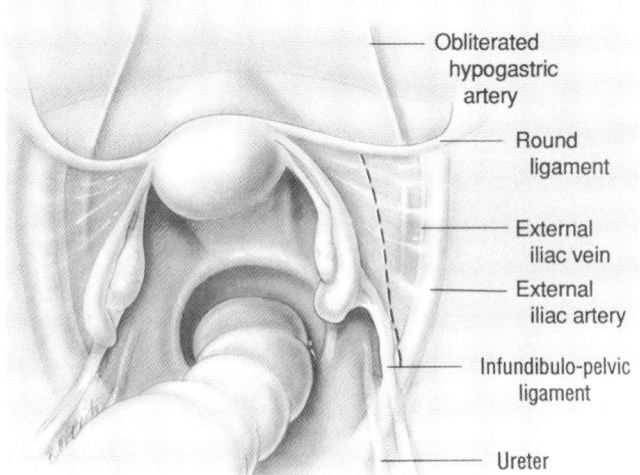

Fig. 39-6 The incision in the pelvic sidewall triangle peritoneum is made along the dashed line.

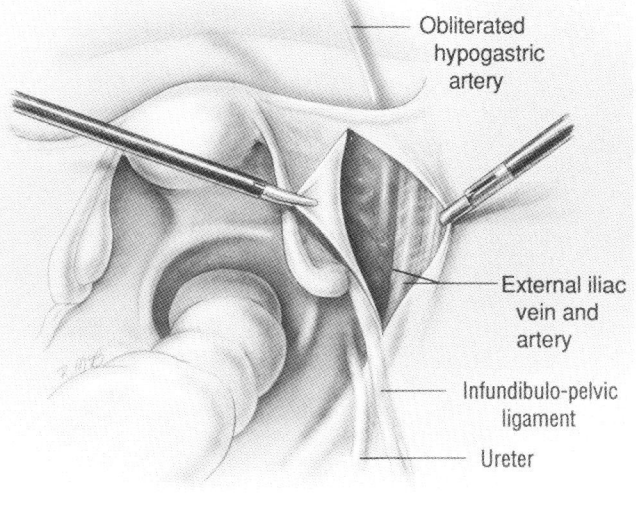

Fig. 39-7 The broad ligament is opened.

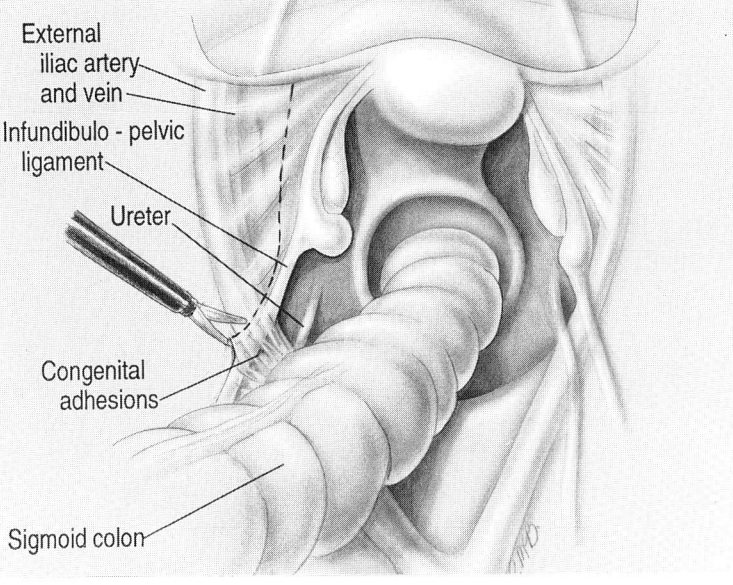

Fig. 39-8 The attachments of the sigmoid colon are divided, and the incision on the left is started at the apex of the pelvic sidewall triangle.

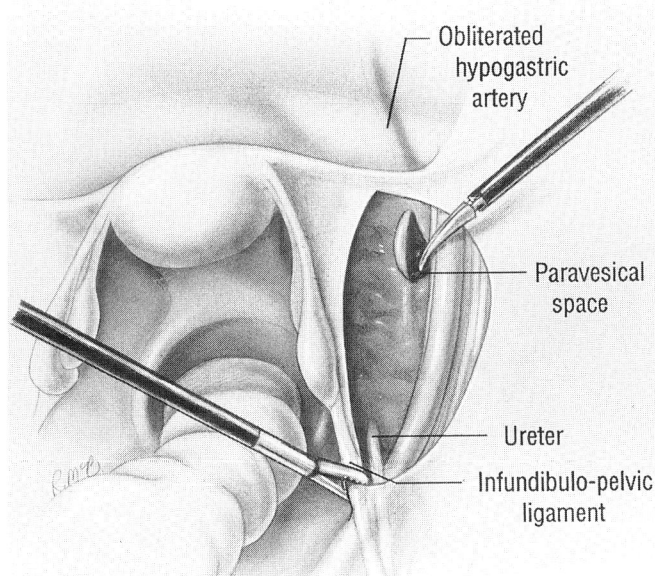

Fig. 39-9 The infundibulopelvic ligament has been pulled medially to expose the ureter at the pelvic brim. The extraperitoneal portion of the obliterated hypogastric artery is identified.

the peritoneal incision is completed; otherwise, the natural anatomic relation between the infundibulopelvic ligament and ureter, which serves to protect the ureter from injury as it lies medial to the infundibulopelvic ligament, is lost.

On the left side, so-called congenital adhesions attach the rectosigmoid to the peritoneum laterally, at or just above the pelvic brim. These usually cover the apex of the pelvic triangle. The dissection on the left side is begun by separating these adhesions from the underlying peritoneum, and the pelvic sidewall triangle is opened at or near its apex (Fig. 39-8). (The external iliac artery will be below the plane of dissection.) The peritoneal incision is then carried distally to the round ligament, which is again not divided at this time.

Step 2. The ureter is identified at the apex of the pelvic triangle

The infundibulopelvic ligament is pulled medially with grasping forceps to expose the ureter at the pelvic brim where it crosses the common or external iliac artery (Fig. 39-9). This is a crucial step, and a good, nontraumatic instrument is invaluable here. It may be necessary to reflect the ureter off the medial leaf of the broad ligament for a short distance to aid in its identification, although this is not always required.

It is important to mobilize the infundibulopelvic ligament adequately; otherwise, it will not be possible to retract its proximal end sufficiently medially to expose the ureter at the pelvic brim. Failure to achieve adequate mobilization of the infundibulopelvic ligament is the most common error in carrying out the dissection. The operator then searches for the ureter distal to the pelvic brim and lateral to the infundibulopelvic ligament, but frequently fails to find it, for the ureter is at that point covered by fatty-areolar tissue or, more distally, by the infundibulopelvic ligament itself, and cannot be seen except in the thinnest pa-

tients. The error stems from the fact that the peritoneal incision has to be extended much further proximally to ensure adequate mobilization of the infundibulopelvic ligament than is required in an open case. The incision frequently has to be extended to where the peritoneum covering the infundibulopelvic ligament blends with the mesentery of the cecum (on the right) or the descending colon (on the left).

The dissection of the apex is more difficult on the left side partly because the ureter is covered by the mesentery of the sigmoid colon, but mainly because it crosses the iliac vessels higher (more proximally), and consequently lies more medial than the right ureter. As a result it is more difficult to expose the left ureter by retracting the infundibulopelvic ligament medially. The peritoneal incision frequently has to be extended to the white line in the paracolic gutter to mobilize the sigmoid colon and, with it, the infundibulopelvic ligament, which at this point lies extraperitoneally, under the mesentery (Fig. 39-10). It is also frequently necessary to mobilize the medial leaf of the broad ligament from the pelvic brim and sacrum. To do this, the operator has to dissect bluntly in a medial direction under the infundibulopelvic ligament, taking care not to perforate the medial leaf of the broad ligament or the right plane of dissection will be lost. Finally, the operator needs to be aware that the external iliac artery will be below the plane of dissection much of the time.

Step 3. The obliterated hypogastric arteries are identified extraperitoneally

The dissection is carried bluntly underneath and caudad to the round ligament, until the obliterated hypogastric artery is identified extraperitoneally (Fig. 39-10). Although the anatomy will be unfamiliar to most general gynecologists, this step is, in fact, the most straightforward part of the dissection. If any difficulty is encountered, the artery should be first identified intraperitoneally where it hangs from the anterior abdominal wall, traced proximally to where it passes behind the round ligament, and then with both its intraperitoneal portion and the dissected space under the round ligament in view, the intraperitoneal part of the ligament should be moved back and forth. It will almost always be possible to detect corresponding movements in the extraperitoneal portion of the ligament.

Step 4. The paravesical spaces are developed

Once the obliterated hypogastric arteries have been identified extraperitoneally, it is simple to develop the paravesical space by bluntly separating the areolar tissue on either side of the artery. The dissection is started lateral to the artery, mindful that the external iliac vein is just lateral to it. The tips of the closed dissecting scissors are placed against the lateral edge of the artery, and the artery is simply pulled medially, whereupon a bloodless plane will open lateral to it (Fig. 39-11). The medial border of the artery is then freed in an identical manner, but working in the opposite direction. During this maneuver the operator must take care not to press on the external iliac vein as the artery is displaced laterally (Fig. 39-12).

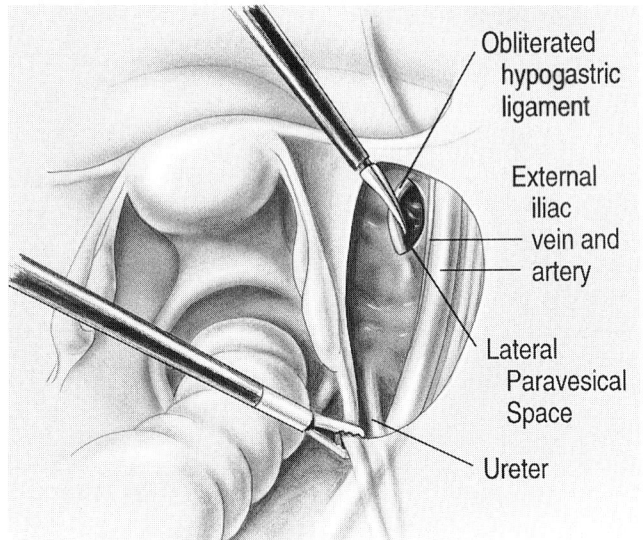

Fig. 39-11 The lateral paravesical space is opened.

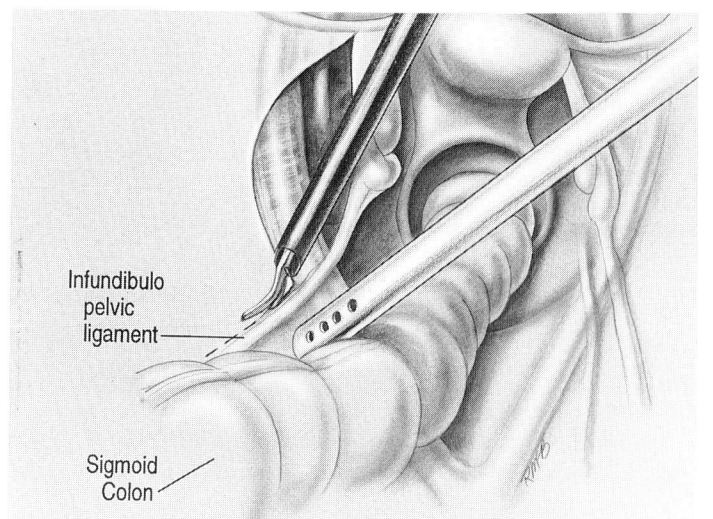

Fig. 39-10 Mobilization of the left infundibulopelvic ligament.

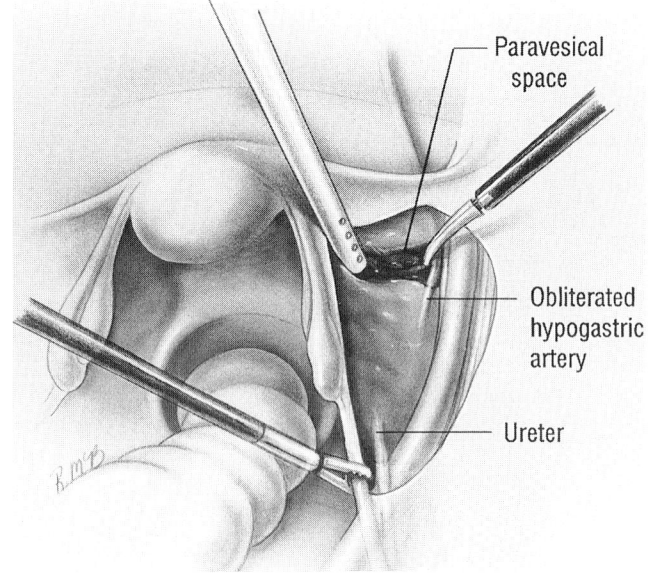

Fig. 39-12 The medial paravesical space is opened.

The purpose of the dissection is to free the obliterated hypogastric artery completely from the surrounding areolar tissues, so that it can be clearly traced proximally. However, it is advantageous to develop the paravesical spaces widely even for a simple hysterectomy; it literally takes only a minute or so, and the uterine arteries and cardinal ligaments will be much better exposed. This is especially helpful if the artery bleeds when it is divided (which can occur despite what appears to be adequate bipolar desiccation) because the bleeding points will be easy to visualize and coagulate.

Step 5. The pararectal spaces are developed

The obliterated hypogastric arteries are next traced proximally to where they are joined by the uterine arteries, and the pararectal spaces are opened by blunt dissection proximal and medial to the uterine vessels, which lie on top of the cardinal ligaments. Once the pararectal spaces have been opened, the ureter on the ipsilateral side is easily identified on the medial leaf of the broad ligament, which forms the medial border of the pararectal space. The uterine artery and cardinal ligament at the distal (caudal) border of the space and the internal iliac artery on its lateral border also become clearly visible at this stage (Fig. 39-13). Starting proximal to the cardinal ligaments, the ureters are then dissected off the medial leaf of the broad ligament for a short distance in preparation for division of the uterosacral ligaments.

Simple hysterectomy

The retroperitoneal dissection will have prepared the stage for a simple hysterectomy, and very little remains to be done. The hysterectomy is completed in three steps (steps 6, 7, and 8).

Step 6. The uterine arteries, round ligaments, and infundibulopelvic ligaments are divided

The uterine arteries are freed from any areolar tissue still covering them and desiccated with bipolar forceps or clipped with the Laprochip (Davis & Geck). The round ligaments and infundibulopelvic ligaments are also desiccated before the arteries are divided to save repeatedly taking the bipolar forceps in and out of the peritoneal cavity. The smoke generated must be continuously suctioned during desiccation. All these structures are then divided starting with the uterine artery (Fig. 39-14). After the round ligament is divided, the incision is continued along the anterior leaf of the broad ligament and the bladder peritoneum to the contralateral side, but the bladder is not dissected off the vagina. After the infundibulopelvic ligament has been divided, the incision is continued along the medial leaf of the broad ligament to where the ureters have been reflected laterally.

Step 7. The uterosacral ligaments are divided, and the posterior vaginal wall is opened

A plane is developed between the peritoneum and the uterosacral ligaments. The peritoneum is incised, and the incision is extended to the pouch of Douglas, which is opened. The incision is continued across the midline to meet a similar incision in the peritoneum of the opposite broad ligament. The ureters are retracted laterally, and the

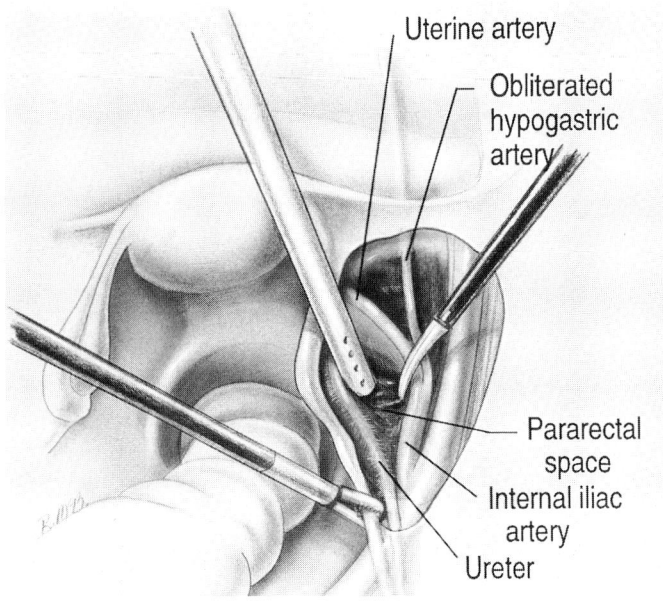

Fig. 39-13 The pararectal space is developed.

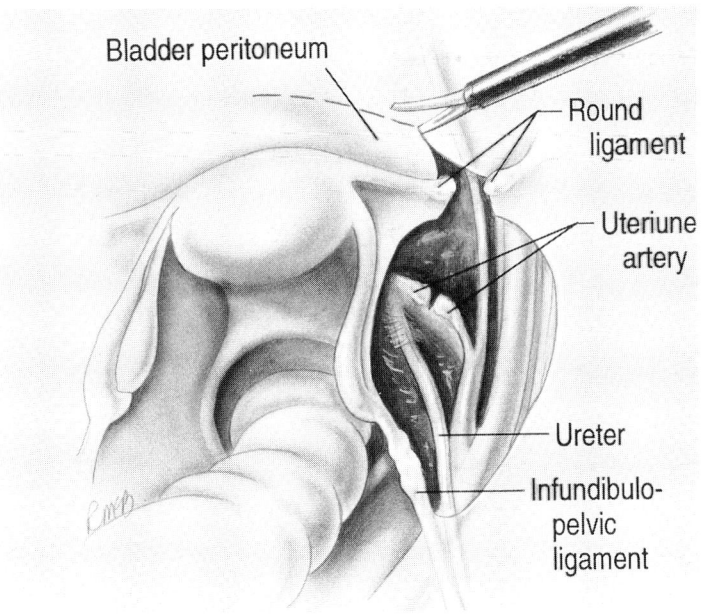

Fig. 39-14 The uterine artery and round ligament have been divided, and the incision is being extended along the anterior broad ligament and bladder peritoneum.

uterosacral ligaments are divided with the closed tips of the dissecting scissors using a monopolar current (Fig. 39-15).

If a Pelosi mobilizer (Nova Endoscopic, Palm, Pa.) is available, the posterior vaginal wall is opened at this time; otherwise, the operation is continued vaginally. To open the posterior vaginal wall laparoscopically, the uterus is sharply anteflexed with the mobilizer to an almost vertical position, whereupon a bulge resembling the cervix will appear at its lower end, which is in fact the hub of the instrument against the posterior vaginal wall. The posterior vaginal wall is then incised against this bulge with the tips of the dissecting scissors closed, using a monopolar current (Fig. 39-16). The incision should not be too close to the cervical attachment of the vagina; otherwise, the incision will be too proximal to facilitate the vaginal part of the procedure.

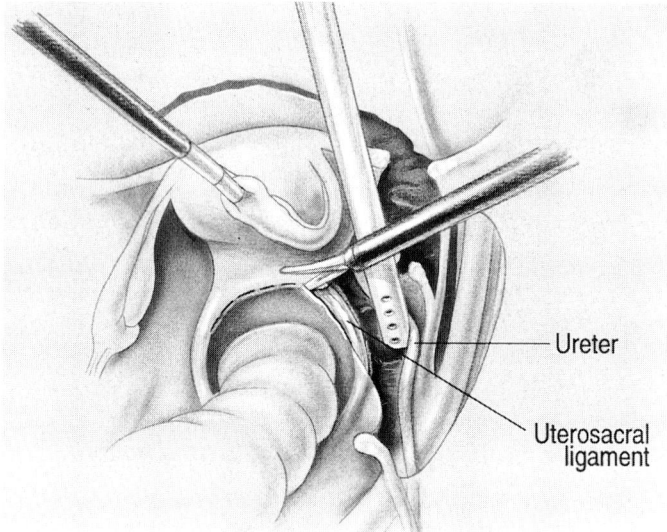

Fig. 39-15 The infundibulopelvic ligament has been divided, and the incision extended along the broad ligament to the uterosacral ligament. The peritoneum is separated from the uterosacral ligament, and the peritoneal incision is continued along the cul-de-sac.

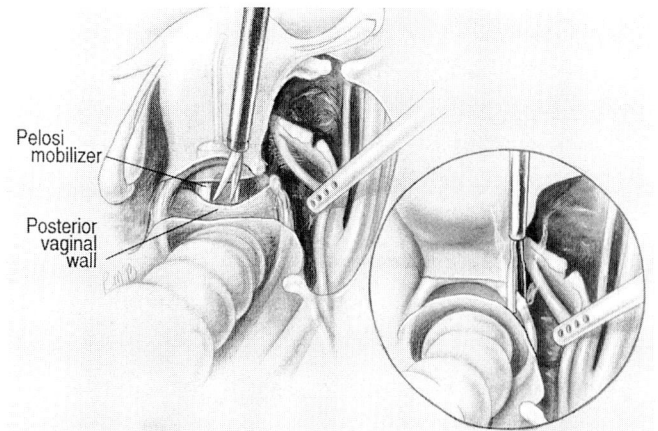

Fig. 39-16 The ureter is retracted laterally as the uterosacral ligament is desiccated and divided. The posterior vaginal wall is opened against the hub of the Pelosi mobilizer.

Step 8. The hysterectomy is completed vaginally

The cervix is grasped with two single-toothed tenacula and is elevated to expose the incision in the posterior vaginal wall. The incision is then continued across the front of the cervix with a scalpel, the bladder is dissected sharply off the cervix, and the anterior cul-de-sac is entered. A Zeppelin clamp is placed on each cardinal ligament, and the ligaments are divided and sutured. The vagina is closed horizontally with a running nonlocking stitch. The pneumoperitoneum is reestablished, and the pelvis is irrigated copiously and checked for hemostasis.

Comment

Once the retroperitoneal dissection has been completed, one must decide which structures, besides the uterine arteries, round ligaments, and infundibulopelvic ligaments (step 6), to divide laparoscopically. Before settling on the uterosacral ligaments and the posterior vaginal wall (step 7), I tried completing the entire hysterectomy laparoscopically, as well as opening the anterior vaginal wall after dissecting the bladder off the cervix and vagina. The following conclusions were reached.

First, it is both tedious and unnecessary to divide the cardinal ligaments laparoscopically. After the uterosacral ligaments have been divided (step 7), the hysterectomy can always be completed vaginally, even in morbidly obese nulligravidas, and completed more easily and quickly than laparoscopically. Rarely, if ever, will situations arise in which laparoscopic completion of the hysterectomy would be preferable.

Second, the vaginal part of the operation is not facilitated very much by opening the anterior vaginal wall laparoscopically. If the vagina is opened from below, the vaginal incision is made distal to the bladder, and the bladder is dissected cephalad. If the vagina is opened laparoscopically, however, the bladder is first dissected in a caudal direction, and the incision is made proximal to the bladder. When the vaginal cuff is then closed from below, the sutures will be placed proximal to the bladder and distal ureter, which can be injured in the process (13).

Third, the posterior vaginal wall used to be rather tedious to open, and the effort did not seem worthwhile. However, this has been rendered so straightforward with the use of the Pelosi mobilizer that I now routinely open the posterior vaginal wall laparoscopically in simple hysterectomies. Laparoscopic incision of the posterior vaginal wall does not have the disadvantages of the anterior incision and does make the vaginal part of the operation much easier, provided the incision is not made too close to the cervix.

Laparoscopic pelvic lymphadenectomy

Once the pelvic spaces have been developed, laparoscopic pelvic lymphadenectomy poses no special problems. Exactly the same approach can be used as with an open technique, but the surgeon will obtain a far better view of the obturator fossa. Sharp scissor dissection is used with the Endo Shears substituting for the Metzenbaum scissors and the Endo Dissect for dissecting forceps.

The first step is to delineate the surgical limits of the dissection which are: the *common iliac artery* proximally (i.e., cephalad), the *psoas muscle* laterally, the *circumflex iliac vein* and pubic bone distally (i.e., caudad), the *obliterated umbilical artery* medially, and the *obturator fossa* inferiorly (i.e., ventrally). During the preceding retroperitoneal dissection, the proximal, distal, medial, and inferior limits of the dissection have already been delineated. All that remains is to separate the external iliac vessels from the psoas muscle.

This is easily done by scoring the dense areolar tissue that attaches the external iliac artery to the psoas muscle very superficially with scissors from the common iliac artery all the way down to the circumflex iliac vein, a branch of the external iliac vein that courses outward and laterally across the lower portion of the external iliac artery. The incision must be very superficial to avoid injury to the external iliac vein, which lies just below the artery. Using blunt dissection with the back of the dissecting scissors or dissecting forceps, the external iliac artery and then the external iliac vein lying under it are successively peeled off the psoas muscle. Once the vein is freed, progressively deeper dissection will gain entry into the obturator fossa, which is identified by the bright yellow fatty-nodal tissue that will come into view. By continuing the plane of dissection lateral to this tissue, the nodal bundle of the obturator fossa will be mobilized medially. There are no branches lateral to the external iliac artery or vein, but very occasionally nutrient muscular branches may be encountered, which can be safely coagulated or clipped.

The lymphadenectomy proper begins after the external iliac vessels and contents of the obturator fossa have been mobilized medially. The first step is to remove the fatty-nodal tissue lying lateral to and in front of the common iliac artery, although sometimes the amount of tissue at this site is very scanty. The nodal tissue is freed by dividing the loose areolar tissue that anchors it to the psoas muscle and common iliac artery, using sharp scissor dissection. The only phase of this dissection requiring special attention is when the uppermost part of the nodal mass is being freed, because an artery is always encountered here deep on the lateral aspect of the common iliac artery. This vessel has to be either cauterized or clipped.

The external iliac artery and vein are next freed from their areolar investments. Each vessel is completely surrounded by its own distinct areolar sheath, and the two sheaths are fused along the entire course of the vessels. The sheath of the external iliac artery is incised with scissors along its dorsal surface from the level of the common iliac artery all the way down to the circumflex iliac vein. There are never any branches of the external iliac artery in this region, but there is usually a hairlike vessel that crosses the artery obliquely at its midportion superficial to its sheath,

and it usually needs to be coagulated. After opening the sheath, its medial border is grasped with dissecting forceps, and the artery is peeled off the inferior surface of the sheath using mostly blunt dissection with the back of the Endo Shears, but cutting areolar attachments as needed. The same process is repeated on the lateral surface of the artery, and this will free it completely from the underlying vein.

At this point, the sheaths of the external iliac artery and vein are still joined along the undersurface of the artery, and the next step is cautiously to incise the sheath of the external iliac vein. This step requires the greatest care in the entire dissection, as the edge of the vessel can easily be compressed and merge imperceptibly with the areolar sheath that covers it. However, once a nick has been made in the sheath, the glistening surface of the vein becomes unmistakably clear and distinct from its areolar covering. The same technique of sharp and blunt dissection can then be used to free the vein circumferentially from its sheath as is used to free the artery. The final step in this part of the dissection is to free the inferior border of the vein, which is tethered by loose areolar tissue to the pelvic sidewall and obturator fossa. This is done not so much because there are any noticeable nodes attached to the sheath, but rather to gain free access to the obturator fossa. Occasionally, an aberrant obturator vein is encountered at this point coursing upward from the obturator fossa to join the external iliac vein on its inferior aspect, rather than the internal iliac vein as is usually the case. An aberrant obturator vein has to be clipped using the Endo Clip and divided to mobilize the external iliac vein completely.

The external iliac nodes are distributed along the course of the external iliac artery in a cephalad-caudad or "north-south" direction, and are attached laterally to the psoas muscle and medially to the sheath of the external iliac artery by loose areolar tissue. Distally, at the level of the circumflex iliac vein, there are prominent nodes lying in a lateral-medial or "east-west" direction across the lower part of the external iliac artery. The lateral-most part of this nodal bundle is about 2 to 3 cm from the artery itself, and there is usually a nutrient branch that has to be coagulated as these nodes are freed from the inferolateral part of the psoas muscle. The medial attachments of these nodes are freed when the external iliac vessels are dissected from their sheaths; all that remains, then, is to free their lateral attachments to the psoas muscle. As this is done, the ileofemoral and genitofemoral nerves are encountered, but can easily be pushed laterally. The nodal tissue and the areolar sheaths of the external iliac vessels to which they are attached can be removed at this point and sent as a separate specimen, or allowed to fall away from the vessels into the obturator fossa and removed later, en block with the remainder of the pelvic nodal tissue.

Finally, the obturator fossa and internal iliac vessels are freed. This is best done by retracting the external iliac vessels laterally, and teasing out the obturator nerve from the inferior-most part of the obturator nodal bundle using the unopened Endo Shears. Once the nerve is freed, the distal attachments of the nodal bundle can be freed from the pubic bone by dividing them with a cutting current to seal the lymphatics. The nodal bundle is then grasped with the grasping forceps, elevated, and placed on tension, and then teased off its ventral-most attachments below the obturator nerve using a gentle sweeping motion with the partly opened scissors. As this nodal tissue is freed in a cephalic direction, residual attachments to the external iliac vein usually need to be freed. Eventually, the internal iliac artery is reached, and the nodal tissue lying anterior, lateral, and medial to it is freed in continuity with the obturator fossa nodal mass. The nodal tissue can be quite adherent in this region because the internal iliac artery does not have an areolar sheath, as do the external iliac vessels. With further dissection in a cephalad direction, the crura or bifurcation of the iliac arteries is reached, and this region must be cleaned with care, ever mindful of the fact that the external and internal iliac veins lie just lateral to these structures. Once the attachments of the nodal bundle in this region are divided, the dissection is complete.

It is essential to use spoon forceps to remove the fatty-nodal tissue, because they will compress tissue into the hollow of their jaws, enabling large chunks of nodal tissue to be removed without fragmenting it. I have used a surgical glove and an "Endobag" in the abdomen to store nodes before their extraction but have not found this to offer any advantages.

Laparoscopic aortic lymphadenectomy

The patient is positioned in a Trendelenburg position and rotated slightly to her left. After the abdomen and pelvis are inspected, washings are taken, the sigmoid colon is retracted laterally, the small bowel is displaced from the pelvis, and the root of the mesentery is elevated. The posterior parietal peritoneum is opened in one of several ways: over the right common iliac artery, medial to the right ureter; parallel to the small bowel mesentery; vertically downward in the midline from the root of the mesentery, or in the reverse direction, starting above the sacral promontory, medial to the sigmoid mesentery. The peritoneum is desiccated with bipolar forceps and incised with scissors, and using mostly blunt dissection, a plane is developed between the peritoneum and the node-bearing fatty areolar tissue overlying the great vessels. It is important to develop this plane properly and widely before carrying the dissection down to the adventitia of the aorta; otherwise, the nodal tissue may be elevated with the bowel mesentery and retroperitoneal fat during retraction, and the tissue will not be removed.

The node-bearing areolar tissue in front of the aorta is then incised, and the incision is carried down to the adventitia of the aorta. This is not always easy because the great vessels are covered by node-bearing tissue and cannot be

seen at this stage except in thin patients without retroperitoneal pathology. There are also no certain landmarks other than the root of the mesentery, which is, however, elevated to retract the bowel, and is not in its normal position. It is usually possible to "feel" the sacrum with a dissecting probe, which is a useful guide to the midline, but the point at which to start the dissection in the superior-inferior plane is not always obvious because the level of the aortic bifurcation above the sacrum is very variable. Often the pulsations of the aorta can be "felt" if it is gently pressed with a probe, but much less clearly than one might imagine. It is much safer to start higher rather than lower (which is the natural tendency) because there are no important structures in front of the aorta below the root of the mesentery, except for the inferior mesenteric artery, which, however, usually lies lateral to the aorta at this point. On the other hand, if the dissection is started too low, there is a danger of injuring the left common iliac vein below the bifurcation of the aorta. Once the plane between the aorta and the overlying nodal tissue has been developed, however, and the glistening surface of the aorta is seen, the dissection is very straightforward, provided one is cautious and knows the anatomy. The only real challenge is to keep the bowel out of the way.

The limits of the dissection are the bifurcation of the aorta inferiorly and the proximal part of the common iliac artery inferolaterally. On the right the dissection is continued across the front of the vena cava until its lateral border is freed. On the left, the plane of dissection is underneath the inferior mesenteric artery distally, and then above the artery more proximally. Although the feasibility of the left-sided dissection has been questioned by some oncologists, it is in fact safer, and no more difficult than the right side, provided the inferior mesenteric artery is dissected free. The superior limit of the dissection is the third part of the duodenum. It is a simple matter to mobilize the duodenum and expose the left renal vein, but this is necessary in cervix cancer only if obvious lymph nodes are present in this area.

Laparoscopic radical vaginal hysterectomy (modified Schauta-Amreich operation)

Radical vaginal operations for cervix cancer offered several advantages over their abdominal counterparts but fell into disuse because they did not allow removal of the pelvic lymph nodes (14). Mitra (15) tried to correct this deficiency by combining the Schauta-Amreich procedure with bilateral extraperitoneal pelvic lymphadenectomy, but his operation never gained popularity because the reduction in morbidity from the vaginal approach was largely lost.

Laparoscopic lymphadenectomy has been developed independently by a number of gynecologic oncologists, and shown to be both feasible and safe (3,16,17). It has been used with frozen section to select patients with stage IB cervix cancer for radical abdominal hysterectomy (those without nodal metastases) or radiation therapy (those with nodal metastases) (16,17). It seemed much more logical to me to try to combine the procedure with a radical vaginal operation, and complete therapy in most patients without the use of pelvic radiation or laparotomy (5).

My original plan was to perform a laparoscopic lymphadenectomy and combine it with laparoscopic division of the proximal attachments of the uterus, the uterine arteries, and the upper portions of the cardinal and uterosacral ligaments, to free the ureter from the broad ligament, and to complete the operation as a Schauta-Amreich procedure but, I hoped, without the need for a Schuchardt incision. This approach was used in the first two cases, but several difficulties were encountered with both the laparoscopic and vaginal parts of the procedure. These were resolved by the development of my technique for retroperitoneal dissection described above, by the use of a more logical partitioning of the operation into laparoscopic and vaginal components, and finally by retracting the ureters out of the pelvis laparoscopically (step 8) throughout the vaginal part of the operation. Only the mature technique will be described.

Laparoscopic phase of the operation

Step 1. The cul-de-sac peritoneum is incised

The pouch of Douglas is incised with dissecting scissors, and the incision is extended proximally on either side of the rectum, below the uterosacral ligaments. It is much more difficult to carry out this step if it is left to last because the tissues become too slack. A rectal probe developed by Reich is used to displace the rectum to the contralateral side (Fig. 39-17). The ureters may or may not be seen on the medial leaf of the broad ligament, but because they always lie above and lateral to the plane of dissection, they are not at risk, and no effort should be expended in trying to identify them at this stage.

Steps 2–7

These steps are almost identical to the steps previously described under dissection of the retroperitoneum and simple hysterectomy, with three exceptions. First, the paravesical and pararectal spaces are developed all the way to the levators. Second, the ureters are reflected off the medial leaf of the broad ligament as far as the pelvic brim. Third, the uterosacral ligaments are not divided, and the vagina is, of course, not opened. Also, the uterine arteries are divided more proximally, where they join the hypogastric arteries, and the distal stumps are dissected free of the underlying tissues and ureter (but the ureteric tunnel is not dissected laparoscopically). Laparoscopic pelvic lymphadenectomy is then carried out as previously described.

To summarize:
Step 2 The pelvic sidewall triangle is opened.

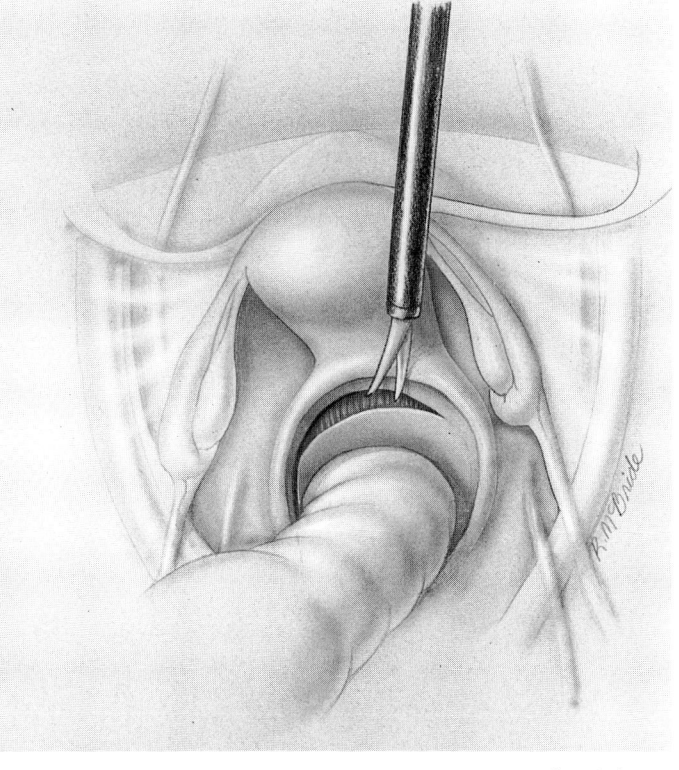

Fig. 39-17 The posterior cul-de-sac peritoneum is incised, and the incision is extended on either side of the rectum, below the uterosacral ligaments.

Step 3 The paravesical and pararectal spaces are developed.
Step 4 The uterine artery and its ureteric branch are coagulated and divided.
Step 5 The ureter is reflected off the broad ligament.
Step 6 The round ligament and adnexal pedicles are coagulated and divided, and the bladder peritoneum is incised.
Step 7 Bilateral pelvic lymphadenectomy is performed.

Step 8. The ureters are retracted out of the pelvis

Before proceeding to the vaginal part of the operation, one end of a vascular tape is inserted through each lateral trocar, passed around the ureters, and withdrawn through the trocars. The trocars are then withdrawn, and the tapes are used to retract the ureters out of the pelvis throughout the vaginal phase of the operation (Fig. 39-18).

Vaginal phase of the operation

Step 9. Formation of the vaginal cuff, division of the supravaginal septum

The vagina is grasped with four Kocher clamps at approximately the 10, 2, 4, and 8 o'clock positions, at the level at which the vagina is to be transected (usually midvagina, or junction of the middle and upper thirds). If the vagina is re-

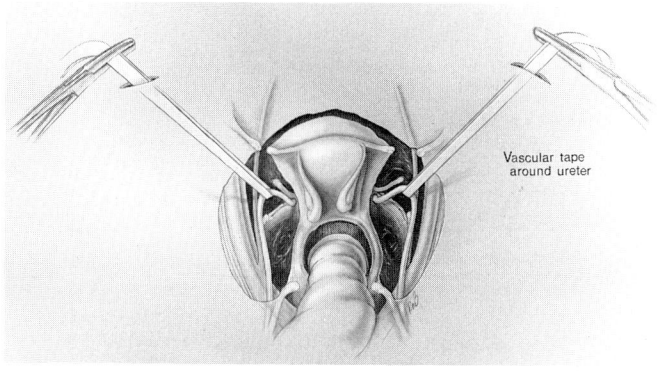

Fig. 39-18 Vascular tapes are passed around the ureters, and they are retracted out of the pelvis laparoscopically.

dundant, more Kocher clamps may need to be used to ensure that it is stretched out flat and there are no ridges in its wall when it is incised. After infiltrating with phenylephrine solution (10 mg in 250 ml saline) just under the vaginal fascia, the vagina is incised circumferentially with cutting diathermy (Figs. 39-19A and 39-19B). The vesicovaginal and rectovaginal spaces are then developed with sharp scissor dissection, and the posterior cul-de-sac is entered. T-clamps are placed on the distal cut edge of the vagina for traction (usually three or four) and a long weighted Auvard speculum is placed in the cul-de-sac.

The anterior dissection proceeds fairly effortlessly until an impasse is reached at the level of the supravaginal septum, which separates the vesicovaginal from the vesicocervical space. This tissue is placed on tension by appropriate traction on the T-clamps and retraction anteriorly. The bladder is pulled up with forceps, and the supravaginal septum is incised. The incision is made approximately 1 cm above the vaginal attachments of the septum, which can usually be discerned. The bladder becomes immediately visible and can be freed further with sharp scissor and then blunt finger dissection to gain entrance into the anterior cul-de-sac (Figs. 39-19C and 39-19D).

Step 10. The paravesical and pararectal spaces are entered, and the vesicocervical ligaments ("bladder pillars") are formed

The cut edge of the distal vagina is pulled laterally (i.e., everted) and rendered taut, and the tissue just under the vaginal fascia is incised with scissors to gain entrance into the paravesical space (Fig. 39-20A). Since the paravesical space has already been opened laparoscopically, this is a surprisingly easy maneuver. Nevertheless, the position of the pubococcygeus muscle should be checked before making the incision to ensure that the dissection is not too lateral; otherwise, some of the muscle fibers can be pulled medially, making the bladder pillars thick and the ureters more difficult to feel. If there is any uncertainty, the pneumoperitoneum can be reestablished and a probe passed laparoscopically into the paravesical space medial to the obliterated hypogastric artery. It will be readily felt vaginally, and the paravesical space can be opened without any further difficulty. The vaginal incision is then enlarged bluntly with the index fingers and extended posteriorly (Fig. 39-20B). The rectum is retracted medially, and the pararectal space is entered. Usually dense bands of connective tissue separate the paravesical and pararectal spaces (the horizontal fascia), and these need to be divided to unite them (Fig. 39-20C). Once the paravesical and pararectal spaces have been united, the entire hand can be placed into the peritoneal cavity, lateral to the uterus and cervix (Fig. 39-20D). The paravesical and pararectal spaces on the contralateral side are then developed in an identical fashion.

Step 11. Division of the uterosacral ligaments (rectal pillars)

Starting on the left side, the uterosacral ligament is placed on tension by pulling the T-clamps upward and to the right. The rectum is retracted medially, and any remaining peri-

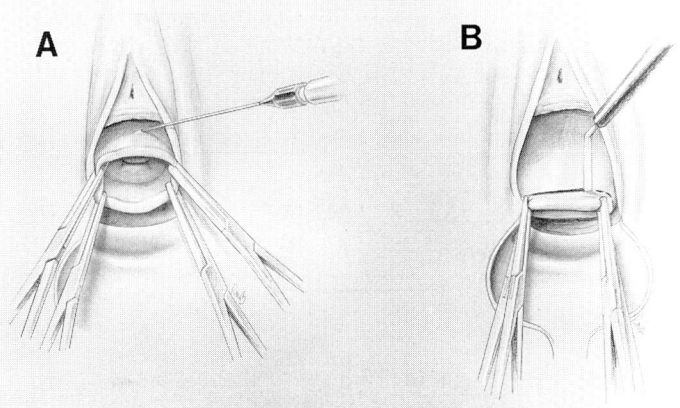

Fig. 39-19 (A) The position of the cuff is demarcated with Kocher clamps, and the vaginal wall is infiltrated with phenylephrine solution. (B) The vaginal wall is incised circumferentially with diathermy, using a cutting monopolar current. (C) The vesicovaginal and recto-

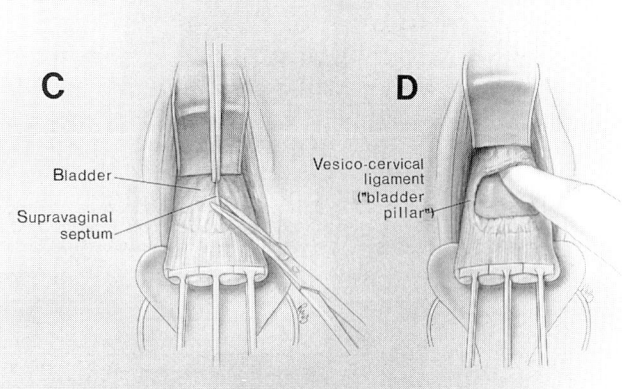

vaginal spaces have been developed, the posterior cul-de-sac entered, T-clamps placed on the vaginal cuff, and the supravaginal septum is being incised. (D) The vesicocervical space is developed with sharp scissor and blunt finger dissection.

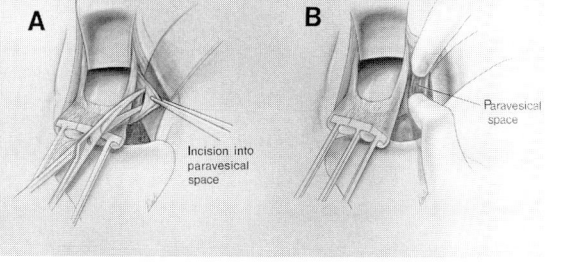
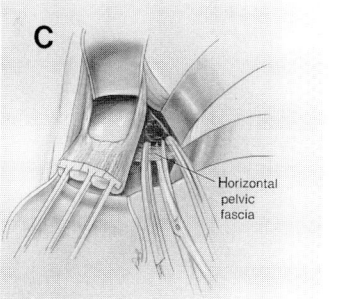

Fig. 39-20 (A) The lateral vaginal wall is incised to enter the paravesical space. (B) The vaginal incision is enlarged. (C) The horizontal pelvic fascia is divided.

toneal attachments not freed laparoscopically are divided at this time. The position of the ureter is verified by palpation, and the uterosacral ligament is clamped close to the rectum with Zeppelin clamps, divided, and suture ligated (Fig. 39-21). The right uterosacral ligament is divided in an identical manner.

The uterus is usually rendered mobile by division of the rectal pillars, and the operation can proceed with either unroofing of the distal ureters or division of the cardinal ligaments, which is the sequence that will be described. Although steps 12 and 13 are largely interchangeable, if access is still suboptimal after the uterosacral ligaments have been divided, it is better to divide the cardinal ligaments first (step 13), but then it will not be possible to deliver the fundus through the anterior vagina. If lateral access is limited, the clamps on the cardinal ligaments can be left in place until the ureters are unroofed and the specimen removed before suturing the pedicles.

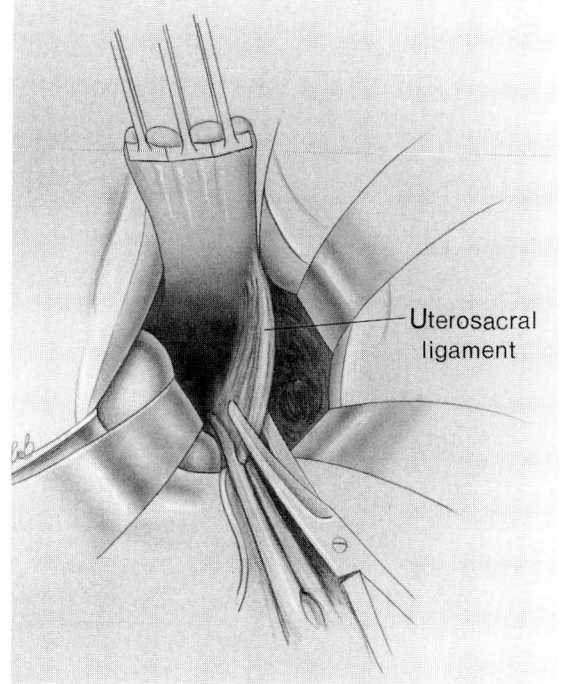

Fig. 39-21 The left uterosacral ligament is being divided.

Step 12. The ureters are freed ("unroofed") from the vesicocervical ligaments

The left bladder pillar or vesicocervical ligament is placed on tension by pulling downward and to the right on the T-clamps, and by using suitable retraction in the vesicocervical and paravesical spaces. The ureter can be easily palpated between the middle and forefingers in the upper part of the ligament distally, and lower down in the ligament more proximally. The relation between the ureter and the uterine artery is different in the vaginal and abdominal approaches because in the vaginal approach the uterus is pulled downward, rather than upward, and the bladder pushed upward rather than downward. A ureteric loop or "knee" is thereby artificially created through which the uterine artery runs obliquely upward from the cervix to the hypogastric artery (Figs. 39-22A and 39-22B). The ureteric tunnel is entered by gradually snipping away the bladder pillar below the bend in the ureter, and once entered, it is enlarged with finger dissection. The lateral wall of the tunnel is clamped with a fine tonsil clamp, divided, and suture ligated (Figs. 39-22C and 39-22D). The medial wall is divided without ligation, but the uterine artery is cauterized medial to the ureteric loop to avoid backbleeding. The right ureter, which tends to be higher, is freed in the same way.

Step 13. Division of the cardinal ligaments

The fundus is delivered through the anterior vagina, and, starting on the left side, the index and middle fingers are placed on either side of the cardinal ligament from above if possible, the uterus and cervix are pulled medially, the bladder and rectum are retracted out of the way, the position of the ureter is checked again, and the ligament is clamped at the pelvic sidewall (or closer to the uterus with smaller lesions), divided, and suture ligated (Fig. 39-23). The right ligament is divided in the same way, and the specimen is removed.

Step 14. The cuff is closed, and the pelvis is inspected laparoscopically

The vagina is closed horizontally with a running, nonlocking chromic suture around a suction drain (hysterovac), which is removed the next day. The pneumoperitoneum is

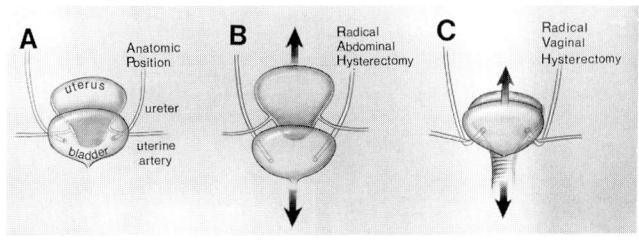

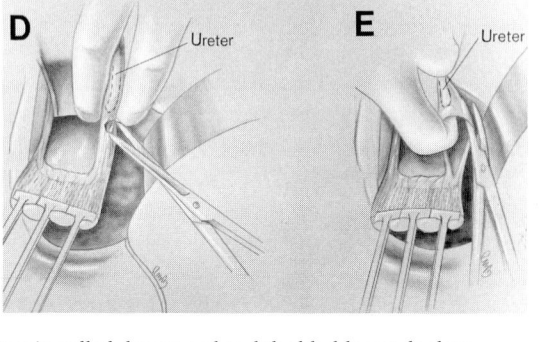

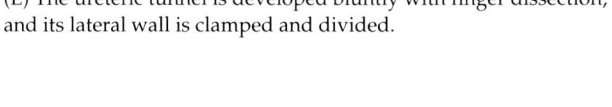

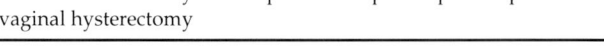

Fig. 39-22 (A) The relation between the ureter and uterine artery: the anatomic position. (B) The relation between the ureter and uterine artery in an abdominal radical hysterectomy after the uterus is pulled upward and the bladder pushed downward. (C) The relation between the ureter and uterine artery in a radical vaginal hysterectomy

after the uterus is pulled downward and the bladder pushed upward. (D) The bladder pillar is held between the index and middle fingers just below the ureters and divided in a series of small snips. (E) The ureteric tunnel is developed bluntly with finger dissection, and its lateral wall is clamped and divided.

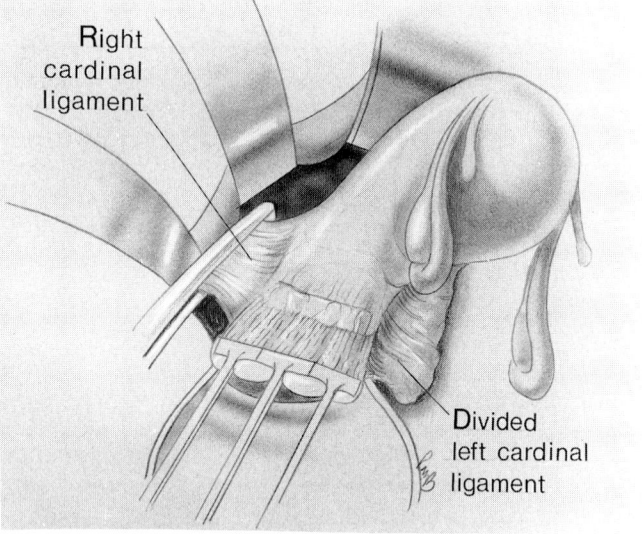

Fig. 39-23 The fundus has been delivered through the anterior vagina, and the left cardinal ligament is being divided.

reestablished, and the pelvis is irrigated copiously and checked for hemostasis. The operative steps are summarized in Table 39-1.

Comment

The rationale for a combined laparoscopic and vaginal approach to radical hysterectomy is compelling. Radical vaginal hysterectomy is an effective but less morbid operation than its abdominal counterpart, and laparoscopic lymphadenectomy complements the operation by correcting its only deficiency vis-à-vis the abdominal operation, the inability to remove the pelvic lymph nodes.

The laparoscopic component contributes much more to the procedure than the lymphadenectomy, for it allows a natural and symbiotic partitioning of the operation into abdominal and vaginal phases. Only those steps of the

Table 39-1 Summary of the operative steps in laparoscopic radical vaginal hysterectomy

Laparoscopic phase

Step 1. The cul-de-sac peritoneum is incised, and the peritoneal incision is carried proximally along each lateral border of the rectum, below the uterosacral ligaments.

Step 2. The pelvic sidewall triangle is opened.

Step 3. The paravesical and pararectal spaces are developed.

Step 4. The uterine artery and its ureteric branch are coagulated and divided.

Step 5. The ureter is reflected off the broad ligament.

Step 6. The round ligament and adnexal pedicles are coagulated and divided, and the bladder peritoneum is incised.

Step 7. Lymphadenectomy is then performed.

Step 8. Each ureter is tagged with vascular tape, and the tape is pulled out through the inferior ports.

Vaginal phase

Step 9. The vaginal cuff is formed, rectovaginal and vesicovaginal spaces are developed, and the supravaginal septum divided.

Step 10. The paravesical and pararectal spaces are developed, the vesicocervical ligament (bladder pillars) is formed, the horizontal pelvic fascia is divided, and the spaces are united.

Step 11. The uterosacral ligaments are divided.

*Step 12. The ureters are unroofed, and the vesicouterine ligament is divided.

*Step 13. The cardinal ligaments are divided, and the specimen is removed.

Step 14. The vagina is closed with a running suture around a suction drain (hysterovac), the pelvis is inspected and irrigated laparoscopically, and trocars are removed.

*Steps 12 and 13 are usually interchangeable.

hysterectomy that are easier to perform vaginally than abdominally are carried out from below—formation of the cuff, division of the cervical ligaments, freeing of the distal ureters—and their execution is greatly facilitated by the preceding abdominal phase of the operation. Strategies that involve either performing the entire hysterectomy laparoscopically (18,19), or following the laparoscopic lymphadenectomy with a radical vaginal hysterectomy (16,20) do not make best use of either the laparoscopic or the vaginal part of the operation, nor do they exploit the potentially symbiotic relationship between them. This is also true of my initial plan to divide the cervical ligaments partly laparoscopically, a tactic that proved to be of no benefit whatsoever (5).

Vaginal entry into the paravesical and pararectal spaces, which can be problematic even for experienced surgeons, is very straightforward after these spaces have been developed laparoscopically. Laparoscopic division of uterine vessels makes it easier to unroof the ureters vaginally because it eliminates the need to ligate the vessels repeatedly, at successively more proximal points, as in the Schauta operation. Finally, the radical hysterectomy is also facilitated by laparoscopic division of the proximal attachments of the uterus, and by freeing the ureters from the broad ligaments. Only distal structures then have to be approached vaginally, and lateral exposure sufficient to divide the cervical ligaments can usually be obtained without a Schuchardt incision. The ureters can be retracted away from the operative field laparoscopically throughout the vaginal part of the operation (step 8), making it possible to divide the uterosacral and cardinal ligaments before the distal ureters are freed. This also makes it easier to unroof the ureters and further reduces the need for a Schuchardt incision.

References

1 Reich H, DeCaprio J, McGlynn F. Laparoscopic hysterectomy. J Gynecol Surg 1989;5:213.
2 Kadar N. A laparoscopic technique for dissecting the pelvic retroperitoneum and identifying the ureters. J Reprod Med (in press).
3 Kadar N. Laparoscopic pelvic lymphadenectomy for the treatment of gynecological malignancies: description of a technique. Gynecol Endosc 1992;1:79–83.
4 Kadar N. Laparoscopic resection of fixed and enlarged aortic lymph nodes in patients with advanced cervix cancer. Gynecol Endosc 1993;2:217–221.
5 Kadar N, Reich H. Laparoscopically assisted radical Schauta hysterectomy and bilateral pelvic lymphadenectomy for the treatment of bulky stage IB carcinoma of the cervix. Gynecol Endosc 1993;2:135–142.
6 Kadar N. An operative technique for laparoscopic hysterectomy using a retroperitoneal approach. J Am Assoc Gynecol Laparosc (in press).
7 Kadar N. An operative technique for laparoscopic radical vaginal hysterectomy and its evolution. Gynecol Endosc 1994;3:109–122.
8 Kadar N, Pelosi MA. Can cervix cancer be adequately staged by laparoscopic aortic lymphadenectomy? Gynecol Endoscopy (in press).
9 Reich H, Kadar N. The laparoscopic treatment of stage III borderline tumor of the ovary. Gynecol Endoscopy (submitted).
10 Kadar N, Homesley H, Malfetano J. Indications for pelvic and aortic lymphadenectomy in the management of endometrial carcinoma. Gynecol Endoscopy (in press).
11 Dembo AJ, Davy M, Stenwig AE, Berle EJ, Bush RS, Kjorstad K. Prognostic factors in patients with stage I epithelial ovarian cancer. Obstet Gynecol 1990;75:263–273.
12 Kadar N. The operative laparoscopy debate: technology assessment of statistical Jezebel? Biomed Pharmacother 1993;47:201–206.
13 Kadar N, Lemmerling L. Urinary tract injuries during laparoscopically assisted hysterectomy: causes and prevention. Am J Obstet Gynecol 1994;170:47–48.
14 Feroze R. Radical vaginal operations. In: Coppelson. Gynecologic oncology. Edinburgh: Churchill-Livingstone, 1981:840–843.
15 Mitra S. The Schauta operation. In: Meigs JV, ed. Surgical treatment of cancer of the cervix. New York: Grune and Stratton, 1954:267–280.
16 Querleu D, Leblanc E, Castelain B. Laparoscopic lymphadenectomy in the staging of early carcinoma of the cervix. Am J Obstet Gynecol 1991;164:579–581.
17 Childers JM, Hatch K, Surwit EA. The role of laparoscopic lymphadenectomy in the management of cervical carcinoma. Gynecol Oncol 1992;47:38–43.
18 Canis M, Mage G, Wattiez A, Pouly JL, Mahnes H, Bruhat MA. La chirugie endoscopique a-t-elle une place dans la chirugie radicale du cancer du col uterin. J Gynecol Obstet Biol Reprod 1990;19:921.
19 Nehzat C, Nehzat F, Welander C. Laparoscopic radical hysterectomy and pelvic and para-aortic lymphadenectomy in the treatment of carcinoma of the cervix. Am J Obstet Gynecol 1992;166:864–865.
20 Dargent D, Roy M, Keita N, Mathevet P, Adeleine P. The Schauta operation: its place in the management of cervical cancer [abstract]. Gynecol Oncol 1993;49:109–110.

Part 6 ◣

Managing Complications of

Gynecologic Surgery

Chapter 40

Managing hemorrhaging complications in obstetrics and gynecology

Luis E. Sanz

When treating the hemorrhaging patient, first consider preservation of life, and second, retention of fertility. Events most frequently associated with bleeding in obstetric patients are uterine atony, ectopic pregnancy, abortion, and lacerations (Table 40-1). In gynecologic patients, myomectomies, vaginal surgery, and cancer surgery are the most common causes of bleeding.

General considerations

It is important to adopt a step-by-step approach in managing the bleeding surgical patient. Always try the most conservative and least invasive means first to avoid major surgical complications: fluid and blood replacement, drug therapy, angiography, and proper tissue oxygenation.

For instance, in the case of a patient bleeding from uterine atony, a common complication after delivery, initial attempts to stop bleeding should include use of oxytocin (Pitocin), methylergonovine maleate (Methergine), prostaglandins, and uterine massage. When needed, concomitant use of fluid and blood replacement is essential. However, if such methods fail, then it is important to select the proper surgical approach to decrease or control bleeding, or to consider the option of angiographic arterial embolization, if available.

Selecting among procedures

Which surgical procedure is most appropriate depends on the type of injury and the patient's condition and parity. For

Table 40-1 Causes of bleeding

Obstetric causes

Abortion

Abruptio placentae

Disseminated intravascular coagulation

Ectopic pregnancy

Lacerations

Molar pregnancy

Placenta accreta or percreta

Placenta previa

Uterine atony

Gynecologic causes

Cancer

Cervical cone biopsy

Dysfunctional uterine bleeding

Hysterectomy

Myomectomy

Ruptured ovarian cyst

Vaginal surgery

Table 40-2 Management options

Hemostasis

Pressure

Repair of vascular laceration

Uterine artery ligation or stapling

Anterior hypogastric artery ligation

Hypogastric artery ligation

Abdominal aorta pressure

Hysterectomy, total

Hysterectomy, supracervical

Pressure pelvic packing

Angiographic embolization

instance, in an older woman with two or more children and no desire for further pregnancy, there is no point in attempting a hypogastric ligation, with its complications, when a supracervical or total hysterectomy can solve the problem faster and permanently (Table 40-2).

Consider the simpler options first, even though these may not be the procedures of choice in all circumstances. One should always try to identify and isolate a particular bleeding vessel and then clamp and tie it. Sometimes there is generalized venous bleeding that can be easily controlled be applying pressure for 5 or 10 minutes with a warm pad. One can also sprinkle a hemostatic agent, such as an absorbable gelatin sponge (Gelfoam), thrombin (Thrombinar, Thrombostat), or Avitene on the bleeding area, which usually stops light venous bleeding.

Uterine artery ligation

If unable to isolate a particular bleeding vessel, try to lessen the blood flow to the uterus by first ligating the hypogastric artery's distal branches to avoid unnecessary interruption of blood to other pelvic areas. Consequently, it is better to try to ligate the uterine artery bilaterally (1). This goal can be achieved either by stapling or suture ligating the uterine artery close to the uterus to avoid damaging the ureters. First, identify and isolate the uterine artery by incising the broad ligament's anterior leaf and dissecting the bladder away from the cervix to displace the ureters (2). Then suture ligate the artery with an absorbable synthetic material, such as polyglycolic acid (Dexon, Dexon-S), by placing a figure-of-eight suture into the lower uterine segment at the insertion of the uterine artery (Fig. 40-1). Better yet, if one can do a good dissection of the uterine artery, staple it with absorbable staples of polydioxanone (Absolok) (3).

There is no need to cut the artery when ligating or stapling it. Not cutting it allows for possible recanalization and future patency. During this procedure, it is important to use absorbable staples because metal staples, unless made of titanium, will interfere with future magnetic resonance imaging studies.

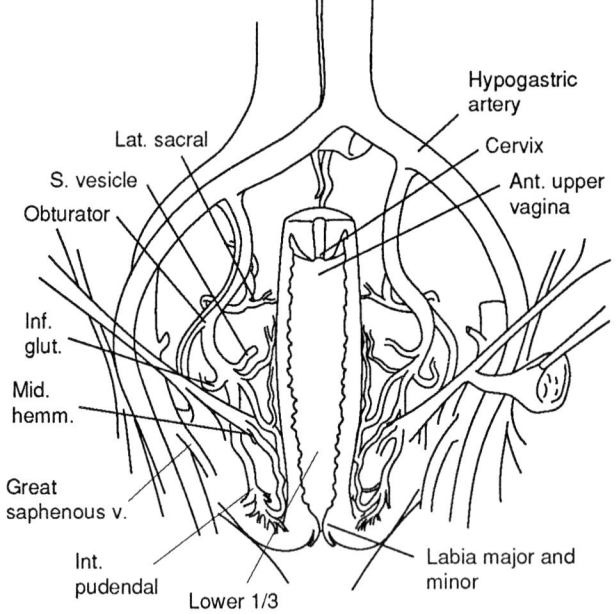

Fig. 40-1 One option in uterine artery ligation is to place a figure-of-eight suture into the lower uterine segment at the insertion of the uterine artery.

Uterine artery ligation is a fast, simple maneuver that will decrease pulse pressure by 60% to 70%. Other advantages are that it interferes only with blood supply to the uterus, sparing other organs. Moreover, because it is done for all hysterectomies, it is easier for the gynecologic surgeon to perform than is a hypogastric ligation.

Uterine artery ligation or stapling is done bilaterally and can take less than 10 minutes. If bleeding persists after a few minutes, ligate the ovarian arteries by the utero-ovarian ligament to avoid compromising the ovaries and the fallopian tubes. Combined bilateral ligation of the uterine and ovarian arteries will decrease arterial pulse pressure by approximately 80%. Collateral flow from the vaginal and internal pudendal artery will continue.

Anterior hypogastric artery ligation

Sometimes, as when the patient bleeds after a hysterectomy, uterine artery ligation is not feasible. It is then necessary to do a bilateral anterior (ventral) hypogastric ligation (4).

One must try to avoid hypogastric ligation. Although it is simpler to perform, morbidity is more serious because flow to the posterior branch, the superior gluteal, is obstructed. The main complication is atrophy of the gluteus maximus, caused by the decreased blood flow from the superior gluteal artery, injury to the internal iliac vein, and ligation by mistake of the external iliac artery, resulting in loss of the isolateral leg (Table 40-3).

To ligate the anterior branch of the hypogastric artery, open the lateral pelvic peritoneum by the bifurcation of the

Table 40-3 Possible complications of ligation

Ligation of external iliac artery

Laceration of external or internal iliac veins

Injury to ureter

Retroperitoneal hematoma

common iliac artery (Fig. 40-2). This area is usually easier to work in because it is away from the bleeding pelvic organs. In this region, the ureter is attached to the peritoneum's medial aspect, making it necessary to clearly identify the ureter before opening the peritoneum.

Open the parietal peritoneum. Leave the ureter attached to the peritoneum but retract it medially. The external and anterior internal hypogastric arteries are then readily visible. Because there are many anatomic variations of these two arteries, always identify both by palpation and visualization to avoid the mistake of ligating the external iliac artery.

Having identified the hypogastric artery, dissect it until the anterior and posterior branches are visible. Be careful when dissecting not to lacerate the internal iliac vein. One can thus avoid having to ligate the posterior trunk of the hypogastric artery and preserve blood flow to the gluteus maximus muscle through the superior gluteal artery. (The same precaution is necessary in angiographic arterial embolization.) Once the anterior branch is identified and isolated, pass a right-angle clamp behind it and ligate it with an absorbable suture but do not cut it. Repeat this step in the contralateral side.

Burchell showed that bilateral anterior hypogastric artery ligation decreases mean arterial pressure by 25% (5). It decreases mean blood flow by 50% and decreases arterial pulse pressure, which is the most important factor in controlling bleeding, by 85%. According to Burchell, the collateral blood supply to the uterus is such that pregnancies have been reported after bilateral anterior hypogastric ligation. The complications of anterior hypogastric ligation

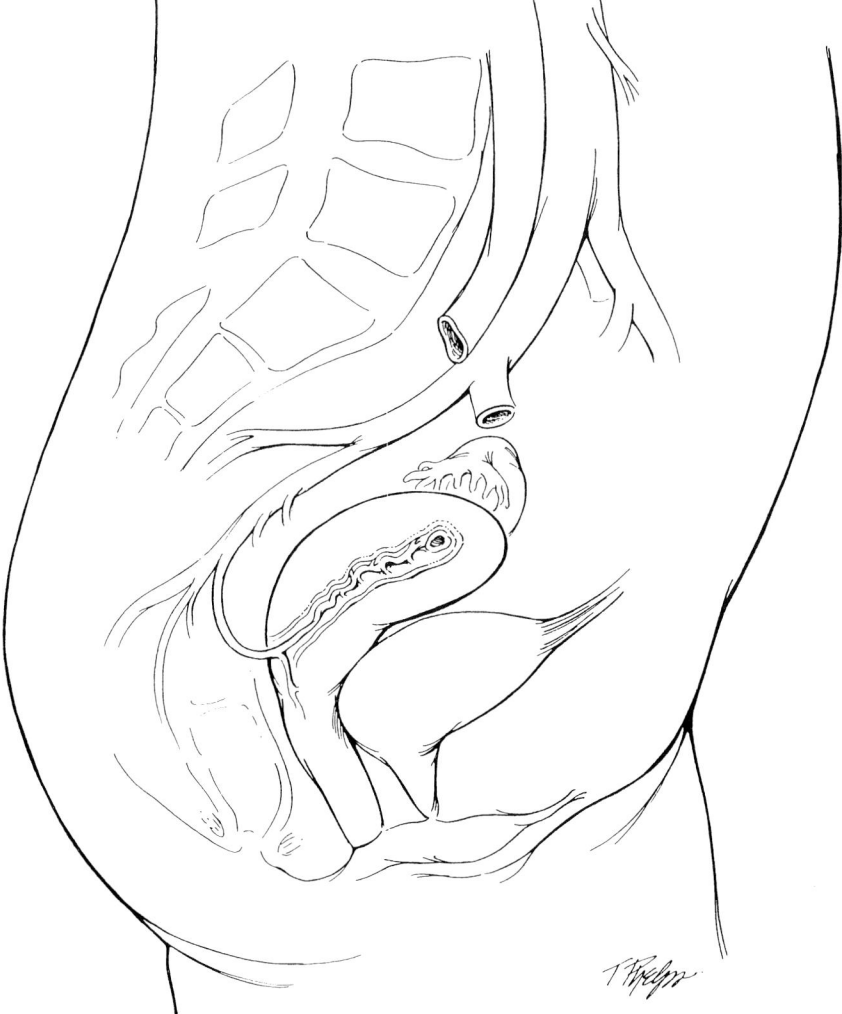

Fig. 40-2 To ligate the anterior hypogastric artery, open the lateral pelvic peritoneum by the bifurcation of the common iliac artery. (Courtesy of artist, Tim Phelps.)

are injury to the ureter, laceration of the anterior hypogastric vein, and retroperitoneal hematoma.

Repairing vascular injuries

It is important to understand how to manage and repair arterial or venous lacerations that can occur during dissection of the hypogastric nodes. Repairing a laceration is more difficult on a vein than on an artery because a vein's thinner wall tends to tear more easily (6).

An arterial or venous injury can be a puncture, laceration, or transection. A venous puncture is best handled by sprinkling a local hemostatic agent on it and applying pressure for at least 10 to 15 minutes. An arterial puncture is best handled by making a figure-of-eight suture with a permanent material like 5-0 or 6-0 polypropylene (Prolene).

Close an arterial or venous laceration with interrupted fine permanent sutures of monofilament polypropylene (Prolene) or multifilament braided-plain polyester (Mersilene). Then apply pressure above and below the vessel to stop blood flow and permit repair. Sometimes vascular clamps are placed above and below the laceration to decrease blood flow and reduce tension on the suture line.

For transection, perform an end-to-end anastomosis by using four-quadrant continuous closure with a permanent suture. Done properly, such closure has a high chance of success. If a vascular surgeon is available, obtain an intraoperative consultation. However, sometimes such expertise is unavailable. Therefore, prepare for situations like this by taking a hands-on microsurgical course that teaches vascular work.

Hysterectomy necessary

Although preservation of fertility is important, do not become so involved in saving the uterus that the patient's life is endangered by massive blood loss or disseminated intravascular coagulation (DIC). Continuous communication with the anesthesiologist is crucial throughout the surgical procedure. Check the amount of fluid and units of blood that the patient has received to avoid fluid overload and DIC.

A hysterectomy may be necessary as a surgical procedure of last resort. The supracervical hysterectomy, although seldom performed today, markedly decreases blood loss and operative time in an emergency situation, which is ideal in a compromised patient. This operation requires ligating only the round ligaments, utero-ovarian ligament, and uterine vessels after dissecting the bladder from the cervix. Amputate the uterine fundus at the level of the internal os, and close the cervical stump with a continuous suture of 2-0 poliglecaprone 25 (Monocryl) or polyglactin (Vicryl).

When supracervical hysterectomy is not feasible (dilated cervix), a total hysterectomy must be performed. In rare cases of massive arterial bleeding, pressure on the distal abdominal aorta can be temporarily used to slow the bleeding and identify the bleeding vessel. Be careful to have someone time the pressure on the aorta to avoid compromising circulation to the lower extremities. Avoid pressing on the aorta distal to the renal arteries for more than 4 or 5 minutes. If one has to press the abdominal aorta—below the renal arteries—for longer than 10 or 15 minutes, inject 5000 U of heparin into the distal aorta to prevent thrombosis in the femoral arteries. Be careful while operating not to block the vena cava because this blockage will decrease venous return to the right side of the heart and may produce hypovolemic shock in an already compromised patient.

The decision to perform a hysterectomy is more common when there exist such obstetric conditions as unresponsive uterine atony, placenta accreta, molar pregnancy, uterine rupture, extension of uterine incisions, and fibroids interfering with proper closure. Complications of postpartum hysterectomy include infection, need for transfusion, DIC, ureteral injury, and maternal death.

Packing technique

Pelvic pressure packing is seldom used today. However, in those rare cases in which extensive venous bleeding cannot be controlled by other means, including angiography, packing can be helpful in decreasing bleeding long enough to allow clotting to occur.

One among several ways to do packing is to impregnate a large quantity of fluffy gauze (Kerlix, Kendall Company, Boston, Mass.) with thrombin and fill the pelvic cavity with it. Then bring a tail through the vaginal cuff and attach a weight to the end for continuous pressure. One can remove the gauze after one to three days under anesthesia to minimize trauma to the area.

Fluid and blood replacement

It is important to properly maintain the patient's plasma volume and its oxygen-carrying capacity. Appropriate for this purpose are volume expanders like lactated Ringer's solution, dextran 70 (Hyskon), and normal saline, as well as whole blood or one of its components, such as packed red blood cells, cryoprecipitate, and fresh frozen plasma (7).

Become aware of the many different approaches to transfusion, including those with autologous, recipient-designated, experimental artificial, and homologous blood. Depending on the circumstance, the transfusion of autologous blood can involve preoperative donation or intrasurgical or preoperative donation or intrasurgical or perioperative autotransfusion (8).

Most hospitals are set up for preoperative donation in which the patient donates her own blood beginning 5 to 6 weeks before elective surgery. A healthy patient can donate up to 5 U of blood during that period but must take iron replacement simultaneously. More units can be donated by the patient if the blood is frozen.

In intrasurgical autotransfusion, blood is aspirated from the noncontaminated field, and the red cells are washed in a high-speed ultracentrifuge (Cell Saver Plus, Haemonetics Corp., Braintree, Mass.) and combined with normal saline for transfusion to the patient. Perioperative autotransfusion involves the removal of 2 U of blood a few hours before surgery, which is stored in standard containers at room temperature for transfusion during the elective procedure. This method diminishes the amount of red blood cells lost during surgery.

The most important research in this area is being done with an artificial red blood cell substitute designed to allow for easy and prolonged storage while eliminating the risk of infection and the need to type and crossmatch. The chemical used is perfluorocarbon (PFC), which carries oxygen in a high-oxygen environment. Fluosol-DA, comprising PFC, emulsifiers, distilled water, and plasma expanders, has been experimentally used in Japan and in the United States, where approval by the Food and Drug Administration is pending (9). Blood substitutes would also be helpful during the perioperative period. A patient's blood could be collected at the start of the operation and replaced by Fluosol-DA. The removed autologous blood could then be used as needed, either during or after the operation, avoiding the use of homologous blood.

Angiographic embolization

Another important treatment method for stopping bleeding is angiographic arterial embolization of the bleeding vessel or the vessel closest to it with pellets of absorbable gelatin sponge, a stainless steel coil 5 cm long holding multiple strands of Dacron polyester (Gianturco spring embolus), or both (10). The angiographer approaches the bleeding pelvic vessel through the contralateral femoral artery (Seldinger technique) under fluoroscopic guidance.

First, a distal aortogram is performed, and the iliac vessels with their branches are identified (Fig. 40-3). Next a guidewire is inserted through the contralateral femoral artery into the bleeding vessel or, if that is difficult, into the anterior hypogastric artery (Fig. 40-4). Then a pigtail catheter is inserted over the guidewire. Finally, the gelatin pellets, mixed with 4 to 5 ml of normal saline, are injected into the selected vessel until the flow through the artery is stopped.

If needed, both anterior hypogastric vessels can be selectively embolized. Computerized digital subtraction radiography is used to eliminate bowel interference patterns. The patient is usually sedated with midazolam (Versed) and fentanyl citrate (Sublimaze), and local anesthetic injected into the puncture site. The procedure usually takes one to two hours.

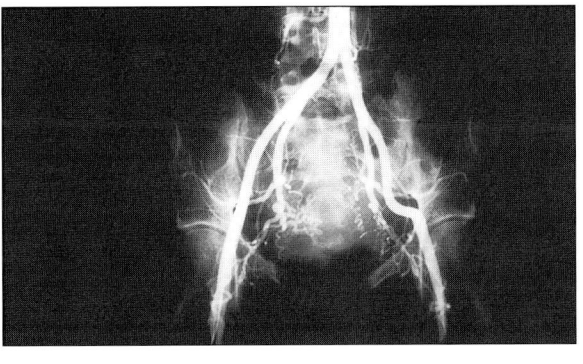

Fig. 40-3 To perform angiographic embolization, first obtain a distal aortogram and identify the iliac vessels and their branches.

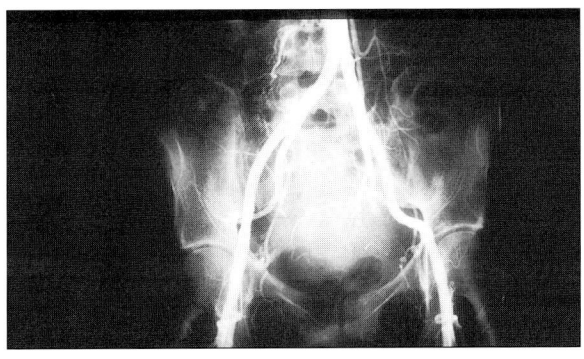

Fig. 40-4 next insert a guidewire through the contralateral femoral artery into the bleeding vessel or anterior hypogastric artery.

To perform angiographic arterial embolization, the hospital must have available a blood bank, vascular surgeon, and intensive care unit in case of an accidental vascular perforation. Chances of success are much better than they were in the past, and morbidity is minimal. The great majority of complications occur in patients with atherosclerosis. However, because we primarily treat healthy women, the likelihood of this situation arising is slight. Rapid arterial blood flow prevents reflux embolization of proximal branches.

One can perform embolization, when appropriate, before surgery, which is less risky for the patient, especially one with a history of previous radiation therapy. Therefore, it is essential to consult the angiographer before taking the patient back to surgery. It is also important that the gynecologist be present during embolization to assist the radiologist, reassure the patient, and be available to take her back to surgery if the procedure fails.

Summary

In managing bleeding, always try the most conservative, least invasive approach first to avoid major complications. Although available procedures range from repair of lacerations through anterior hypogastric ligation to hysterectomy, it is important to realize that concomitant use of fluids, oxygen, blood, and blood components is very important in helping prevent shock while trying to control bleeding. Finally, angiographic embolization can complement surgical management and, in many cases, make surgery unnecessary.

References

1 O'Leary J. Effects of bilateral ligation of the uterine and ovarian vessels in dogs. Int J Gynaecol Obstet 1980;17:460.
2 O'Leary J. Uterine artery ligation for hemorrhage. In: Sanz L, ed. Gynecologic surgery. Oradell, NJ: Medical Economics, 1988:385.
3 Harjola PT, Ala-Kulju K, Heikkinen L. Polydioxanone in cardiovascular surgery. Thorac Cardiovasc Surg 1984;32:100.
4 Clark S. Postpartum hemorrhage and technique for hypogastric ligation. In: Sanz L, ed. Gynecologic surgery. Oradell, NJ: Medical Economics, 1988:377.
5 Burchell RC. Physiology of internal iliac artery ligation. Obstet Gynecol 1964;24:737.
6 Gomes M. Vascular complications in gynecologic surgery. In: Delgado G, Smith J. Management of complications in gynecologic oncology. New York: Wiley, 1982.
7 Silberstein L, Kruskall RL, Stehling LC, et al. Strategies for the review of transfusion practices. JAMA 1989;262:1993.
8 Owings D, Kruskall RL, Thurer LM, et al. Autologous blood donations prior to elective cardiac surgery. JAMA 1989;262:1963.
9 Baranowski J. Your hematocrit is zero. Diagn Med 1980;12:61.
10 Rosenthal D. Angiographic embolization for postoperative hemorrhage. Contemp Obstet Gynecol 1987;30(S87):111.

Suggested readings

Goodnough L. Autologous donation—a safe transfusion alternative. Contemp Obstet Gynecol 1993;27.

Pearl M, Braga C. Percutaneous transcatheter embolization for control of life threatening pelvic hemorrhage from gestational trophoblastic disease. Obstet Gynecol 1992;80:571.

Winslow R. Blood substitutes minireview. In: International Conference on Red Cell Metabolism and Function. New York: Alan R. Liss, 1988.

Winslow R. Hemoglobin based red cell substitutes. Baltimore: Johns Hopkins University Press, 1992.

Chapter 41

Recognizing injuries to the urinary tract

Larry C. Kilgore and Hugh M. Shingleton

Injury to the urinary tract, a rare complication of abdominal and pelvic surgery, may be almost unavoidable in some circumstances, even for the experienced. It occurs more often in women, in whom it is most frequently associated with hysterectomy. In men it occurs most commonly during colorectal surgery. Bladder injuries are most likely to occur during vaginal hysterectomy in attempts to open the anterior peritoneal fold. Abdominal hysterectomy may also be associated with bladder injuries in women undergoing difficult operations or with distorted anatomy.

The great majority of ureteral injuries are associated with total abdominal hysterectomy performed for benign indications (1–3). Many injuries to the ureters and some to the bladder are not recognized intraoperatively (1,2,4). However, in one series, 84% of the injuries were recognized during the procedure. Most experienced surgeons would agree that these injuries can be avoided or recognized. Physicians in training should be taught to assess possible urologic injuries and manage them in the perioperative period.

Incidence of urologic injury

In one teaching-hospital series of more than 5500 patients undergoing gynecologic surgery, there was an overall 0.4% incidence of urologic injury (5). Injuries to the bladder and ureter occurred in a ratio of 5.3 to 1. The incidence of bladder damage associated with vaginal hysterectomy was 1.3%; with abdominal hysterectomy, 0.4%.

In studies that appeared before 1963, two authors, with a total of more than 7800 patients, reported ureteral damage rates of 0.5%, according to Symmonds (6). However, another three series, with a total of 750 patients, reported an incidence of 2.5%. Symmonds accepts the higher figure, because he believes many ureteral injuries are silent.

The incidence of ureteral injuries in association with gynecologic cancer surgery has changed dramatically in the last quarter century. A tabulation of a series of 4716 patients operated on between 1973 and 1983 resulted in an overall incidence rate of 2.3% for ureteral fistulas associated with radical hysterectomy and pelvic node dissection for cancer of the cervix (7). Earlier series had reported rates of 8% to 15%. Bladder fistulas (overall rate 0.57%) rarely occurred.

Bladder injuries

Fistulas most often are associated with hysterectomy (8), but also occur after urologic procedures, pelvic cancer and its therapy, and obstetric and pelvic trauma. It is said that it is no sin to cut the bladder; the sin is not to recognize the damage. When the bladder dome or base is opened and recognized at surgery, a simple layered closure followed by adequate bladder drainage for a few days allows healing in most cases (Fig. 41-1). Lacerations to the trigone are more

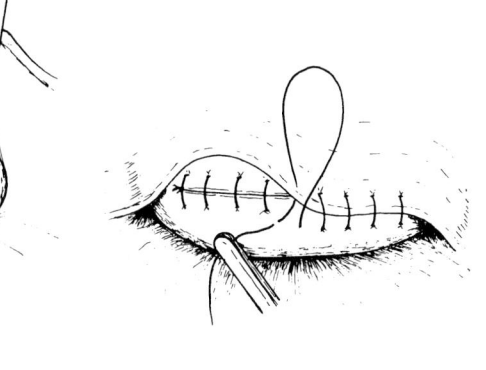

Fig. 41-1 To close a laceration in the bladder dome or base place a 3-0 absorbable running suture in the muscularis to invert the bladder mucosa (A); bring the bladder peritoneum over the first suture line and secure it with a second running 3-0 suture (B). (Adapted from Shingleton HM. Repairing injuries to the urinary tract. Contemp Obstet Gynecol 1984;March:76.)

Table 41-1 Causes of bladder damage during abdominal hysterectomy

Damage occurs most often while:

grasping the vaginal vault with clamps or suturing the cut edges of the vagina, the two most common causes of unrecognized bladder injuries;

separating the bladder from the cervix and from the upper vagina, especially when distorted anatomy and abnormal adhesions are present.

Damage occurs less often while:

incising the parietal peritoneum, especially after previous pelvic surgery;

developing the bladder flap, especially with distorted anatomy or after previous cesarean section;

entering the vagina anteriorly without sufficient mobilization of the bladder; and

indiscriminate use of cautery around bladder base.

Adapted from Shingleton HM. Repairing injuries to the urinary tract. Contemp Obstet Gynecol 1984;March:76.

Table 41-2 How to avoid bladder injury during abdominal hysterectomy

Open the parietal peritoneum high.

Develop the bladder flap high.

Use sharp rather than blunt dissection in developing the plane between the bladder and the cervix.

Free the bladder below the level of the cervix both centrally and laterally to avoid damage (see Fig. 41-2). Avoid use of right-angle clamps at the vaginal angles. These clamps are often responsible for bladder and ureteral injuries.

Suture the vault under direct visualization with the bladder retracted.

Leave the vagina open and draining, unless the vault area is dry. Bladder injury plus infected hematoma equals fistula.

Use suprapubic bladder drainage in difficult cases with dissection around the bladder.

Adapted from Shingleton HM. Repairing injuries to the urinary tract. Contemp Obstet Gynecol 1984;March:76.

complicated in that layered closure could compromise the ureteral orifices. In this circumstance, bilateral ureteral stent placement is advised to support the layered closure.

A variety of circumstances or operative maneuvers can lead to bladder damage during abdominal hysterectomy (Table 41-1). However, various techniques can reduce bladder injuries (Table 41-2). A combination of good exposure, instrumentation, and sharp dissection of tissue planes can reduce the incidence of bladder lacerations. Filling the bladder with sterile milk or dilute methylene blue after a difficult operation can help reveal unrecognized injuries. Before excising the specimen, a wise surgeon always verifies that the cervix and upper vagina are clear of the bladder and rectum (Fig. 41-2). In cases of extensive bladder dissection placing the bladder at risk of fistula formation, extended drainage via transurethral or suprapubic catheter is advised.

Urinary leakage into the vagina within the first 10 to 12 postoperative days usually indicates bladder injury. Contemporary Ob/Gyn's "Update on General Surgery 1983" has a summary of the diagnostic procedures for confirming and repairing bladder fistulas (9).

Virtually all posthysterectomy fistulas are small and occur just anterior to the vaginal cuff in the bladder base. Once the cuff is healed, a simple repair can be done using the Latzko technique, which avoids excision of the fistulous tract. This can be done relatively early in the postoperative period. A layered repair may require a delay of 2 to 4 months before the fistula site is edema free and the edge is smooth. In nonirradiated patients, successful results with both Latzko and layering techniques have ranged from 88% to 100%.

Ureteral injuries

Most of the injuries to the ureters associated with gynecologic surgery used to involve the pelvic ureter, but now that more para-aortic node dissections are being done,

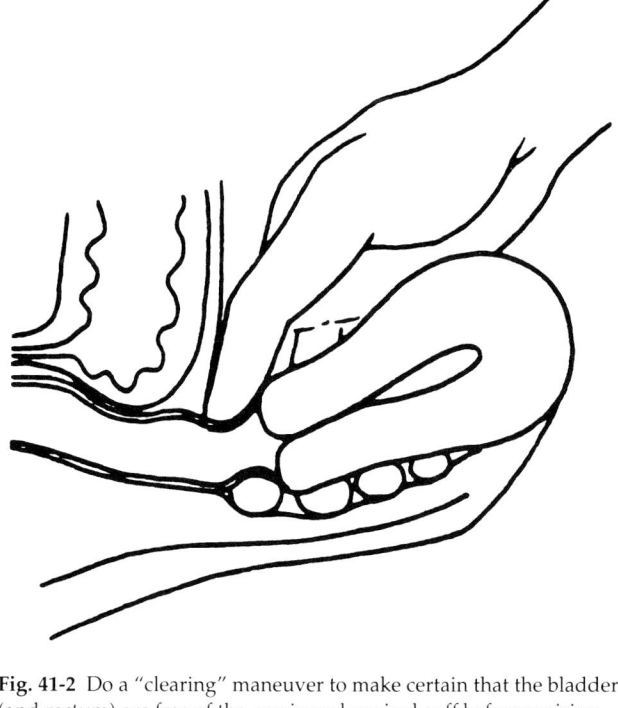

Fig. 41-2 Do a "clearing" maneuver to make certain that the bladder (and rectum) are free of the cervix and vaginal cuff before excising the specimen after sharp dissection. (Reproduced by permission from Shingleton HM. Repairing injuries to the urinary tract. Contemp Obstet Gynecol 1984;March:76.)

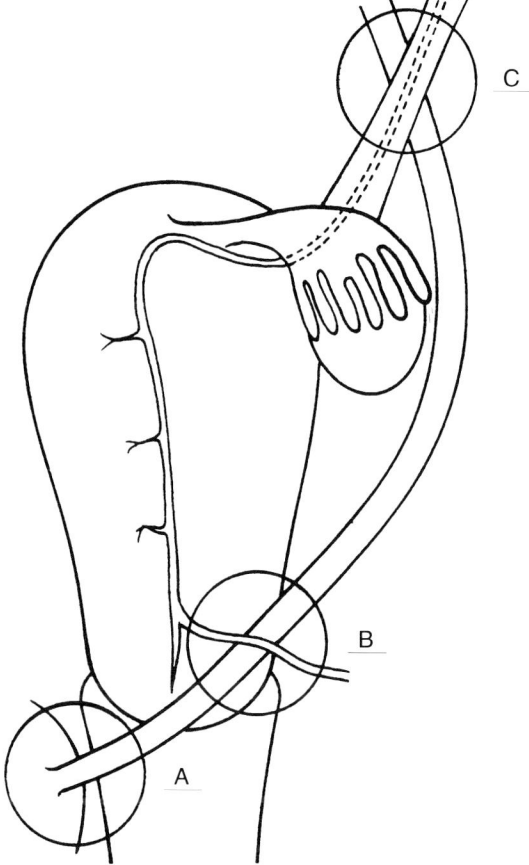

Fig. 41-3 Common sites of ureteral injury associated with hysterectomy are ureterovesical junction (A); junction of uterine artery and ureter (B); and infundibulopelvic ligament (C). (Adapted from Shingleton HM. Repairing injuries to the urinary tract. Contemp Obstet Gynecol 1984;March:76.)

more injuries above the pelvic rim are noted. In surgery for benign conditions, the most likely points of injury are in the vicinity of the infundibulopelvic ligament, the uterine artery, and at the ureterovesical junction (Fig. 41-3). Hazardous maneuvers that lead to ureteral injury are clamping and oversewing to stop bleeding associated with loss of the uterine artery or ovarian pedicle; kinking or obstructing the ureter at the pelvic brim when reperitonealizing the pelvis; obstruction during cul-de-sac obliteration by the Moskowitz technique; and injury or obstruction at or near the ureterovaginal junction associated with clamping or suturing the vaginal cuff. The Wertheim hysterectomy is most often responsible for injuries at this last site. Tunneling of the ureter near the bladder during this procedure may result in direct trauma to the ureteral sheath or in ischemic injury to the lower ureter.

Other operations that put the ureter at high risk are those associated with major pelvic infection, endometriosis, ovarian masses, and leiomyoma uteri, especially those involving the broad ligament or cervix. Vaginal hysterectomy—especially for major uterine prolapse—may also result in ureteral damage, as may anterior colporrhaphy, Marshall-Marchetti-Krantz and Burch procedures, and cesarean section, especially low transverse incisions, cesarean section hysterectomy, and abdominal hysterectomy with a wide vaginal cuff.

An axiom of surgery is that adequate exposure should reduce or prevent injury to contiguous organs (3). All sur-

geons must be capable of opening the pararectal and paravesical retroperitoneal spaces and tracing the ureter throughout its pelvic course to keep it free from injury. It is equally important to visualize the ureter directly during difficult operations and to recognize any intraoperative damage. If necessary, inject indigo-carmine dye intravenously to confirm extravasation from the ureter. If a simple visual check of the pelvic ureter before reperitonealization reveals marked dilation, look for a ligature near the cuff as the cause of the obstruction. Or one can open the dome of the bladder to see if urine passes into the bladder from both ureteral orifices. If there is doubt, insert a small Silastic catheter through the ureteral orifice to determine patency (Fig. 41-4). Some suggest using a carbon dioxide urethroscope inserted through the dome of the bladder, or transurethrally, as another method of observing ureteral patency.

Bleeding from the uterine artery pedicle puts the ureter at special risk. In one study, investigators found that 79% of ureteral injuries occurred at the junction of the uterine artery and the ureter (1). Compression of the hypogastric

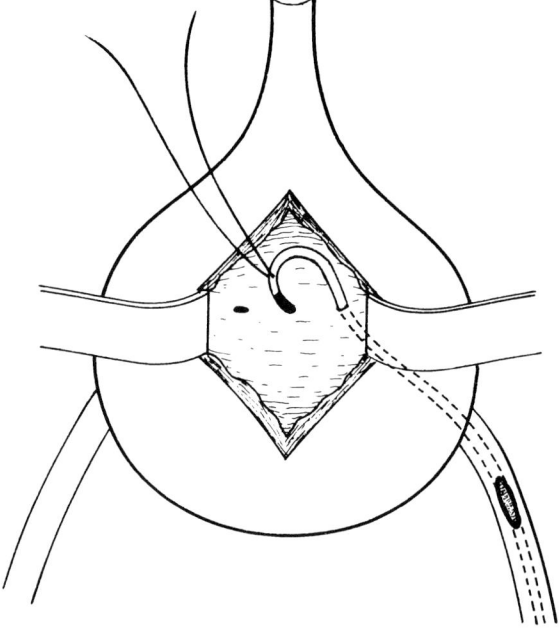

Fig. 41-4 A cystotomy will allow the passage of a Silastic stent beyond the site of injury to check patency. (Adapted from Shingleton HM. Repairing injuries to the urinary tract. Contemp Obstet Gynecol 1984;March:76.)

artery may allow better exposure of the bleeding vessel, which can be dissected out and clamped under direct vision (10). The skilled pelvic surgeon will use smaller clamps often placed parallel to the ureter to avoid a crush injury. Size 3-0 or 4-0 absorbable sutures should also be used to avoid unnecessary kinking of periureteral tissue. It may be necessary to ligate the anterior branch of the hypogastric artery to control bleeding. To carry out these maneuvers, one should have extensive familiarity with the retroperitoneal space and know the position of the ureter at all times.

Some surgeons advocate a routine preoperative intravenous pyelogram (IVP). An IVP provides information about ureteral displacement, dilation, or duplication. Others suggest prophylactically placing a ureteral catheter before difficult pelvic surgery. However, excessive manipulation of a ureter containing a rigid catheter can cause damage. In general it is much better to *visualize* the ureter and to hold it out of harm's way than to depend on feeling it, with or without a stenting catheter. It is one thing for a skilled pelvic surgeon to "snap" or feel a ureter; it is quite another for an inexperienced surgeon to depend on palpation alone. Resident physicians should be required to open the retroperitoneal space routinely on benign abdominal cases and to visualize the ureter's course in the pelvis directly. At the same time they should expose and demonstrate the anterior branch of the hypogastric artery. These simple maneuvers take very little time but will guarantee a knowledge of the appropriate anatomy when it is needed during difficult procedures.

Unrecognized ureteral injuries

Certain signs and symptoms will identify the patient who has an undiagnosed ureteral injury postoperatively (Table 41-3). Fever, ileus, and abdominal distention are clues to an intra-abdominal urinary leak, as are flank pain and tenderness, urinomas, anuria, abnormal IVPs in the early postoperative period, and urinary leaks (11). Leaks do not always occur immediately, but may be delayed. Some leaks can be diagnosed only by the use of postoperative IVPs following difficult surgery.

Many factors must be considered in managing the ureteral injury (Table 41-4). Intraoperative recognition allows immediate correction and may not substantially extend the patient's hospital stay. Stenting of the injured ureter at surgery, with or without suturing, is effective in a number of instances, including ligation, clamping, or sheath injuries (Fig. 41-5). Ureteral stents come in various sizes and may be straight or pigtailed. Most pelvic surgeons prefer the pigtail variety to avoid suturing the stent in place. Straight stents must be sutured in place to avoid peri-

Table 41-3 Symptoms and signs of postoperative ureteral injury

Symptoms	Signs
Flank pain, tenderness	Urinoma
Fever, sepsis	Abnormal pyelogram Urine leak Obstruction
Ileus, abdominal distention	Anuria Silent loss of kidney
Urinary leak Vaginal Cutaneous	

Adapted from Shingleton HM. Repairing injuries to the urinary tract. Contemp Obstet Gynecol 1984;March:76.

Table 41-4 Factors to consider in managing ureteral injury

If recognized intra-operatively	*If recognized post-operatively*
Mobility of ureter and bladder	Time interval to diagnosis
Time required to repair damage	Degree of impairment of renal function

Common to both

Age and general condition of patient

Underlying condition leading to original surgery

Level of and extent of injury

Associated pathology in area of injury

Adapted from Shingleton HM. Repairing injuries to the urinary tract. Contemp Obstet Gynecol 1984;March:76.

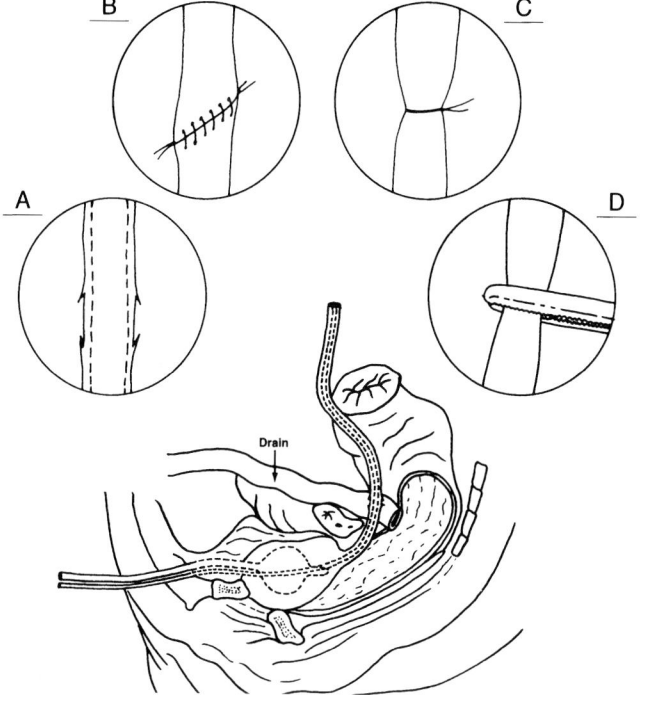

Fig. 41-5 For ureteral injuries, place stent in the affected ureter and bring it out with a Foley catheter. Procedure is suitable for injuries of the ureteral sheath (A); transections, repaired by end-to-end anastomosis (B); ureteral ligation (C); and clamp injuries (D). (Reproduced by permission from Shingleton HM. Repairing injuries to the urinary tract. Contemp Obstet Gynecol 1984;March:76.)

staltic advancement into the bladder. Newer pigtail stents have a long suture through the distal end. This can be brought out of the bladder alongside the Foley catheter for later stent removal without cystoscopy. Most stents used in this setting can be removed in 3 to 6 weeks.

In managing clamping injuries to the ureter, the surgeon should determine whether the ureter is vital or devitalized. It is easy to underestimate ureteral damage. If there is concern about possible extravasation through the clamp site, use indigo-carmine dye intravenously and observe the ureter for a leak. If the ureteral color is good and there is no obvious severe damage or leakage, the ureteral sheath may be approximated with several 5-0 chromic sutures. The ureter should be stented, and the injury site should be drained extraperitoneally (10).

If a segment of ureter is damaged, reimplantation into the bladder is strongly preferred (Fig. 41-6). If reimplantation is not feasible, an end-to-end anastomosis may be in order, depending on the site of the injury. Most ureters can be reimplanted if the injury is within 6 cm of the bladder, whereas above that level, an end-to-end anastomosis or a transureteroureterostomy may be advisable (Figs. 41-7 and 41-8) (12). Reimplantation of the ureter into the bladder may require a psoas hitch or, in the nonirradiated patient, a bladder flap. Excellent illustrations of a number of these procedures are available (12). Transureteroureterostomy is potentially hazardous to both urinary tracts and should be used as a last resort (6). Extraperitoneal drainage of the anastomosis site is expedient, preferably with closed suction drainage. Injuries to the upper ureter may require downward mobilization of the kidney or transureteroureterostomy.

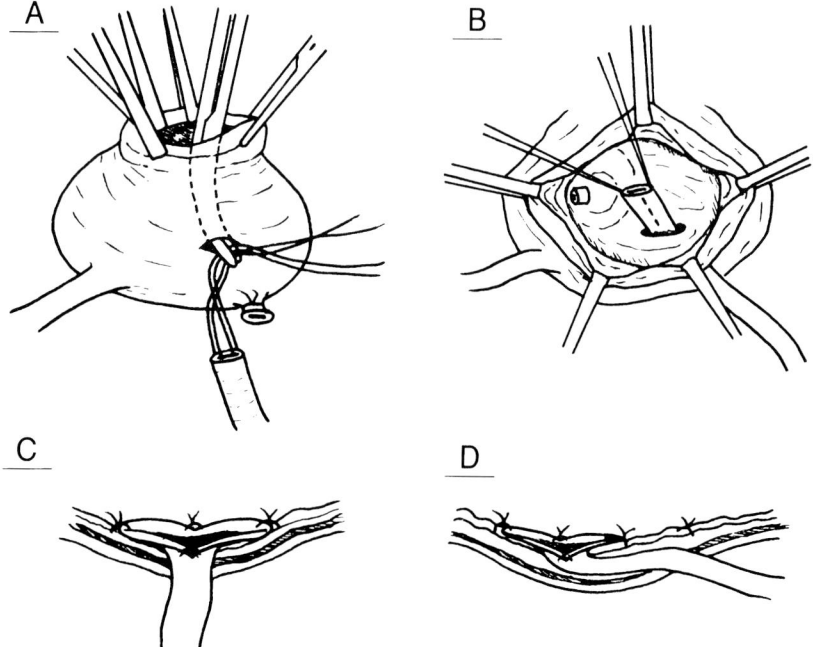

Fig. 41-6 When following the technique for ureteral reimplantation, bring the ureter through an incision adjacent to the ligated ureteral stump (A and B); fishmouth the ureteral end, and sew it into position using 4-0 chromic catgut interrupted sutures (C). (D) A tunneled anastomosis may be used; this antireflux technique is not mandatory in adults. (Reproduced by permission from Shingleton HM. Repairing injuries to the urinary tract. Contemp Obstet Gynecol 1984;March:76.)

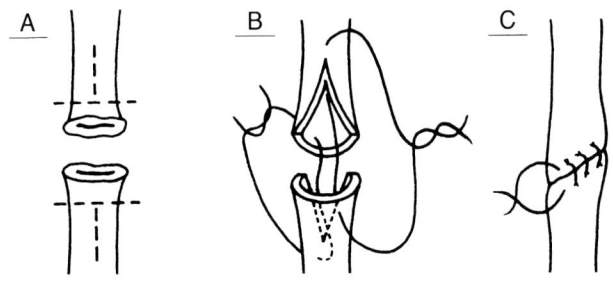

Fig. 41-7 In end-to-end anastomosis technique, freshen the cut ends (A) and spatulate the ureter (B) to allow an oblique anastomosis (C) formed with interrupted 4-0 chromic catgut sutures. (Reproduced by permission from Shingleton HM. Repairing injuries to the urinary tract. Contemp Obstet Gynecol 1984;March:76.)

Once a postoperative diagnosis of ureteral injury is made, various factors should be considered before any action is taken (Table 41-4). The time interval before diagnosis, the patient's general condition, and the degree of impairment of renal function are especially important, as is the underlying condition that led to the original surgery, the level and extent of the ureteral injury, and the associated pathology (especially infection) in the area of the injury.

Once a ureteral obstruction or fistula is documented postoperatively, every effort should be made to stent the ureter and allow healing without surgery. The majority of ureteral fistulas in the nonirradiated patient will heal after stent placement only. Retrograde pyelography with cystoscopy and stent placement should be the first maneuver. If this is unsuccessful, antegrade stent placement may be accomplished after percutaneous nephrostomy. In certain cases, 2 to 4 weeks of percutaneous nephrostomy drainage may be necessary followed by second attempts at stent placement. If circumstances prevent stent placement, surgery with planned reimplantation of the ureter is in order.

Summary

Skilled gynecologic surgeons should have the technical ability to prevent and recognize most bladder and ureteral injuries (Table 41-5). They should be able to repair lacerations that occur during abdominal or vaginal hysterectomy, the latter from the vaginal approach. Gynecologists, with good training, also can repair simple posthysterectomy bladder fistulas, especially if they use the Latzko technique. However, the practicing gynecologist is wise to seek consultation with a gynecologic oncologist or experienced urologic surgeon in more complicated situations. These include ureteral reimplantation with or without bladder hitches, bladder-flap procedures, transureteroureterostomies, fistulas associated with pelvic-vaginal irradiation, and transvesical closures of large complex bladder fistulas, especially recurrent fistulas after failed repairs (Table 41-6). In a number of such repairs, omental pedicles or flaps can

Table 41-5 Procedures for which the gynecologic surgeon should be prepared

Exploring the retroperitoneal space

Opening the pararectal and paravesical spaces

Exposing the ureter in the pelvis to keep it "out of harm's way"

Recognizing intraoperative bladder or ureteral injury

Stenting the ureter after partial injury by clamps and ligatures

Repairing the bladder laceration from the abdominal or vaginal approach

Repairing a posthysterectomy bladder fistula by the Latzko or layered techniques

Calling for help

Adapted from Shingleton HM. Repairing injuries to the urinary tract. Contemp Obstet Gynecol 1984;March:76.

Table 41-6 Corrective operations to be performed by skilled* pelvic surgeons

Bladder flaps

Complex urologic fistulas involving bowel or other organs

Transureteral ureterostomy

Transvesical closures of bladder fistula

Ureteral end-to-end anastomoses or reimplantations

Urinary diversions

Vaginal or abdominal repairs of bladder fistula irradiation

*Urologists, gynecologic oncologists, and gynecologists with additional training in general surgery or urology qualify as skilled. Adapted from Shingleton HM. Repairing injuries to the urinary tract. Contemp Obstet Gynecol 1984;March:76.

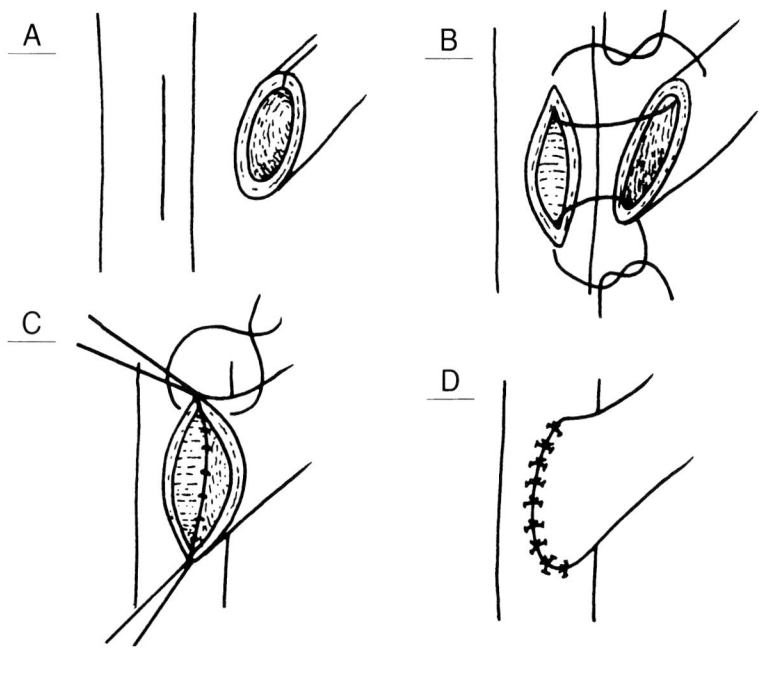

Fig. 41-8 For transureteral ureterostomy, bring ureter from contralateral side (A) and anastomose it to an incision made in the recipient ureter (B, C). Make the anastomosis in oblique fashion to prevent stricture, using interrupted sutures of 4-0 chromic catgut (D). (Reproduced by permission from Shingleton HM. Repairing injuries to the urinary tract. Contemp Obstet Gynecol 1984;March:76.)

be used to bring in additional blood supply to the anastomosis. A combination of good surgical skill, familiarity with retroperitoneal anatomy, and the ability to suspect and recognize urinary tract injury will minimize perioperative morbidity and allow good surgical outcomes even with difficult cases.

References

1 Flynn JT, Tiptaft RC, Woodhouse CRJ, et al. The early and aggressive repair of iatrogenic ureteric injuries. Br J Urol 1979;151:453.

2 Hoch WH, Kursh ED, Persky L. Early aggressive management of intraoperative ureteral injuries. J Urol 1975;114:530.

3 Symmonds RE. Prevention and management of genitourinary fistula. J Continuing Ed Obstet/Gynecol 1979;21:13.

4 Zinman LM, Libertino JA, Roth RA. Management of operative ureteral injury. Urology 1978;12:290.

5 Miyazawa K. Urological injuries in gynecologic surgery. Hawaii Med J 1980;39:11.

6 Symmonds RE. Ureteral injuries associated with gynecologic surgery: prevention and management. Clin Obstet Gynecol 1976;19:623.

7 Shingleton HM, Orr JW Jr. Cancer of the cervix: diagnosis and treatment. Edinburgh: Churchill-Livingstone, 1983:77.

8 Graber EA, O'Rourke JJ, McElrath T. Iatrogenic bladder injury during hysterectomy. Obstet Gynecol 1964;23:267.

9 Bresette JF, Patterson JA. Strategy for repairing vesicovaginal fistulas. Contemp Obstet/Gynecol 1983;21:68.

10 Smith AM. Injuries of the pelvic ureter. Surg Gynecol Obstet 1975;140:761.

11 Bright TC III, Peters PC. Ureteral injuries secondary to operative procedures. Urology 1977;9:22.

12 Fry DE, Milholen L, Harbrecht PJ. Iatrogenic ureteral injury. Arch Surg 1983;118:454.

13 Belan G. Early treatment of ureteral injuries found after gynecological surgery. J Urol 1977;118:25.

Chapter 42

Repairing the bladder during gynecologic surgery

John B. Wheelock, Hans-B. Krebs, and

W. Glenn Hurt

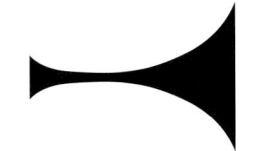

In women, the urinary bladder lies on the anterior lower uterine segment and upper vagina. Reflected pelvic peritoneum and loose areolar connective tissue attach the bladder to these organs in a way that allows the two organ systems to function independently. Genital tract diseases often involve the bladder, predisposing it to injury during gynecologic surgery. However, poor surgical technique during procedures for benign gynecologic disease is also responsible for many bladder injuries.

Incidences, sites, and causes

Our review of records at the Medical College of Virginia Hospitals showed bladder injuries occurring in at least 1.8% of abdominal hysterectomies and 0.4% of vaginal hysterectomies. Tancer reported bladder fistulas in 4 (0.17%) of 2400 abdominal hysterectomies performed over 7 years (1).

Failure to recognize and repair bladder injuries increases morbidity and may lead to formation of vesicovaginal fistulas, whereas immediate repair followed by catheter drainage for about 10 days will prevent significant complications. Investigators at the Johns Hopkins Hospital found that of 77 patients with bladder injuries none suffered untoward sequelae when lacerations were recognized during surgery and managed appropriately (2).

During abdominal surgery, the most frequent sites and times of bladder injury are the dome, during entry of the peritoneal cavity; the fundus, during dissection and displacement from pelvic masses or from the anterior surface of the uterus; the lateral corpus, during clamping and suturing of the cardinal ligaments; and the base or trigone, during excision of the cervix and suturing of the vaginal cuff (3). During vaginal hysterectomies, almost all bladder injuries involve damaging the base or trigone while attempting to enter the anterior cul-de-sac. Those associated with surgery for such benign diseases as endometriosis and leiomyomata usually occur during separation of dense adhesions between the bladder and adjacent pelvic structures (Table 42-1) (4).

General recommendations

The first step in preventing bladder injury during pelvic laparotomy is to make certain the bladder is free of urine. For uncomplicated cases, some gynecologic surgeons recommend transurethral catheterization during preparation, while others favor suprapubic extraperitoneal needle aspiration after incising the abdominal wall. For utmost safety, one should insert a transurethral Foley catheter after preparing the vagina and connect it to a closed system to permit constant drainage of urine. This will keep the bladder empty and out of the operative field. During vaginal surgery, initially empty the bladder by transurethral suprapubic catheterization to allow adequate decompression.

Table 42-1 Predispositions to bladder injury

Endometriosis

Ovarian tumors

Pelvic inflammatory disease associated
with leiomyomata, pelvic abscess, or tubo-
ovarian abscess

Uterine leiomyomata adherent to bladder
or located low on anterior uterus

Some gynecologists have recommended routinely in-stilling dyes into the bladder to disclose penetrating blad-der injuries immediately. Although this step may help for difficult pelvic dissections, it is usually not necessary for routine gynecologic surgery.

Prerequisites for avoiding bladder injury are adequate exposure of the operative field, a thorough knowledge of pelvic anatomy, and strict adherence to the following basic surgical practices:

• Carefully isolate and ligate bleeding vessels rather than use blind clamping and suturing techniques that might damage the bladder.

• Use clean, sharp dissection to open tissues along anatomic planes while applying steady traction to the uterus.

• Keep in mind that previous cesarean sections, pelvic infec-tions, endometriosis, and distortion by tumors complicate bladder dissections and predispose the patient to injury.

Abdominal operations

Lower abdominal incisions

The bladder is at risk of injury every time one incises the lower abdominal wall and enters the peritoneal cavity. Risk is somewhat higher if the bladder adheres to the anterior abdominal wall as a result of previous procedures. When using a midline incision, enter the peritoneal cavity through the incision's most cephalad portion. Maylard and other transverse incisions of the peritoneum are safest when started lateral to the midline.

Obese patients with thick layers of preperitoneal fat are at particular risk of bladder injury. Preperitoneal fat is rel-atively avascular compared with bladder muscularis. Therefore, brisk bleeding during dissection of preperi-toneal fat in the vicinity of the vesical dome is a warning that one may be about to incise the bladder. If this happens, try to enter the abdomen through a more cephalad part of the incision.

Abdominal hysterectomy

The bladder is often easy to locate, but sometimes difficult to dissect from the anterior lower uterine segment and up-per vagina because of fibrosis caused by previous pelvic in-fection, endometriosis, or cesarean sections. To prevent injury to the fundus, begin mobilizing the bladder by en-tering the vesicocervical space through bilateral incisions of the vesicouterine fold of pelvic peritoneum. Next exert trac-tion on the uterus and the cut edge of the bladder peri-toneum to visibly expose the loose connective tissue between the bladder and the anterior lower uterine seg-ment (Fig. 42-1).

Carefully dissect the supravaginal septum, which is formed by fusion of the cervical and vesical fascia and sep-arates the vesicouterine and vesicovaginal spaces. Enter the vesicovaginal space, which also contains areolar connective tissue, and dissect the bladder from the anterior lower uter-ine segment and upper vagina with Metzenbaum scissors, directing their tips toward the cervix and away from the bladder. Exert steady traction cephalad during dissection to help identify the tissue planes.

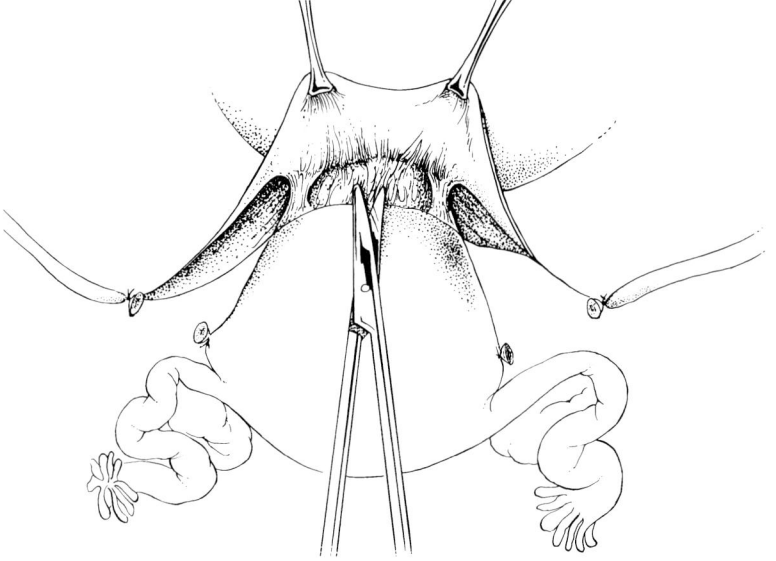

Fig. 42-1 Opening the vesicovaginal space. Pulling the bladder peritoneum upward with Allis clamps exposes the areolar tissue between the bladder base and the cervix. The bladder pillars are seen on each side of the cervix.

While clamping the cardinal ligaments, protect the bladder's lateral aspects from injury by adequately mobilizing the bladder from the cervix and other adjacent structures. Before cutting the cardinal ligaments, place a clamp parallel to the side of the cervix so that it will slide lateral to clamp that portion of the cardinal ligament adjacent to the cervix. Once this clamp is applied, do not place any more clamps lateral to it. If troublesome bleeding occurs, avoid blind clamping or blind suturing.

Displace the bladder downward sufficiently to protect the base and trigone during excision of the cervix and ensure safe suturing of the vaginal cuff. For optimal exposure, retract the uterine specimen or vaginal cuff cephalad while gently lifting the bladder anteriorly with a small retractor placed in the vesicovaginal space.

Vaginal hysterectomies

Fewer bladder injuries are associated with the vaginal route, probably because candidates for vaginal hysterectomy are carefully screened to rule out genital tract disease, dense adhesions, and gross anatomic distortions. Lacerations that do occur are most often due to poor surgical technique. Typically, persistent attempts to enter the anterior cul-de-sac in the face of difficult situations result in inadvertent cystotomy and a gush of urine into the operative field. One can prevent such accidents by carefully identifying planes of dissection and the vesicouterine fold.

After applying a tenaculum to the portion and providing downward traction, incise the anterior vaginal wall approximately 1 cm distal to the bladder sulcus, the grooved depression of the vaginal wall that marks the attachment of the bladder to the cervix. Carry this incision through all layers of the anterior vaginal wall.

Use scissors with the tips pointed toward the cervix to enter the vesicovaginal space and dissect this space further by inserting the closed scissors up the midline against the anterior uterine segment, opening them, and withdrawing

them while slightly open. Many gynecologists use a gauze-tipped index finger to push the bladder further cephalad once proper planes are identified.

Evaluating the bladder will usually reveal a transverse double fold of peritoneum, the vesicouterine fold. Elevate this fold's superior layer with thumb forceps or an Allis clamp and incise the fold under direct vision. Next, immediately enter the anterior cul-de-sac and elevate the bladder out of the operative field using a small Deaver retractor with modified curve or some similar instrument.

If the vesicouterine fold does not become visible, do not enter the anterior cul-de-sac until the uterosacral and paracervical ligaments have been clamped, cut, and ligated. This gives the bladder more mobility, permitting it to be displaced further cephalad.

Evaluating bladder injury

If one suspects injury, instill 10 ml of indigo-carmine or methylene blue dye diluted in 500 ml of normal saline into the bladder through a transurethral catheter. Some prefer to use sterile milk or pediatric formula because it does not stain tissues surrounding the laceration. Reinstillation of dye or milk following repair will help reveal further lacerations and ensure watertight closure.

To avoid compromising the ureteral orifice, check how close the injury is to the trigone before starting repair. If one does a cystotomy to obtain adequate exposure, make a longitudinal incision of 3 to 4 cm between two Allis clamps extraperitoneally in the anterior bladder wall (Fig. 42-2). Because of the anatomic distribution of bladder wall vessels, this approach is less likely than a transverse incision to cause bleeding. Cystostomies are also helpful in dissecting the bladder from the posterior symphysis during repeat retropubic procedures. They are useful as well in trachelectomies or other difficult cases in which gynecologic disease has caused fusion of tissue planes between cervix and bladder.

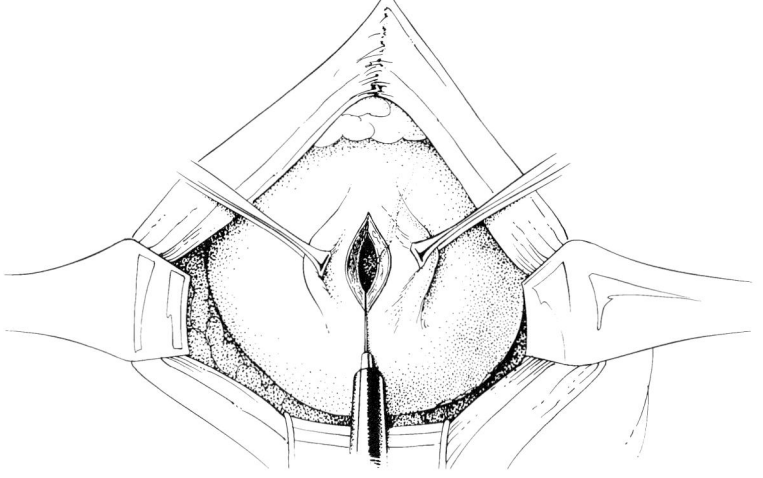

Fig. 42-2 Cystotomy. Make a median incision of the bladder with a Bovie knife between two Allis clamps.

Repair

Do not use permanent suture material to repair bladder lacerations because it may act as a nidus for stone formation. Rather, use 2-0 or 3-0 absorbable suture material. To prevent stone formation, some practitioners recommend not placing any suture through the bladder mucosa. In our experience, incorporating the mucosa within a catgut suture allows better approximation of the wound edges, facilitates a watertight closure, and does not promote stone formation. However, polyglycolic sutures, which are not absorbed as readily as catgut sutures, should not be allowed to penetrate the mucosa (5).

Minor injury

Bladder lacerations involving the serosa or superficial seromuscular layers may be repaired with one layer of interrupted or continuous sutures of a 3-0 chromic catgut (Fig. 42-3). Prolonged, continuous bladder drainage is not necessary. Small lacerations penetrating the bladder mucosa should be closed using two layers.

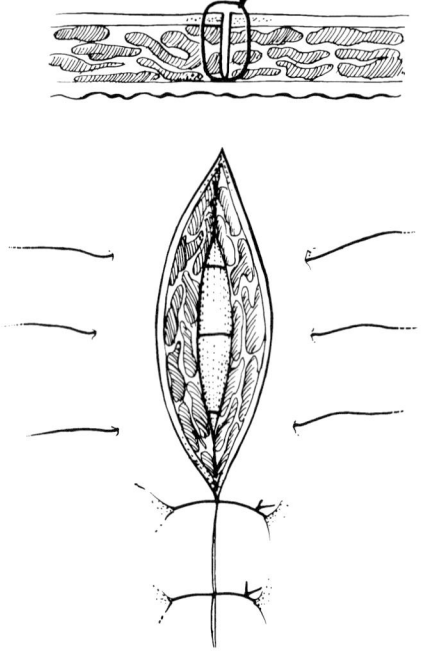

Fig. 42-3 Partial-thickness injury. Place interrupted stitches of 3-0 chromic catgut through the bladder's muscular and serosal layer.

Major injury

Large lacerations that involve all bladder wall layers sometimes require mobilizing the bladder to promote tension-free repair. After one has identified the laceration's limits, one can simplify exposure by placing traction sutures at either end. Then close the bladder in two layers with 2-0 or 3-0 chromic catgut.

In the first layer, incorporate the full thickness of the bladder wall on either side of the laceration, including the mucosa (Fig. 42-4, left). For the second layer, use an imbricating Lembert suture approximating the more superficial muscular and serosal layers overlying the first row of sutures (Fig. 42-4, right).

As a rule, close both layers with interrupted stitches. However, continuous stitches are satisfactory when the wound edges are clean and the bladder wall is thick, healthy, and vascular.

Crushing injuries of the bladder wall may cause necrosis and fistula formation. Excise the damaged area and close the defect in two layers.

After repairing a large laceration, decompress the bladder with continuous drainage, using a 16 or 18 Fr Foley or Malecot suprapubic catheter inserted through a separate extraperitoneal cystotomy incision and secured to the anterior bladder wall with an absorbable purse-string suture (Fig. 42-5). Generally continue drainage for 7 to 10 days. In a healthy patient with an uncomplicated bladder injury, one may want to discontinue it earlier. In a debilitated patient whose bladder may have been within the field of radiation therapy for pelvic malignancy, it is wise to continue drainage for longer than 10 days.

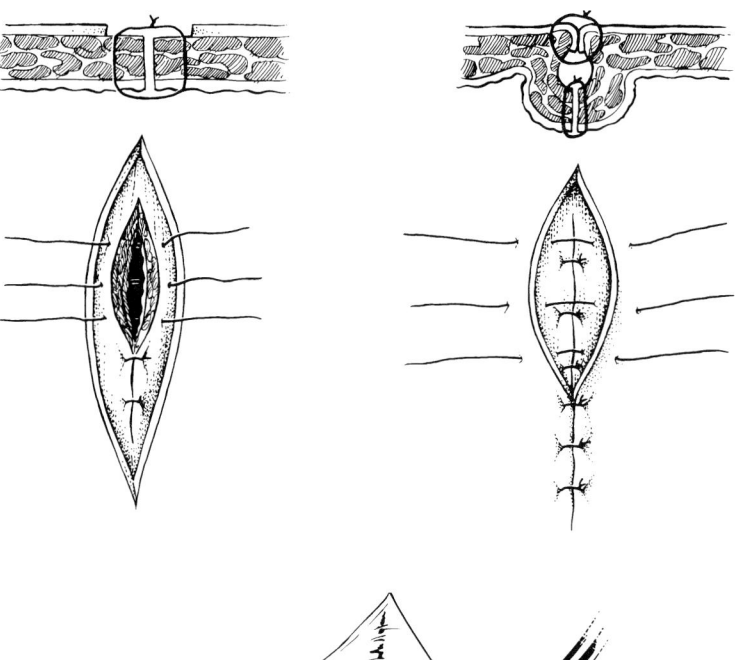

Fig. 42-4 Full-thickness injury. Use two layers. In the first layer, use interrupted stitches of 3-0 chromic suture to incorporate the muscular and mucosal layers (*left*). In the second layer, use interrupted Lembert sutures through the serosa and muscular layer to imbricate the deep layer (*right*).

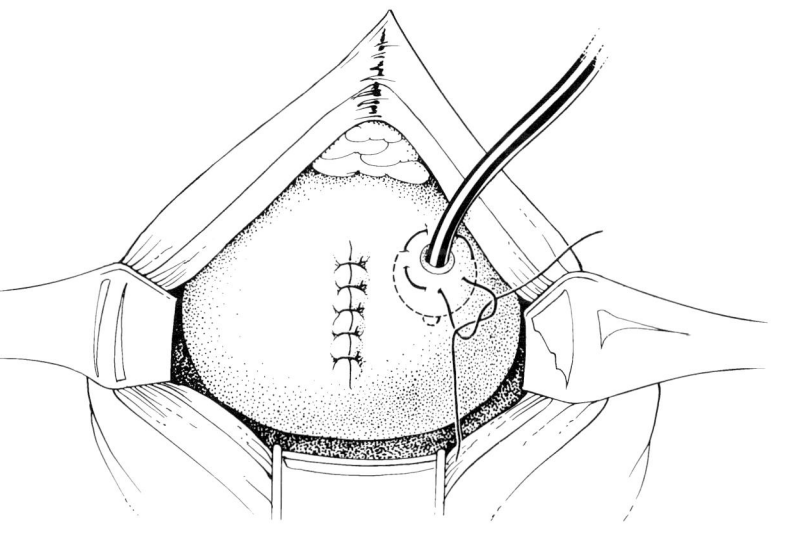

Fig. 42-5 Postoperative drainage. Insert a suprapubic catheter through a separate stab wound outside the repaired bladder laceration and secure it with a purse-string suture to decompress the bladder with continuous drainage.

References

1 Tancer ML. Urologic injuries: bladder and urethra. In: Schaefer G, Graber EA, eds. Complications in obstetric and gynecologic surgery. Hagerstown, Md: Harper & Row, 1981:399.

2 Everett HS, Mattingly RF. Urinary tract injuries from pelvic surgery. Am J Obstet Gynecol 1956;71:502.

3 Hurt WG, Dunn LJ. Complications of gynecologic surgery and trauma. In: Greenfield LJ, ed. Complications in surgery and trauma. Philadelphia: JB Lippincott, 1984:790–799.

4 Benson RC, Hinman F. Urinary tract injuries in obstetrics and gynecology. Am J Obstet Gynecol 1955;70:467.

5 Vaselli AJ, Bennett AH. Suture material in urologic and gynecologic surgery. Infect Surg 1983;2:522.

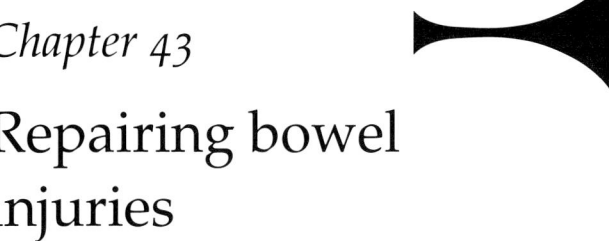

Chapter 43

Repairing bowel injuries

John B. Wheelock and Hans-B. Krebs

Intestinal tract injuries as complications of gynecologic surgery, although uncommon, are potentially lethal. Occurrence is most likely when dealing with endometriosis, pelvic inflammatory disease, or cancer. But many other gynecologic procedures, from simple hysterectomy to uterine curettage, can also cause bowel injury.

Pelvic surgeons should be able to recognize and repair any intestinal injuries they might inadvertently cause or contribute to. To do this successfully requires knowledge of bowel anatomy and use of correct suture material and instruments. The techniques described here should provide guidance.

Injury incidence and types

The true incidence of intestinal tract injury associated with surgery for benign gynecologic conditions is difficult to determine, because superficial injuries are rarely documented. At our institution, during the past decade, 128 bowel injuries requiring surgical repair were recorded. Of all lacerations, 37% occurred during entrance into the peritoneal cavity, 35% while lysing adhesions or performing pelvic or abdominal dissections, 10% during laparoscopy, 9% during vaginal surgery, and 9% during dilation and curettage (D & C) and dilation and evacuation (D & E). Bowel injuries may involve either the small or large bowel, and may be superficial, minor, or major. A superficial injury involves the serosal or superficial muscular layer of the intestine, a minor injury completely penetrates the muscularis or mucosa of the bowel in circumscribed areas, and a major injury interrupts the intestinal mucosa in several areas or in large areas, or actually transects the bowel completely.

Procedures permitting injuries

Entering the peritoneal cavity

If one enters the peritoneal cavity directly through an abdominal incision created by previous surgery, one could injure bowel adhering to the anterior abdominal wall as a result of that surgery. Obese patients are also at risk for intestinal injury during incision when, because of poor exposure, one grasps the small bowel with forceps in an attempt to elevate the peritoneum.

Lysis of adhesions and intra-abdominal and pelvic dissections

One may also cause intestinal injury while lysing adhesions caused by previous abdominal surgery or pelvic infections. Even when performed by experienced hands, dissecting malignant masses and endometriosis involving the bowel carries a high risk of bowel laceration.

Laparoscopy

One may damage the intestinal tract during blind entry into the peritoneal cavity with the Veress needle or trocar. In addition, electrocoagulation can thermally injure the bowel.

Vaginal surgery

The rectum is the bowel site most likely to be injured during vaginal surgery. It may be entered inadvertently during dissection of a rectocele or while attempting to enter the space of Douglas to drain an abscess or for vaginal hysterectomy, transvaginal tubal ligations, or culdoscopy. During such procedures, one may also lacerate small bowel fixed in the posterior cul-de-sac.

Dilation and curettage

D & C and, in particular, D & E for termination of first- and second-trimester pregnancies may result in uterine perforation, and the bowel may be injured by the suction curette.

Preventing bowel injury

When entering the peritoneal cavity

To avoid bowel injury when entering the peritoneal cavity through an abdominal incision created by previous pelvic surgery, extend the new incision above the old one. One may then safely enter the peritoneum in the apical part of the incision. In obese patients who have had no previous abdominal surgery, carefully dissect the preperitoneal fat down to the peritoneum. Grasp the peritoneum with smooth forceps and roll it between the thumb and index finger, separating bowel and abdominal wall serosal surfaces. Then regrasp the peritoneum with the smooth forceps.

When lysing adhesions and doing intra-abdominal pelvic dissections

Always use sharp dissection rather than blunt dissection with fingers or gauze-tipped clamps whenever the dissected tissues do not separate readily. This approach will help to avoid tearing into the bowel wall. It is extremely important to keep dissected tissues under tension and to follow anatomic planes. If dissection of a particular area fails to advance, reevaluate the anatomy and continue dissection at another point where anatomic planes are apparent.

When performing laparoscopy

One can avoid inflicting bowel injury by using an open laparoscope technique when one suspects adhesions. Nasogastric suction to deflate a potentially dilated stomach will decrease the chance of gastric perforation. Use bipolar co-agulation to decrease the risk of bowel burns associated with unipolar instruments. Another way to avoid thermal injury is to make use of clips or bands rather than electrocoagulation for tubal occlusion.

During vaginal surgery

Declining use of culdoscopy and transvaginal tubal ligation has lowered the incidence of bowel complications stemming from vaginal surgery. Inadvertent entrance into the rectum during posterior repair is usually a result of poor technique. One can avoid this problem almost entirely by careful dissection that respects anatomic planes.

During D & C

Correctly determining gestational age and uterine size and position will help to prevent uterine perforation during D & C and D & E, and will thereby reduce the possibility of bowel injury with the suction curette.

Management program

General pointers

Repair all lacerations as soon as they are recognized. When the bowel's full thickness is involved, isolate the injured portion from the rest of the peritoneal cavity to prevent spillage and contamination. Wall the lacerated area off with a moist gauze pack, and place rubber-shod clamps on both sides of the laceration to prevent further contamination.

Coverage against anaerobes with a second- or third-generation cephalosporin for 24 to 48 hours seems logical if an unprepared colon has been penetrated. Remove spilled feces immediately, thoroughly lavage the abdominal cavity after repair, irrigate the abdominal cavity after repair, irrigate the abdominal incision, and consider delayed wound closure.

If one anticipates bowel complications before surgery because of known abscess, endometriosis, extensive adhesions, or tumor, cleanse the bowel mechanically and consider giving antibiotics before proceeding further.

Use fine sutures of chromic or silk (usually 3-0) on an atraumatic needle. Silk sutures, being permanent and stronger, are commonly used in the outside layer of a bowel repair. In contrast with chromic sutures, they should not penetrate the bowel mucosa and should be cut close to the knot. In general, use interrupted rather than continuous ("running") stitches, as they contract the suture line less and reduce risk of lumen stenosis. Continuous stitches are usually satisfactory for suturing the colon because stenosis is less likely.

Place a nasogastric tube during surgery to keep the bowel decompressed, and leave it in place until the patient has active bowel sounds or has passed flatus. Advance the diet after surgery in the usual sequence for a major abdominal procedure. Special feeding precautions are unnecessary.

Superficial injury

One need not repair small superficial tears in the bowel limited to the serosa, as serosal agglutination occurs in a few hours and the bowel heals readily. Small but deeper lacerations are easily repaired with a 3-0 chromic catgut or silk purse-string inverting suture (Fig. 43-1). Place the stitches through the serosal, muscular, and submucosal layer but avoid the mucosa. Then tie the suture and invert the defect.

Close larger superficial tears in the large or small bowel with a single seromuscular layer of interrupted 3-0 silk sutures (Fig. 43-2).

Minor injury

If the injury penetrates the full thickness of the muscularis, or even the mucosa, close it in two layers. An internal row of interrupted 3-0 chromic catgut stitches should include all bowel layers (Fig. 43-3). After tying the sutures, invert the laceration and the first row of stitches with a row of interrupted 3-0 silk Lembert stitches.

Longitudinal lacerations of the small intestine are best repaired transversely to the bowel to prevent luminal stenosis. One can easily convert a longitudinal to a transverse laceration by placing traction sutures into the middle of the tear (Fig. 43-4). However, longitudinal lacerations of the colon may be repaired longitudinally because luminal stenosis is less likely.

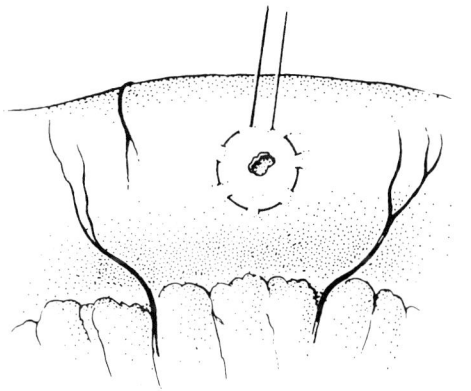

Fig. 43-1 Repair of small bowel laceration with purse-string suture.

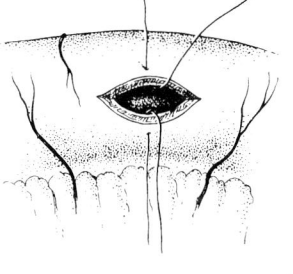

Fig. 43-4 Repair of longitudinal bowel lacerations. Sutures are placed in middle of wound edges. Traction on suture converts direction of laceration from longitudinal to transverse.

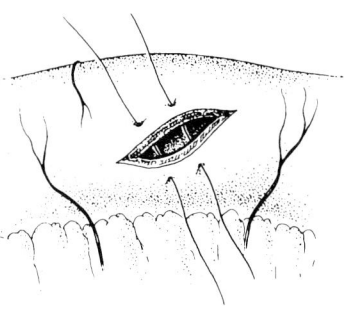
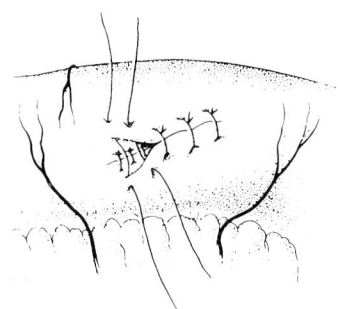

Fig. 43-2 Repair of superficial bowel laceration with a single layer of interrupted 3-0 silk or catgut sutures, showing placement of sutures and sutures tied.

Fig. 43-3 Repair of minor bowel lacerations penetrating entire thickness of bowel wall. Internal layer of interrupted 3-0 chromic catgut sutures includes all three bowel layers. External layer of interrupted 3-0 silk Lembert sutures inverts first suture line.

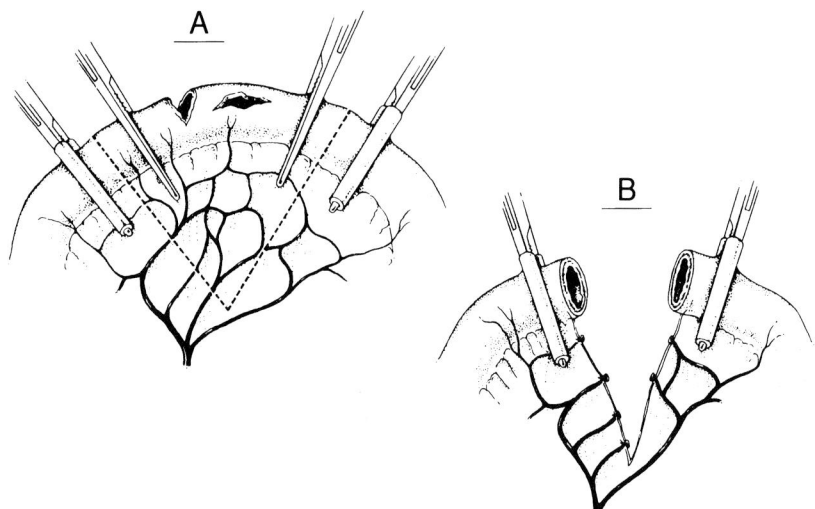

Fig. 43-5 Major injury repair. Preparation and resection of lacerated bowel segment. (A) Note placement of crushing and non-crushing clamps. (B) Lacerated bowel segment excised.

Major injury

Unless inadvertent separation of the bowel with straight wound edges has occurred, repair includes segmental resection before intestinal tract continuity can be restored. First, suction the bowel contents from the injury site. Prevent further spillage of stool by placing crushing (for example, Kocher) clamps on each side of the laceration (Fig. 43-5). Then carefully dissect the mesentery of the injured intestinal segment from the bowel and individually ligate vessels as one encounters them. Place rubber-shod clamps near each end of the intact bowel, and transect the bowel between the clamps.

Gambee anastomosis

In 1951, Gambee described "a single-layer open intestinal anastomosis" applicable to both the small and large intestine (1). The technique, popularized by Wheeless, is easy to learn and results in stronger anastomoses than do alternative suturing procedures (2,3). Size 3-0 chromic catgut may be used for all necessary sutures (Fig. 43-6).

With a Lembert suture, pick up the serosa and muscularis approximately 5 mm from the bowel's edge on the mesenteric side. After tying it on the side, approximate the serosal surfaces of the afferent and efferent loops and invert the bowel mucosa. Place simple through-and-through stitches penetrating the intestinal wall's entire thickness inside the bowel lumen approximately 5 mm apart. Tie all knots on the inside. Because the lumen is inaccessible in the final phase, begin, end, and tie the final stitch on the outside of the anastomosis.

The final stitch should penetrate the bowel wall completely with each maneuver: far outside-in, near inside-out. This done, place Lembert sutures in the 3, 9, and 12 o'clock positions. Together with the one placed earlier at the

mesenteric site (6 o'clock position), these will secure the anastomosis in all quadrants. Finally, check the adequacy of the lumen by palpating the inside of the anastomotic ring between thumb and index finger.

Anastomosis with stapling

Intestinal anastomosis with surgical stapling instruments, a modern alternative to the Gambee technique, appears to offer better healing, because less tissue handling means less edema and inflammation. Because blood supply is interrupted less, the anastomoses are stronger and function sooner than with manual suturing. Also, operating time is reduced. Therefore, the stapling technique is always preferable to manual techniques, provided the surgical instruments are available.

To anastomose the small or large bowel, one will need both a gastrointestinal anastomosis (GIA) and a thoracoabdominal (TA) instrument. The GIA stapler is useful for sealed transection or division of spurs, as it can cut and staple at the same time. The TA stapler, which produces a double staggered row of staples 30, 55, and 90 mm in length but does not transect the bowel, is used to close the incisions and cut ends in the gastrointestinal tract.

To use the two staplers for resection and functional end-to-end enteroanastomosis of the bowel as described by Steichen, transect the lacerated bowel segment with the GIA instrument after dissecting the mesentery (4). Then activate it and divide the bowel, leaving the two ends closed with a double staggered staple line (Fig. 43-7). Excise a corner from the antimesenteric end of the stapled bowel loops just large enough to accommodate the prongs of the GIA instrument (Fig. 43-8). Insert the stapler limbs and align the bowel ends evenly. Close the instrument and simultaneously divide the double wall between the two bowel loops,

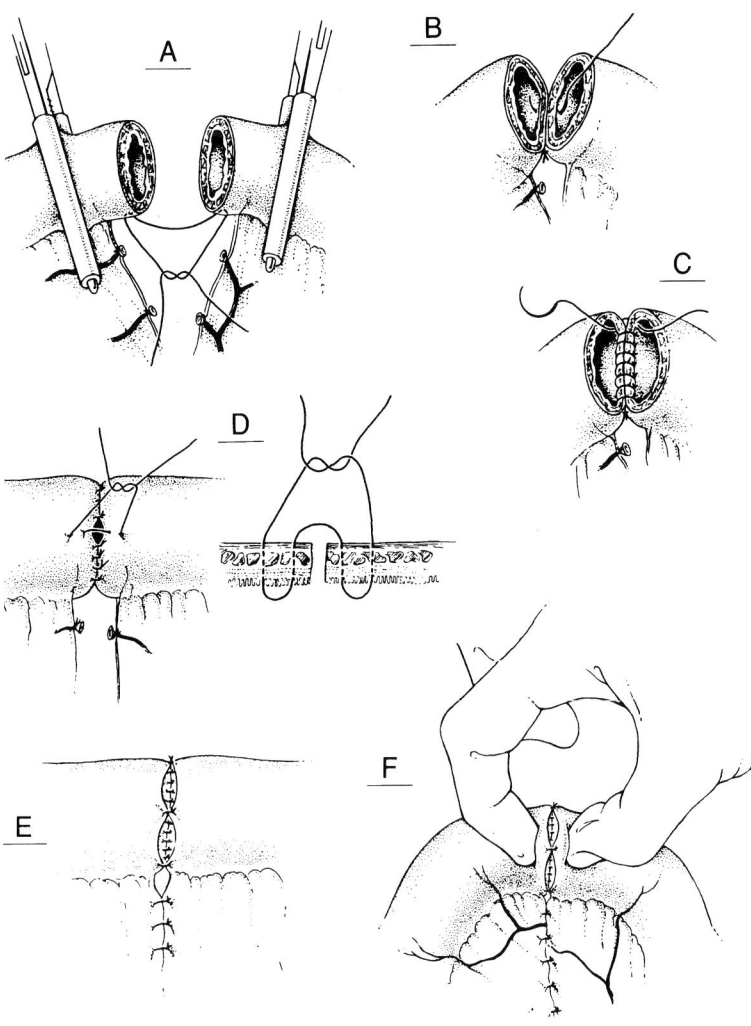

Fig. 43-6 Gambee anastomosis. (A) Lembert suture at mesenteric border. Tying of Lembert suture results in serosa-to-serosa approximation of proximal and distal bowel ends. (B) The first Gambee stitch is placed, and the posterior row of Gambee sutures is completed. (C) All knots are tied on the inside. (D) Final stitch in Gambee anastomosis runs outside-in, inside-out, outside-in, inside-out. Suture goes through all three intestinal wall layers and is tied on outside. Lembert stitches are placed for reinforcement of anastomosis in all bowel quadrants. (E) Mesenteric defect is closed. (F) Adequacy of lumen is checked.

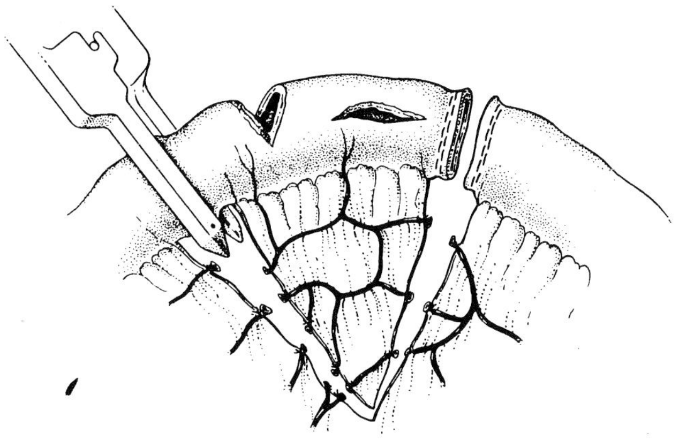

Fig. 43-7 Anastomosis with stapling. Resection of lacerated bowel segment with GIA stapler. A double staggered staple line is placed on specimen and on patent side.

joining the opposed walls by a double staggered staple line on either side of the division.

Withdraw the GIA instrument, leaving a common opening through which one can inspect the anastomotic staple line for hemostasis. Then close the opening with one application of the TA 30 or TA 55 instrument.

Transverse loop colostomy

One should act to protect a large-bowel anastomosis by a proximal temporary colostomy under the following conditions:
• if the bowel was inadequately prepared;
• if closure of the two segments was accomplished under tension;
• if blood supply of the reanastomosed bowel is questionable (for example, because of previous radiation therapy); and
• when reanastomosis is performed in an infected area.
The colostomy provides an exit for feces while placing the distal bowel at rest. This ensures wound healing and decreases the possibility of anastomotic leakage and subsequent breakdown.

A transverse loop colostomy, which is most commonly used, may be brought out through the upper end of the ab-

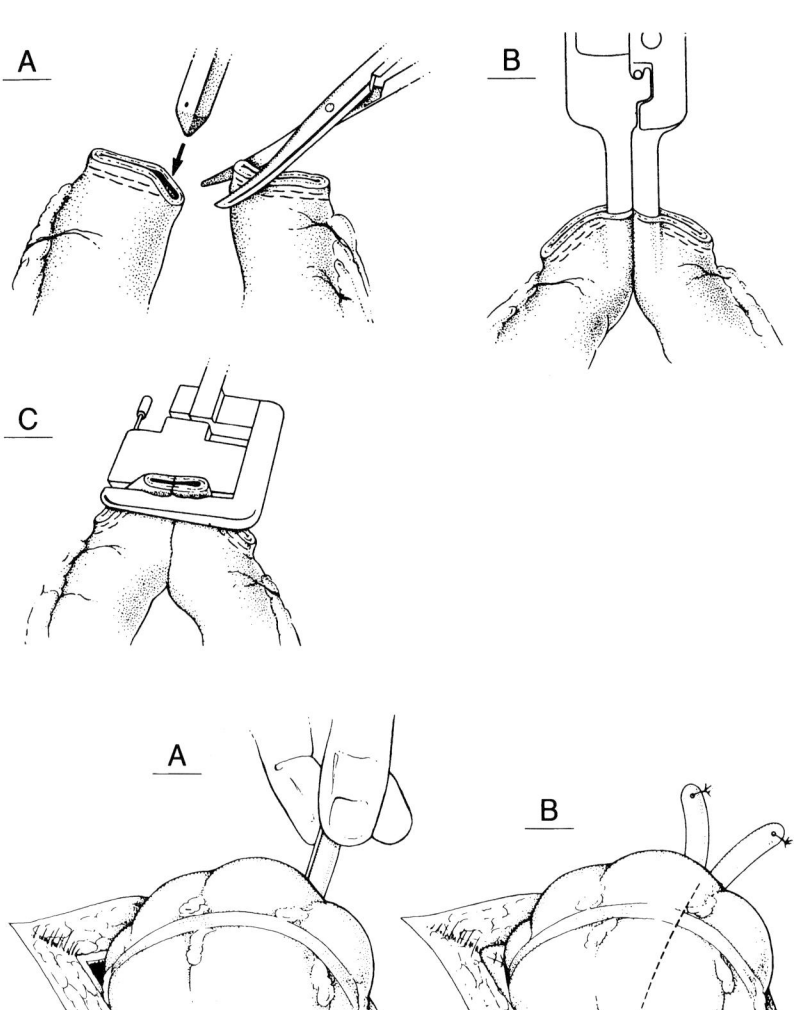

Fig. 43-8 Functional end-to-end anastomosis of bowel. (A) Excision of a corner from antimesenteric end of stapled bowel loops. GIA instrument is inserted into antimesenteric ends of stapled bowel loops. (B) Stapler limbs are aligned and instrument divides double wall between two loops; simultaneously, two double staggered staple lines join bowel wall. (C) Common opening is closed with single application of TA 30 or TA 55.

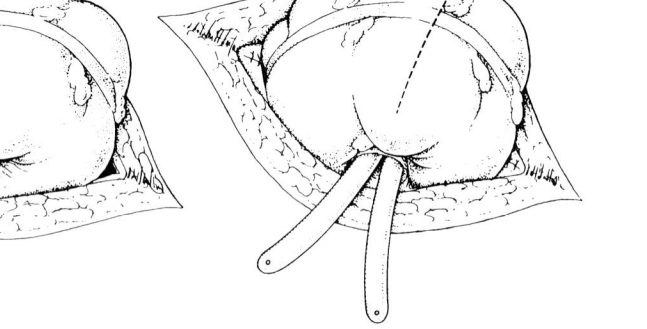

Fig. 43-9 Transverse loop colostomy. (A) Insertion of Hollister bridge through opening in mesocolon in exteriorized bowel segment. (B) Hollister bridge is unfolded and fixed with sutures to the skin. Bowel loop is opened 48 to 72 hours postoperatively by hot cautery along line indicated.

dominal incision above the umbilicus. Generally, the colostomy will be closed within a few weeks, so the patient will not experience any significant long-term problem with herniation.

Alternatively, one may make a small transverse incision in the upper abdomen, on either the right or left side, as circumstances indicate. Identify the omentum and bring it into the wound. One can easily recognize the transverse colon by its haustral markings and can bring the taenia coli into the field without difficulty. Carefully dissect fatty tags and omental attachments off its surface. Then make an opening in the mesocolon immediately adjacent to the bowel, insert a Hollister bridge (Fig. 43-9), unfold it, and allow it to rest on the skin, which will prevent retraction of the exteriorized segment into the peritoneal cavity. One need not stitch the bowel to the abdominal wall.

In closing the peritoneum, fascia, subcutaneous tissue, and skin, take care that sufficient room is left on either side of the bowel to avoid strangulation.

If one desires immediate decompression of the colon, insert a larger catheter (for example, a Malecot) through a stab wound into the bowel. Secure it with a purse-string suture and connect it to a drainage bag. In most cases, one may temporarily cover the loop with Vaseline gauze and leave it closed for 2 to 3 days until the wound has sealed.

Then open the bowel transversely to the axis with hot cautery. Fit a disposable bag around the stoma.

Summary

As can be seen, minor lacerations of the small and large bowel, once recognized, can be repaired with relative ease, while major small-bowel lacerations usually require intestinal resection and reanastomosis. The Gambee technique and, even more so, stapling devices have removed the complexity from intestinal anastomosis. Major large-bowel injury is repaired similarly, but temporary colostomy may be necessary. For this, transverse loop colostomy is most appropriate.

References

1 Gambee LP. A single-layer open intestinal anastomosis applicable to the small as well as the large intestine. West J Surg Obstet Gynecol 1951;59:1.

2 Wheeless CR. The Gambee intestinal anastomosis in gynecologic surgery. Obstet Gynecol 1975;46:448.

3 Hamilton JE. Reappraisal of an open intestinal anastomosis. Ann Surg 1967;165:917.

4 Steichen FM. The use of staples in anatomical side-to-side and functional end-to-end enteroanastomosis. Surgery 1968;64:948.

Chapter 44

Preoperative and postoperative management

Alexander F. Burnett

Preoperative and postoperative care for gynecologic surgery cannot be completely described within the confines of a single book chapter. Rather, this chapter will discuss preoperative radiographic and laboratory evaluations, bowel preparations, and prophylaxis against thromboembolic phenomena.

Preoperative evaluation in benign gynecology

The patient who is to be taken to the operating room with a presumed benign pelvic mass, dysfunctional bleeding, or any other gynecologic complaint worthy of surgical exploration requires judicious use of the minimal amount of laboratory and radiographic tests to potentially identify abnormalities that could alter the approach to the patient. A complete blood count and basic chemistry analyses are inexpensive tests that will yield necessary information preoperatively. All operative candidates require at least a type and screening of a blood sample, with the majority of patients undergoing laparotomy requiring crossmatching for 2 to 4 U of blood. Information about autologous blood donation should be provided. All women of reproductive age should also undergo pregnancy testing, especially before elective surgery.

In the patient with a history of any pulmonary compromise, an arterial blood gas analysis preoperatively on room air can serve two valuable functions. First, it may reveal previously undiagnosed poor pulmonary function, which may alter anesthetic approaches to the patient. Second, it may serve as a baseline from which to compare postoperative values in patients suspected of having acute pulmonary deterioration.

An electrocardiogram and chest radiogram are required before anesthesia in many hospitals for patients over 40 years of age.

Several radiographic studies are available to evaluate women before surgery. One should select those tests that will give specific answers to preoperative questions. For evaluating pelvic architecture and morphology, ultrasonography can be very helpful, particularly with the addition of vaginal-probe ultrasound. Computed tomography and magnetic resonance imaging can also delineate pelvic pathology, but at a much higher cost than ultrasound. An intravenous pyelogram (IVP) is important in defining the course of the ureters, possible duplications within the urinary system, the presence of a pelvic kidney, and the morphology of the ureters, which may indicate obstruction or lack of function of urinary tract organs. The intimate anatomic relation between the ureters and the gynecologic organs underscores the importance of identifying the ureteral course—this is particularly true in anticipated surgeries involving endometriosis, pelvic inflammatory disease, oncologic surgery, irradiated patients, or repeat pelvic surgeries, as all of these conditions may insinuate the ureters to even closer proximity to the pelvic organs.

Preparation for the operating room

An adequate discussion of the planned surgical procedure with the patient preoperatively is paramount. A reasonable explanation of potential complications must be included. Informed consent dictates that all reasonable therapeutic options be presented to the patient in such a way that she can make an intelligent decision about treatment course.

Bowel preparation

All patients undergoing abdominopelvic surgery should undergo bowel preparation preoperatively. Mechanical and antibiotic bowel preparations reduce fecal load within the bowels and reduce bacterial load within the feces. The advantages to these properties are many. For simplicity in operating in the pelvis, bowels that are emptied of their contents may be packed out of the field more easily. More importantly, the risks to the patient in the event of inadvertent puncture of the bowel lumen are greatly reduced. Small punctures in a well-prepared colon may be easily handled by oversewing the defect in one or two layers as determined by the size of the defect (1). Larger defects and coagulation injuries to the bowel may require resection of the damaged portion of the bowel. Most often, resections of well-prepared bowel may be satisfactorily reanastomosed without radically altering the patient's postoperative course. However, significant compromise of the unprepared sigmoid colon and subsequent fecal spill often necessitate a colostomy (2). Adequate bowel preparation is the best insurance that, should inadvertent injury occur during gynecologic surgery, a colostomy will not have to be performed.

Many bowel problems mimic gynecologic illness. A pelvic mass may be discovered at laparotomy to be colonic in origin, such as one related to Crohn's disease or a colonic carcinoma. Conditions that may mimic acute gynecologic disease, including acute pelvic inflammatory disease or torsion of the adnexae, include appendicitis, Meckel's diverticulitis, diverticulitis or diverticular abscess, and volvulus. All these conditions would be more safely operated on with a prepared intestinal tract. In an emergent situation in which there is the possibility of perforating a viscus (such as a suspected perforated ectopic pregnancy), bowel preparation would be unwarranted as a waste of valuable time.

There are several methods of mechanically preparing the bowel. The two most common procedures are the 3-day mechanical preparation and the one-day mechanical preparation. The 3-day preparation that we use involves having the patient take in only clear liquids for 3 days before surgery. The night before surgery the patient drinks 10 ounces of magnesium citrate, and, if the fecal stream is not mostly clear at this point, we may administer a small enema in the morning before surgery. This procedure can be done completely on an outpatient basis and is generally well tolerated by the patient. Appropriate counseling of a specific clear liquid diet must be provided for patients with dietary

restrictions. The one-day procedure, which we use in the majority of our patients, involves administration of an oral polyethylene glycol solution (GoLytely) that lavages the gut. The patient drinks approximately 4 L of the solution over 2 to 3 hours beginning in the late afternoon before surgery. The fecal stream should be clear at the completion of this preparation, and rarely are further evacuation methods necessary. This preparation is well tolerated by patients, provides less intestinal cramping than magnesium citrate overall, and provides a superior cleansing of the gut with reduced bacterial content (3). Preparation with polyethylene glycol does not significantly alter the patient's electrolytes or hematologic parameters (4).

Some advocate the addition of oral antibiotics in the preparation of the bowel. The usual regimen involves an erythromycin-based antibiotic and neomycin taken within 12 hours of surgery. We routinely administer parenteral antibiotics at the time of surgery, generally a first- or second-generation cephalosporin, which has been shown to diminish the postoperative wound infection rate (5). Parenteral antibiotic prophylaxis may also include a third-generation cephalosporin (such as ceftriaxone) and metronidazole in those cases in which colonic surgery is highly anticipated. As with any genital tract surgery, antibiotic prophylaxis for subacute bacterial endocarditis must be performed when indicated.

Thromboembolic prophylaxis

Venous thrombosis and pulmonary embolism can be a significant problem following gynecologic surgery. Studies have shown up to 46% of postoperative deaths from gynecologic procedures for benign disease are due to pulmonary embolism (6). In the United States, pulmonary embolism is the most frequent medical cause of maternal mortality associated with live births (7). Overall women are at an increased risk of pulmonary embolism, with a prevalence of 4.5 occurrences per 10,000 women per year in the United States compared with 1.75 occurrences per 10,000 men per year (8). Virchow's three factors predisposing to venous thrombosis are hypercoagulability, venous stasis, and vessel injury. Prophylaxis for deep venous thrombosis and pulmonary embolism therefore is directed at preventing all three from developing. Patients with gynecologic malignancies are at particular risk because their cancer contributes to a hypercoagulable state, their pelvic surgeries tend to be long, and their recovery time tends to be prolonged.

Vessel injury can be minimized with good surgical technique. Avoidance of prolonged retraction along the pelvic vessels is critical, and this is achieved by careful placement of retractors, particularly self-retaining retractors, away from the area of the vessels. Direct injury to major vessels should be repaired immediately. One should also avoid placement in the lithotomy position with the hips hyperflexed for prolonged periods of time, as this will impede venous return from the legs.

Two types of therapy are used for the prevention of pulmonary embolism: pharmacologic and nonpharmacologic. To significantly decrease fatal pulmonary embolism, all large prospective trials of preventive techniques have documented the necessity of initiating the techniques before surgery and continuing them for the duration of the postoperative stay (9). The most common pharmacologic prophylaxis used is heparin therapy, typically given as 5000 U subcutaneously 2 hours preoperatively and every 8 hours thereafter for up to 7 days. This regimen has demonstrated a decrease in venous thrombosis and pulmonary emboli (10). There is a nonsignificant increase in the incidence of postoperative wound hematomas in patients treated with this regimen (11). In the event of postoperative bleeding while on heparin, the half-life of the drug is very short, and anticoagulation should be reversed within approximately 4 hours. If anticoagulation must be reversed rapidly, protamine sulfate will neutralize heparin. The other potential side effect of heparin therapy is thrombocytopenia secondary to an immune phenomenon (12). This typically will occur 6 to 14 days after the initiation of heparin; however, milder forms of thrombocytopenia may occur as shortly as 2 days after beginning therapy. Therefore, all patients on heparin should have their platelet counts monitored routinely. Other pharmacologic agents used for prophylaxis include dextran, which reduces platelet function, and warfarin, which interferes with the clotting cascade.

Nonpharmacologic prophylaxis

In the high-risk patient (history of recent deep venous thrombosis or previous documented pulmonary embolism), one may consider placement of a filter in the inferior vena cava preoperatively. These devices will trap any significantly sized clot from proceeding to the lungs while maintaining patency of the inferior vena cava.

In all of our patients we utilize pneumatic compression stockings preoperatively, during surgery, and postoperatively until the patient is ready for discharge from the hospital. These stockings typically extend to the knee, with the compression bladder over the gastrocnemius muscles. These periodically inflate to a pressure of 25 to 35 mm Hg. This compression of the calf serves two purposes: first, it prevents venous stasis in the legs, which has been documented to augment flow in the femoral veins and the inferior vena cava; second, it increases the patient's own fibrinolytic activity, reducing the incidence of deep venous thrombosis (13). Studies have shown that even with the compression devices placed on patient's arms, there is a significant reduction in deep venous thrombosis, attributable to increased fibrinolytic activity (14).

Controlled studies have revealed that use of pneumatic compression stockings only during the first 24 hours postoperatively is ineffective in reducing the risk of thromboembolism and pulmonary embolism. When applied preoperatively and used for the duration of the postoperative stay, the pneumatic compression stockings have shown a significant prevention of deep venous thrombosis and pulmonary embolism (13).

Combining pharmacologic and nonpharmacologic regimens theoretically may afford synergistic prophylaxis against pulmonary embolism. The World Health Organization's task force on the prevention of pulmonary embolism suggests that for high-risk patients (defined as patients undergoing orthopedic surgery or surgery for gynecologic malignancies), there may be an additive benefit to combining use of pneumatic compression stockings and low-dose heparin (15). One or a combination of these methods should be utilized in any patient undergoing abdominopelvic surgery to prevent the development of deep venous thrombosis or pulmonary embolism.

References

1 Delgado G. Complications related to the nonradiated gastrointestinal tract. In: Delgado G, Smith JP, eds. Management of complications in gynecologic oncology. New York: Wiley, 1982:45.

2 Cohn I, Nance FC. Intestinal antisepsis and peritonitis from perforation. In: Sabiston DS, ed. Textbook of surgery. Philadelphia: WB Saunders, 1986:991.

3 Fleites RA, Marshall JB. The efficacy of polyethylene glycol–electrolyte lavage solution versus traditional mechanical bowel preparation for elective colonic surgery: a randomized, prospective, blinded clinical trial. Surgery 1985;98:708.

4 Huddy SP, Rayter Z. Preparation of the bowel before elective surgery using a polyethylene glycol solution at home and in hospital compared with conventional preparation using magnesium sulphate. J R Coll Surg Edinb 1990;35:16.

5 Schoetz DJ, Roberts PL. Addition of parenteral cefoxitin to regimen of oral antibiotics for elective colorectal operations. A randomized prospective study. Ann Surg 1990;212:209.

6 Amirikia H, Evans TN. Ten-year review of hysterectomies: trends, indications, and risks. Am J Obstet Gynecol 1979;134:431.

7 Centers for Disease Control. CDC Surveillance Summaries. MMWR 1991;40:1.

8 Quinn DA, Thompson BT. A prospective investigation of pulmonary embolism in women and men. JAMA 1992;268:1689.

9 Koppenhagen K, Adolf J. Low molecular weight heparin and prevention of postoperative thrombosis in abdominal surgery. Thromb Haemost 1992;67:627.

10 Clarke-Pearson DL, DeLong ER. A controlled trial of two low-dose heparin regimens for the prevention of postoperative deep venous thrombosis. Obstet Gynecol 1990;75:684.

11 Clarke-Pearson DL, DeLong ER. Complications of low-dose heparin prophylaxis in gynecologic oncology surgery. Obstet Gynecol 1984;64:689.

12 Walls JT, Curtis JJ. Heparin-induced thrombocytopenia in patients who undergo open heart surgery. Surgery 1990;108:686.

13 Clarke-Pearson DL, Synan IS. Prevention of postoperative venous thromboembolism by external pneumatic calf compression in patients with gynecologic malignancy. Obstet Gynecol 1984;63:92.

14 Knight MTN, Dawson R. Effect of intermittent compression of the arms on deep venous thrombosis in the legs. Lancet 1976;2:230.

15 Goldhaber SZ, Morpurgo M. Diagnosis, treatment, and prevention of pulmonary embolism. Report of the WHO/International Society and Federation of Cardiology Task Force. JAMA 1992;268:1727.

Chapter 45

Management and prevention of pelvic adhesions

Shawky Z. A. Badawy and

Christina M. Drollette

During the past two decades, several investigators evaluated the various causes of pelvic adhesions and the means of their prevention and treatment. The results of these studies suggest that pelvic adhesions lead to serious problems: namely, pelvic pain, intestinal obstruction, and infertility. However, little is still known about the mechanisms involved in their formation and prevention. This also suggests that more research is needed to achieve optimum results in prevention and treatment of pelvic adhesions.

Operations on the female pelvic organs present a unique set of circumstances with regard to the formation of adhesions. There is relatively little intrinsic motility in the female reproductive organs, and blood tends to pool in the pelvis; both circumstances tend to promote the formation of adhesions. Certainly, gynecologic surgeons recognize the prevalence of such pelvic adhesions from their clinical practice. Therefore, the prevention of postoperative adhesions is a pertinent topic for all gynecologists, especially for those specializing in infertility (1).

In the era before abdominal and pelvic surgical procedures had become common, adhesions were of little importance. Rarely mentioned in standard surgical textbooks, they found their place only in the writings of pathologists. As the frequency of abdominopelvic surgery has increased over the last century, the incidence of pelvic adhesions has risen in direct proportion (2).

The incidence of pelvic adhesions in the general population is not known. The incidences reported pertain to studies in special groups of symptomatic patients. In a retrospective review by Rapkin of 100 consecutive laparoscopies performed to evaluate chronic pelvic pain, 26 (26%) of 100 patients had pelvic adhesions. In the same study, 34 (39%) of 88 infertility patients undergoing laparoscopy had pelvic adhesions (3). These two subsets should not be used, however, to estimate the incidence of adhesions in the general population, because pelvic pain and infertility are associated with pelvic adhesions, and therefore the studies include biased populations. Women undergoing laparoscopy for tubal ligation are perhaps a better representation of the general population. In a study by Kresch and associates, out of 50 asymptomatic women who underwent a tubal ligation via the laparoscope, 12% had adhesions (4). The incidence is therefore significant, and the topic is worthy of consideration. It is only through fundamental knowledge that treatment can be instituted and adhesions and their complications prevented.

Etiology

The etiology of pelvic adhesions is multifactorial. Tissue trauma due to surgery or improper handling, introduction of foreign bodies, and inflammatory disease play important roles. In a study by Stovall, Elder, and Ling, it was found that a history of previous pelvic surgery was significantly associated with the presence of adhesive disease ($p < 0.001$)

343

(5). Postoperative adhesions have been described in 55% to 100% of patients at the time of second-look laparoscopy following laparotomy for pelvic surgery (6–8). These included both re-formed and de novo adhesions. Adhesion development has also been described following laparoscopic surgery. It is known that trauma damages the peritoneal tissue and underlying vascular structures, which leads to the release of various inflammatory cells, fibrinogen, histamine, and vasoactive kinins. These substances increase vascular permeability with more exudation of fibrinogen and inflammatory cells. If the peritoneum is capable of producing plasminogen activator, then the fibrinous deposits break down and resolve without adhesion formation. On the other hand, lack of production of plasminogen activator by the peritoneal cells allows the persistence of fibrinous deposits and adhesion formation. A vast number of both experimental and clinical observations confirm that any circumstance which produces ischemic tissue can cause the development of adhesions to such tissue (2). Buckman and associates discovered that plasminogen activator activity is normally present in the mesothelium and submesothelial blood vessels of peritoneum. This activity results in the spontaneous lysis of many fibrinous attachments within 72 to 96 hours of development of the fibrin. Grafts can greatly diminish this activity if the underlying peritoneum is made ischemic upon application of the graft. Tight suturing can also create ischemia and hence result in decreased availability of plasminogen activator. The peritoneum not only loses its ability to lyse fibrin, but it may also actively inhibit fibrinolysis by normal tissues (9). Mechanical abrasion of peritoneal surfaces also reduces plasminogen activator activity and hence may explain the association between adhesion formation and abrasion (10).

Foreign bodies such as powders from the surface of gloves, lint from packs, drapes, or gowns, wood fibers from disposable paper items, and suture materials have been found in a large percentage of postoperative adhesions. In a study by Weibel and Majno, foreign bodies were observed in two-thirds of the cases of postoperative adhesions found at autopsy (11). The presence of foreign bodies is suggestive of a cause-effect relationship for the formation of adhesions. Recent data suggest, however, that in the absence of an additional peritoneal injury, foreign bodies are an infrequent cause of adhesion formation (12). Holtz investigated the importance of suture size, suture reactivity, and peritoneal injury concurrent with suturing and found that the use of microsuture might reduce postoperative adhesion formation. This study failed to show that the histologic reactivity of suture materials was a significant variable in adhesion induction. The experiment also confirmed that suture placement infrequently induces adhesion formation when no concurrent peritoneal injury exists (13).

Ryan, Grobety, and Majno, using male and female Wistar rats, tested the effect of two relatively minor insults that commonly occur in the surgical setting—drying of the serosal surface and bleeding—on the formation of adhesions. The results of their study showed that drying alone has little effect, but drying along with bleeding consistently produced adhesions to the dried area. Fresh blood alone also produced adhesions (14). These observations may explain why the posterior cul-de-sac, where blood tends to gravitate, is so frequently involved in postoperative adhesions.

Pelvic adhesions may result from any inflammatory process that irritates the peritoneum. Such conditions include pelvic inflammatory disease (PID), appendicitis, peritonitis, endometriosis, and the previous use of an intrauterine contraceptive device (5). In PID, the presence of inflammatory cells, their secretions, and peritoneal injury lead to adhesions. The relation between appendicitis and infertility is variable. Geerdsen and Bech Hansen compared 39 women who had surgery in childhood for acute perforated appendicitis with 39 women who had surgery in childhood for acute nonperforated appendicitis with respect to sterility and found no statistically significant difference in the incidence of sterility between the two groups (15). Mueller and colleagues studied the importance of a history of appendectomy for appendicitis in 279 women with laparoscopically or surgically diagnosed tubal infertility and a control group of 957 fertile women. No excess risk of tubal infertility was associated with a simple appendectomy without rupture. However, when the operation was reportedly for a ruptured appendix, the relative risk of tubal infertility was 4.8 for women who had never been pregnant and 3.2 for women with one or more previous pregnancies. The authors concluded that early diagnosis and treatment of suspected appendicitis in girls and women of reproductive age may reduce the incidence of tubal infertility resulting from the sequelae of a ruptured appendix (16).

Peritonitis of an infectious form is clearly associated with adhesion formation. The mechanisms by which infection induces adhesions have not been clearly established; however, bacteria release numerous enzymes that may damage tissue and produce substantial inflammatory exudates. In addition, bacteria secrete substances that may limit blood flow to the tissues and attract inflammatory cells (12).

Much work has been done recently in trying to elucidate the role of cytokines and tissue plasminogen activator, and how they relate to the formation of pelvic adhesions. Heinonen, Aine, and Seppala studied the concentrations of peritoneal fluid leukotriene B_4 and prostaglandin E_2 in women with acute salpingitis confirmed by laparoscopy. The mean levels in the peritoneal fluid of women with acute salpingitis were significantly higher than the respective levels in the peritoneal fluid of control subjects. The authors suggested that these chemical mediators may therefore have a role in the development of peritoneal adhesions after acute salpingitis (17).

Thompson and coworkers studied the effect of inflammation and ischemia on plasminogen activator activity. They reported that inflamed peritoneum had significantly less plasminogen activator activity than did normal peritoneum and that visceral ischemia also resulted in a significant decrease in plasminogen activator activity. These data support the hypothesis that plasminogen activator activity is needed to prevent the production of fibrous adhesions, because fibrous adhesions are so often found after inflammation and ischemia of the peritoneum (18).

Vipond and associates also found that plasminogen activator activity was significantly lower in inflamed peritoneum than in control tissue. In addition, they found that plasminogen activator inhibitor-1 was not detectable in control peritoneum, but was detectable in inflamed tissue, and hence might be another explanation for the reduction in fibrinolytic activity in inflamed tissue (19).

To investigate the usefulness of recombinant tissue plasminogen activator as an agent in reducing postoperative pelvic adhesions, Doody, Dunn, and Buttram applied recombinant tissue plasminogen activator to a rabbit uterine horn injury model. On second laparoscopy, it was found that treatment with recombinant tissue plasminogen activator significantly reduced both adhesion quantity and density (20). Menzies and Ellis also found that recombinant tissue plasminogen activator applied topically is an effective inhibitor of adhesion formation in the rabbit model (21).

Decreased plasminogen activator activity has been suggested as a mechanism of pelvic adhesion formation in women with endometriosis. However, currently available data do not support this suggestion. In a study by Batzofin and associates, the peritoneal fluid level of plasminogen activator activity was assayed. In 45 patients studied, there were no discernible differences between the level in patients with and that in patients without endometriosis or pelvic adhesions. If such differences exist, they may be present in the tissues, but apparently are not detectable in the peritoneal fluid (22).

Perforation of the uterus is one of the complications of the use of an intrauterine device that can result in the inadvertent introduction of the device into the peritoneal cavity. Badawy and Iskander examined the omental reaction to "Lippes Loop" intrauterine contraceptive devices that perforated the uterus. Microscopic examination of the omental tissues surrounding the perforated loop was consistent with foreign body granulomatous reaction (23).

Therefore, trauma to the peritoneal surface, either during surgery or due to foreign material, results in inhibition of plasminogen activator and increased production of leukotriene B_4 and prostaglandin E_2. These reactions mediate adhesion formation.

Pathogenesis

The peritoneum is a thin layer of loose connective tissue covered by a layer of mesothelium (Fig. 45-1). Destruction of the serosa results in the outpouring of fibrinogen; a fibrin clot forms, causing the adherence of adjacent structures; this fibrin clot, if not absorbed, eventually becomes organized by fibroblast proliferation to produce collagenous adhesions (Fig. 45-2).

Milligan and Raftery followed the development of adhesions microscopically after abdominal surgery in the rat (24). On the first postoperative day, capillary dilatation and margination were noted at the visceral surfaces of the adhesions, with an outpouring of mainly polymorphonuclear leukocytes and fibrin. Approximately 3 to 4 days after surgery the macrophage was the predominant inflammatory cell and the fibrin began to disappear. On postoperative day 5 fibroblasts and bundles of collagen constituted the adhesions. They increased in amount between 2 weeks and 2 months after surgery.

The continuity of the mesothelium has been considered the key to fibrin absorption and the prevention of adhesion formation (25). Raftery, in an electron microscopic study to determine the origin of new mesothelium (26), concluded that the contribution of detached mesothelial cells to peri-

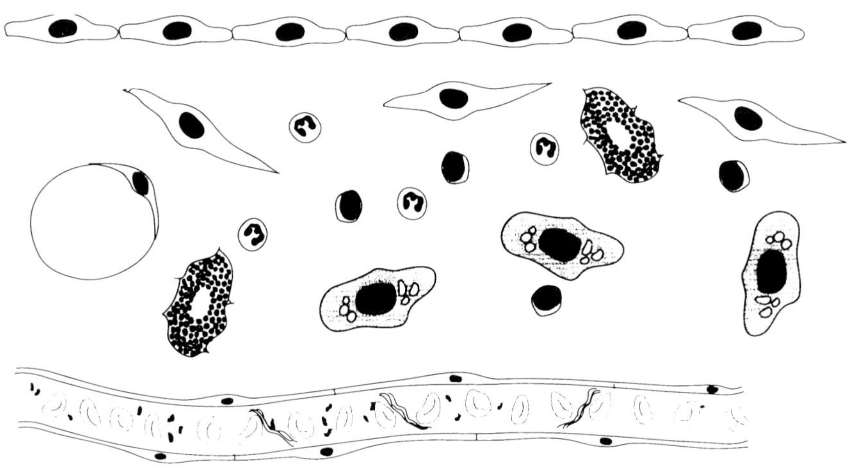

Fig. 45-1 Normal peritoneum consists of a layer of mesothelial cells overlying loose connective tissue containing lymphocytes, macrophages, adipocytes, fibroblasts, plasma cells, mast cells, and blood vessels.

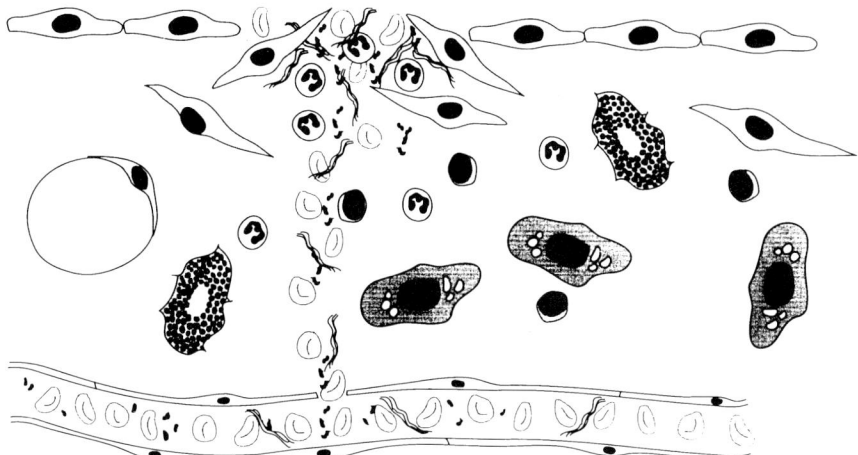

Fig. 45-2 Adhesions form when there is destruction of the serosa. The connective tissue vasculature transports various cell types to the injured area, including polymorphonuclear leukocytes, platelets, and fibrin. A sticky fibrinous exudate forms, causing adherence of adjacent structures.

toneal wound healing is negligible. It appears that mesothelial cells which become detached at the time of operation instead enter the peritoneal fluid, and probably undergo necrosis subsequently (26). It is known that large defects heal as rapidly as smaller ones, perhaps because mesothelization occurs from the base of the defect (25). Raftery, in his electron microscopy study, tried to elucidate the origin of the "new" mesothelial cells. He concluded that the new mesothelium arises from subperitoneal connective tissue cells but could not determine conclusively whether the "new" cells arise from primitive mesenchymal cells or fibroblasts present in the perivascular connective tissue. It was clear that mesothelial cells were present at the base of the wound within 2 days of peritoneal injury, with complete healing by a single layer of mesothelial cells occurring in 5 days (26).

All these studies address the peritoneal factors leading to formation of new adhesions. Recurrence of adhesions following adhesiolysis is probably a different process related to impaired healing as a result of decreased blood supply and preexisting fibroblastic reaction. The study of the peritoneal fluid changes in patients with pelvic adhesions may lead to understanding of the various biological factors associated with these adhesions. Various cytokines are present in peritoneal fluid. Interleukin-1 and tumor necrosis factor were demonstrated in the peritoneal fluid of patients with endometriosis. Interleukin-6 was demonstrated in high concentrations in patients with nonendometriotic pelvic adhesions. Peritoneal macrophages are known to produce interleukin-1, tumor necrosis factor, and interleukin-6. It has been suggested that elevated peritoneal levels of interleukin-6 may be due to the presence of subclinical infection. In addition, interleukin-1 and tumor necrosis factor in peritoneal fluid may stimulate the production of interleukin-6 by vascular endothelium (27). The role of the various interleukins in the etiology of adhesions or the symptoms related to the presence of these adhesions needs further studies.

Clinical significance

Pelvic adhesions are a significant cause of mechanical small-bowel obstruction (5,28), infertility (5,25,26), and pelvic pain (5,29,30).

Adhesions have been implicated as a cause of pelvic pain by their restriction of movement of pelvic organs (4). In a study by Kresch and coworkers, laparoscopy was used to evaluate women who consistently reported pelvic pain in the same location for a minimum of 6 months, versus asymptomatic women who underwent laparoscopy for tubal ligation. In the control group, adhesions found were loose, allowing free and unrestricted movement of the organs. In the patients complaining of chronic pain, adhesions appeared to restrict motion or expansibility of one or more organs. It was suggested that adhesions that restrict mobility or distensibility of organs are more likely to cause pelvic pain than those adhesions that do not (4). Further studies are indicated to investigate the location and type of nerve endings contiguous to the adhesions. It also would be interesting to study the levels of bradykinin, histamine, and other autocoids that are able to stimulate pain receptors in order to rule out other factors as the cause of the chronic pelvic pain.

Questions have also been raised about the effect of adhesions on follicular development. With respect to infertility, the effect of periovarian adhesions on ovarian response to gonadotropins has been the subject of several studies. In a study by Diamond and colleagues, the effect of periovarian adhesions on follicular development was assessed by the estradiol response to ovarian stimulation, by the sonographic appearance of the ovaries on the day of human chorionic gonadotropin (hCG) administration, and by the number of follicles aspirated and the number of mature oocytes recovered at laparoscopy. The ability to aspirate ovarian follicles did not correlate with serum estradiol level on either the day of or the day after hCG administration. Similarly, the total number of follicles 1.0 to 1.4 cm or larger than 1.5 cm did not correlate with the number of follicles aspirated. It appeared that periovarian adhesions are not a major determinant of the ovarian response to gonadotropin stimulation (31).

Similarly, a study by Mahadevan and colleagues also examined the effect of periovarian adhesive disease upon folliculogenesis. Forty-one stimulated cycles of women taking clomiphene citrate, human menopausal gonadotropin, and hCG for in vitro fertilization and embryo transfer were studied. Each patient was assessed by ultrasound before laparoscopic oocyte recovery. The follicles in each ovary larger than 1.2 cm were counted. By laparoscopy it was possible to determine the degree of periovarian adhesive disease. In total, 116 follicles were collected from 45 adhesion-free ovaries, and 59 follicles were collected from 37 adhesed ovaries. These numbers are, statistically, significantly different. In contrast to the study by Diamond and coworkers, these data suggest that the presence of periovarian adhesive disease inhibits folliculogenesis by a yet undetermined mechanism (32). A possible explanation for poor folliculogenesis may be ovarian entrapment. It may be that the mechanical pressures of adhesions around the ovaries inhibit adequate follicular growth. If an optimum follicular diameter of 1.8 cm is to be reached, then space must exist for follicles to develop (33). Molloy and coworkers evaluated the effect of inducing ovulation in 23 patients with severe adhesions and in 48 patients with adhesion-free ovaries in 51 treatment cycles. A significantly higher number of cancelled oocyte retrievals, a significantly lower rate of estradiol rise, and a lower peak value of estradiol before and after the administration of hCG were found in patients with severe adhesions. These patients took longer to respond to a hyperstimulation regimen, and when a response finally occurred, they formed fewer follicles. Fewer oocytes were aspirated from the study group and resulted in lower pregnancy rates in the patients with adhesions. The majority of these patients had a history of severe PID as the cause of their adhesions. Oophoritis as well as salpingitis may have been present. Such severe infection may compromise ovarian blood supply and, with resultant ovarian capsule scarring, diminish optimum follicular growth (33). Hence, perhaps intrinsic disease, rather than the adhesions themselves, was partially or wholly responsible for the poor performance of these patients.

In humans, the ovulated oocytes adhere with their cumulus mass of follicular cells to the surface of the ovary. The fimbriated end of the tube sweeps over the ovary to pick up the ovum (29). Entry of ova into the tube is facilitated by muscular movements that bring the fimbria into contact with the surface of the ovary (34). Any periovarian or peritubal adhesions may interfere with this mechanism and result in infertility (29).

Ectopic pregnancies have been implicated as a possible sequela of peritubal adhesions (30). Tubal pregnancy can result from a delay in the passage of the conceptus through the fallopian tube. Peritubal adhesions may reflect the presence of endosalpingeal damage, or they may alter tubal motility and theoretically could predispose a patient to the occurrence of a tubal pregnancy. In a study by Tulandi and colleagues, 69 women found to have periadnexal adhesions on laparoscopic examination underwent subsequent laparotomy and salpingo-ovariolysis, and 78 women found to have periadnexal adhesions on laparoscopic examination did not undergo subsequent adhesiolysis. There was no difference in the ectopic pregnancy rate between the treated group and the nontreated group, but the incidence was increased above that in women without pelvic adhesions. In this study salpingo-ovariolysis did not decrease the incidence of ectopic pregnancy, suggesting that endosalpingeal damage plays a more important role in the development of ectopic pregnancy than do peritubal adhesions (35).

Diagnosis

A diagnosis of pelvic adhesions can be reached by a combination of predictive factors in the history, physical examination of a patient, direct vision, and radiographic adjuncts.

Stovall, Elder, and Ling undertook a prospective study to determine if the presence of pelvic adhesions at subsequent laparoscopy could be predicted by the preoperative history and physical examination. They analyzed 273 patients undergoing laparoscopy. At the time of the preoperative history and physical examination, the only historical predictor significantly associated with adhesive disease was previous pelvic surgery. Physical examination predictors significantly associated with the presence of adhesions included uterine immobility, a right adnexal mass, and right adnexal tenderness. Other historical predictors not significantly associated with pelvic adhesions included a history of PID, endometriosis, previous pelvic adhesions, previous tubal occlusions, and chronic pelvic pain. Physical examination predictors not significantly associated with adhesive disease at laparoscopy were cervical motion tenderness, uterine tenderness, left adnexal tenderness, and left adnexal mass. It is noteworthy that a right adnexal mass and right adnexal tenderness were significantly associated with pelvic adhesions, but a left adnexal mass and left adnexal tenderness were not. The authors theorize that perhaps this is because most examiners use the right hand to perform a pelvic examination, thereby making the right adnexa easier to palpate. Also, the sigmoid colon may interfere with palpation of the left adnexa. This is contradicted, however, by the fact that in this study the most frequent physical finding was left adnexal tenderness. This study also revealed a 25.6% false-negative rate for patients with both a negative history and a normal physical examination. Hence, the approach to the patient with chronic pelvic pain or infertility could be guided, to some extent, by a history of previous pelvic surgery or uterine immobility, but reservations must still be held (5).

Hysterosalpingography is a useful radiologic adjunct in diagnosing pelvic adhesions. Karasick and Goldfarb studied the efficacy of hysterosalpingography in the detection of peritubal adhesions without tubal occlusion and used laparoscopy to verify their results. Peritubal adhesions were diagnosed on hysterosalpingography by using the following radiographic criteria alone or in combination: convoluted fallopian tube, loculation of spillage of contrast medium into the peritoneal cavity, ampullary dilatation, peritubal halo effect (double contour appearance of the tubal wall), and vertical fallopian tube. Of patients with the hysterosalpingographic diagnosis of peritubal adhesions, 75% had this diagnosis confirmed by subsequent laparoscopy, resulting in a 25% false-positive rate of diagnosis of peritubal adhesions using hysterosalpingography. These findings suggest that hysterosalpingography can be a useful diagnostic procedure in the initial investigation of infertility due to peritubal adhesions, but confirm that laparoscopy and laparotomy are the only definitive procedures in identifying peritubal adhesions (36).

Hydrogynecography is a new technique to visualize pelvic adhesions by the use of transvaginal ultrasonography following introduction of fluid medium in the cul-de-sac via the uterine cavity. Maroulis and associates evaluated 38 patients for infertility and pelvic pain using this technique. The examination was conducted with the patient in the dorsal lithotomy position following careful cleaning of the vagina and cervix using iodine-povidone (Betadine) and saline solutions. Saline was injected through a uterine balloon catheter inserted into the uterus. The amount of saline used varied between 150 and 300 ml per patient to create enough fluid medium in the cul-de-sac. The ultrasonographic examination showed adhesions in 9 of 38 patients, and these were confirmed by laparoscopy. The ultrasonography failed to diagnose adhesions in four of the remaining patients. The overall predictive value of hydrogynecography was 84%. The problems related to this method include pelvic pain during the procedure due to uterine contractility. Also, tubal occlusion limits the value of this technique because fluid cannot be introduced into the pelvic cavity. All these problems can be avoided by injecting the fluid directly into the cul-de-sac. Again, small periovarian and peritubal adhesions may not be diagnosed by this technique, and laparoscopy remains the ultimate method for the diagnosis of pelvic adhesions (37).

Laparoscopy has become the gold standard by which to diagnose pelvic adhesions (36) owing to its speed, simplicity in qualified hands, lack of need of major surgery, absence of lengthy hospital stays, and the tiny incision required. Laparotomy is also another direct visualization method to diagnose pelvic adhesions, but this requires major surgery with its increased risks.

The need for a standard classification scheme of pelvic adhesions is obvious. It would alleviate inconsistencies in the medical literature of describing pelvic adhesions, and lead to a more uniform understanding of the adhesions described by any author in any study. Also, a standard classification would enable clinicians to keep more accurate records of the stage of their patients' diseases, and therefore eliminate speculation during future treatment, second-look procedures, and various interventions as to how the patient's disease had advanced or regressed since last treatment. For these reasons, the American Fertility Society has created a standard classification scheme to describe the stages of pelvic adhesions (38,39). The variables that are "scored" include whether the adhesions are filmy or dense, and the degree to which the ovaries or tubes are enclosed or the cul-de-sac obliterated. Some authors still do not use this standard classification scheme in their reports, however, but find it more appropriate to create their own staging system based on whether the adhesions found are filmy or dense, vascular or avascular, and whether or not they have extended to the pelvic wall or bowel (30).

The use of a uniform, internationally accepted classification for pelvic adhesions allows investigators to compare results of treatment. It also allows infertility surgeons to give a prognosis in a given case during preoperative counseling. The American Fertility Society classification is adequate and fulfills these criteria.

Laparoscopic evaluation of patients with infertility or pelvic pain may reveal on occasion the presence of perihepatic adhesions. This finding is referred to as the Fitz-Hugh and Curtis syndrome. It is a well-known sequela of PID. However, this syndrome has been described in a group of patients without history of pelvic infection. These patients were also fertile, and the perihepatic adhesions were discovered following tubal sterilization. This may suggest that perihepatic adhesions are the only residual effect of pelvic infection and should not be considered to be of unfavorable outcome in infertile patients (40).

Pelvic adhesions with or without tubal obstruction may suggest endosalpingeal disease. Evaluation of the endosalpinx may help the reproductive surgeon to formulate a prognosis about the overall outcome with regard to infertility. Salpingoscopy has been performed during laparoscopy and laparotomy for such cases. Various endoscopes have been used including flexible, duodenal fiberscope, bronchofibroscope, and rigid endoscope. In a study by Shapiro and colleagues, salpingoscopy for 12 patients with adhesions revealed abnormal findings in the endosalpinx in 8 patients. In their study pregnancy occurred in two patients with normal salpingoscopic findings (41). Previous studies have shown that salpingoscopy findings correlate better with subsequent pregnancy rate than do either hysterosalpingography or external examination of the fallopian tubes at laparoscopy (42).

Treatment

Treatment decisions involve the use of macrosurgery versus microsurgery. In gynecologic microsurgery, the magnification intensifies the surgeon's awareness of impending trauma, and facilitates the use of unipolar microelectrodes or bipolar microforceps for the attainment of precise hemostasis. It also makes lysis of adhesions easier because the interface between the adhesions and the peritoneal tissue is easier to visualize. Manipulation of tissue with fine atraumatic instruments reduces serosal abrasion. The use of fine suture material with minimum tissue reaction decreases the likelihood of tissue damage. Foreign body contamination is also made more obvious, and therefore can more easily be avoided (12). Fayez and Suliman compared the results of macrosurgical and microsurgical tuboplasty procedures performed on infertility patients after other causes of infertility had been ruled out. Use of the microscope improved results in all categories, particularly in anastomosis procedures. These authors concluded that the microscopic techniques have a definite advantage and are recommended for use in all tuboplasty procedures (43). This study is a significant contribution, and it suggests that the use of magnification and microsurgical principles has improved the fertility outcome following infertility surgery.

Tulandi et al. evaluated the effect of salpingo-ovariolysis using microsurgical or laser techniques on pregnancy occurrence. There were 147 cases diagnosed by laparoscopy as periadnexal adhesions. The adhesions were rated by the modified international classification sanctioned by the International Federation of Fertility Societies; 69 cases were treated, and 78 cases were not treated. There was no statistically significant difference in the degree of adhesions between the two groups. The cumulative pregnancy rate at 12 and 24 months' follow-up was 32% and 45% in the treated group, and 11% and 16% in the nontreated group, respectively. The study suggests that salpingo-ovariolysis is associated with a higher pregnancy rate. This study is a controlled one comparing two groups with nearly the same degree of adhesions. This aspect is lacking from many other studies. The use of life table analysis and cumulative pregnancy rate in this study is a better approach to statistical analysis than the use of absolute figures given in other studies (35).

Recently, laparoscopic surgery has been used by experienced gynecologists for treatment of many pelvic conditions including lysis of adhesions. In support of laparoscopy, Reich reports the viable pregnancy rate for four groups of women: it was 78% for 27 women who underwent laparoscopic salpingo-ovariolysis, 28.5% for 7 women who underwent laparoscopic salpingostomy, 75% for 12 women who were treated by laparotomy with microsurgical salpingo-ovariolysis, and 13% for 15 women who were treated by laparotomy with microsurgical salpingostomy in a nonrandomized study (44). Thus, the pregnancy rate following laparoscopy or laparotomy may be basically the same for lysis of adhesions or salpingostomy in skilled hands, but controlled trials are lacking.

In a study by Fayez, 83 patients had tuboplasty by means of operative laparoscopic techniques. The procedures and their respective patency and pregnancy rates were salpingolysis, 100%, 67%; ovariolysis, 100%, 72%; salpingo-ovariolysis, 100%, 50%; fimbrioplasty, 64%, 35%; and neosalpingostomy, 31%, 10%. The author suggests that operative laparoscopy may be the method of choice for tubal operations that involve any of the first three procedures, whereas perhaps laparotomy with use of microsurgical techniques would be more appropriate for the last two procedures (45). It is difficult to reach that conclusion on the basis of this study, however, because a laparotomy control group was not included.

All these studies suggest that operative laparoscopy for lysis of adhesions and tuboplasty are almost equal in fertility outcome. However, these studies are not randomized, and the authors are skilled in the use of laparoscopy and biased in its use. Also, the degree of adhesive process is not known because the authors have not used a standard classification.

Another choice in the treatment of infertility-related pelvic adhesions involves whether to use laser laparoscopy or conventional laparoscopy. Donnez states that there are at least three advantages of laser laparoscopy over conventional operative laparoscopy: precise destruction of diseased tissue, minimal bleeding, and minimal damage to the adjacent normal tissue (46). In a study by Filmar, Gomel, and McComb, the relative effectiveness of the carbon dioxide (CO_2) laser versus electromicrosurgery in lysis of adhesions was assessed in the female white rat. The results suggest that electromicrosurgery and the CO_2 laser are equally effective in lysis of adhesions in the rat model (47). One must take into account, however, that this adhesion model was induced rather than being a natural by-product of surgery, that the model used is a rat instead of human, and that the amount of adhesions induced varied widely from animal to animal, necessitating a large number to arrive at valid conclusions. Bellina and associates conducted a study designed to compare the effect of wound healing after the use of the CO_2 laser and the electrosurgical unit on the peritoneal membrane of the New Zealand White rabbit. The effects compared were tissue damage, adhesion formation, and healing time. The laser, when compared with the electrosurgical scalpel in this study, produced no adhesion formation and less tissue injury, immediately and throughout the healing phase ($p < 0.0039$) (48). This has been confirmed by other studies suggesting that the use of the CO_2 laser with a high power density has minimal thermal damage effect, and that tissue healing is proper (49,50).

Tulandi compared the effect of salpingo-ovariolysis with the use of CO_2 laser or microdiathermy needle on the occurrence of subsequent pregnancy. The study was prospective and randomized. Thirty patients were treated with the use of a CO_2 laser, and 33 patients were treated with a microdiathermy needle. There was no significant difference in the duration of infertility or the degree of periadnexal adhesions between the two groups. The pregnancy rates at 2-year follow-up were not statistically different: 53.3% for the laser group and 51.5% for the microdiathermy group. The surgery–conception interval was shorter in the laser-treated group. However, this interval was not significantly different from that in the other group. The study suggested that perhaps a larger series of patients is needed to determine if the use of the laser shortens the time to pregnancy. This is a solid study and gives credence to the evaluation of the methods of treatment because it is prospective and randomized (51).

Postoperative tubal occlusion and adhesion formation are important factors in failure rates following reconstructive tubal surgery (12). Diamond and coworkers performed second-look laparoscopies to determine the effectiveness of initial laparotomy lysis of adhesions. At both operative procedures the adhesions were scored by type (0, none; 1, filmy, avascular; 2, organized, vascular), at each of nine locations: both ovaries, both fimbriae, omentum, small bowel, colon, pelvic sidewall, and cul-de-sac. Adhesion re-formation was independent of the initial type of adhesion. Neither the rate nor the type of adhesion recurrence was determined by the variable amount of time between the initial and second-look operative procedures. It was concluded that reproductive pelvic surgical procedures are frequently complicated not only by adhesion re-formation but also by de novo adhesion formation (52). The results of this study may have been affected by differences in the skill of the surgeons involved, variation in technique, multiple observers scoring the adhesions, and severity of disease.

Trimbos-Kemper and associates went one step further than Diamond and colleagues. Not only did they evaluate the initial lysis of adhesions and use second-look laparoscopy to evaluate its effectiveness, as did Diamond and colleagues, but they also employed third-look laparoscopy to evaluate the effectiveness of the adhesiolysis during second-look laparoscopy. A second-look laparoscopy on the eighth day after salpingostomy, fimbrioplasty, or adhesiolysis was performed in 188 patients. Of the 188 patients, 64 had a third-look laparoscopy 2 years following the previous second-look. To compare, laparoscopy was performed 2 years after surgery on 127 patients who had not had a previous second-look laparoscopy with lysis of adhesions. When adnexal adhesions in this group were compared with those in the 64 patients who underwent the second-look and third-look laparoscopies, significantly more of those in whom a second-look laparoscopy with lysis of adhesions was performed were found to have no adhesions. It was concluded that a second-look laparoscopy significantly reduced the occurrence of permanent pelvic adhesions (53). Other investigators have had the same experience, especially if second-look laparoscopy was done before the fourth postoperative week (54,55). One must also keep in mind that intrauterine pregnancy is the final endpoint for which infertility surgeons strive to keep the incidence of postoperative adhesions low. In this study, although the second laparoscopy significantly reduced the number of permanent pelvic adhesions, the cumulative intrauterine pregnancy rates after 3 years in the patients who did and in those who did not have a "second-look" laparoscopy were similar (43). Hence, one must decide whether the additional laparoscopy would really be necessary, as the pregnancy endpoint is the same. Furthermore, these studies are not randomized. The effect of the degree of initial adhesions on the outcome is not stated. Also patients may not submit to several laparoscopic procedures to evaluate the results of surgery.

Furthermore, Tulandi and coworkers in a randomized study evaluated the effect of second-look operative laparoscopy one year following reproductive surgery. Of 38 patients who had salpingo-ovariolysis by laparotomy, 19 had second-look laparoscopy, and adhesions were found in 13 patients. Lysis of adhesions was done in only 10 patients. The remaining 19 patients were followed expectantly. At 12, 24, and 36 months, the cumulative pregnancy rate was 27%, 67%, and 67% in the group that had second-look laparoscopy, and 27%, 45%, and 52% in the group that received expectant management, respectively. The difference between the two groups was not significant. There was also no significant difference in the occurrence of ectopic pregnancy. The same group of investigators evaluated the effect of second-look laparoscopy for patients who had salpingostomy for bilateral hydrosalpinx. The patients were divided into a group that had the laparoscopy and lysis of adhesions, and a group that was followed expectantly. Again the cumulative pregnancy rate at 12, 24, and 36 months' follow-up was not statistically different between the two groups. This study is very significant because it is a randomized controlled one. It also suggests that second-look operative laparoscopy following reproductive surgery for adhesions and salpingostomy does not increase the pregnancy rate or decrease the incidence of tubal pregnancy in these circumstances. It also suggests that there is no need for a third-look or fourth-look laparoscopy following such surgical procedures (56).

Aboulghar, Mansour, and Serour describe an ovarian hyperstimulation medical treatment to circumvent the difficulties regarding fertility caused by periadnexal adhesions. Forty-two women with peritubal and periovarian adhesions as the only cause of infertility were hyperstimulated with clomiphene citrate and human menopausal gonadotropin in 103 cycles. The subsequent pregnancy rate per cycle in patients who underwent controlled ovarian hyperstimulation was statistically greater than that in patients with no ovarian hyperstimulation. The authors suggest that the achievement of pregnancy with this line of treatment is possibly due to more than one factor. The increase in ovarian size may bring the ovary close to the fimbria. Multiple ovulation may increase the chance of ovum pick-up, and hyperstimulation may have an effect on tubal vascularity and motility that may enhance the ovum pick-up mechanism. The authors believe that this line of treatment could be attempted before microsurgery or in vitro fertilization and embryo transfer in patients with peritubal and periovarian adhesions with at least one patent tube (29). The pregnancy rate per cycle correlated with the degree of adnexal adhesions, as it was 36.4% with minimal adhesions, 22% with mild adhesions, and 6.7% with moderate adhesions. However, the number was too small to be statistically significant. Until the pregnancy rate following ovarian hyperstimulation is shown to be significantly related to the degree of periadnexal adhesions, no firm conclusions can be drawn.

Pelvic adhesions are found in approximately 30% to 50% of chronic pain cases. Lysis of adhesions laparoscopically or by laparotomy leads to pain relief in only a limited number of patients (57). Some patients experience relief for a few months and then a recurrence of pain, suggesting a placebo effect. Another study be Peters et al. suggested a beneficial effect of adhesiolysis for pelvic pain in patients with severe adhesions involving the intestinal tract (58).

Prevention

Since the beginning of this century there have been many efforts to develop effective strategies to prevent development of postoperative adhesions. To prevent deposition of fibrin in the peritoneal exudate, agents such as sodium citrate, heparin, and other anticoagulants have been used. To remove fibrin already formed, enzymes such as trypsin, papain, pepsin, hyaluronidase, streptokinase, and streptodornase have been used. Peritoneal lavage has been used to remove fibrin mechanically. In attempts to prevent the fibrin-coated peritoneal walls from coming into contact with one another, the abdomen has been distended with oxygen or filled with saline, paraffin, olive oil, lanolin, vitreous of calf eye, amniotic fluid, macromolecular solutions of all sorts, and silicones. The following barrier methods have been attempted to prevent peritoneal contact: Cargile membrane, oiled silk, silver foil, gold beater's skin, calf peritoneum, and free grafts of omentum. Vigorous defecation has been encouraged by cathartics and enemas. It has even been suggested that patients consume iron filings after surgery, and then undergo the passage of a magnet over their abdomen in order to move the fibrin-coated, iron-laden loops of intestine away from each other. Prevention of fibroblastic proliferation has been attempted with the use of adrenocorticotrophic hormone, steroids, and cytotoxic agents (2). Several agents are being used currently in efforts to prevent adhesion formation (Table 45-1).

Table 45-1 Agents currently used for adhesion prophylaxis

Intended mechanism	Agent
Inhibit inflammatory reaction	Corticosteroids
	Promethazine
	Nonsteroidal anti-inflammatory drugs
	Progestins
	Calcium-channel blockers
	Pentoxifylline
Prevent fibrin deposition	Heparin
Promote fibrin lysis	Urokinase
Prevent tissue damage	Dextran 70, 32%
	Povidone
Mechanical separation	Dextran 70, 32%
	Amnion
	Silicone
	Surgicel
	Gore-Tex
	Interceed
Augment plasminogen activator	Pentoxifylline
	Recombinant tissue plasminogen activator

Corticosteroids continue to be commonly used agents in the prophylaxis of postoperative adhesion formation. They reduce the initial inflammatory response to tissue injury, decreasing vascular permeability, stabilizing lysosome membranes, and inhibiting the synthesis and release of histamine and other factors (59). They also have been reported to inhibit fibroblast migration and proliferation in animal models (60). However, recent studies have indicated that corticosteroids may actually stimulate fibroblast growth (61). At best the evidence remains conflicting. If there is any preventive effect of steroid therapy on postoperative formation of peritoneal adhesions, it is probably not due to inhibition of fibroblast growth, but rather to limiting the initial phase of the inflammatory response. Steroids can reduce the effectiveness of the immune system and therefore make the possibility of infection a risk. They also have been known to reduce wound healing (12). This danger of iatrogenic complications must be kept in mind, but, thus far, the wide acceptance of dexamethasone use postoperatively indicates that frequent serious complications are uncommon.

Corticosteroids are frequently used in conjunction with promethazine (Phenergan), an antihistamine that uniquely blocks the release of histamine from mast cells. Promethazine also inhibits the increased vascular permeability associated with histamine and other mediators and protects the cellular lysosome system, thereby reducing the degree of secondary cellular damage that follows the release of intracellular enzymes, and may inhibit fibroplasia (59).

Ibuprofen (Motrin) also has been studied. It has been shown to inhibit prostaglandin biosynthesis, platelet aggregation and secretory activity, leukocyte migration and phagocytosis, and to suppress lysosome release (62). Holtz failed to find ibuprofen effective in reducing peritoneal adhesion formation or re-formation in the New Zealand White rabbit model. It must be recognized that the tissue drug levels were unknown in this study. Perhaps the therapeutic regimen would have yielded more favorable results if adjusted (63). Other studies have found nonsteroidal anti-inflammatory drugs effective in reducing peritoneal adhesion formation or re-formation (64,65).

Indomethacin has been tried in several studies for prevention of adhesions. Indomethacin is a potent inhibitor of cyclooxygenase; therefore, it leads to inhibition of prostaglandin synthesis. It also leads to inhibition of platelet aggregation and function. In a controlled animal study by DeLeon and colleagues, ibuprofen and indomethacin were found to be equally effective in reducing adhesion formation by 30% (66). In another controlled study, DeSimone and coworkers used indomethacin in a single preoperative dose or four perioperative doses in the rat to evaluate the effect on carrageenan-induced peritoneal adhesions. Indomethacin was found to decrease the adhesion formation rate to 49% (67).

Progestins also have been shown to have immunosuppressive actions. They have been reported to decrease antibody production and to inhibit human mixed lymphocyte culture and leukocyte migration. Progestins also decrease vascular permeability and aid in the involution of granulation tissue (12). Holtz and associates examined the effect of intramuscular injections of medroxyprogesterone acetate on adhesion formation and found that the medroxyprogesterone acetate did not reduce the amount of adhesion formation in the New Zealand White rabbit model. In fact, there was a statistically significant increase in adhesion scores in the medroxyprogesterone-acetate-treated group. One must consider the possibility of sampling error, however, because only eight animals were used in this study. Also, it must be kept in mind that medroxyprogesterone acetate is a synthetic hormone. Perhaps the results would have been different had a natural progestin been used in this study (68).

Steinleitner, Kazensky, and Lambert developed a model to test the efficacy of adhesion prophylaxis mediated by calcium channel blockade after lysis of established pelvic adhesive disease in the New Zealand White rabbit. Verapamil-treated animals formed significantly fewer adhesions than did control animals after adhesiolysis (69). Although this work appears promising, a different verapamil delivery method would be needed in women, because the placement of a small osmotic pump on the anterior abdominal wall is a rather invasive method and would require another surgery for its removal. Data from the literature on calcium channel blockade suggest that these agents have the potential to modulate sequential as-

pects of the peritoneal repair process, including protection against ischemic or traumatic cell injury, inhibition of vasoactive mediator release, decrease in exudation of fibrin-rich plasma as substrate for clot formation, reduction of phagocyte activation, and inhibition of fibroblast penetration into fibrin matrices (69).

The Adhesion Study Group conducted a study to examine the effect of 250 ml of 32% dextran 70 on reducing postoperative adhesion formation. Infertility patients of reproductive age requiring an operation for distal tubal disease, endometriosis, or pelvic adhesions were recruited from nine study centers. An overall reduction in adhesion formation was found to occur more frequently in the group treated with 32% dextran 70 ($p < .05$), although in the patients whose initial extent of adhesion scores were "moderate" or "mild," no difference was found in the total change and extent of adnexal adhesions with regard to treatment (70). The fact that 32% dextran 70 was associated with reduced adhesion formation in the dependent portions of the pelvis in this study supports the hydroflotation mechanism theory for dextran's prevention of postoperative adhesions. Presumably, floating tissues would not come into direct apposition with each other for long periods of time such that peritoneal reepithelialization may occur without fibrin bridge and subsequent adhesion formation (70). Another explanation for the beneficial effect of 32% dextran 70 is that it coats the raw surfaces and retards two major causes of adhesion formation: peritoneal abrasions and blood clot adherence (71).

Jansen performed a prospective, randomized, controlled study that conflicts with the belief that 32% dextran 70 is an effective antiadhesion agent. In 164 female patients who underwent operations for infertility, 32% dextran 70 or 0.5% hydrocortisone sodium succinate or both were instilled into the peritoneal cavity. All of the patients had a subsequent laparoscopy 12 to 24 days postoperatively to diagnose and treat adhesions that may have been forming. Jansen concluded from this study that there is no empiric basis for the use of intraperitoneal 32% dextran 70 or 0.5% hydrocortisone in the attempt to prevent peritoneal adhesions (72).

The side effects of the intraperitoneal use of 32% dextran 70 include infection (73), anaphylactic reactions (74), transient increase in bleeding time, increased central venous pressure, increased body weight, and unilateral vulvar edema (70,75). It is also believed that as fluid is shifted into the peritoneal cavity to equilibrate the hyperosmotic dextran load, the potential exists for intravascular electrolyte imbalance (70). Indeed, in a study by Utian, Goldfarb, and Starks, three of seven rabbits experienced an early death after the intraperitoneal administration of 32% dextran 70, thought to be due to postoperative fluid imbalance secondary to the hyperosmolarity of the 32% dextran (71). Bernstein and colleagues investigated the effect of dextran solutions on the growth of different bacterial species. The study showed that dextran's potential as a medium for bacterial growth is significant (76). Weinans and coworkers evaluated the effect of 32% dextran 70 on serum glutamic oxalacetic transaminase (SGOT) and serum glutamic phosphorus transaminase (SGPT) concentrations in patients postoperatively. Postoperative SGOT and SGPT values increased. The use of 32% dextran 70 in combination with corticosteroids or halothane leads to an increased risk of liver function disturbances. The alterations of the SGOT and SGPT values may be explained by the perioperative administration of 200 ml of 32% dextran 70, which equates to administering 50 grams of glucose. After resorption of the glucose, the hepatocytes may be damaged by enhanced glycogen deposition or lipid accumulation in the liver (75). The need to use 32% dextran 70 should always be weighed against the possible risks.

Goldberg, Sheets, and Habal, using dog and rat models, conducted exploratory laparotomies to examine the effect of applying hydrophilic polymer solutions (povidone [polyvinylpyrrolidone] and dextran) to tissue surfaces, surgical gloves, and sponges before contact with internal organs and tissues. An important aspect of this set of experiments was the evaluation of these polymeric agents as protective coatings to prevent tissue damage before organ manipulation, rather than for treatment of damage that had already been produced by manipulation during surgery. They concluded that the addition of hydrophilic polymer solutions and coatings to tissue and surgical material surfaces minimizes adhesions by providing a lubricating boundary for protection (77). Many questions remain to be answered concerning the use of polymers, such as differences in performance as a function of molecular structure, molecular weights, concentrations, osmolarity, buffering, and general polymer bioacceptance.

Another new drug that is being evaluated for its efficacy in preventing adhesion reformation in pentoxifylline, a methylxanthine analogue currently used to treat peripheral vascular disease. The data demonstrate a marked inhibition of adhesion re-formation after lysis of pelvic adhesions under the influence of subcutaneously administered pentoxifylline in rabbits ($p < .001$). It is suggested that this drug may modulate peritoneal repair through multiple interventions in the adhesion-formation cascade, including decreased granulocyte-mediated tissue damage during the acute postinjury phase, improved perfusion of damaged structures, and augmented plasminogen activator production resulting in enhanced fibrinolysis (78).

Prevention of fibrin deposition and enhancement of fibrinolysis have been attracting attention for many years in the attempt to limit development of peritoneal adhesions. To investigate the prevention of fibrin deposition and how it relates to postoperative adhesion formation, operations on the pelvis for infertility were performed on patients irrigated with either lactated Ringer's solution or lactated Ringer's plus heparin at 5000 IU/L. Laparoscopy was performed within 12 days to diagnose and treat pelvic adhesions. Analysis of adhesion improvement scores in relation to initial adhesion scores showed that no significant benefit was obtained from the use of heparin (79).

To investigate fibrinolysis and its effect on prevention of adhesions, Gervin, Puckett, and Silver instilled urokinase at 10,000 to 20,000 U/kg of body weight intraperitoneally into adult mongrel dogs and found that it was effective in preventing adhesions in 80% of the animals. Although no wound healing or coagulation defects were encountered in this study (10), such potential complications make the use of intraperitoneal urokinase less attractive in human surgery.

Various barrier methods have been tried in the attempt to prevent postoperative adhesions. Natural and synthetic materials that have been used include gelfilm, Silastic, Gelfoam, amnion, peritoneum, omentum, and Surgicel, among others (1). An ideal barrier designed to prevent adhesions should perform a variety of functions. First, its use must be associated with a low risk of complications and side effects. This would necessitate low tissue reactivity, thereby minimizing the establishment of a tissue inflammatory reaction. Second, the barrier should be easy to handle and apply. Third, it should adhere on its own, not requiring sutures or foreign material to hold it in place. Fourth, the barrier should be absorbable so as not to require another surgical intervention to remove it. Finally, the barrier must be efficacious in reducing the formation or re-formation of adhesions (80).

In a study by Badawy and coworkers, the amniotic membrane was used as a graft intra-abdominally in nulliparous female Sprague-Dawley rats to study the healing process and the graft's efficacy in preventing postoperative adhesions. The study showed no evidence of rejection, infection, or necrosis of the intra-abdominal amniotic membrane graft. There was no significant difference in the incidence of adhesions between the control and graft sites of the uterine horns, but the difference between the control and graft site adhesions on the anterior abdominal wall peritoneum was statistically significant. This finding may reflect differences in tissue response (81), which must be accounted for when trying to develop an ideal barrier method.

Yemini and colleagues studied the efficacy of silicone sheeting in preventing postoperative formation of adhesions after an adhesiolysis procedure in the female rabbit model. It was concluded that the application of silicone sheeting for 5 days appears to be an effective method of reducing adhesion formation during the healing process in injured pelvic organs in rabbits (82). A silicone barrier interferes with the formation of the fibrinous network and, hence, the formation of adhesions. This method of adhesion prophylaxis would unfortunately necessitate another operation to remove the silicone sheeting 5 days after its placement.

Surgicel is a knitted fabric made from oxidized regenerated cellulose. Galan and associates considered the effect of this barrier method in rabbits. When the effect of Surgicel was tested within suture groups, a significant difference was noted in the polyglycolic acid (Dexon-S) group but not in the polyglactin (Vicryl) group. Hence, the question remains whether Surgicel is useful in the prevention of postoperative adhesions or whether the choice of suture material is of equal importance (83).

Boyers, Diamond, and DeCherney used Gore-Tex surgical membrane, a nonreactive expanded polytetrafluoroethylene, to cover ischemic defects in the pelvic sidewall peritoneum to reduce postoperative adhesion formation in a rabbit pelvic sidewall and uterine horn injury model. The total adhesion score for Gore-Tex-covered lesions was significantly lower than the total score for control lesions. It was concluded that Gore-Tex surgical membrane is an effective barrier for reducing primary adhesions in this pelvic injury model and offers promise for adhesion reduction in human pelvic surgery (84). These results were confirmed in a recent study by the surgical membrane study group. In this study patients with extensive adhesions and myomata had Gore-Tex surgical membranes placed following adhesiolysis and myomectomy. There was significant reduction in adhesion formation and re-formation (85). It is unfortunate that it requires suturing to hold it in place, because an ideal barrier should adhere on its own. Gore-Tex polytetrafluoroethylene has been used successfully as a pericardial membrane substitute for more than 10 years (86). In contrast to the Gore-Tex vascular graft and Gore-Tex cardiovascular patch, which are designed to encourage cellular penetration and tissue adhesion, the Gore-Tex surgical membrane has an extremely small pore size (≤ 1 μm), which discourages tissue attachment (84). On the contrary, a similar study design was carried out by Goldberg, Toledo, and Mitchell using 15 New Zealand White rabbits. In this study, the Gore-Tex mean adhesion score was 2.3 times higher than the control, a statistically significant difference. The Gore-Tex surgical membrane did not appear to be an effective adjuvant for postoperative adhesion prophylaxis in this animal model. This study illustrates the importance of surgical design, because the Gore-Tex surgical membrane was held in place with several sutures, but no sutures were placed around the control sites, compromising their model (87).

Interceed (TC7) is a fabric composed of oxidized, regenerated cellulose specifically designed as a surgical adjuvant to reduce the formation of postoperative adhesions. To test the effectiveness of this new antiadhesion barrier, the Adhesion Barrier Study Group studied 74 infertility patients with bilateral pelvic sidewall adhesions at treatment laparotomy and second-look laparoscopy (88). Pelvic sidewalls covered with Interceed had a 90% improvement over control sidewalls in preventing adhesion formation. Sekiba and the obstetrics and gynecology adhesion prevention committee evaluated Interceed in a randomized multicenter study. Sixty-three infertility patients with pelvic sidewall adhesions due to pelvic inflammatory disease after surgery or to endometriosis were treated by laparotomy and adhesiolysis. The pelvic sidewalls were randomly selected for Interceed application. The results showed that Interceed was eight times more effective than surgery alone in preventing adhesion re-formation. This prevention of adhesions occurred regardless of the initial size of deperitonealized area. Furthermore, Interceed was effective in preventing adhesions after surgical treatment of severe endometriosis (89).

Hemostasis is essential in prevention of adhesions in general and before application of Interceed. Wiseman and associates demonstrated in the rabbit model that the Interceed barrier alone did not reduce adhesions at sites of bleeding. Application of Interceed after achieving hemostasis with thrombin significantly reduced adhesion formation. These investigators also showed that the results were improved by using heparin to moisten Interceed (90). In another study Wiskind and colleagues evaluated Interceed for prevention of adhesion formation following ovarian surgical wounds in rabbits. In this study the ovary was bivalved microsurgically and covered with Interceed in a randomized fashion with one ovary as control. In a second-look laparotomy 4 weeks later, the adhesions score for the Interceed-treated ovaries was not significantly different from that for controls (91). It is difficult to extrapolate the results of these animal studies to clinical situations.

Interceed rapidly forms a gelatinous mass that provides a protective coating around healing tissue during the initial 7 to 10 days after application (80). During this time, re-epithelialization of damaged surfaces is completed. Interceed, because it forms a gelatinous mass, does not require subsequent surgical intervention for its removal.

Luciano and colleagues compared the effect of using the CO_2 laser versus electrocautery in preventing postoperative adhesions in the female rabbit model. There were no differences in the depth of thermal damage, in the extent of collagen formation, or in postoperative adhesion formation between CO_2-treated animals and electrocautery (92). Tulandi drew the same conclusions in a study comparing adhesion formation following CO_2 laser or microdiathermy for salpingo-ovariolysis procedures in humans (51).

The lack of uniformity in experimental models makes assessment of the efficacy of any prophylactic regimen difficult. Variables include the animal model used, the method of inducing adhesion formation, the location of the induced adhesions, whether the same surgeon performs all of the operations, the dosage and route of administration of the therapeutic agent, and whether adhesion formation or re-formation is being evaluated (12). Areas of future investigation will probably continue with barrier methods, which appear to be the most promising.

Summary

As we learn more about the reaction of intraperitoneal tissues to injury, ischemia, and foreign bodies, the mechanisms of healing of the peritoneum, and the mechanisms by which adhesion development can be circumvented, our approach to this everyday problem of postoperative adhesion formation can change from arbitrary rules and intuition to rational management. At this stage, reproductive surgeons should continue to follow the principles of microsurgical techniques during each procedure. This includes gentle handling of tissues, intermittent tissue irrigation, and proper hemostasis. The use of adjuvants such as steroids, antihistamines, and high molecular weight dextran solutions may be of value in some cases. More research studies of various barrier methods to prevent adhesions must be conducted. A second-look operative laparoscopy done one year after surgery to evaluate the site of the previous surgery and for lysis of re-formed adhesions is feasible.

References

1 Soules MR, Dennis L, Bosarge A, et al. The prevention of postoperative pelvic adhesions: an animal study comparing barrier methods with dextran 70. Am J Obstet Gynecol 1982;143:829–834.

2 Ellis H. The cause and prevention of postoperative intraperitoneal adhesions. Surg Gynecol Obstet 1971;133:497–511.

3 Rapkin A. Adhesions and pelvic pain: a retrospective study. Obstet Gynecol 1986;68:13–15.

4 Kresch AJ, Seifer DB, Sachs LB, et al. Laparoscopy in 100 women with chronic pelvic pain. Obstet Gynecol 1984;64:672–674.

5 Stovall TG, Elder RF, Ling FW. Predictors of pelvic adhesions. J Reprod Med 1989;34:345–348.

6 Surrey MW, Friedman S. Second-look laparoscopy after reconstructive pelvic surgery for infertility. J Reprod Med 1982;27:658–660.

7 Daniell JF, Pittaway DE. Short-interval second-look laparoscopy after infertility surgery: a preliminary report. J Reprod Med 1983;28:281–283.

8 DeCherney AH, Mezerh HC. The nature of post tuboplasty pelvic adhesions as determined by early and late laparoscopy. Fertil Steril 1984;41:643–646.

9 Buckman RF, Buckman PD, Hufnagel HU, et al. A physiologic basis for the adhesion-free healing of deperitonealized surfaces. J Surg Res 1976;21:67–76.

10 Gervin AS, Puckett CL, Silver D. Serosal hypofibrinolysis: a cause of postoperative adhesions. Am J Surg 1973;125:80–88.

11 Weibel MA, Majno G. Peritoneal adhesions and their relation to abdominal surgery: a postmortem study. Am J Surg 1973;126:345–353.

12 Holtz G. Prevention and management of peritoneal adhesions. Fertil Steril 1984;41:497–507.

13 Holtz G. Adhesion induction by suture of varying tissue reactivity and caliber. Int J Fertil 1982;27:134–135.

14 Ryan GB, Grobety J, Majno G. Post operative peritoneal adhesions: a study of the mechanisms. Am J Pathol 1971;65:117–140.

15 Geerdsen J, Bech Hansen J. Incidence of sterility in women operated on in childhood for perforated appendicitis. Acta Obstet Gynecol Scand 1977;56:523–524.

16 Mueller BA, Daling JR, Moore DE, et al. Appendectomy and the risk of tubal infertility. N Engl J Med 1986;315(24):1506–1508.

17 Heinonen PK, Aine R, Seppala E. Peritoneal fluid leukotriene B$_4$ and prostaglandin E$_2$ in acute salpingitis. Gynecol Obstet Invest 1990;29(4):292–295.

18 Thompson JN, Paterson-Brown S, Harbourne T, et al. Reduced human peritoneal plasminogen activating activity: possible mechanism of adhesion formation. Br J Surg 1989;76(4):382–384.

19 Vipond MN, Whawell SA, Thompson JN, et al. Peritoneal fibrinolytic activity and intra-abdominal adhesions. Lancet 1990;335:1120–1122.

20 Doody KJ, Dunn RC, Buttram VC Jr. Recombinant tissue plasminogen activator reduces adhesion formation in a rabbit uterine horn model. Fertil Steril 1989;51:509–512.

21 Menzies D, Ellis H. Intra-abdominal adhesions and their prevention by topical tissue plasminogen activator. J R Soc Med 1989;82:534–535.

22 Batzofin JH, Holmes SD, Gibbons WE, et al. Peritoneal fluid plasminogen activator activity in endometriosis and pelvic adhesive disease. Fertil Steril 1985;44:277–279.

23 Badawy SZ, Iskander S. Omental reaction in cases of uterine perforation by the IUCD. Contraception 1974;10(1):73–77.

24 Milligan DW, Raftery AT. Observations on the pathogenesis of peritoneal adhesions: a light and electron microscopical study. Br J Surg 1974;61:274–280.

25 Holtz G. Prevention of postoperative adhesions. J Reprod Med 1980;24:141–146.

26 Raftery AT. Regeneration of parietal and visceral peritoneum: an electron microscopical study. J Anat 1973;115:375–392.

27 Bayloo RP, Funari VA, Azziz R, Watson JM, Martinez-Maza O. Elevated interleukin-6 levels in peritoneal fluid of patients with pelvic pathology. Fertil Steril 1992;58:302–306.

28 Coletti L, Bossart PA. Intestinal obstruction during the early postoperative period. Arch Surg 1964;88:774–778.

29 Aboulghar MA, Mansour RT, Serour GI. Ovarian superstimulation in the treatment of infertility due to peritubal and periovarian adhesions. Fertil Steril 1989;51:834–837.

30 Mecke H, Semm K, Freys I, et al. Incidence of adhesions in the true pelvis after pelviscopic operative treatment of tubal pregnancy. Gynecol Obstet Invest 1989;28:202–204.

31 Diamond MP, Pellicer A, Boyers SP, et al. The effect of periovarian adhesions on follicular development in patients undergoing ovarian stimulation for in vitro fertilization–embryo transfer. Fertil Steril 1988;49:100–103.

32 Mahadevan MM, Wiseman D, Leader A, et al. The effects of ovarian adhesive disease upon follicular development in cycles of controlled stimulation for in vitro fertilization. Fertil Steril 1985;44:489–492.

33 Molloy D, Martin M, Speirs A, et al. Performance of patients with a "frozen pelvis" in an in vitro fertilization program. Fertil Steril 1987;47:450–455.

34 Diaz-Infante A Jr, Virutamasen P, Connaughton J, et al. In vitro studies of human ovarian contractility. Obstet Gynecol 1974;44:830–839.

35 Tulandi T, Collins JA, Burrows E, et al. Treatment-dependent and treatment-independent pregnancy among women with periadnexal adhesions. Am J Obstet Gynecol 1990;162:354–357.

36 Karasick S, Goldfarb AF. Peritubal adhesions in infertile women: diagnosis with hysterosalpingography. AJR Am J Roentgenol 1989;152:777–779.

37 Maroulis GB, Parsons AK, Yeko TR. Hydrogynecography: a new technique enables vaginal sonography to visualize pelvic adhesions and other pelvic structures. Fertil Steril 1992;58:1073–1075.

38 The American Fertility Society. The American Fertility Society classifications of adnexal adhesions, distal tubal occlusion, tubal occlusion secondary to tubal ligation, tubal pregnancies, mullerian anomalies and intrauterine adhesions. Fertil Steril 1988;49:944–955.

39 The American Fertility Society. Classification of endometriosis. Fertil Steril 1979;32:633–634.

40 Hanjani SA, Neely T, Chatwani A. Perihepatic adhesions: not necessarily pathognomonic of pelvic infection. Am J Obstet Gynecol 1992;167:115–116.

41 Shapiro BS, Diamond MP, DeCherney AH. Salpingoscopy: an adjunctive technique for evaluation of the fallopian tube. Fertil Steril 1988;49:1076–1079.

42 Cornier E. Ampullosalpingoscopy. In: Siegler A, ed. The fallopian tube: basic studies and clinical contribution. Mount Kisco, NY: Futura Publishing, 1986:383–390.

43 Fayez JA, Suliman SO. Infertility surgery of the oviduct: comparison between macrosurgery and microsurgery. Fertil Steril 1982;37:73–78.

44 Reich H. Laparoscopic treatment of extensive pelvic adhesions, including hydrosalpinx. J Reprod Med 1987;32:736–742.

45 Fayez JA. An assessment of the role of operative laparoscopy in tuboplasty. Fertil Steril 1983;39:476–479.

46 Donnez J. CO_2 laser laparoscopy in infertile women with endometriosis and women with adnexal adhesions. Fertil Steril 1987;48:390–394.

47 Filmar S, Gomel V, McComb P. The effectiveness of CO_2 laser and electromicrosurgery in adhesiolysis: a comparative study. Fertil Steril 1986;45:407–411.

48 Bellina JF, Hemmings R, Voros JI, et al. Carbon dioxide laser and electrosurgical wound study with an animal model: a comparison of tissue damage and healing patterns in peritoneal tissue. Am J Obstet Gynecol 1984;148:327–334.

49 Badawy SZA, ElBakry MM, Baggish MS. Comparative study of continuous and pulsed CO_2 laser on tissue healing and fertility outcome in tubal anastomosis. Fertil Steril 1987;47:843–847.

50 Badawy SZA, ElBakry MM, Baggish MS, et al. Pulsed CO_2 laser versus conventional microsurgical anastomosis of the rat uterine horn. Fertil Steril 1986;46:127–131.

51 Tulandi T. Salpingo-ovariolysis: a comparison between laser surgery and electrosurgery. Fertil Steril 1986;45:489–491.

52 Diamond MP, Daniell JF, Feste J, et al. Adhesion reformation and de novo adhesion formation after reproductive pelvic surgery. Fertil Steril 1987;47:864–866.

53 Trimbos-Kemper TCM, Trimbos JB, van Hall EV. Adhesion formation after tubal surgery: results of the eighth day laparoscopy in 188 patients. Fertil Steril 1985;43:395–400.

54 Jansen RPS. Early laparoscopy after pelvic operations to prevent adhesions: safety and efficacy. Fertil Steril 1988;49:26–31.

55 Raj SG, Hulka JF. Second-look laparoscopy in infertility surgery: therapeutic and prognostic value. Fertil Steril 1982;38:325–329.

56 Tulandi T, Falcone T, Kafka I. Second-look operative laparoscopy 1 year following reproductive surgery. Fertil Steril 1989;52:421–424.

57 Steege JF, Stout AL. Resolution of chronic pelvic pain after laparoscopic lysis of adhesions. Am J Obstet Gynecol 1991;165:278–283.

58 Peters AAW, Trimbos-Kemper GCM, Admiral C, Trinbos JB. Br J Obstet Gynecol 1992;99:59–62.

59 Replogle RL, Johnson R, Gross RE. Prevention of postoperative intestinal adhesions with combined promethazine and dexamethasone therapy. Ann Surg 1966;163:580–588.

60 Holden M, Adams LB. Inhibitory effects of cortisone acetate and hydrocortisone on growth of fibroblasts. Proc Soc Exp Biol Med 1957;95:364–368.

61 Granat M, Schenken JG, Mor-Yosef S, et al. Effects of dexamethasone on proliferation of autologous fibroblasts and on the immune profile in women undergoing pelvic surgery for infertility. Fertil Steril 1983;39:180–186.

62 Gernaat CM, Stubbs DF. Clinical brochure for investigators studying ibuprofen and myocardial infarction. Kalamazoo, Mich: The Upjohn Company, 1980.

63 Holtz G. Failure of a nonsteroidal anti-inflammatory agent (ibuprofen) to inhibit peritoneal adhesion reformation after lysis. Fertil Steril 1982;37:582–583.

64 Siegler AM, Kontopoulos V, Wang CF. Prevention of postoperative adhesions in rabbits with ibuprofen, a nonsteroidal anti-inflammatory agent. Fertil Steril 1980;34:46–49.

65 Larsson B, Svanberg SG, Swolin K. Oxyphenbutazone—an adjuvant to be used in prevention of adhesions in operations for fertility. Fertil Steril 1977;28:807–813.

66 DeLeon FD, Toledo AA, Sanfilippo JS, Yssman MA. The prevention of adhesion formation by nonsteroidal anti-inflammatory drugs: an animal study comparing ibuprofen and indomethacin. Fertil Steril 1984;41:639–642.

67 DeSimone JM, Meguid MM, Kurzer M, Westervelt J. Indomethacin decreases carrageenan-induced peritoneal adhesions. Surgery 1988;104:788–795.

68 Holtz G, Neff M, Mathur S, et al. Effect of medroxyprogesterone acetate on peritoneal adhesion formation. Fertil Steril 1983;40:542–544.

69 Steinleitner A, Kazensky C, Lambert H. Calcium channel blockade prevents postsurgical reformation of adnexal adhesions in rabbits. Obstet Gynecol 1989;74:796–798.

70 Adhesion Study Group. Reduction of postoperative pelvic adhesions with intraperitoneal 32% dextran 70: a prospective, randomized clinical trial. Fertil Steril 1983;40:612–619.

71 Utian WH, Goldfarb JM, Starks GC. Role of dextran 70 in microtubal surgery. Fertil Steril 1979;31:79–82.

72 Jansen RPS. Failure of intraperitoneal adjuncts to improve the outcome of pelvic surgery in young women. Am J Obstet Gynecol 1985;153:363–371.

73 King IR. Candida albicans pelvic abscess associated with the use of 32% dextran 70 in conservative pelvic surgery. Fertil Steril 1989;51:1050–1052.

74 Borten M, Seibert CP, Taymor ML. Recurrent anaphylactic reaction to intraperitoneal dextran 75 used for prevention of postsurgical adhesions. Obstet Gynecol 1983;61:755–757.

75 Weinans MJ, Kauer FM, Klompmaker IJ, et al. Transient liver function disturbances after the intraperitoneal use of 32% dextran 70 as adhesion prophylaxis in infertility surgery. Fertil Steril 1990;53:159–161.

76 Bernstein M, Mattox JH, Ulrich JA, et al. The potential for bacterial growth with dextran. J Reprod Med 1982;27:77–79.

77 Goldberg EP, Sheets JW, Habal MB. Peritoneal adhesions: prevention with the use of hydrophilic polymer coatings. Arch Surg 1980;115:776–780.

78 Steinleitner A, Lambert H, Kazensky C, et al. Pentoxifylline, a methylxanthine derivative, prevents postsurgical adhesion reformation in rabbits. Obstet Gynecol 1990;75:926–928.

79 Jansen RPS. Failure of peritoneal irrigation with heparin during pelvic operations upon young women to reduce adhesions. Surg Gynecol Obstet 1988;166:154–160.

80 Linsky CB, Diamond MP, Cunningham TJ, et al. Adhesion reduction in the uterine horn model using an absorbable barrier, TC7. J Reprod Med 1987;32:17–20.

81 Badawy SZ, Baggish MS, ElBakry MM, et al. Evaluation of tissue healing and adhesion formation after an intraabdominal amniotic membrane graft in the rat. J Reprod Med 1989;34:198–202.

82 Yemini M, Shoham Z, Katz Z, et al. Effectiveness of silicone sheeting in preventing the formation of pelvic adhesions. Int J Fertil 1989;34:71–73.

83 Galan N, Leader A, Malkinson T, et al. Adhesion prophylaxis in rabbits with Surgicel and two absorbable microsurgical sutures. J Reprod Med 1983;28:662–664.

84 Boyers SP, Diamond MP, DeCherney AH. Reduction of postoperative adhesions in the rabbit with Gore-Tex surgical membrane. Fertil Steril 1988;49:1066–1070.

85 The Surgical Membrane Study Group. Prophylaxis of pelvic sidewall adhesions with Gore-Tex surgical membrane: a multicenter clinical investigation. Fertil Steril 1992;57:921–923.

86 Revuelta JM, Garcia-Rinaldi R, Val F, et al. Expanded PTFE surgical membrane for pericardial closure. J Thorac Cardiovasc Surg 1985;89:451–455.

87 Goldberg JM, Toledo AA, Mitchell DE. An evaluation of the Gore-Tex surgical membrane for the prevention of post operative peritoneal adhesions. Obstet Gynecol 1987;70:846–848.

88 Interceed (TC7) Adhesion Barrier Study Group. Prevention of postsurgical adhesions by Interceed (TC7), an absorbable adhesion barrier: a prospective randomized multicenter clinical study. Fertil Steril 1989;51:933–938.

89 Sekiba K, and the Obstetrics and Gynecology Adhesion Prevention Committee. Use of Interceed (TC7) absorbable adhesion barrier to

reduce postoperative adhesion reformation in infertility and endometriosis surgery. Obstet Gynecol 1992;79:518–522.

90 Wiseman DM, Gottlick LE, Diamond MP. Effect of thrombin-induced hemostasis on the efficacy of an absorbable adhesions barrier. J Reprod Med 1992;37:766–770.

91 Wiskind AK, Rice VM, Dudley AG. Evaluation of adhesion formation using Interceed (TC7) absorbable adhesion barrier on ovarian surgical wounds in the rabbit model. Obstet Gynecol 1993; 81:1025–1028.

92 Luciano AA, Whitman G, Maier DB, et al. A comparison of thermal injury, healing patterns, and postoperative adhesion formation following CO_2 laser and electromicrosurgery. Fertil Steril 1987; 48:1025–1029.

Chapter 46

Geriatric gynecologic surgery

Edward A. Graber

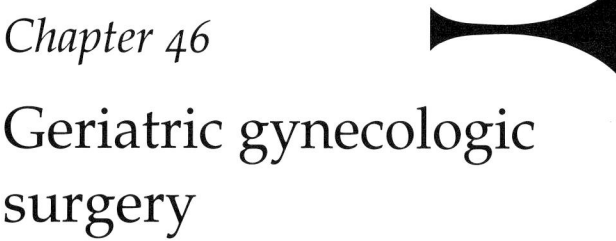

By the year 2000, 31 million people in the United States will be over 65. They will occupy 35% of the nation's hospital beds and will account for about the same percentage of the national medical expenditures. The majority of the recipients of medical care will be women. Furthermore, women between the ages of 60 and 69 have the highest incidence of major surgery, much of it gynecologic (1).

Life itself has been described as a terminal disease. We have managed to postpone the inevitable with better disease prevention, changes in lifestyle, more effective medication, better anesthesia, safer blood transfusions, and new surgical innovations. Age-related pathologic changes, however, still march on. Accumulating random DNA-specific mutations, deleterious changes in the enzyme systems, and genetically programmed deterioration all produce diseases. The basic product with which the physician who contemplates geriatric gynecologic surgery is presented is a compromised individual. The surgeon must be familiar with her unique problems and the variations in diagnosis and care that the geriatric patient requires.

Preoperative considerations

Before undertaking surgery, the physician must carefully weigh the answers to the following critical questions:
- Is the proposed surgery clearly indicated?
- What is the risk-benefit ratio?
- Is the patient's general condition good enough to withstand the stress of the surgery and its possible complications?
- Will the procedure be curative or merely palliative?
- Will the proposed operation clearly improve the quality of the patient's remaining years of life?

One must also factor in the lifestyle of many older women. In our mobile society, families are widely dispersed, and children are not available as backup providers of daily care. As a woman gets older, her spouse and old friends may no longer be alive. Many of these patients have been retired from their careers, their social security payments may be inadequate, and their pensions may not measure up to previous expectations. The patient is subject to greater immobility and isolation. Injuries and falls are more common, and depression may become a major problem (2).

By and large, elderly women tolerate surgery well, especially if it is vaginal surgery. Even when major medical problems exist, if they can be treated and stabilized, then a good outcome can still be anticipated. Age itself is less important than the patient's general health. If elective surgery is not feasible, nonoperative measures can be substituted.

Pathophysiology

Generally the elderly patient does not fare well in emergency situations. Her ability to maintain homeostasis is compromised, and her capacity to respond quickly and adequately to an acute insult precipitates a rapid decline in her physical, neurologic, and intellectual status.

Age-related changes in almost every organ system must be taken into account. Anemia, hypertension, heart disease, diabetes, changes in the major enzyme systems, altered membrane permeability, changes in protein synthesis, cerebral ischemia, dehydration, hormonal changes, lowered liver efficiency, diminished lung effectiveness, and compromised kidney competence all must be factored in (3).

Nervous system

The nervous system in the elderly undergoes marked changes. The brain is reduced in size with particular loss of gray matter. There is neuronal depletion as well as changes in synapses and nerve networks. The brain stem also shows deterioration of vulnerable areas. This results in major or minor memory defects, depression, and balance problems. Decreased sympathetic nervous system reactivity also occurs, which produces reflexive anomalies and learning difficulties. There is also a greater reliance on others for emotional and physical help. Cognitive impairment, agitation, and sleep disturbances are common. It does not take much to decompensate a system that is invariably compromised to a lesser or greater degree. If the patient presents any symptoms of significant neurologic impairment, preoperative consultation may save both the patient's family and the physician a great deal of aggravation. Acute surgical stress may have a devastating effect on the woman's neurologic responses, control of body functions, memory, and thinking (4,5).

Immunity

Age-related diminution of immunity probably results from glandular atrophy, helper T cell dysfunction, and lessened antibody formation. The decline in immune response is variable in onset, severity, and manifestations. This results in increased susceptibility to infection. Good antiseptic surgical technique is obligatory. Nosocomial infections are more common in this age group, especially with the use of catheters, drainage tubes, and intubation tubes. A muted immune response may mask the usual signs of this complication. If one is not aware of this, and increased vigilance is not instituted, infection may be missed, and then even vigorous delayed therapy may fail (6).

Autoimmunity increases with age. This is a major etiologic factor in the increase of malignancy, diabetes, arthritis, amyloidosis, emphysema, and other autoimmune diseases characteristic of the elderly.

Cardiovascular system

The cardiovascular system in the geriatric population is characterized by a rise in total peripheral resistance. Hy-

pertension is present in 35% to 50% of persons over the age of 60. This is of the low renin type, and generally geriatric patients seem to respond better with the use of calcium channel blockers. If there is concomitant heart disease, angiotensin-converting enzyme medications and beta-blockers may also be useful.

There are basically four problems associated with the aging heart: 1) decreased cardiac output; 2) thickened and more rigid valves, resulting in calcific aortic stenosis or mitral regurgitation; 3) deficiencies in coronary circulation; and 4) conditions requiring a cardiac pacemaker. Cardiac risks in gynecologic surgery increase with signs of heart failure, valvular disease, a history of myocardial infarction in the past 6 months, or a significantly abnormal electrocardiogram (7).

The aging heart and blood vessels respond poorly to hemorrhage, shock, or sepsis. These realities are manifested by the fact that 70% of surgical deaths among the elderly are due to strokes, kidney failure, or cardiac failure.

The likelihood of thrombophlebitis or thromboembolism is increased in the elderly, especially with prolonged immobilization or venous damage or stasis. One must consider early ambulation, elastic support stockings, pneumatic pressure boots, or prophylactic use of heparin.

Lungs

Lung surface decreases 20% to 30% with aging. There is a decrease in lung volume and gas exchange. Residual volume is increased. The respiratory muscles are weaker and more rigid. Alveoli are fewer in number and larger in size.

In the elderly, there may be lung damage from chronic infection, obstructive lesions, smoking, chronic emphysema, asthma, or tumors. A complete preoperative evaluation, including spirometry when indicated, will pay huge dividends in anticipating postoperative problems. Good pulmonary toilet after surgery may prevent postoperative complications. Smoking before and after surgery should be forbidden.

Shock, sepsis, pulmonary edema, aspiration, or pulmonary embolism may lead to adult respiratory distress syndrome (ARDS). This is the leading cause of death in surgical intensive care units. ARDS results in severe dyspnea and hypoxia, deterioration of oxygen transport, and perfusion difficulties. Treatment is difficult and is characterized by a significant failure rate. Mechanical ventilation, Swan-Ganz catheterization to guide fluid and electrolyte therapy, dopamine to augment cardiac output, diuretics to reduce preload forces, and antibiotics are the usual therapeutic modalities (8,9).

Kidneys

The kidney loses mass with age. There is decreased blood flow, perfusion, and glomerular filtration. Creatinine clearance decreases 10% per decade after the age of 30. Fifty percent of renal function is compromised before there is an evaluation of blood urea nitrogen or creatinine. The kidney becomes progressively insensitive to antidiuretic hormone. Chronic infection is increasingly present with advancing years.

The aging kidney has a greater tendency to fail. Once shutdown occurs, restoring normal function becomes increasingly difficult. The postoperative urinary output requires assiduous monitoring, and underlying problems must be diagnosed and corrected early. Damage to the drainage system may produce permanent kidney inadequacy (10).

Gastrointestinal tract

The gastrointestinal tract usually functions adequately in the elderly. There are, however, several changes that are significant. There is an increased gastric pH, decreased absorption surface, decreased motility, and decreased splanchnic blood flow. All these interfere with absorption of food, drugs, or any substances taken by mouth. In some patients the absorption of many foods, vitamins, and other necessary elements may be less than optimal. Such women may require preoperative nutritional supplementation.

Postoperatively, intestinal function may return slowly. One can anticipate normal function within a reasonable time. If feeding is instituted before bowel sounds return, ileus is more prevalent. With intra-abdominal pathology, there is generally an impaired inflammatory response. There may be diminished sensitivity to pain, little or no fever, a normal white blood cell count, and absence of expected signs and symptoms. Serious problems such as postoperative intestinal obstruction, peritoneal inflammation, and intra-abdominal abscess may occur without any of the characteristic signs or symptoms.

Despite a benign presentation, the intensity of the underlying process may be undiminished. Appendicitis, pancreatitis, or any other intra-abdominal pathology may be difficult to diagnose as well. The surgeon should foresee the possibility of misdiagnosis before the operation and take steps to manage unanticipated conditions (11,12).

Drug adjustments

The elderly consume at least 25% of all prescription drugs. They usually take several medications. It is estimated that 30% of the recipients of prescriptions do not fill them. This is probably because patients are unable to pay the high cost of medication, they have memory problems, or they just do not believe the medications are necessary. Even if the prescription is filled, older patients with their memory loss, confusion in following instructions, diminished attention span, and eyesight difficulties may not take the medication correctly.

Most drugs are lipid soluble. Fat deposits in the elderly increase considerably, taking the place of muscle. Also the lack of exercise and a high-carbohydrate diet contribute to this phenomenon. Excess fat deposition causes the retention of fat-soluble drugs and results in changes in their excretion and metabolism. There is also a decrease in body water, decrease in cardiac output, and decrease in serum albumin resulting in less drug binding. This combination results in abnormal drug distribution. Finally, excretion may be diminished due to decreased liver mass with diminished liver enzyme capacity, as well as changes in the renal blood flow and glomerular filtration rate. All these make excretion unpredictable. Drug doses must be curtailed and changed accordingly. Doses should be adjusted on the basis of the patient's response. Abnormal reactions are four times greater in the elderly than in the general population.

Certain medications should be stopped altogether before an operation, or their side effects may interfere with operative homeostasis. Monoamine oxidase inhibitors and clonidine, for example, should be stopped at least one week before surgery because they potentiate pressor agents that may be necessary during administration of anesthesia. Surgeons should emphasize the importance of stopping alcohol and tobacco preoperatively. Anticoagulants should be terminated and reversed before operation. Beta-blockers may be continued if the anesthetist is made aware of their use. Note all drug allergies carefully and be certain that warning signs are displayed prominently on the patient's chart (13,14).

All analgesics, sedatives, and other potentially depressing medication should be given in half-dosages. These medications require frequent nursing attention. Doses are repeated on an as-needed schedule rather than as routine time orders. If not monitored carefully, patients may be overdosed and become irrational, confused, and difficult to control. Cardiovascular and respiratory depression are possible occurrences.

Local anesthesia is safest. Some suggest that epidural anesthesia is second best according to safety evaluations. This is true if small, intermittent, meticulously supervised doses are given and expert technique is practiced. Otherwise, general anesthesia is the next safest, and finally spinal anesthesia. Marked hypotension is undesirable in the older woman.

Hypothermia is a major problem in the elderly. A cold room, inadequate blankets, cold intravenous fluids and blood, or heat loss from an open peritoneal cavity may lower core temperature. The geriatric patient may not shiver or be aware that she is cold. Body temperature is best monitored by frequent rectal temperatures. Corrective measures must be undertaken before the temperature falls below 97°F. Uncontrolled hypothermia results in hypotension, cardiac arrhythmia, depression of all body functions, and even in death.

Homeostasis

Electrolyte homeostasis in the elderly is altered by the decrease of intracellular water. In addition, the kidney loses some of its ability to concentrate fluid, resulting in the overall loss of total body water. Measures to correct this tendency of dehydration and hyperosmolality may precipitate pulmonary edema and cardiac failure, especially when fluids are administered too rapidly or in excessive amounts (2).

Many older people are anemic and have very low red blood cell reserves. Hemorrhage may become a major problem. Early adequate replacement of blood is mandatory.

Serum potassium levels are usually diminished in the older population. This is especially true if the patient is on digitalis or is taking diuretics. Sodium remains normal. Fluid and electrolyte values must be carefully monitored. Because normal functional reserves are compromised, any therapy that is instituted must be attempted slowly and carefully. Correcting severe acidosis may take days of close observation, and the physician should not attempt to correct abnormal values with massive doses.

Malignant disease

With aging the incidence of malignancy increases. This must be kept in mind in the evaluation of the geriatric gynecologic patient. Careful examination of the vulva, vagina, cervix, uterine body, adnexa, cul-de-sac, and rectum should be routine. In addition, one must rule out cancer of the breast, colon, and lungs because of their frequency.

In women over age 60, carcinoma of the colon is more frequent than any other malignancy except those of the breast and lung. A mass arising from the colon may easily be mistaken for an ovarian tumor on pelvic examination. Before undertaking any gynecologic surgery in the older patient with a left adnexal mass, one should order a complete colonoscopy as well as a barium enema.

Primary tumors of the breast may be small and nonpalpable. A routine mammogram should be done at least yearly after the age of 50. Tumors of the breast, stomach, and colon frequently metastasize to the ovary. If there are any symptoms or signs of involvement in these organs, a full preoperative evaluation is indicated. One should be especially suspicious of metastasis when bilateral ovarian tumors are palpated or visualized.

For women over 65, the mortality rate resulting from radical surgery is somewhat higher than that for younger women. This is especially true in the presence of obesity, hypertension, cardiac or lung compromise, or severe complicating diseases of other organs.

Intraoperative and postoperative complications are relatively common. These include pneumonia, myocardial infarction, urinary tract infection, thrombophlebitis, and the unstable vasomotor response to bleeding. There is an increased incidence of postoperative urinary and rectal fistulas. If the patient has a gynecologic malignancy, and there

is a reasonable chance of cure, everything possible should be done within the bounds of appropriate risk-benefit considerations. If only short-term palliation is possible, methods other than surgery can make the patient's remaining life easier and her death less painful and more dignified. Repeated major surgical procedures are definitely not indicated if they only give the patient a few extra months of life. Surgery should not just extend dying (15,16).

General principles

Most underlying gynecologic surgery in the elderly is undertaken electively to correct such conditions as uterine prolapse, urinary dysfunction, cystorectocele, or urinary and rectal fistulas. These conditions impair the quality of life, but do not threaten survival. If surgery is chosen, it should have a reasonably high chance of success and a low risk of creating postoperative failure that may be worse than the original condition. There are cases in which medical alternatives may give equal or even superior results without the potential morbidity or even mortality of surgery.

Major surgery is indicated without question if it is potentially lifesaving or will relieve major suffering. Older patients take extra time for healing and repair. Morbidity is higher. Hospitalization may be longer. The surgeon must also take into account the social, family, and financial problems associated with environmental changes. After radical surgery, months may be necessary for recovery and, in the event of recurrence, months to die. All of this must be considered before borderline indications for surgery are followed cavalierly. Extensive surgery that has a minimum chance of cure is not recommended.

Gynecologic surgery, especially if it is major, requires adequate support teams. This includes the immediate family, a good intensive care unit, hyperalimentation and metabolic teams, good anesthesiologists, and informed internists (17).

Preoperative workup

Physicians should use all the diagnostic aids available to them for the preoperative workup. Cervical biopsy, colposcopy, endometrial sampling, ultrasonography, computed tomography, magnetic resonance imaging, complete blood studies, individual system evaluation, and consultation with appropriate specialists should all be used when indicated.

It is most disconcerting to find an unexpected lesion at surgery that involves a system other than the genital tract. If there is any uncertainty about the diagnosis after an adequate preoperative workup, one should institute a prophylactic bowel preparation and have a competent general surgeon on call. This will prevent opening and closing without definitive surgery, and consequently a second operation, repeated anesthesia, and a great deal of explanation and embarrassment on the part of the gynecologic surgeon (18).

Vaginal operations

Older patients tolerate vaginal surgery better than the abdominal approach. There is minimal packing, less handling of bowel, earlier gastrointestinal mobility, normal breathing, and less distention.

Pelvic floor operations

Pelvic floor relaxation problems are the most frequent benign abnormalities. Cystorectoceles need not be corrected just because they are present. Most women who have delivered children vaginally have a certain amount of pelvic fascia injury, which is compounded during the menopause by estrogen deficiency and further fascial deterioration. Unless the damage is severe enough to permit the bladder or rectum to prolapse through the external vaginal opening, or if it severely hinders intercourse, surgery is not indicated. Estrogen therapy and reassurance may be all the treatment necessary.

If surgical correction is necessary, a good posterior repair is important. Recurrence of the cystocele is fairly common after operation, and the posterior repair, which usually holds better, will prevent significant descent of the anterior vagina. If operation is not feasible, the use of a Smith-Hodge pessary is quite adequate.

Uterine prolapse

The standard operation for uterine prolapse is vaginal hysterectomy, anterior and posterior repair, and the repair of an enterocele. In experienced hands the operation is relatively brief, and there is only a minimal chance of operative complications. For the older patient with medical compromise, vaginal hysterectomy may not be the operation of choice. Technically, this operation requires uterine mobility, adequate descent, adequate vaginal fornices, lack of local infection and ulceration, good assistance, good exposure, good lighting, and blood on call. Before surgery, cervical infection must be resolved, urinary tract infections controlled, and biopsies of suspicious lesions examined to rule out malignancy. The McCall technique for closure and support of the vaginal vault may help prevent postoperative enterocele and vaginal prolapse, complications to which the elderly are especially prone.

A recurring question is how serious the uterine prolapse must be to warrant surgery in the elderly. It is the opinion of most gynecologists that there is no reason to operate if the prolapse is minimal. When the cervix projects through the vaginal introitus or when cervical ulceration becomes a problem, surgery is indicated.

If the woman's health is compromised, lesser surgery than a vaginal hysterectomy should be considered. A Manchester-Fothergill operation with cervical amputation under sedation as well as local anesthesia is an excellent and viable option. This procedure has a 95% success rate, produces minimal complications, permits a short hospitalization, and allows the patient to lead a normal life thereafter. An anterior and especially posterior pelvic repair is added if indicated.

Finally, if a patient is debilitated or severely ill, other alternatives such as the Le Fort operation with cervical amputation or a high perineorrhaphy under local anesthesia should be considered. Finally, the use of a vaginal pessary may be adequate.

Prolapse of the vaginal vault sometimes follows hysterectomy (abdominal or vaginal) or after Marshall-Marchetti-Krantz or Burch operations. It is frequently accompanied by an enterocele. Treatment of this annoying condition is abdominal suspension of the vault to the sacrum with polyester strips (Mersilene) (abdominal sacropexy), sacrospinal ligament fixation, a high perineorrhaphy, a Le Fort vaginal closure, or vaginectomy. If a nonocclusive operation is undertaken, it should include correction of the enterocele, cystorectocele repair, and perineorrhaphy. The choice of procedure undertaken should be based on the experience of the operator and the general condition of the patient (19).

Urinary incontinence

Urinary incontinence of the elderly may be a diagnostic mine field. Clinical evaluation is mandatory, and one must understand that aging in itself may be the problem. Infection, local changes in the bladder or urethra, brain pathology, psychiatric problems, neurologic changes due to diabetes, and various other diseases producing neuropathology, urethral pressure instability, hypoestrogenism, stress incontinence, detrussor incontinence, abnormal pressure transmission, damaged pelvic support, and many other factors may be of etiologic importance.

The extent and complexity of the urologic workup is still not universally accepted. Consultation with a competent urologist may be helpful. Cystometry, urinary culture, determination of residual urine, and tests for leakage are basic. If surgery is decided upon for stress urinary incontinence, the most effective operations are the Marshall-Marchetti-Krantz or the Burch operations. Each is relatively simple, and their postoperative cure rates are excellent. Suture suspension of the proximal urethra has not withstood the test of time compared with the suprapubic approach.

Many patients with incontinence respond to nonsurgical treatment such as vaginal estrogens, Kegel's exercises, bladder training, correction of poor voiding habits, and voiding by the clock. In patients with medical complications, pessaries, which correct the urethrovesical angle, catheterization with Silastic catheters, or protective diapers may be necessary.

Infection, trauma, malignancy, or radiation may cause sigmoidorectal, rectovaginal, or vesicovaginal fistulas. One should not rush to repair them. Clean granulation tissue and eradication of local infection are necessary for success. Slight, intermittent leakage may well be observed and treated with local cleansing (20).

Intraoperative management and postoperative care

With abdominal as well as vaginal operations, attention to hydration including constant monitoring of the urinary output is mandatory. Oximeter evaluation and arterial blood gas analysis, electrocardiographic monitoring, careful replacement of blood to maintain blood volume, water and electrolyte testing and correction, and central venous or pulmonary wedge pressure determination all are helpful.

The incision in abdominal operations should be transverse if possible. If, however, there is any doubt about the diagnosis or if there is a malignancy, a vertical incision is mandatory in anticipation of possible extension demanded by the findings. A Maylard incision may also be adequate. Closing the incision with Smead-Jones sutures will help prevent evisceration (2,21,22).

The operation should be concluded as quickly as feasible, and the patient should be sent to the recovery room for intensive care. The support team should be available for early consultation should complications occur. A working laboratory must be available for immediate tests for clotting problems, gas analysis, and so forth. The same holds for emergency radiologic or other laboratory procedures.

Prophylactic antibiotics and miniheparinization should be started preoperatively and continued postoperatively for a set period. This helps considerably to control thrombophlebitis, pulmonary embolization, and infection. In addition to those listed, other major complications of the postoperative period are wound and soft tissue infections, fever, atelactasis, pneumonitis, cuff infection, hematomas, intra-abdominal abscess, electrolyte imbalance, and confusion. These are discussed elsewhere in this book.

Correction of complications is extremely important. Once the patient becomes severely ill, it becomes much more difficult to reverse the course in the elderly. Lung complications are especially frequent. To correct this, secretions should be removed as frequently as necessary. Intubation and oxygen with mucolytic agents and humidification should be instituted early. If intubation is required for more than one week, a tracheotomy may be necessary.

Myocardial infarction frequently occurs in this age group. There may be few of the usual symptoms or signs. The only early signs may be tachycardia, arrhythmia, or congestive heart failure. Early cardiac consultation will help control the potentially life-threatening complication (23).

Summary

Scrupulous preoperative evaluation, reasonable risk-benefit analysis, meticulous surgical technique, and vigilance in the postoperative period are the keys to successful geriatric gynecologic surgery. Most geriatric gynecologic procedures are elective. Before recommending surgery in this age group, one should consider viable nonsurgical alternatives. However, one should not deny surgery, because of age alone, to a woman who is healthy and a good risk. The quality of life is much more important than the years.

References

1 Kennedy AW, Flagg JS, Webster KO. Gynecological cancer in the very elderly. Gynecol Oncol 1989;32:49.
2 Barber HRK. Perimenopausal and geriatric gynecology. New York: Macmillan Publishing Co., 1988:2,247.
3 Lang WR, Aponte GE. Gross and microscopic anatomy of the aged female reproductive organs. Clin Obstet Gynecol 1967;10:454.
4 Schneider J, Benito R. Extensive gynecologic surgical procedures in patients more than 75 years of age. Surg Gynecol Obstet 1988; 167:497.
5 Bussey EW. The brain in aging. Clin Obstet Gynecol 1987;29:374.
6 Trofalter K. Immune response to aging. Obstet Gynecol 1986; 29:384.
7 Hooyman N, Cohen HJ. Medical problems associated with aging. Clin Obstet Gynecol 1986;29:353.
8 Schleuter DP. Pulmonary risks. Clin Obstet Gynecol 1973;16:91.
9 Piscitelli J, Parker RT. Gynecological surgery in the elderly patient. Clin Obstet Gynecol 1986;29:453.
10 Lewis EJ, Kark RM. Renal disease. In: Practical geriatric medicine. New York: Churchill Livingstone, 1985:368.
11 Mattingly RF. Surgery in the aging female. Clin Obstet Gynecol 1964;7:573.
12 Clark SL, Hornestein M, Phelan JP. Experience with pulmonary catheter in obstetrics and gynecology. Am J Obstet Gynecol 1985;152:374.
13 O'Malley K, Meagher F. Pharmacologic aspects of therapeutics. In: Practical geriatric medicine. New York: Churchill Livingstone, 1985:51.
14 Montamont SC, Cusack BJ, Vestel RE. Management of drug therapy in the elderly. N Engl J Med 1989;321:303.
15 Pierson AL, Figge PK, Buchsbaum HJ. Surgery for gynecological malignancy in the aged. Obstet Gynecol 1975;46:523.
16 Crichlow RW, Rubin A. General surgical lesions confused in older patients with gynecological lesions. Clin Obstet Gynecol 1967; 10:544.
17 Allen CM, Becker PM. Random controlled trial of geriatric consultation team. JAMA 1986;255:2617.
18 Breen JL. Gynecological oncology in the aged. Clin Obstet Gynecol 1067;10:498.
19 McKeithen WS. Major gynecological surgery in the elderly female 65 years of age or older. Am J Obstet Gynecol 1975;126:59.
20 Graber EA. Gynecology in the elderly. In: Practical geriatric medicine. New York: Churchill Livingstone, 1985:397.
21 Cherico A, Rubin A. Medical complications of the preoperative and postoperative care in elderly women. Clin Obstet Gynecol 1967;10:481.
22 Weksler ME. Evaluation of elderly patients for surgery. In: Practical geriatric medicine. New York: Churchill Livingstone, 1985:24.
23 Wallace D, Hernandez W, Schlaerth JB. Prevention of abdominal wound disruption utilizing Smead-Jones closure technique. Obstet Gynecol 1980;56:226.

Index